Kumar & Clark's
Cases in Clinical Medicine

FIFTH EDITION

Kumar & Clark's Cases in Clinical Medicine

PHILIP XIU

MA (Cantab), MB BChir, MRCP, MRCGP, MScClinEd, FHEA, MAcadMEd, RCPathME
Honorary Senior Lecturer
Leeds University School of Medicine
Medical Examiner
Leeds Teaching Hospitals Trust
UK

NICHOLAS AVEYARD

BM BCh, MA (Oxon)
Anaesthetic Registrar
Royal Devon University Healthcare
NIHR Academic Clinical Fellow
University of Exeter
UK

MICHAEL L. CLARK

MD, FRCP
Honorary Senior Lecturer
Barts and The London School of Medicine and Dentistry,
Queen Mary University of London, and Princess Grace Hospital
London, UK

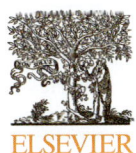

ELSEVIER

First edition 2000
Second edition 2006
Third edition 2013
Fourth edition 2021
Fifth edition 2026

The right of Philip Xiu and Nicholas Aveyard to be identified as authors of this work has been asserted by them in accordance with the Copyright, Designs and Patents Act 1988.

Content Strategist: Alex Mortimer
Content Project Manager: Supriya Barua
Design: Amy Buxton
Illustration Manager: Akshaya Mohan
Marketing Manager: Deborah J. Watkins

ISBN: 978-0-4432-6189-3

Printed in India
Last digit is the print number: 9 8 7 6 5 4 3 2 1

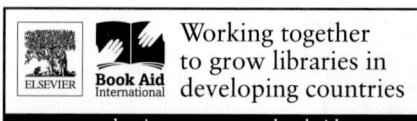

Working together to grow libraries in developing countries

www.elsevier.com • www.bookaid.org

CONTENTS

1   Emergency Medicine and Toxicology   1

2   Cardiology   24

3   Respiratory Disorders   78

4   Gastroenterology   131

5   Liver and Biliary Tract Disorders   157

6   Kidney and Urinary Tract Disease   175

7   Neurologia   211

8   Psychiatry   259

9   Rheumatology and Bone Disease   281

10   Endocrinology and Diabetes   311

11   Haematology and Oncology   355

12   Dermatology   417

13   Infectious Diseases   444

14   Sexually Transmitted Infections   457

15   Care of the Elderly and Palliative Care   469

Index   511

ACKNOWLEDGEMENTS

This edition is based on the original contributions of skilled clinicians who were regularly on the take for acute general medicine; their expertise is warmly acknowledged.

We would like to thank the original contributors:

Jane Anderson PhD FRCP
Simon Aylwin MA MB BChir PhD MRCP
Mark Caulfield MB MD FRCP FAHA
Charles R A Clarke MA FRCP MB BCh
David P D'Cruz MD FRCP
Ramesh C Joshi MD FRCP
Karim Meeran MD FRCP
David G Paige MA MB BS FRCP
Drew Provan MD FRCP FRCPath
Martin J Raftery MD FRCP
Gurcharan S Rai MD MSc FRCP
Armine Sefton MB BS MSc MD FRCP(Edin) FRCPath
David Watson BSc (Hons) MB BS FRCA
Mark Weaver MBBS MRCPsych
James R Wilkinson MRCP(UK) MB BS BSc (Hons)
Mahummad M Yaqoob MDFRCP

The field of medicine is constantly evolving, and with it, the methods of teaching and learning must adapt. This latest edition of *Kumar and Clark's Cases in Clinical Medicine* reflects this evolution, having been thoroughly updated to meet the needs of today's medical students and practitioners.

As new editors, we are honored to build upon the excellent foundation laid by Parveen Kumar and Michael Clark. We have maintained their vision of creating an engaging, easy-to-read format that makes learning both enjoyable and effective. The core principle of following a patient's journey from initial symptoms to diagnosis remains at the heart of this book.

This edition has been comprehensively refreshed to align with the content requirements of key examinations, including the Medical Licensing Assessment (MLA), Applied Knowledge Test (AKT), and PLAB (Professional and Linguistic Assessments Board) exams. We have expanded our collection to over 200 high-yield, real-life clinical cases, covering a wide range of acute symptoms and conditions encountered in medical practice.

Significant updates have been made to reflect the latest guidelines and management approaches across various specialties. Notably, we have enhanced our coverage of Dementia and added new sections on Elderly Care, Palliative Care, Metabolic Bone Diseases, and a fully expanded Dermatology chapter.

The case-based approach continues to be a cornerstone of this book, allowing readers to develop their clinical reasoning skills in a structured, step-by-step manner. Each case guides you through the process of narrowing down a broad differential diagnosis to the most likely conditions, mirroring the thought process required in real-world clinical scenarios.

We believe that this latest edition will prove to be an invaluable resource for medical students, junior doctors, and practitioners preparing for examinations or seeking to refresh their knowledge of acute presentations in medicine.

As we carry forward the legacy of Kumar and Clark, we remain committed to the principle that learning medicine should be both challenging and enjoyable. It is our hope that this book will not only aid in your studies but also reinforce the privilege and satisfaction that comes with caring for patients.

We wish you the very best in your medical careers and hope that this book serves as a trusted companion on your journey.

Philip Xiu and Nicholas Aveyard

CHAPTER 1

Emergency Medicine and Toxicology

Shock

CASE HISTORY (1)

A 60-year-old bank manager presents with crushing central chest pain. This started 45 minutes ago and has remained constant ever since.

On examination, he is pale and clammy. His pulse is 100/min and poor volume, and his blood pressure (BP) is 90/60.

Diagnosis

Shock – cardiogenic; history suggestive of myocardial infarction (MI).

CASE HISTORY (2)

A 50-year-old male who works in a bar has been brought to hospital, vomiting a large amount of blood. He gave no history of upper abdominal pain but did admit to drinking a bottle of whisky a day.

He also reveals a previous hospital admission with abdominal swelling, which was due to alcoholic liver disease. He was told that his liver disease was bad and that he must stop drinking and take propranolol regularly, as he had varices on endoscopy. He had not stopped drinking, nor was he taking his propranolol.

On examination, he is sweating profusely with visible shaking of his extremities. His pulse rate is 120/min with a BP of 85/50.

Diagnosis

Shock – hypovolaemia due to blood loss, probably from oesophageal varices

PHYSIOLOGY OF SHOCK (FIG. 1.1)

Shock is an acute life-threatening condition of circulatory failure, causing inadequate oxygen delivery to meet cellular metabolic needs. It can be:

- Cardiogenic: failure of the heart to maintain adequate cardiac output
- Hypovolaemic: reduction in the volume of blood within the circulation
- Distributive: loss of vasoregulation
- Obstructive: physical obstruction to cardiac flow or filling

CAUSES OF SHOCK

- Cardiogenic: MI, arrhythmias, acute valvular incompetence, myocarditis, cardiomyopathy
- Hypovolaemia: profound dehydration, haemorrhage
- Obstructive: pulmonary embolism, cardiac tamponade, tension pneumothorax
- Distributive shock: anaphylaxis, sepsis, neurogenic

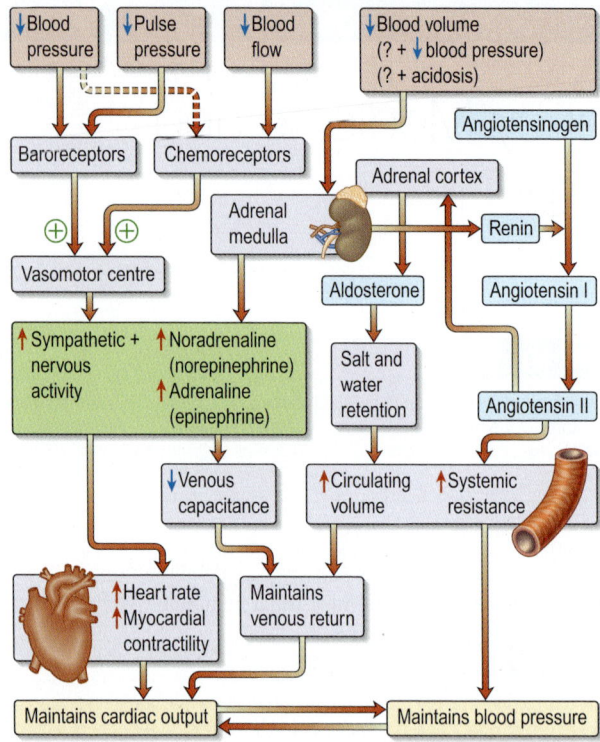

Fig. 1.1 The sympathoadrenal response to shock, showing the effect of increased catecholamines on the *left* of the diagram and the release of angiotensin and aldosterone on the *right*. Both mechanisms result in maintaining the blood pressure (BP) and cardiac output in shock.

REMEMBER

A patient might have more than one cause of shock, for example, Case 2 may have alcoholic cardiomyopathy (pump failure), as well as haematemesis (decreased blood volume).

CLINICAL EXAMINATION

In assessing the shocked patient, the following indices should be monitored:
- Pulse rate and respiratory rate (RR)
- Peripheral venous filling/capillary refill time
- Temperature
- Arterial BP (consider arterial cannulation if critically ill)
- Consider dynamic central venous pressure (CVP) and cardiac output monitoring in the intensive care unit (ICU)
- Urinary output
- Mental status

INFORMATION

Patients at risk of further deterioration will have one or more of the following vital signs, which would indicate transfer to an ICU:
- Heart rate (HR) >120 beats per minute (bpm)
- Heart rate <40 bpm

- Systolic BP <80 mm Hg
- Respiratory rate >30/min
- Respiratory rate <8/min
- Oxygen saturation <90%
- Glasgow coma scale (GCS) <8
- Core temperature >39°C
- Core temperature <35°C
- Urine output <0.5 mL/kg per h for 2 consecutive h

INVESTIGATIONS

- Haemoglobin (Hb) and haematocrit, urea and electrolytes (U and Es), liver biochemistry, coagulation studies, troponin (if cardiac cause suspected), glucose
- Serum lactate
- Electrocardiogram (and consider continuous monitoring)
- Arterial blood gas (ABG) analysis: in hypovolaemic shock (as in all shock states), there is a metabolic acidosis with a high hydrogen ion concentration and low bicarbonate concentration. In cases with respiratory complications, the PO_2 and PCO_2 values will help indicate the need for ventilatory support
- Imaging: chest X-ray (CXR) can help assess for treatable pathology (e.g. pneumothorax/haemothorax, pneumonia), CT scans can be helpful in assessing patients with trauma or excluding a pulmonary embolism (PE), bedside echocardiography can assist with the assessment of cardiac function (and excluding potential causes e.g. tamponade)

HOW WOULD YOU TREAT THESE PATIENTS? (FIG. 1.2)

Case 1

In cardiogenic hypotension, the key issues are pain relief, arrhythmia management, and the treatment of pulmonary oedema. Pain relief with incremental doses of intravenous (IV) opiates will aid reduction in myocardial oxygen consumption. Correcting electrolyte disturbances and hypoxia, and controlling angina pain might assist in arrhythmia management. If bradycardic, consider IV atropine, isoprenaline, adrenaline or temporary transvenous pacing (if refractory). Intravenous diuretics (e.g. furosemide) are needed for pulmonary oedema (consider adding further vasodilators, e.g. glyceryl trinitrate). Acute revascularisation (e.g. percutaneous coronary intervention) will likely be indicated. In the context of persistent hypotension, infusion of inotropic agents such as dobutamine might be necessary while correctable abnormalities are sought (e.g. acute mitral regurgitation following papillary muscle rupture). Percutaneous insertion of an intraaortic balloon counterpulsation pump may be necessary for refractory cardiogenic hypotension following transfer to a specialist centre as a prelude to surgical intervention.

Progress. This patient initially improved on inotropes, diuretics and vasodilator therapy. However, he remained hypotensive, with a BP <90 and poor output. He was transferred to the cardiac centre for the insertion of an intraaortic balloon pump. He did not respond and died 3 days later (mortality can be as high as 80% in cardiogenic shock).

Case 2

In hypovolaemic hypotension, the principal priorities are the reduction of further fluid loss and the simultaneous restoration of fluid volumes via wide-bore IV cannulae. Transfuse blood products in line with local major haemorrhage protocols. Infusion of red cells improves oxygen transport capacity (a target of 70–90 g/L is broadly accepted). Consider giving fresh frozen plasma, especially for patients who are actively bleeding and have a prothrombin time (PT),

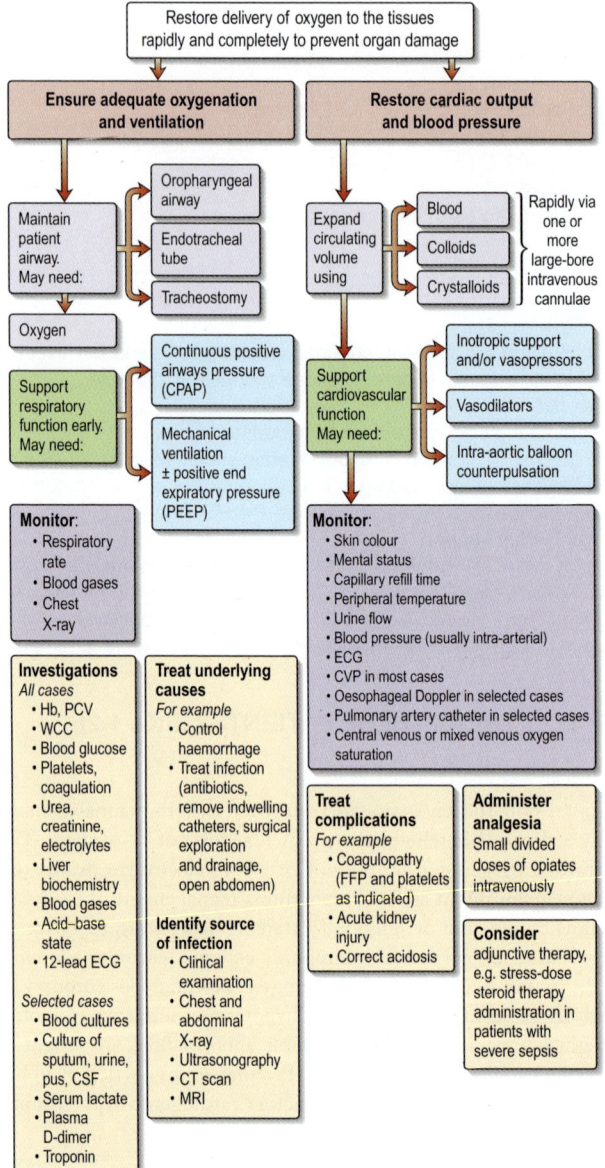

Fig. 1.2 Management of shock. Patients require intensive nursing care. FFP: fresh frozen plasma.

international normalised ratio (INR), or activated partial thromboplastin time (aPTT) greater than 1.5 times normal. If the fibrinogen level remains less than 1.5 g/L despite this, consider cryoprecipitate.

Consider platelet transfusion for patients who are actively bleeding and have a platelet count of less than 50×10^9/L. Reverse any anticoagulants, for example, prothrombin complex concentrate if taking warfarin.

At the earliest opportunity, the patient with haematemesis will require an endoscopy to find the bleeding lesion and treat it.

Progress. This patient was successfully resuscitated, and variceal banding was performed at endoscopy. He left the hospital after 7 days and was referred to the local liver unit for consideration of liver transplantation (Child Grade C alcoholic liver disease).

CASE HISTORY (3)

A 68-year-old male is brought to the emergency department by ambulance. His wife says that he developed abdominal pain 4 days ago, which has grown progressively worse. He has always suffered from indigestion and pain in the stomach area after food, for which he has taken antacids with some relief.

On this occasion, the pains became worse, and she said her husband had refused to get out of bed and appeared to be confused and disorientated. She had called an ambulance, which brought him to the hospital.

On examination, he was pyrexial at 39°C. He was pale, unsure of his surroundings and moaning about his abdominal pain. His pulse was 125 bpm with a BP of 90/40, and he had cold peripheries. He was breathless, and his O_2 saturations were 90%.

Abdominal examination revealed a distended abdomen, tender to touch, with absent bowel sounds.

WHAT IS THE CAUSE OF SHOCK IN THIS PATIENT?

This patient most likely has septic shock secondary to intraabdominal infection. He will need fluid resuscitation, urgent investigations and probably a laparotomy.

PATHOPHYSIOLOGY OF SEPTIC SHOCK

In sepsis, hypotension primarily results from impaired vascular tone. Sympathetic activation often leads to high cardiac output with low systemic vascular resistance. Hypovolaemia can occur from interstitial fluid losses due to widespread endothelial dysfunction and reduced venous tone. In more profound sepsis, myocardial depression also occurs due to circulating cytokines, such as tumour necrosis factor (TNF).

DISTRIBUTIVE SHOCK: SEPSIS, SEVERE SEPSIS AND SEPTIC SHOCK

Definition of Sepsis (from 3rd International Consensus: Sepsis-3)

- Sepsis is defined as life-threatening organ dysfunction caused by a dysregulated host response to infection
- Organ dysfunction (severe sepsis) can be identified as an acute change in total sequential organ failure assessment (SOFA) score of >2 points consequent to the infection:
  - The baseline SOFA score can be assumed to be 0 in patients not known to have preexisting organ dysfunction.
  - A SOFA score of >2 reflects an overall mortality risk of approximately 10% in a general hospital population with suspected infection. Patients presenting with modest dysfunction can deteriorate further.
- Patients with suspected infection who are likely to have a prolonged ICU stay or to die in the hospital can be promptly identified at the bedside with quick SOFA (qSOFA), that is alteration in mental status, systolic BP ≤100 mm Hg, or RR of ≥22/min
- Septic shock is a subset of sepsis in which underlying circulatory and cellular/metabolic abnormalities are profound enough to increase mortality substantially
- Patients with septic shock can be identified by a clinical construct of sepsis with persisting hypotension requiring vasopressors to maintain mean arterial pressure (MAP) ≥65 mm Hg and having a serum lactate level >2 mmol/L (18 mg/dL) despite adequate volume resuscitation. Based on these criteria, hospital mortality can be as high as 40% (Table 1.1)

TABLE 1.1 ■ The Relationship of Lactate Level in Sepsis to Mortality

Lactate (mmol/L)	Mortality
<2	15%
2–4	25%
>4	38%

From Trzeciak S, Dellinger RP, Chansky ME, et al. Serum lactate as a predictor of mortality in patients with infection. *Intensive Care Medicine*. 2007;33:970–977.

Symptoms and Signs

- Pyrexia and rigors, or hypothermia (unusual but more common in the elderly and associated with worse prognosis)
- Nausea, vomiting
- Vasodilatation, warm peripheries
- Bounding pulse
- Hypotension, low diastolic pressure, widened pulse pressure
- Can present with signs of cutaneous vasoconstriction
- Other signs include:
  - Jaundice
  - Coma, stupor
  - Bleeding due to coagulopathy
  - Rash and meningism
  - Hyper- or hypoglycaemia

HOW WOULD YOU MANAGE THIS CASE? (SEE FIG. 1.2)

Immediate Action

- Comprehensive ABCDE approach
- Correct hypoxaemia: titrate controlled supplemental oxygen
- Determine cause: examination, CXR and abdominal X-ray (AXR), ECG, ABGs, full blood count (FBC), U and Es, amylase, blood cultures
- Wide-bore IV access
- Intravenous crystalloid fluid resuscitation then reassess, consider vasopressors in critical care setting if minimal response to fluid resuscitation
- Early empirical broad-spectrum IV antibiotics (e.g. piperacillin/tazobactam) guided by local antibiotic protocols and resistance patterns, likely causative organism, and the patient's immune function
- Insert a urinary catheter and monitor urinary output

Shock is a medical emergency. The longer it persists, the lower the chance of recovery because secondary injury, from coexistent hypoxaemia and delayed reperfusion, is now recognised to cause further cytokine activation and the development of multiple organ failure (MOF).

> **INFORMATION**
>
> There is often progressive evidence of impending circulatory collapse in septic patients – increasing HR, oliguria, tachypnoea or confusion. *Act before shock has become established!*

FURTHER MANAGEMENT

- Consider early intubation and intermittent positive-pressure ventilation (IPPV) if there is evidence of respiratory distress, reduced consciousness (GCS <8), severe hypoxaemia or severe acidosis
- Goal-directed fluid resuscitation to provide adequate cardiac output with good urine output
- Vasopressors, such as noradrenaline, should be considered to maintain a MAP >65 mm Hg if unresponsive to fluid resuscitation (these patients should have an arterial catheter inserted to ensure accurate monitoring of intraarterial BP)
- Consider adding inotropic support, such as a dobutamine or adrenaline infusion, as this presentation is consistent with a low cardiac output and peripheral vasoconstriction
- Central venous access to facilitate vasopressors, inotropes, electrolyte replacement and CVP measurement
- Early recourse to stress-dose steroid therapy (e.g. IV hydrocortisone) if requiring vasopressors
- Attempted early control of the source of infection: seek a surgical opinion for treatment of the abdominal condition

SUMMARY

Timely intervention in patients with sepsis might prevent the progression of shock. Fluid resuscitation and treatment aimed at the primary cause should be instituted rapidly. Prognosis is dependent on the cause and response to treatment. For instance, mortality from urinary sepsis has a better prognosis than a similar clinical situation resulting from peritonitis.

Progress. This patient had peritonitis secondary to a perforated ulcer. He was resuscitated and admitted to the ICU. He later had a laparotomy with washout of the peritoneum and oversewing of the ulcer and an omental patch. He remained in the ICU, needing inotropic support and ventilation for 4 days, and was then transferred to the ward. He eventually made a good recovery. Helicobacter pylori eradication was given subsequently.

Anaphylaxis

CASE HISTORY

A 24-year-old female had been cleaning a pond in the summer when she was stung by a wasp. A few minutes later, she felt unwell and had to lie down as she felt faint. She then noticed some difficulty in breathing and felt a 'tightening' of her face. She felt very flushed, sweaty and lightheaded. Her partner called an ambulance, and on scene, they recorded her BP as 75/32 mm Hg with an HR of 105 bpm.

Diagnosis

Anaphylactic shock – due to wasp sting.

INFORMATION

Anaphylactic Reactions Can Be Fatal
- Reactions to penicillin: 1 death in every 7.5 million injections
- Bee and wasp stings: severe reactions in 1:200 stings
(United States 60–80 deaths per year)
(United Kingdom 5–10 deaths per year)

ANAPHYLACTIC SHOCK

Typically follows a second or third exposure to trigger (allergen).

History

- Exposure to insect bite, bee or wasp sting, seafood, nuts, drugs (e.g. penicillin, NSAIDs) or contrast media
- Dizziness, wheeze and facial swelling
- Past history of allergy

Examination

- Erythema, urticaria, angio-oedema, pallor, cyanosis
- Oedema of the face, pharynx and larynx
- Stridor due to laryngeal oedema
- Signs of profound vasodilatation: warm peripheries, low BP, tachycardia
- Bronchospasm
- Pulmonary oedema
- Nausea, vomiting, abdominal cramps, diarrhoea

HOW WOULD YOU MANAGE THIS PATIENT?

- Concurrently assess and treat using ABCDE approach
- Remove trigger if possible and keep patient supine or semirecumbent
- Ensure clear airway and administer oxygen if hypoxic (be wary of the potential for airway difficulties and call anaesthetics early if concerned)
- Establish large-bore venous access
- Administer 0.5 mg adrenaline (epinephrine) IM to create depot support for the circulation
- Perform serial cardiorespiratory assessments
- Repeat IM adrenaline after 5 min if still hypotensive
- Obtain three blood samples (using a serum or clotted blood test tube) to measure mast cell tryptase concentrations: one as soon as possible after resuscitation, a second between 1 and 4 hours after the onset of symptoms and a third after 24 hours (to provide baseline levels)

FURTHER MANAGEMENT

- If persistent hypotension, give rapid bolus of IV crystalloid and commence IV adrenaline infusion with critical care support
- Consider salbutamol 2.5 to 5 mg nebulised for bronchospasm
- Consider nebulised adrenaline for persistent stridor
- After initial management, give a nonsedating oral antihistamine (e.g. cetirizine) if persisting urticaria
- Consider IV hydrocortisone for refractory reactions, shock, or refractor bronchospasm
- Always confirm precipitant through allergy testing
- Advise on Medic-Alert bracelet
- Provide the patient with an adrenaline (epinephrine) 0.3 mg autoinjector (e.g. EpiPen) and tuition to inject into the thigh in the event of exposure to allergen

PREVENTION

- Avoid triggering factors, for example, food, stings
- Patient education is vital
- Patients should always carry preloaded syringes for adrenaline self-administration

Acute Respiratory Distress Syndrome (ARDS)

CASE HISTORY

You are called urgently to the emergency department as a 35-year-old known drug user has been sent to the hospital having been found unconscious. Their GCS is 5, they have a noninvasive blood pressure (NIBP) of 100/60, an RR of 20/min with an oxygen saturation of 85% despite high-flow O_2 therapy.

WHAT ARE THE POSSIBLE CAUSES OF DEPRESSED CONSCIOUSNESS, AND WHAT ARE YOUR IMMEDIATE ACTIONS?

- You need to consider primary neurological causes, such as intracranial haemorrhage, space-occupying lesions, postictal state or infection
- You must also consider other causes, such as alcohol intoxication, drug overdose, hypoglycaemia, severe electrolyte derangement, hepatic encephalopathy, respiratory failure, and hypothermia
- **On examination**, look for evidence of focal neurological signs, pinpoint pupils, trauma to the head or evidence of seizures such as tongue laceration or incontinence
- Ensure the airway is not obstructed, establish IV access, and take blood gases, blood glucose, and blood and urine for toxicology

Arterial blood gas analysis reveals pH 7.2, PaO_2 6.4, $PaCO_2$ 2.5 and lactate 4.1 mmol/L.

WHAT DO THESE RESULTS INDICATE?

Acute **type 1 respiratory failure** with a metabolic (lactic) acidosis.

There is vomitus around the patient's mouth and on his clothing. The CXR shows patchy shadowing at the right base.

Following naloxone administration, he becomes agitated, moving all limbs but does not respond purposely to command.

WHAT IS THE IMMEDIATE MANAGEMENT?

Respiratory failure is probably related to aspiration of vomitus. Intubation and IPPV are indicated. Continuous positive airway pressure (CPAP) or noninvasive ventilation is contraindicated because of the danger of further vomiting and lack of cooperation.

The patient was transferred to the ICU. On the ward round next morning, ventilatory pressures are high for standard tidal volumes and he remains hypoxic.

KEY FEATURES OF ARDS

The diagnosis of ARDS is based on fulfilling three main criteria:

1. Acute onset (within 1 week)
2. Bilateral opacities on chest radiography or CT (see Fig. 1.3), or bilateral B lines and/or consolidations on ultrasound not fully explained by effusions, atelectasis or nodules/masses

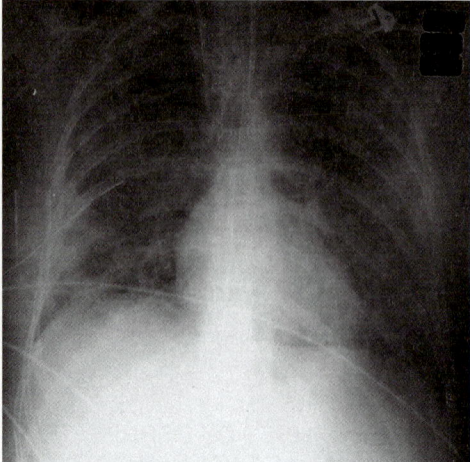

Fig. 1.3   Chest X-ray (CXR) appearances in acute respiratory distress syndrome (ARDS). Bilateral diffuse alveolar shadowing with air bronchograms and no cardiac enlargement. (From Feather A, Randall D, Waterhouse M, eds. *Kumar and Clark's Clinical Medicine*, 10th ed. Elsevier, 2021; Fig. 10.30.)

3. PaO_2/FiO_2 (arterial to inspired oxygen) ratio of ≤300 mm Hg or SpO_2/F_iO_2 (pulse oximetric saturation to inspired oxygen) ratio of ≤315

CAUSES

- Severe sepsis usually with pulmonary origin, for example, bacterial pneumonia, COVID-19
- Pulmonary aspiration (as in this case)
- Multiple trauma and massive transfusion
- Postcardiac bypass syndrome
- Pancreatitis
- Toxic fume exposure, including smoke inhalation
- Cerebral injury such as subarachnoid haemorrhage

PATHOPHYSIOLOGY

Profound hypoxaemia results from venous admixture or shunting of deoxygenated blood through poorly ventilated or unventilated lung units. This arises because:

- Endothelial dysfunction leads to widespread interstitial oedema and impaired alveolar capillary perfusion
- The stiff (low-compliance) lungs result in reduced tidal volume and reduced end-expiratory lung volume; this then causes small airway collapse
- Once the airways are collapsed, Laplace's law explains why it is difficult to reexpand them (consider the difficulty in initially blowing up a balloon)
- Additional small airway pathology is present, particularly with direct lung injury, for example smoke inhalation
- The lung can be likened to a wet sponge: the dependent sponge is waterlogged and the air spaces collapsed, so only the nondependent areas of the lung will contribute to gas exchange
- The additional component of airway inflammation in some causes of ARDS explains the high mortality associated with direct lung injury (>60%)

MANAGEMENT

The high mortality of ARDS is critically dependent on resolution of the primary cause. Treatment of the lung is essentially supportive. Further injury must be avoided by tolerating relative hypoxaemia (aiming to limit oxygen toxicity by keeping the fraction of inspired oxygen F_iO_2 <70%) and allowing permissive hypercapnia (limiting tidal volume to avoid barotrauma – overdistension of functioning lung and risk of pneumothorax). Ventilatory techniques include:

- Deep sedation and neuromuscular paralysis to increase chest wall compliance; a semirecumbent bed position unless contraindicated
- Small tidal volumes (e.g. initially 6 mL/kg of predicted body weight) and prolonged inspiratory time to maintain an inspiratory plateau pressure <30 cm H_2O
- Titrate PEEP to recruit lung units
- Prone positioning to improve ventilation/perfusion V/Q matching and clearance of lung secretions

EXPERIMENTAL METHODS

- Inhaled nitric oxide to overcome hypoxic pulmonary vasoconstriction, improve V/Q matching and reduce pulmonary hypertension
- Rescue therapy with steroids to limit the proliferative fibrotic process of lung repair
- High-frequency ventilation
- Extracorporeal membrane oxygenation

OUTLOOK

Mortality from ARDS remains high (overall 30%–40%). Lung remodelling might, however, result in considerable eventual recovery. Progression of the underlying disease, hospital-acquired infection, or the development of cardiogenic shock secondary to right ventricular (RV) failure significantly increase mortality.

Progress. The patient developed multiorgan failure with impaired hepatic synthesis, including coagulopathy, cholestatic jaundice and acute tubular necrosis requiring haemofiltration. IV cefuroxime and metronidazole were started initially but subsequently *Pseudomonas* was cultured from respiratory secretions and IV piperacillin/tazobactam was commenced. A week later, a tracheostomy was performed and ventilatory support was progressively weaned over the next 3 weeks. He was discharged from the hospital 6 weeks after admission.

Self-Poisoning

Poisoning is a major health problem worldwide. The WHO estimates that a million people a year die of self-harm. Drugs, alcohol and chemicals (e.g. copper sulphate used in agriculture) are the major causes with over 700,000 deaths every year worldwide.

GENERAL POINTS

- 80% of patients seen in the emergency department will be conscious
- There is a poor correlation between the history of the amount, type and timing of poisons consumed and blood toxicology
- Frequently, more than one drug will have been consumed
- Alcohol is the most commonly consumed second agent
- Carefully assess suicide risk

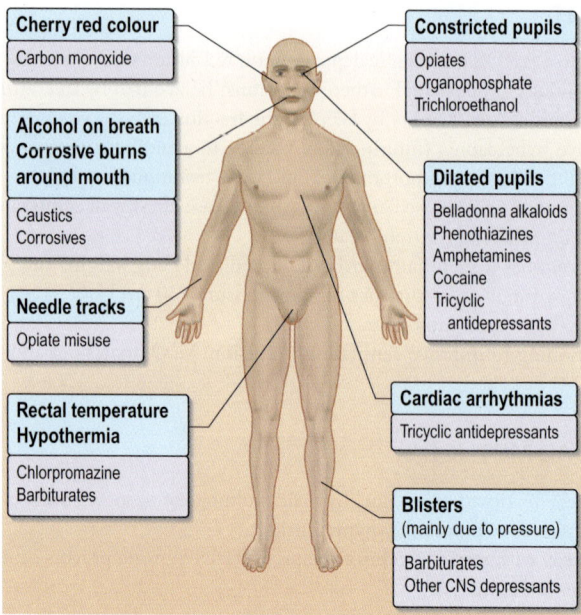

Fig. 1.4 Physical signs of poisoning.

WHAT PARTICULAR POINTS DO YOU NEED TO ASSESS ON PHYSICAL EXAMINATION (FIG. 1.4)?

- Assess and record conscious level using the GCS (see Chapter 7)
- Document RR and cyanosis (use pulse oximetry)
- Measure BP and pulse
- Record pupillary size (small with opiates) and reactivity to light
- Measure temperature
- If consciousness is depressed, check for signs of coexistent head injury
- Look for needle tracks or signs of drug use

CASE HISTORY (1)

A 25-year-old female is admitted semiconscious and smelling of alcohol, having taken an indeterminate amount of an unknown drug at some point earlier that evening.

On examination, she has depressed consciousness (GCS 11), an RR of 12/min, a BP of 95/70 and small, reactive pupils.

WHAT SHOULD YOU DO?

- Comprehensive ABCDE approach to assessment and treatment
- Ensure no airway compromise, apply oxygen if hypoxic
- Serial physical observations – HR, NIBP, RR, oxygen saturation (SaO_2), temperature
- Thorough physical examination as previously discussed
- Baseline investigations: venous blood gas, FBC, U and Es, liver biochemistry
- Paracetamol and salicylate levels at 4 h or thereafter post overdose

- Blood and urine samples for toxicology: particularly useful in seriously ill patients with altered consciousness
- Consider ABGs if hypoxic or altered respiration

INFORMATION

Take advice from the 24-h National Poisons Information Service (see 'Significant Websites' section) in all serious overdoses: there might have been recent advances in management of the specific poisoning you are dealing with.

Some common drugs used for overdose exhibit delayed action, for example, aspirin, paracetamol, tricyclic antidepressants, iron (more common in children), cophenotrope, and all modified-release preparations.

GENERAL MANAGEMENT

- Nurse in left lateral position
- Clear mouth of vomitus, debris and obstructing objects
- Intravenous access
- Nursing care of mouth and pressure areas
- Maintain normothermia

RESPIRATORY SUPPORT

- Protect airway because vomiting is a risk: vomiting is particularly associated with opiates, benzodiazepines, alcohol and tricyclic antidepressants
- Respiratory depression might occur with opiates, benzodiazepines, alcohol or tricyclic antidepressants
- Monitor with continuous pulse oximetry
- Administer oxygen if hypoxic
- Reducing GCS (<8), loss of gag or cough reflex is a strong indication for intubation

CARDIOVASCULAR SUPPORT

- Watch for hypotension (systolic BP <80 mm Hg):
  Mild: raise the end of bed
  Severe: rapid IV crystalloid bolus and reassess
  Very severe: critical care support, insertion of arterial and CVP lines
- Measure urine output: aim for 0.5 mL/kg per hour. Urine output is a useful guide to adequacy of the circulation
- Monitor ECG for arrhythmias

WHAT OTHER PROBLEMS MIGHT OCCUR?

Blood Pressure

- Watch for hypotension (see earlier)
- Less commonly, transient hypertension might be seen with amphetamine and cocaine

Arrhythmias

- Might arise from hypoxia or metabolic acidosis
- Bradycardia might occur with beta-blockers, digoxin and organophosphorus compounds

- Ventricular and supraventricular tachycardias occur due to theophyllines, tricyclic antidepressants/phenothiazines (due to prolonged QT interval), cocaine, ecstasy and amphetamine

Hypothermia

- Can occur due to unconsciousness, especially with phenothiazines and barbiturates
- Measure temperature regularly
- Nurse under a forced-air warming blanket if required

Hyperthermia

- Can occur with amphetamines, ecstasy and cocaine, selective serotonin reuptake inhibitors (SSRIs), salicylates and tricyclic antidepressants

WHAT SPECIFIC MANAGEMENT PROCEDURES ARE THERE FOR OVERDOSES?

Reducing Absorption

- Gastric lavage: should only be used for life-threatening overdoses and only within the first hour for significant recovery of poison. Avoid lavage if corrosives, paraffin or petrol have been taken because of the risk of inhalation. Always intubate if the patient is unconscious
- Induced emesis: should **not** be used because it is ineffective at removal of poison and delays the use of activated charcoal
- Activated charcoal: binds drugs in the intestine and is valuable for adsorbing most poisons with the greatest effect on aspirin, tricyclic antidepressants and theophyllines. For most drugs, do not use more than 1 h post ingestion of poison or with an oral antidote

Active Elimination

- Repeated doses of charcoal might enhance elimination for selected drugs even after the drug has been absorbed. This works for aspirin, barbiturates, quinine, theophylline and carbamazepine
- Urine alkalinisation is mainly used for salicylate overdose
- Haemodialysis helps in severe salicylate poisoning, barbiturates, ethylene glycol, alcohol and lithium poisoning

Antagonising the Influences of Poisons

- Acetylcysteine or methionine replenishes cellular glutathione stores in paracetamol poisoning
- Ethanol is a competitive inhibitor of alcohol dehydrogenase and is given in ethylene glycol (antifreeze) poisoning. Fomepizole is also useful when ethanol is contraindicated, for example, previous excess alcohol user or liver disease
- Naloxone and opiates compete at the same receptor

Progress. The partner of this 25-year-old patient attended the hospital shortly after admission. He had found two empty boxes of diazepam that the patient had been taking for acute anxiety over the last few months. He said that her drug misuse might be related to her being made redundant a week ago. She did not require ventilation and woke up gradually. She was reviewed by the mental health team once medically fit (Box 1.1).

BOX 1.1 ■ Benzodiazepine Overdose

Clinical Features
- Drowsiness, ataxia, slurred speech, coma
- Respiratory depression and hypotension might occur

Management – the Problems

Respiratory depression or – in combination with alcohol – vomiting and aspiration

Treatment – Supportive
- Protect airway and neurological observations
- Gastric lavage is not required
- Flumazenil is a benzodiazepine antagonist that can be used in severe overdose with marked respiratory depression only
- Beware: seizures have followed flumazenil administration
- Patients are usually fit to be discharged at 24 h

Paracetamol (Acetaminophen) Poisoning

REMEMBER

- Paracetamol is consumed in 45% of overdoses in the UK
- As little as 7.5 to 15 g (15–30 tablets) can cause severe hepatic necrosis

CASE HISTORY (2)

A young female, aged 18, was brought into A and E by her boyfriend who had found her drowsy. A packet – possibly containing paracetamol tablets – and half a bottle of wine were found near her. They had argued the previous night, and she had threatened suicide. He thought that she had taken the tablets 6 hours ago. A past history of an eating disorder was elicited.
On examination, she was very thin and had a GCS of 10. There were no other physical signs.

INVESTIGATIONS

- Venous blood gas to assess for acidosis (consider ABG if hypoxic)
- Baseline U and Es
- Liver biochemistry
- Coagulation studies
- Paracetamol and salicylate levels
- Glucose

This patient's paracetamol level was 140 mg/L and her salicylate level was <10 mg at 6 h post overdose. She was admitted to the medical assessment unit (MAU).

REMEMBER

- Nausea and vomiting are extremely common in the first 24 h
- Abdominal pain usually develops after 24 hours
- Persistent nausea with subcostal pain usually indicates significant hepatic necrosis
- Chronic alcohol excess or other enzyme-inducing drugs increase the metabolism of drugs
- Hypoglycaemia may occur
- Paracetamol is a constituent (with an opiate) of coproxamol or codydramol

PHYSICAL EXAMINATION

- Check RR in case a compound preparation (e.g. codydramol) or other drugs have been consumed
- Haematuria, proteinuria and loin pain after the first 24 h might indicate acute kidney injury (AKI)
- Later: liver flap and altered consciousness might develop after 3 days

HOW SHOULD YOU MANAGE THIS PATIENT?

Paracetamol can cause hepatic necrosis, with maximum damage sustained 72 to 96 h after ingestion. Renal damage occurs even without major liver damage.

Treatment Nomogram (Fig. 1.5)

- Plot measured serum paracetamol concentration against the time since ingestion on your local treatment nomogram, for example, the National Poisons Information Service nomogram for the UK
- If any doubt, treat with acetylcysteine
- If suggestion of acute liver injury, give acetylcysteine even if paracetamol is below treatment line
- To avoid underestimating in obese patients (>110 kg), use a body weight of 110 kg (rather than their actual body weight) when calculating the total dose of paracetamol ingested

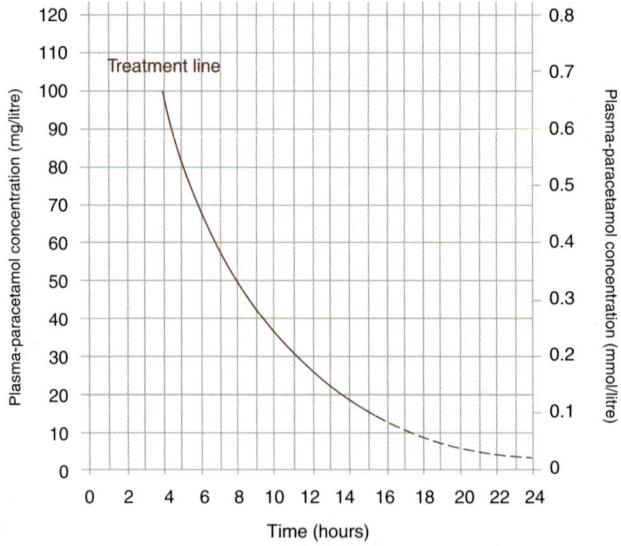

Fig. 1.5 Example nomogram for treatment of paracetamol poisoning. The nomogram is unreliable if the timing of overdose (OD) is uncertain or if they have taken a modified-release preparation – if in doubt treat. Although the *line* is often extended to 24 h (*dotted lines*), the concentrations are not based on clinical trial data. (From Hamilton P. *Blood Tests Made Easy.* Elsevier, 2023; Fig. 13.3)

> **INFORMATION**
> - Severe liver or renal damage: always seek specialist advice
> - Refer to a specialist liver unit if acidotic (pH <7.3), INR >3.0 at 48 h or >4.5 at any time, oliguric or creatinine >300 micromole/L, or if there is evidence of encephalopathy or hypoglycaemia or hypotension with systolic BP <60 mm Hg
> - There is evidence that administration of acetylcysteine in patients with established hepatic encephalopathy can still improve prognosis

ANTIDOTES – REGIME FOR TREATMENT

Acetylcysteine by Infusion

Example regime (always check local guidelines):
- Acetylcysteine 150 mg/kg in 200 mL 5% glucose over 15-60 min (ceiling weight of 110 kg)
- Then 50 mg/kg in 500 mL 5% glucose over 4 h, followed by 100 mg/kg in 1 L over 16 h
- Total dose 300 mg/kg over 21 h

What Are the Adverse Reactions to Acetylcysteine?

- Local itching and rashes at infusion sites
- Systemic effects include nausea, flushing, angio-oedema, bronchospasm and hypotension
- Treatment is with discontinuation of the infusion and an antihistamine
- Once these effects have been resolved, the acetylcysteine infusion can be resumed at 100 mg/kg in 1 L over 16 h

With a GCS of 10, opiate ingestion was also suspected and naloxone was given. As she responded well to this, a naloxone infusion was started with the rate adjusted to clinical response as a single IV naloxone dose lasts only 30 min.

Intubation and ventilation were not required; pulse oximetry showed no impaired oxygenation.

SUMMARY: HOW WOULD YOU TREAT A PARACETAMOL OVERDOSE?

If a Patient Presents Within 8 h (As in This Case)

- Consider administration of activated charcoal if the patient presents within 1 hour of paracetamol ingestion and has ingested more than 150 mg/kg of paracetamol (caution if reduced GCS)
- Use treatment nomogram at 4 h or later to guide the use of acetylcysteine (see Fig. 1.5)
- If there is doubt about the timing and if ≥150 mg/kg body weight has been ingested, then treat with acetylcysteine immediately
- If the 4-h paracetamol level is below the treatment line, discontinue acetylcysteine if the patient is not at high risk of liver toxicity, for example, asymptomatic, INR and ALT within the normal range
- If acetylcysteine is started within 8 h, the prognosis is good and patients can be considered for discharge at the end of the infusion if blood tests are normal
- Prior to discharge, check that INR and plasma creatinine are normal
- Ensure liaison with psychiatric services deliberate overdose

If a Patient Presents at 8 to 24 h Post Ingestion

- Patients presenting more than 8 h post ingestion are at greater risk of hepatotoxicity; the efficacy of treatment with acetylcysteine declines
- Give acetylcysteine to all patients who present 8 to 24 h after ingestion of an acute overdose of more than 150 mg/kg of paracetamol, even if the plasma-paracetamol concentration is not yet available
- Individual response to paracetamol overdose can be variable, and the validity of the treatment line beyond 15 h post ingestion is not clear
- At the end of the infusion, check that the INR and plasma creatinine are normal. If so, the risk of damage is negligible and discharge can be planned
- If INR or creatinine is abnormal, or the patient develops symptoms, continue to monitor these blood tests till normal

If a Patient Presents Over 24 h Post Ingestion

- Start acetylcysteine without waiting for blood results if ≥150 mg/kg paracetamol has been ingested as an acute overdose (within 1 h) or there is clinical evidence of liver injury (e.g. jaundice, encephalopathy, hepatic tenderness)
- If asymptomatic and ingested <150 mg/kg, wait for blood results before starting acetylcysteine
- Acetylcysteine is indicated if alanine aminotransferase (ALT) is above the upper limit of normal, INR >1.3 (in the absence of another cause), or the paracetamol concentration is detectable
- All should have liver biochemistry, INR, creatinine, glucose and arterial pH monitored regularly

Progress. This patient was given acetylcysteine, and her INR remained within the normal range. She was discharged after being seen by liaison psychiatry who completed an urgent referral to the community mental health team.

Salicylate Overdose

CASE HISTORY

A 16-year-old female was brought to the emergency department by her parents after an episode of nausea, followed by severe vomiting. Her parents then found packs of aspirin tablets in her bedroom, which she said she had taken because of difficulties with friends at school. She also complained of tinnitus and deafness. The parents think the aspirin ingestion occurred about 4 h ago.

On examination, she is hyperventilating with peripheral vasodilatation, profuse sweating and tachycardia suggesting a moderate/severe **salicylate overdose.**

- Aspirin is rapidly absorbed: usually peaks at 4 h
- <150 mg/kg body weight causes mild toxicity
- 150 to 130 mg/kg body weight causes moderate toxicity
- 300 to 500 mg/kg body weight causes severe toxicity
- Beware modified-release formulations: these can prolong absorption
- Aspirin itself might delay gastric emptying

WHAT ARE THE POTENTIAL CLINICAL FEATURES OF SALICYLATE OVERDOSE?

- Early features include nausea, vomiting, tinnitus or deafness (severe overdose), sweating and hyperventilation
- Later features include Kussmaul's respiration, hyperpyrexia, confusion, coma, fits and renal impairment

INVESTIGATIONS

- Blood gases typically show a mixed respiratory alkalosis and metabolic acidosis with normal or high arterial pH (anion gap is usually increased in severe cases)
- Plasma salicylate measured after 2 hours in symptomatic patients (4 hours if asymptomatic)
- Check U and Es, FBC and coagulation studies (can cause disseminated intravascular coagulation (DIC))
- Monitor blood glucose levels
- ECG - tachycardia is common and can cause ventricular dysrhythmias in severe cases

WHAT ARE THE CHALLENGES IN MANAGING SALICYLATE OVERDOSE?

- Aspirin delays gastric emptying
- People who appear well initially might have very high salicylate levels
- Early hypokalaemia and respiratory alkalosis may be replaced after 4 to 6 hours by metabolic acidosis
- Hypo-prothrombinaemia might occur (increased prothrombin time/INR)

HOW WOULD YOU MANAGE THIS PATIENT?

- Consider activated charcoal if ingested <1 h previously (caution if GCS reduced)
- IV fluids with potassium supplements to correct dehydration and hypokalaemia (and to improve urine flow)
- Treat hyperthermia, for example, cooled IV fluids or ice packs
- Forced alkaline diuresis should not be used
- Urine alkalinisation if plasma salicylate levels >500 mg/L: 8.4% bicarbonate (~225 mL) in 1 h with careful monitoring
- Haemodialysis should be used only when the salicylate level is >700 mg/L

Progress. This young patient had a salicylate level of 620 mg/L. She was treated with IV fluids and urine alkalinisation. She was kept in the hospital for 3 days, during which time she fully recovered and her blood gases and electrolytes returned to normal. She was seen with her parents by the mental health team, but further counselling was not thought to be necessary.

INFORMATION

Risk factors for mortality from salicylate poisoning:

- Age >70 years
- Central nervous system features
- Metabolic acidosis
- Hyperpyrexia

- Late presentation
- Pulmonary oedema
- Salicylate concentrations >700 mg/L (5.07 mmol/L)

Tricyclic Antidepressant Overdose

These have become less common since (much safer) SSRIs became available. Features of overdose are mainly due to antimuscarinic and alpha-blocking adverse effects. Arrhythmias occur due to prolongation of the QT interval.

Clinical Features

- Drowsiness, confusion but rarely unconsciousness
- Blurred vision due to fixed dilated pupils
- Sinus tachycardia with long QT interval
- Ventricular arrhythmias
- Hypotension
- Hypothermia
- Hyperreflexia and extensor plantars
- Agitation, visual and auditory hallucinations: common during recovery
- Seizures: in <5%

Treatment – Supportive

- Activated charcoal (if <2 h since ingestion): reduces absorption of tricyclics, anticholinergic action delays gastric emptying
- Cardiac monitor and watch for hypotension
- Neurological observations
- If QRS >100 milliseconds or pH <7.45, give IV sodium bicarbonate bolus followed by infusion (requires regular monitoring of pH and electrolytes, target pH between 7.45 and 7.55)
- Sodium bicarbonate can treat tachyarrhythmias and bradyarrhythmias even if the patient is not acidotic
- Ventricular arrhythmias (despite treatment with sodium bicarbonate) should not be treated with antiarrhythmics but with under-drive or over-drive temporary pacing
- Seizures: treat with IV benzodiazepines

Cocaine

Cocaine (Fig. 1.6) can be inhaled (snorted), injected, swallowed, or separated from its hydrochloride base and melted as crack.

> **CASE HISTORY**
>
> A 32-year-old male is brought to the emergency department by his friends who were all at a party together. A large amount of alcohol was drunk and some drugs had been used. The patient had been found semiconscious, and when his friends tried to move him, he seemed to have no movement on the left side of his body.
>
> **On examination**, he has a GCS of 9. He has signs of left hemiparesis.

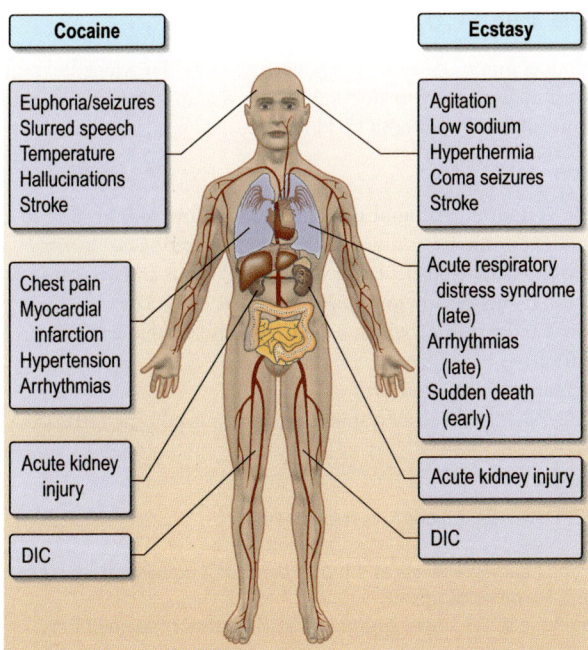

Fig. 1.6 Features of cocaine and Ecstasy misuse. DIC: disseminated intravascular coagulation.

If a young person presents with a stroke or MI, cocaine overdose should always be looked for.

WHAT ARE THE POTENTIAL CLINICAL FEATURES OF COCAINE TOXICITY?

- Euphoria, slurred speech, dilated pupils
- Pyrexia, sinus tachycardia and hallucinations (auditory, tactile and olfactory)
- Hypertension (may be severe), rarely causing haemorrhagic stroke
- Hyperventilation
- MI may occur in 6% of those with chest pain
- Ventricular arrhythmias
- Seizures
- Later features – kidney injury, DIC

HOW WOULD YOU MANAGE THIS PATIENT?

- ABCDE approach to assessment and treatment
- Admit to high dependency unit (HDU)
- Blood tests (Hb, white cell count [WCC], U and Es, glucose, INR)
- Arrange urgent CT scan

Progress. In this patient, the CT provided evidence of cerebral haemorrhage, and he was transferred to the stroke unit.

Ecstasy (See Fig. 1.6)

Ecstasy is an amphetamine derivative known as 3,4-Methylenedioxy-methamphetamine (MDMA), which stimulates the sympathetic nervous system and prevents neuronal reuptake of catecholamines, dopamine and serotonin (5-HT).

Clinical Features

- There may be agitation, profound dehydration and low sodium due to excess water consumption and inappropriate antidiuretic hormone secretion
- Early arrhythmias (supraventricular or ventricular) occur and can cause sudden death
- Nausea, vomiting, muscle pain and rhabdomyolysis can occur
- Hypertension (can be severe), which can rarely cause a haemorrhagic stroke
- Hyperventilation
- Visual hallucinations, coma, seizures
- Late features – AKI, DIC, acute respiratory distress syndrome (ARDS)

INVESTIGATIONS

- Baseline: FBC, U and Es, glucose, liver biochemistry
- 12-lead ECG
- Paracetamol and salicylate levels at 4 h or thereafter if coexistent overdose is suspected
- Urine screening for other drugs
- Consider imaging (e.g. CT brain) if reduced GCS or abnormal neurology

Treatment – Supportive

- Activated charcoal reduces absorption within 1 h
- Early hyponatraemia due to excessive water consumption following ecstasy use should be looked for before giving any IV fluids
- Cardiac monitor and watch for hypertension
- Treat agitation or seizures with IV benzodiazepines
- Hyperthermia >39°C can be reduced by 1 L of cold saline - if temperature does not respond, IV dantrolene might help
- Ventricular arrhythmias should be treated with antiarrhythmics

Gamma Hydroxybutyric Acid (GHB)

GHB has been used for bodybuilding and weight reduction. It was sold as a salt, which forms a colourless liquid in water but is no longer available legally. The seaweed-like taste can be impossible to detect when added to an alcoholic drink. GHB has been used to facilitate 'date rape'.

Clinical Features

- History might indicate no intent or knowledge of consumption of any drug
- Initial euphoria, disinhibition, agitation, confusion, nausea and diarrhoea progressing within 1 h to drowsiness and unconsciousness (potentiated by alcohol)
- Nausea, vomiting, muscle pain, sinus tachycardia, and rarely, seizures
- Bradycardia, respiratory depression and even Cheyne–Stokes respiration might rarely occur
- Be alert to the possibility that such patients might have suffered sexual assault

Treatment of GHB Consumption – Supportive

- Activated charcoal reduces absorption within 1 h: observe for a minimum of 2 h, even if apparently much improved clinically
- Monitor BP, HR and pulse oximetry
- Treat seizures with IV benzodiazepines
- Bradycardia associated with hypotension should be treated with IV atropine

Significant Websites

https://www.toxbase.co.uk Toxbase – database of UK National Poisons Information Service
https://www.toxinz.com Database of the New Zealand Poisons Centre
https://www.nlm.nih.gov/enviro/index.html Environmental health, toxicology and chemical information from the National Library of Medicine
https://www.who.int/ipcs/poisons/centre/directory/en Contact details of all poisons centres worldwide
https://www.wikitox.org Home of the Clinical Toxicology Teaching Resource Project

Further Reading

Academy of Medical Royal Colleges. Statement on the initial antimicrobial treatment of sepsis. Oct 2022 [internet publication].

Faculty of Intensive Care Medicine. Guidelines on the management of ARDS. 2018. https://www.ficm.ac.uk/news-events-education/news/guidelines-management-ards.

Herridge, M.S., Tansey, C.M., Matte, A., et al., 2011. Functional disability 5 years after acute respiratory distress syndrome. N. Engl. J. Med. 364, 1293–1304.

Matthay, M.A., et al., 2024 Jan 1. A new global definition of acute respiratory distress syndrome. Am J Respir Crit Care Med. 209 (1), 37–47.

NICE CKS, 2020. Anaphylaxis: assessment and referral after emergency treatment.

NICE CKS, 2024. Suspected sepsis: recognition, diagnosis and early management.

Resuscitation Council (UK), 2021. Emergency treatment of anaphylactic reactions.

Singer, M., et al., 2016 Feb 23. The Third International Consensus Definitions for Sepsis and Septic Shock (Sepsis-3). JAMA 315 (8), 801–810.

Taylor Thompson, B., Chambers, R.C., Liu, K.D., et al., 2017. Acute respiratory distress syndrome. N. Engl. J. Med. 377, 562–572.

CHAPTER 2

Cardiology

Syncope

Simple faints are a common and benign condition. However, anyone witnessing a faint will know that patients can look very unwell, and it is not surprising that they are often brought to the hospital for assessment. Patients who faint are often sat in a chair or even stood up – in both cases causing a recurrence or delaying recovery.

> **CASE HISTORY (1)**
>
> A 25-year-old male is brought to the hospital having fainted at work. He still appears pale, but his clinical examination is normal. He had a similar episode 2 years earlier. His resting 12-lead ECG is normal.

WHAT ARE THE KEY QUESTIONS IN ESTABLISHING THE DIAGNOSIS?

- Reliable eye-witness account: if not available, make a phone call to the patient's workplace
- Prodromal symptoms: nonspecific but almost always present for some minutes before a vasovagal attack (faint)
- Precipitating cause: anything from the sight of blood to a hangover!
- Circumstance of event, frequently in:
  - Pub (even without alcohol)
  - Restaurant: before or after food
  - Church, mosque or synagogue
  - Warm environment

In the absence of any abnormal investigations, the most likely diagnosis is vasovagal syncope (see Table 7.5). You should be aware of some other specific forms of vasovagal syndrome:

- Carotid sinus syncope: commonly on turning the head or shaving the chin, due to carotid sinus hypersensitivity, usually in the elderly
- Cough syncope: after a paroxysm of coughing, usually in a patient with obstructive airway disease
- Micturition syncope: more common in men, usually occurs in the night when going to pass urine or during micturition itself

WHAT IS THE DIFFERENTIAL DIAGNOSIS?

There are many other causes of syncope and all might need to be excluded.
- Cardiac:
  - Arrhythmia: associated with either profound bradycardia or tachycardia, symptomatic palpitations can be a pointer but often are not present
  - Structural: for example, outflow obstruction (notably aortic stenosis or hypertrophic cardiomyopathy), ischaemia, tamponade, pulmonary embolism (PE)
- Neurological: seizures, cerebrovascular disease, transient ischaemic attack (TIA), cerebrovascular accident (CVA) or vertebrobasilar ischaemia are the most common causes. A good

eyewitness account is key to the diagnosis. **Note:** Some jerky movements of the limbs, and even incontinence, can occur in a prolonged vasovagal attack, especially if the patient remains upright

- Metabolic:
  - Hypoglycaemia: well known in diabetics, spontaneous hypoglycaemia from an insulinoma is a rare cause
  - Drugs/alcohol
- Hyperventilation/anxiety (if suspected, symptoms can often be readily reproduced by voluntary hyperventilation): usually associated with a tachycardia, symptomatic palpitations, and the patient might feel light-headed or have a feeling of being distanced from the surroundings. They may experience chest pain and/or paraesthesiae with numbness in their arms, hands or lips. Pallor and peripheral cyanosis can be striking in a full-blown attack. Circumstances provoking an attack can often be the same as for a faint (e.g. warm room, stressful situation)
- Orthostatic hypotension: especially in elderly patients. This is often caused by drugs, for example, for hypertension (HTN), but do not forget autonomic neuropathy and Parkinson disease

Progress. This patient was sent home, having made a full recovery from his 'faint'.

CASE HISTORY (2)

A 68-year-old male passed out suddenly at the wheel of his car and ran into the car in front. His wife reports that he was pale and sweaty, but that loss of consciousness was brief and he recovered quickly.

His pulse is 78/min, blood pressure (BP) 140/85, and there is no abnormality found on examination. His ECG showed a left bundle branch block (LBBB).

REMEMBER

- Sudden loss of consciousness without warning must be assumed to have a cardiac cause until proved otherwise
- Altered consciousness when driving has legal implications and the patient must be warned not to drive again until the diagnosis is established

INVESTIGATIONS

- The history of the event is the key to further investigation and blanket investigations are unrewarding without some clinical pointers as to the cause
- Complete a full systematic physical examination and observations, including a supine-standing BP if possible
- A 12-lead ECG should be performed on every patient presenting with syncope
- Arrange blood tests based on presentation: consider troponin if signs are suggestive of myocardial infarction (MI), full blood count (FBC) if suggestive of anaemia, urea and electrolytes (U and Es) if concerns about potential seizure activity and blood glucose if risk of hypoglycaemia
- If cardiac cause is suspected, arrange transthoracic echocardiography and electrophysiology (EP) studies, for example, Holter monitor
- If neurally mediated (vasovagal) syncope is suspected, consider a tilt test. This is usually carried out with a mechanised tilt table giving a head-up tilt of 60 degrees for 45 min, with continuous ECG and BP monitoring. Although false-positive results can occur, if the prodrome before the faint reproduces the symptoms, it provides strong support for the diagnosis

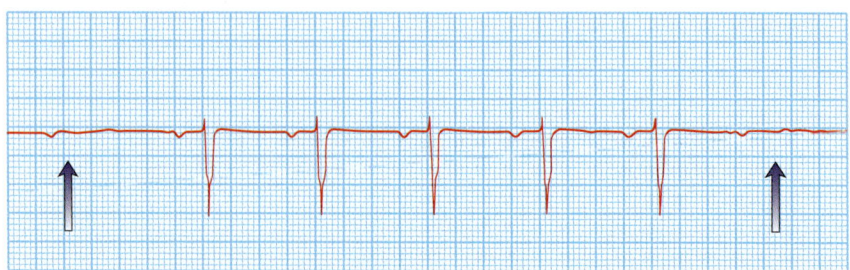

Fig. 2.1   Mobitz type II atrioventricular (AV) block. The P waves that do not conduct to the ventricles (*arrows*) are not preceded by gradual PR interval prolongation. (From Feather A, Randall D, Waterhouse M, eds. *Kumar and Clark's Clinical Medicine*, 10th edn. Elsevier, 2021; Fig. 30.41.)

This patient required admission, cardiac monitoring and further investigation as the LBBB indicates cardiac disease.

Progress. This patient's echocardiogram (echo) showed no abnormality. However, his ambulatory ECG monitoring subsequently showed periods of asymptomatic **Mobitz type II second-degree heart block** (Fig. 2.1). A pacemaker was implanted, and he had no further problems.

CASE HISTORY (3)

A 48-year-old physiotherapist presents with an episode of unconsciousness that occurred when she was at a party with her medical team. A nursing colleague thought she was pulseless at the time of the collapse. She reports two previous similar episodes requiring overnight admission to the hospital. A 12-lead ECG and cardiac enzymes are normal. She was previously investigated with 24- and 48-h ECG tapes, echo and CT scanning of the head, but no abnormalities were found.

An electrophysiological study was therefore performed to exclude the possibility of tachyarrhythmia. During this study, she spontaneously became bradycardic and hypotensive, but no arrhythmias were induced. A tilt table test performed the following day produced profound bradycardia, hypotension and syncope on 60-degree head-up tilting.

REMEMBER

In a tilt test, syncope is often accompanied by 10 to 20 s of asystole. This recovers as soon as the patient is returned to the flat; for this reason, a doctor should always be present.

WHAT IS THE LIKELY DIAGNOSIS?

Neurally mediated syndromes are due to a reflex (called Bezold–Jarisch) that may result in both bradycardia (sinus bradycardia, sinus arrest and atrioventricular (AV) block) and reflex peripheral vasodilatation. These syndromes usually present as syncope or presyncope (dizzy spells).

Progress. A dual chamber pacemaker (DDD) pacing system was implanted and programmed to produce a tachycardic response to counter any detected bradycardia of sudden onset. So far, she has had no more syncopal attacks.

A Clinical Approach to Patients With Tachycardia

The main reason that people have difficulty assessing tachyarrhythmias is that they concentrate on the ECG changes without thinking about the patient.

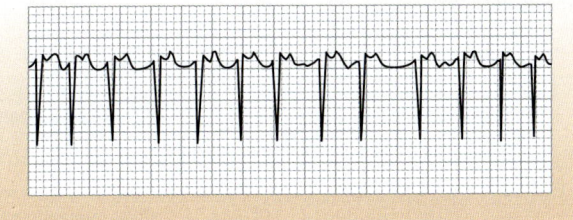

Fig. 2.2 Narrow-complex tachycardia.

CASE HISTORY (1)

A 35-year-old male presents with tachycardia at a rate of 180 beats per minute (bpm). He is not seriously compromised by his tachyarrhythmia and the BP is 128/64. His ECG is shown in Fig. 2.2.

There are three simple questions you need to ask yourself as you approach a patient with an acute tachyarrhythmia:

What Is the Heart Rate and Rhythm?

180 bpm and regular in this patient for example.

Has the Patient Collapsed?

In other words, is the patient clinically compromised by the tachycardia or not? In assessing the degree of cardiovascular collapse, take the heart rate (HR) into account. Remember that the maximal HR you would expect a patient to achieve on the treadmill is 220 minus age.

Someone with an HR at this level (180 bpm) is going at the same rate you would expect if they had just hurried up several flights of stairs.

This patient is not compromised by the tachycardia, so it is likely that he has a healthy ventricle. People with HRs substantially above their predicted maximum, who tolerate the situation well, are more likely to be suffering from a primary electrophysiological problem than from an arrhythmia secondary to left ventricular (LV) disease.

Are the ECG Complexes Broad or Narrow?

Take a 12-lead ECG of the arrhythmia. Divide tachycardias into broad complex (QRS complex of >120 ms or three small squares on the standard ECG) and narrow complex rather than try to split them into supraventricular tachycardia (SVT) and ventricular tachycardia (VT) at first glance. If you follow this approach, you will not treat VT as SVT, which is an error to avoid.

A 12-lead ECG is also valuable in sorting out the mechanisms in narrow-complex tachycardias; the retrograde P waves can be seen in the ST–T segments in reentrant tachycardias, but they may be seen only in some leads. *Don't be fooled into thinking you can diagnose and manage arrhythmias with rhythm strips alone.*

Having answered these questions, you should decide who needs admission to the hospital (Table 2.1).

REMEMBER

Think about the underlying state of the ventricle.

TABLE 2.1 ■ Patients With Tachycardia: Who to Admit

	Broad Complex	Narrow Complex
Collapsed	Usually need immediate cardioversion and must be admitted. Do *not* give verapamil or other negatively inotropic drugs	Usually need admission to hospital, especially if in heart failure
Did not collapse	Require further investigation	Can probably go home if tachycardia stops on treatment (Case 1)
	Need admission to establish diagnosis	Need rapid outpatient assessment
	Irregular tachycardia in this group may be due to WPW with AF, so do *not* give verapamil	If this is a recurrent problem, need a referral to a cardiologist to be considered for EPS, as may benefit from radiofrequency ablation of their pathway or their arrhythmia focus

AF, atrial fibrillation; *EPS*, electrophysiological studies; *WPW*, Wolff–Parkinson–White syndrome.

To be safe:

- Always assume that a broad-complex tachycardia is VT until proved otherwise
- If in doubt, use direct current (DC) cardioversion rather than drugs
- Seek advice if your first drug does not work
- Beware of verapamil (which should not be used as first-line therapy) and other negatively inotropic drugs
- Check the electrolytes and correct them appropriately before using drugs, but do not delay treatment in a patient who is compromised because you are waiting for results. Remember, in an emergency, K^+ levels can be roughly measured using blood gas machines in the emergency department and used to guide replacement therapy

WHAT IS THE LIKELY DIAGNOSIS FOR THIS PATIENT?

Narrow-complex SVT.

SUPRAVENTRICULAR TACHYCARDIA (SVT)

These are narrow-complex tachycardias (Fig. 2.2) unless there is a bundle branch block. Adenosine is very useful for their diagnosis and will terminate some SVTs:

- Atrial tachycardia: an SVT from a focus in the atrium, rather than due to reentry
- Atrial flutter (Afl): look for regular rhythm, often with a rate of 150. Adenosine will help in the diagnosis, often revealing underlying flutter waves
- Atrial fibrillation (AF): look for lack of P waves, irregular rhythm, and baseline; this can be very hard to see with very fast rates, in which case adenosine will help
- Reentrant tachycardias:
  - Wolff–Parkinson–White (WPW) is the classic example of a reentrant tachycardia. The depolarisation wavefront 'reenters' the atrium through the bundle of abnormal conducting tissue between the ventricle and atrium. In some cases, a bundle is present but is not visible on the resting ECG, so that it is a 'concealed pathway'. Never treat AF in WPW with digoxin or verapamil – this can cause dangerous retrograde conduction down the accessory pathway, leading to ventricular fibrillation (VF)
  - Atrioventricular nodal reentry tachycardia (AVNRT)

WHAT ECG FEATURES SUGGEST THAT A TACHYCARDIA IS AN SVT?

- Normal LBBB or right bundle branch block (RBBB) morphology but be careful: VT from right ventricular (RV) outflow tract with LBBB morphology can look like SVT. A small, stubby R wave in V_1–V_2 is characteristic of VT
- You might be able to see evidence of both atrial and ventricular activity. A constant relationship between the P waves and the QRS complexes suggests a supraventricular origin
- The frontal and horizontal QRS axes are in the same general direction as that in the sinus rhythm
- It slows with manoeuvres designed to increase vagal tone, for example, carotid sinus massage
- If the onset is witnessed, you might see a P wave that is premature

HOW WOULD YOU MANAGE THIS PATIENT?

This rhythm responded to adenosine 6 mg IV going up in 6-mg aliquots to a maximum of 18 mg. Intravenous beta-blockade (esmolol has a very short half-life of seconds and can be very useful) can also be used. Synchronised DC cardioversion (start with 50–70 J) should be used if medication fails.

CASE HISTORY (2)

A 57-year-old female presents with a tachycardia at a rate of 132 bpm.
On examination, she is hypotensive (90/50), looks pale and distressed, and has bibasal crackles. The 12-lead ECG shows an axis of –120 degrees, and the complexes are predominantly positive across the chest leads (Fig. 2.3).

WHAT IS THE LIKELY DIAGNOSIS?

This is broad-complex tachycardia with gross axis deviation, probably VT (Box 2.1). The patient needs urgent treatment.

VENTRICULAR TACHYCARDIA (VT)

This causes a broad complex regular tachycardia (Fig. 2.3), often called monomorphic VT. However, a broad complex pattern can be caused by any tachycardia if there is a preexisting abnormality of the conduction system (usually bundle branch block). So, for example, AF with bundle branch block can cause a broad-complex tachycardia that is irregular. Although adenosine can be useful for diagnostic purposes, do not waste time using it if the patient is compromised.

> **BOX 2.1 ■ Distinction Between Supraventricular Tachycardia With Bundle Branch Block and Ventricular Tachycardia**
>
> VT is more likely than SVT with bundle branch block where there is:
> - a very broad QRS (>0.14 s)
> - extreme left axis deviation
> - AV dissociation
> - a bifid, upright QRS with a taller first peak in V_1
> - a deep S wave in V_6
> - a concordant (same polarity) QRS direction in all chest leads (V_1–V_6)
> - presence of capture or fusion beats
> - no response to adenosine
>
> ---
>
> *VT*, ventricular tachycardia; *SVT*, supraventricular tachycardia

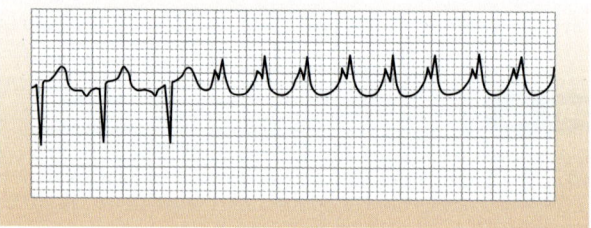

Fig. 2.3   Broad-complex tachycardia after three normal beats.

WHAT FEATURES SUGGEST THAT A TACHYCARDIA MIGHT BE VT?

- A **QRS duration** of >140 ms strongly suggests a ventricular origin
- The frontal and horizontal **axes** are grossly discordant with that seen in sinus rhythm. Most people are used to looking at the frontal QRS axis in the limb leads. The horizontal axis is estimated by seeing where the predominantly negative QRS complexes become equiphasic as you look across from V_1 towards V_6. This equiphasic point is called the zone of transition and is usually at V_3 or V_4. In VT, there might be no transition zone or it might be far to the right, or left, of V_4
- **QRS morphology:** the pattern is not typical of LBBB or RBBB. These are specific appearances that strongly suggest VT, for example, concordance; seek help if unsure
- **Fusion beats:** these are beats where there is simultaneous activation of the ventricles from a focus of arrhythmia and from the atria via the AV node at the same time. These beats will look like a cross between the standard VT complex and the patient's normal complexes in the sinus rhythm
- **Capture beats:** occasionally, the atria 'capture' a normal complex in the midst of a tachycardia
- You might be able to see evidence of both atrial and ventricular activity. If there is no constant relationship between the P waves and the QRS complexes, it suggests a ventricular origin, and this is called AV dissociation

A Word About Torsade de Pointes

Torsade de pointes is an uncommon form of VT with a characteristic ECG pattern (often called polymorphic VT; Fig. 2.4). The complexes appear to twist around the baseline by virtue of their

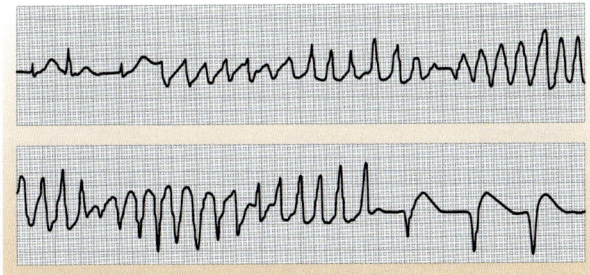

Fig. 2.4 Torsade de pointes showing the complexes twisting around the baseline.

changes in amplitude. It is particularly associated with syndromes, involving a long QT interval. Correct diagnosis of torsade de pointes is necessary because the treatment is very different from VT, and treating the underlying cause can often have a marked effect.

ACUTE TREATMENT OF ARRHYTHMIAS

Always think about the underlying state of the ventricle when treating an acute arrhythmia.
There are problems with the use of any antiarrhythmic drugs:

- Many arrhythmias arise due to preexisting LV disease; you need to be aware of any drugs that you give, which could further suppress LV function and make matters worse
- A drug that is ineffective for the rhythm in question might depress ventricular function without alleviating the rate-related stress on the ventricle
- Ischaemia might alter the electrophysiological activity of drugs that are antiarrhythmic under normal circumstances (Fig. 2.5), making them potentially proarrhythmic in ischaemic myocardium. This limits the use of drugs in many patients because it is often difficult to exclude the possibility of coexisting ischaemia. It is therefore often safer to use DC cardioversion than drugs
- Both digoxin and verapamil can be dangerous in WPW; if you are uncertain, it is safer to use DC cardioversion

Adenosine

Intravenous adenosine should be used in most SVTs and is safe because of its very short half-life. The major limitation is that it should not be used in asthmatics. It will not usually cardiovert AF or flutter but will slow the rate transiently (often for only one or two complexes – have the ECG running) and enable you to see the baseline, helping you make the diagnosis. It will cardiovert most other SVTs. Although it is safe to give adenosine to patients in VT, it will not usually cardiovert the problem, although it might slow the rate. Remember to give it as a rapid bolus; warn the patient, he/she will feel *terrible* transiently, and remember that he/she might become transiently asystolic.

HOW WOULD YOU MANAGE THIS PATIENT?

- This patient has a VT with severe hypotension and pulmonary oedema - she requires emergency DC cardioversion
- Measure and correct any electrolyte abnormality while preparing for DC cardioversion. If in doubt, give empirical IV magnesium sulphate, 8 mmol over 10–15 min (it is not appropriate

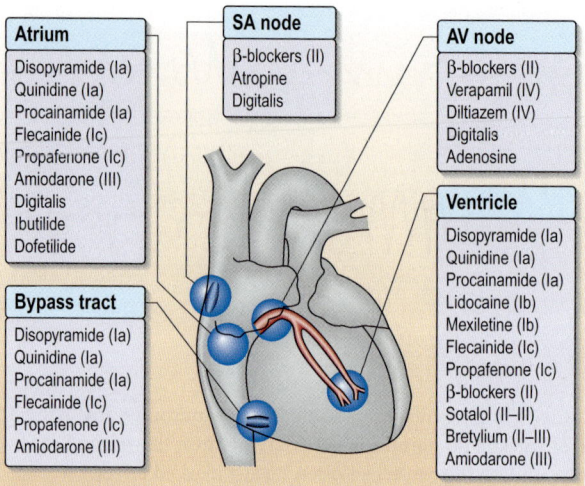

Fig. 2.5   Drugs used to treat arrhythmias. The *numbers* in brackets refer to the Vaughan-Williams classification.

to give K^+ because hypo- or hyperkalaemia can be arrhythmogenic, so you must know the serum K^+ before treating it)

- The arrhythmia did not settle with the DC shock, and IV amiodarone was started with a view to repeat DC cardioversion
- This patient has clinical evidence of poor LV function, but in someone who has a good LV, a beta-blocker, such as sotalol, might be used
- Finally, in patients refractory to treatment, remember the possibility of torsade de pointes, with low magnesium and potassium levels

Progress. Repeat DC cardioversion was successful and this patient improved. However, she remains at risk of sudden death, and therefore she was referred to cardiology for further management. She was given an implantable cardioverter–defibrillator.

Atrial Fibrillation

PREVALENCE AND RISKS

Atrial fibrillation (AF) remains one of the most common and challenging of arrhythmias. It is estimated that 10% of the population will suffer from AF at some stage of their lives. Patients who remain in AF after their hospital admission face a long-term risk of embolism and stroke. This is reduced by the use of anticoagulation, but long-term anticoagulation also carries a risk. In an ideal world, all patients would be cardioverted to sinus rhythm, but this might not be possible when there is underlying heart disease.

CASE HISTORY (1)

A 76-year-old female with a history of HTN presents with a 6-week history of worsening palpitations accompanied by breathlessness.

On examination, she is breathless on minimal exertion and has a raised jugular venous pressure (JVP) with bibasal crackles; BP is 98/58 and HR is 160 bpm. The ECG is compatible with AF (Fig. 2.6).

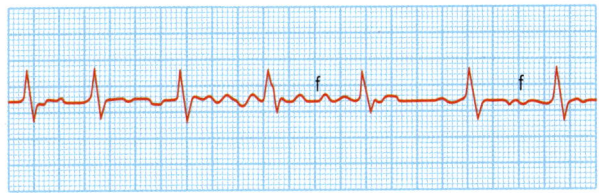

Fig. 2.6 Atrial fibrillation. Note the absolute rhythm irregularity and baseline undulations (*f waves*). (From Kumar P, Clark M, eds. *Kumar and Clark's Clinical Medicine*, 9th edn. Edinburgh: Elsevier; Fig 23.46A.)

HOW WOULD YOU MANAGE THIS PATIENT?

This patient has AF in association with acute heart failure. The chest X-ray (CXR) shows evidence of pulmonary oedema. You need to treat the decompensated heart failure with diuresis (e.g. IV furosemide) and rate control (e.g. digoxin). Remember that a tachycardia might be an indication of poorly controlled heart failure or the AF might have tipped her into heart failure. Occasionally, poor LV function is secondary to poor rate control, but more commonly, poor rate control is secondary to poor control of congestive cardiac failure (CCF). In such cases, where digoxin fails to control the rate (as in this patient), use amiodarone in the acute setting to improve rate control and the chance of cardioversion. The long-term use of amiodarone should be avoided.

Calculate thromboembolic risk with the CHA_2DS_2-VASc score (Table 2.2) against bleeding risk – HAS-BLED (Table 2.3) or ORBIT score. Commence appropriate anticoagulation, for example, low-molecular-weight heparin (LMWH) at acute presentation transitioning to direct oral anticoagulant (DOAC) or warfarin once stable.

Progress. She was anticoagulated and proceeded to cardioversion as an outpatient. She converted to sinus rhythm but had to continue anticoagulation for a further 3 months.

REMEMBER

Atrial fibrillation alone, without evidence of heart failure, can cause breathlessness.

CASE HISTORY (2)

A 70-year-old female with a history of HTN presented to the hospital with a history of 6 h of palpitations. She had been taking 75 mg of aspirin, prescribed by her general practitioner (GP), for 2 years. The ECG showed AF at a rate of 132 bpm. The patient looked well and had a BP of 142/78; there was no cardiomegaly on the X-ray. She was clear that the symptoms started acutely 6 h previously.

HOW WOULD YOU MANAGE THIS PATIENT?

This patient reverted to sinus rhythm in response to a single DC shock (200 J). She remained in sinus rhythm at follow-up 6 months later.

Clinicians have several choices when faced with a patient in AF.

TABLE 2.2 ■ **CHA$_2$DS$_2$-VASc Scoring System for Nonvalvular Atrial Fibrillation**

	Risk Factors	Score/Points
C	Congestive heart failure	1
H	Hypertension	1
A$_2$	Age ≥75	2
D	Diabetes mellitus	1
S$_2$	Stroke/TIA/thromboembolism	2
V	Vascular disease (aorta, coronary or peripheral arteries)	1
A	Age 65–74	1
Sc	Sex category: female	1
Annual risk of stroke		
0 points = 0% risk: No prophylaxis		—
1 point = 1.3% risk: Consider oral anticoagulant in men		—
2+ points = 2.2% risk: Oral anticoagulant		—

TIA, transient ischaemic attack. (From Feather A, Randall D, Waterhouse M, eds. *Kumar and Clark's Clinical Medicine*, 10th edn. Elsevier, 2021; Box 30.15.)

TABLE 2.3 ■ **HAS-BLED Score for Bleeding Risk on Oral Anticoagulation in Atrial Fibrillation**

Clinical Characteristic	Score/Points
Hypertension (systolic ≥160 mm Hg)	1
Abnormal renal function	1
Abnormal liver function	1
Stroke in past	1
Bleeding	1
Labile INRs	1
Elderly: age ≥65 years	1
Drugs as well	1
Alcohol intake at same time	1

INRs, International normalised ratios. (From Feather A, Randall D, Waterhouse M, eds. *Kumar and Clark's Clinical Medicine*, 10th edn. Elsevier, 2021; Box 30.16. From European Society of Cardiology Clinical Practice Guidelines. *European Heart Journal*. 2012;**33**:2719–2747.)

WHEN SHOULD CARDIOVERSION BE ATTEMPTED?

Generally, DC cardioversion is always worth trying at least once provided there are no contraindications. Cardioversion can also be achieved with medications but don't forget that there is nearly as much of a risk of a thromboembolic event as with DC cardioversion. These patients should therefore be appropriately anti-coagulated. Amiodarone (200 mg × 3 daily for 1 week then 200 mg maintenance per day) and class 1c drugs (e.g. flecainide) both promote cardioversion. Fig. 2.5 shows the sites of action of drugs on the heart (N.B. flecainide should not be used in the presence of ventricular disease).

Direct current conversion (using a biphasic defibrillator) reverts AF to sinus rhythm in 80% of patients. This is the best treatment for AF of less than 24 h duration (see Case history 2).

WHAT PRECAUTIONS SHOULD BE TAKEN TO PREVENT EMBOLISM DURING CARDIOVERSION?

The risk of cerebral embolism can be markedly reduced by anticoagulation; patients who have been in AF for more than 24 h should be adequately anticoagulated with warfarin or a DOAC for a minimum of 3 weeks before and 4 weeks after elective cardioversion.

With a transesophageal echo (TOE)-guided approach, patients do not need formal anticoagulation prior to cardioversion but should be covered with a full therapeutic dose of subcutaneous (SC) heparin before and during the procedure. If this is successful, they need another 4 weeks of formal anticoagulation with warfarin (or a DOAC) post procedure.

Remember, a patient suffering a stroke because of lack of anticoagulation in AF is a case of negligence. A common misconception is that aspirin is as effective as warfarin or DOACs, but this is not true. You need to make a careful risk-benefit analysis of the use of oral anticoagulants in elderly patients, but in most of them, the benefits will outweigh the risks (Tables 2.2 and 2.3).

WHAT SHOULD BE DONE TO PROMOTE GOOD RATE CONTROL IN THE LONG TERM IF CARDIOVERSION FAILS?

Digoxin alone is often not effective in rate control and a second drug often needs to be added – beta-blockers or verapamil is usually effective. There is no good evidence that digoxin promotes conversion to sinus rhythm, and it should not be used in paroxysmal AF. The only good way to assess rate control is with a 24-h tape.

If this strategy fails, amiodarone is an excellent second-line treatment: it helps with rate control, makes cardioversion more likely, and can be used with poor LV function, but remember that it does have long-term side effects. However, it can sometimes be effectively used at a lower dose (100 mg daily), with a lower risk of side effects, especially in the elderly.

SHOULD I GIVE PROPHYLACTIC MEDICATION TO PREVENT AF IF SINUS RHYTHM IS ACHIEVED?

This depends on numerous clinical factors, you should discuss this with a cardiologist.

WHICH PATIENTS SHOULD I REFER TO AN ELECTROPHYSIOLOGIST?

Patients without evidence of underlying heart disease and who have either failed drug therapy or do not want to take any medication (usually young patients) should be referred for EP studies with a view to a definitive EP procedure to prevent further AF. However, any patient might potentially benefit from this approach; if in doubt, discuss any case with your cardiologist.

REMEMBER

Atrial fibrillation becomes more stable over time; it might be less easy to cardiovert, the longer you wait.

Bradycardia and Pacing

Bradycardia due to increased vagal tone is a common finding in health and is also seen in an extreme form in vasovagal attacks when periods of asystole can occur.

Bradycardia is an increasing problem in the elderly and very elderly and can reflect degenerative disease of the conducting system at all levels:

- Sinus node: sick sinus syndrome
- AV node: complete heart block, slow AF
- His–Purkinje system: bifascicular block (left axis deviation and RBBB)

CASE HISTORY (1)

A 78-year-old male without any prior cardiac disease was brought to the hospital after collapsing at home with a brief loss of consciousness. On arrival, he had fully recovered and the ECG showed a bifascicular block. During monitoring overnight, he was shown to have periods of **complete heart block**, he had a further syncopal episode, and his HR dropped to 32 bpm.

DIAGNOSIS

- Difficulties often arise in establishing arrhythmia as a cause of dizzy spells when the condition is intermittent, as it often is in the early stages
- Twenty-four-hour ECG is the best investigation, but repeat tapes might be needed to demonstrate an abnormality when the history is very suggestive. Occasionally, in a patient with persistent symptoms and no findings on repeat ambulatory ECG monitoring, an implantable ECG recording device can help

HOW WOULD YOU ACUTELY MANAGE THIS PATIENT?

Bradycardia with any evidence of shock, syncope, MI, heart failure or risk of asystole (Mobitz type 2, complete heart block, recent asystole or ventricular pauses >3 s) requires prompt treatment. Give atropine 1st line (500 mg IV boluses up to 3 mg), then consider an isoprenaline or adrenaline infusion. If this is ineffective, start transcutaneous pacing.

WHAT DEFINITIVE MANAGEMENT DOES THIS PATIENT NEED?

Insertion of a dual-chamber pacemaker (DDD)

HOW ARE PACEMAKERS CLASSIFIED?

Notation is by the following abbreviations:
- Chamber paced (0 = none, A = atrial, V = ventricular, D = both or dual)
- Chamber sensed (0 = none, A = atrial, V = ventricular, D = both or dual)
- Response to sensing (0 = none, I = inhibited, T = triggered, D = both T + I)
- Rate response (0 = none, R = rate modulation)
- Antitachycardia function (0 = none, P = antitachycardia pacing, S = shock, D = pace and shock)

For example, VVI = ventricular pacing, ventricular sensing, inhibition of pacing when a beat is sensed; DDD(R) = dual pacing, dual sensing, inhibition and triggered as appropriate when a beat is sensed, rate response mode available.

WHICH TYPES OF PACEMAKERS ARE COMMONLY USED?

- VVI: usually for AF with slow ventricular rate and/or pauses
- DDD: for complete heart block

Rate response (R) is used when a patient has lost the chronotropic response, that is, cannot increase the HR with exercise/stress. The cardiologist inserting the pacemaker will decide this but will need to know the patient's usual level of activity/independence to make this decision. Atrial pacing and sensing (AAI) pacemakers are not often used in practice because a small proportion of these patients go on to develop coexisting AV nodal disease; in anticipation of this, DDDs are usually implanted.

WHAT ARE THE POTENTIAL COMPLICATIONS OF PACEMAKERS?

All problems with pacemakers need to be referred to the pacing clinic; they will check the pacemaker and adjust its function as necessary. They will also refer to a cardiologist when necessary.

Surgical Problems

- Infection is potentially very serious. Even slight redness around the scar should be treated promptly with antibiotics, for example, flucloxacillin 0.5-1 g × 4 daily; if relevant, send swabs first. This usually occurs early after implantation
- Haematoma can predispose to infection or technical problems

Technical Problems

- Fibrosis occurring around the pacemaker tip can cause pacemaker thresholds to rise, which can affect pacemaker function
- Lead displacement will cause pacemaker malfunction, usually manifesting as failure to capture. It is most common in the first 6 weeks after implantation
- Lead or pacemaker erosion through the skin usually occurs in the long term
- Pacemaker syndrome refers to vague feelings of weakness or dizziness in patients with VVI pacemakers and complete heart block. This is caused by loss of synchrony between atrial and ventricular contraction, leading to episodic falls in BP and retrograde conduction of pacing impulse from the ventricle to atria, which cause simultaneous atrial and ventricular contraction. It is not seen with dual-chamber pacing and is treated by upgrading to a dual-chamber system

---

REMEMBER

If you suspect a pacemaker problem, always send the patient to a pacing clinic that day to have the function checked. The clinic will consult with a cardiologist if necessary. Out of hours, call the cardiologist on call.

CASE HISTORY (2)

A 78-year-old male is admitted for a routine hip replacement. You are quickly bleeped to the orthopedic ward; when you arrive the orthopaedic trainee tells you the patients ECG shows 'VT'. You rush to see the patient, who is sitting up reading his newspaper. His rhythm strip from his preoperative ECG as shown in Fig. 2.7.

WHAT DO YOU TELL THE TRAINEE DOCTOR AND WHAT DO YOU DO?

- This is a paced rhythm, but there is evidence of failure to capture
- You ask the pacing clinic to check his pacemaker; they find that the sensing threshold has risen, but all other parameters are fine
- They increase his pacemaker output, and his pacemaker function returns to normal

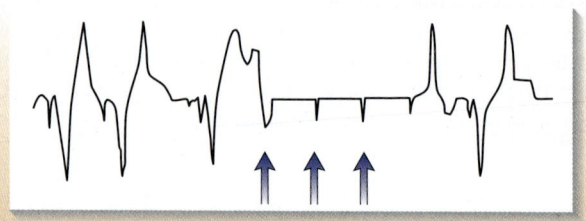

Fig. 2.7   Electrocardiogram showing pacing spikes (*arrows*) with failure to capture.

REMEMBER

- Bradycardia and even transient conduction disturbance (first-degree and Mobitz type I or Wenckebach) can occur in healthy people during sleep. Great caution is needed when interpreting rhythm disturbances at night
- Always take dizzy spells in a patient with a pacemaker seriously. Formal evaluation and an urgent pacing clinic check are required

---

Cardiac Arrest and Basic Life Support

CASE HISTORY

You are walking alone along an isolated corridor of your hospital. Just ahead, you observe someone collapse to the ground. As you approach, you notice he is one of the hospital porters. He is lying motionless.

WHAT SHOULD YOU DO?

- Check for danger, and then shake and shout to check responsiveness
- Call for help if unresponsive
- Open the airway and check for signs of breathing

WHAT TWO METHODS COULD YOU USE TO OPEN THE AIRWAY?

1. Head tilt, chin lift
2. Jaw thrust in suspected cervical spine injury

THERE ARE NO SIGNS OF BREATHING AND YOU REMAIN ALONE. WHAT MUST YOU DO NOW?

You must leave the patient and go to the nearest place where you can initiate the cardiac arrest call
   You have initiated the emergency call from a telephone further along the corridor

WHAT SHOULD BE YOUR NEXT ACTION?

There are no signs of circulation after your assessment. The patient is cyanosed and motionless.
   Commence basic life support (see Fig. 2.8).

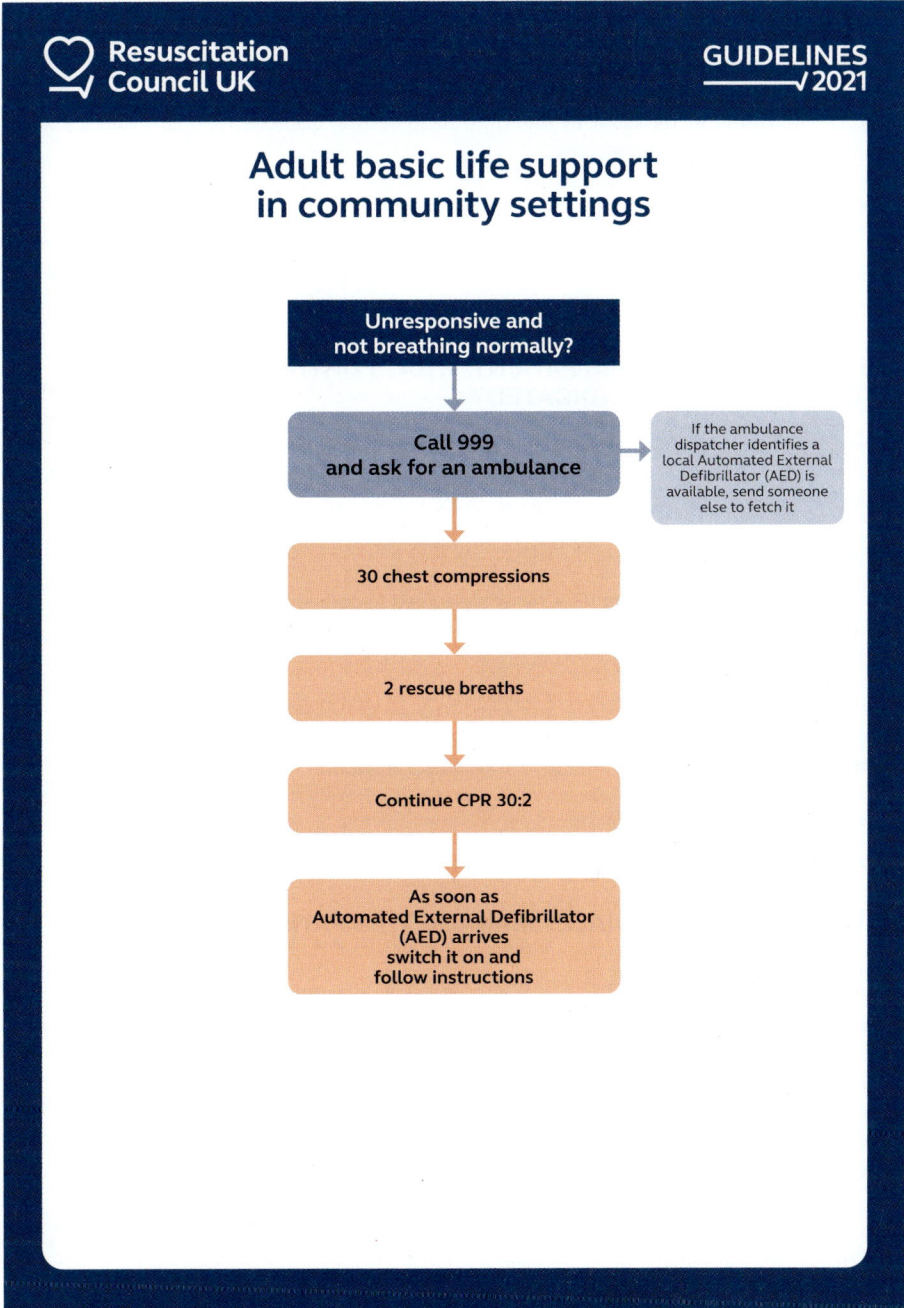

Fig. 2.8 Adult basic life support (out of hospital). AED, automated external defibrillator; CPR, cardiopulmonary resuscitation. (Reproduced with the kind permission of Resuscitation Council UK.)

Commence chest compressions – carefully noting the following:

- Hand position: place the heel of the hand on the sternum, two fingers' breadth above where the rib margins meet
- Arm position: lock the elbows and lean directly over the patient
- Rate: aim to maintain a rate of 100 to 120/min
- Depth: compress the chest by one-third of its resting diameter (5–6 cm), and allow full recoil in between compressions
- Give cardiopulmonary resuscitation (CPR) at a ratio of 30:2 (30 compressions to 2 breaths)
- Continue this until the defibrillator arrives (Fig. 2.9)

Progress. The patient showed VF on the defibrillator and was successfully brought back into sinus rhythm with DC cardioversion, and he now has a palpable pulse.

AFTER STABILISING THIS PATIENT, WHAT FURTHER INTERVENTIONS ARE INDICATED?

He will need further investigations to rule out structural heart disease (echo and angiogram). He will then require EP studies and an automatic implantable cardioverter–defibrillator (AICD; Box 2.2) to prevent recurrence because he has, in effect, had an 'out of hospital' VF arrest.

> **REMEMBER**
>
> - The chance of survival from VF is generally agreed to deteriorate by 5% to 10%/min
> - Early defibrillation is crucial

Chest Pain and Acute Coronary Syndromes

CASE HISTORY (1)

You are called to assess a 73-year-old female who gives a 40-min history of sudden-onset severe dull central chest pain radiating down her left arm. She has a history of treated HTN and has not smoked for 15 years.

HOW WOULD YOU INITIALLY MANAGE THIS PATIENT?

Immediately, when she arrives:

- Targeted history
- Risk factor profile (smoking, HTN, lipids, diabetes, family history, age, gender, ethnic origin)
- Systematic examination (BP, pulse, murmurs, chest signs)
- Serial 12-lead ECG and continuous cardiac monitoring
- Give aspirin 300 mg orally
- Relieve pain – titrate IV morphine to effect and give an antiemetic
- Serial cardiac biomarkers – high sensitivity troponin (usually begins to rise 2 to 3 h after onset of myocardial)
- Send U and Es (correct any electrolyte abnormalities to reduce arrhythmia risk), FBC, lipid panel, glucose and glycated haemoglobin (HbA1c) (important risk factors)

Cardiac Markers in the Early Assessment of a Patient With Chest Pain (Fig. 2.11)

Troponins start to be released within minutes of myocardial damage and are very useful. Apart from in the patient with known LBBB, though, they rarely play a role in initial management

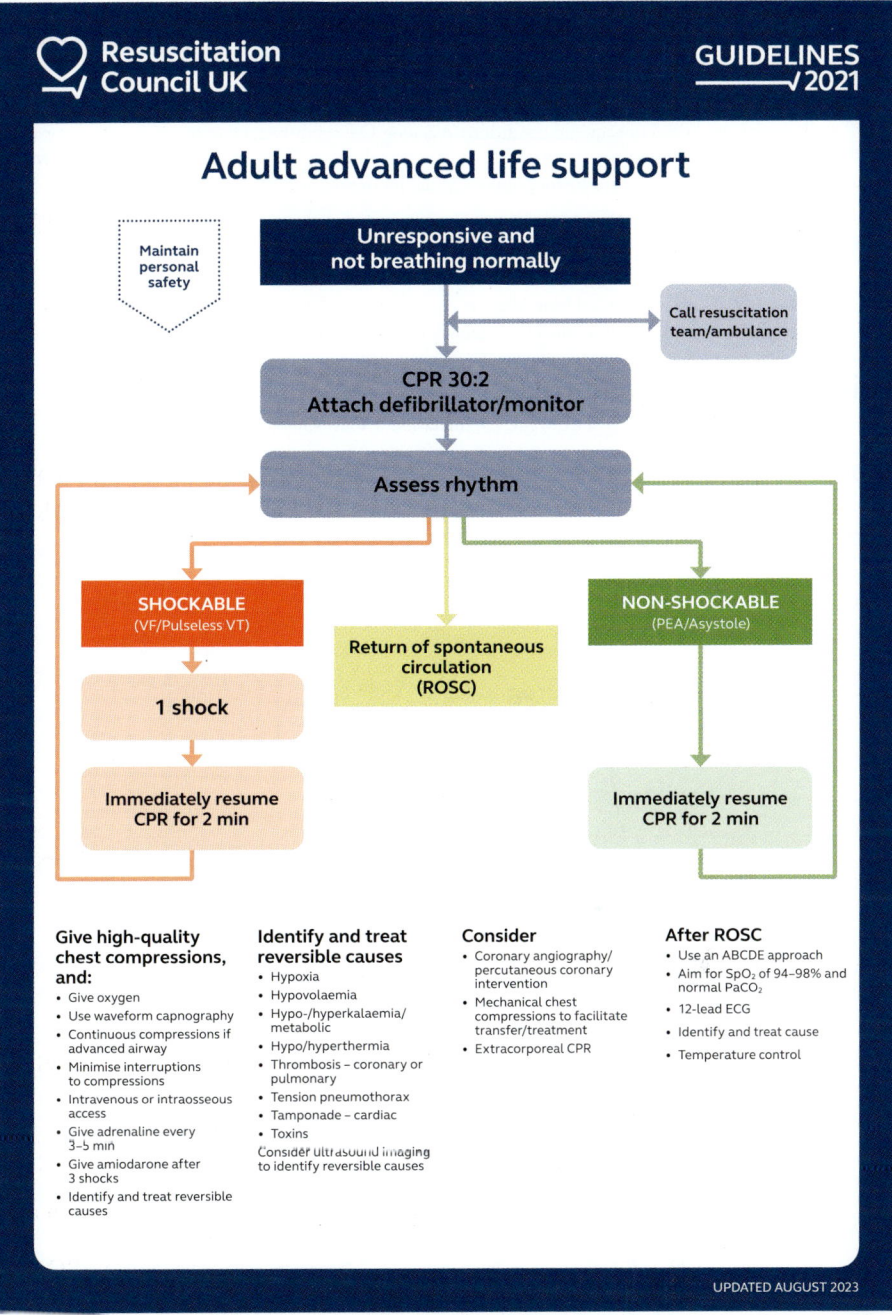

Fig. 2.9 Adult advanced life-support algorithm. ABCDE, Airway, Breathing, Circulation, Disability, Exposure; CPR, cardiopulmonary resuscitation; PEA, pulseless electrical activity; VF, ventricular fibrillation; VT, ventricular tachycardia. (Reproduced with the kind permission of Resuscitation Council UK.)

BOX 2.2 ■ AICDs – Indications for Implantation

Primary Prevention

- Coronary disease, LV dysfunction (EF ≤35%) and inducible VT
- High-risk, inherited or acquired conditions, e.g. long QT syndrome, hypertrophic cardiomyopathy, Brugada syndrome
- Chronic coronary disease, a history of myocardial infarction, and LVEF ≤30%: from MADIT II trial

Secondary Prevention

- Cardiac arrest due to VT/VF
- Sustained VT with structural heart disease
- Unexplained syncope with inducible sustained VT or VF with advanced structural heart disease and no other identifiable cause

AICD Plus Biventricular Pacing

- Any of the above with QRS ≥130 ms, LV dilatation, LVEF ≤30%, and advanced heart failure

AICD, automatic implantable cardioverter–defibrillator; *EF*, ejection fraction; *LV*, left ventricular; *VF*, ventricular fibrillation; *VT*, ventricular tachycardia; *LVEF*, left ventricular ejection fraction.

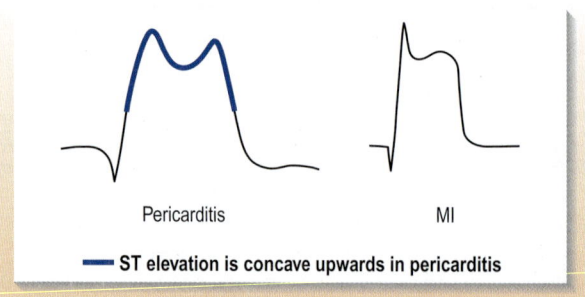

Fig. 2.10   ECG changes in pericarditis and myocardial infarction (MI).

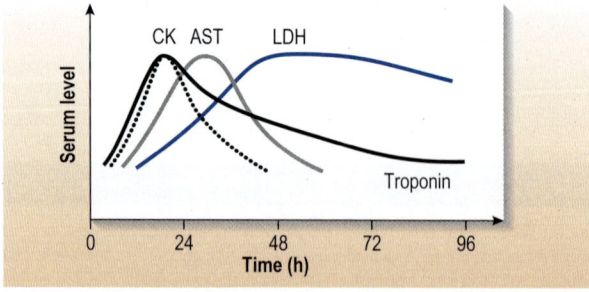

Fig. 2.11   Enzyme and troponin profile in acute myocardial infarction. *AST*, aspartate aminotransferase; *CK*, creatine kinase; *LDH*, lactate dehydrogenase.

decisions at the time of admission in patients with acute coronary syndrome (ACS). They should, however, be measured both at admission and at 4 to 12 h in all patients with a suspected ACS. Most other cardiac markers take several hours to rise and might be misleading; they are therefore used much less, given the availability of troponin assays.

REMEMBER

Every year patients are inappropriately discharged from emergency departments with ACS because their initial investigations are normal. If in doubt admit the patient and repeat.

WHAT ARE THE ACUTELY LIFE-THREATENING CAUSES OF CHEST PAIN TO CONSIDER?

- Aortic dissection
- Acute coronary syndrome (ACS)
- Pericarditis and pericardial tamponade
- Pulmonary embolism
- Pneumothorax
- Boerhaave perforation

Note: Many episodes of chest pain do not fit easily into any category and patients are often admitted and treated for acute ACS. Their symptoms should be assessed in conjunction with their risk factor profile. If in doubt, it is safer to admit.

WHAT FEATURES WOULD MAKE YOU SUSPECT AORTIC DISSECTION?

- Pain tends to radiate to the back, starts abruptly, and is often intense and described as tearing
- On examination: absent arm or leg pulses, murmur of aortic regurgitation (AR), different BP in the arms, neurological signs
- Electrocardiogram might be normal or show inferior ischaemia or MI
- As the dissection in the aortic wall extends proximally, it disrupts the origin of the sub-clavian arteries (affecting arm BP) first, then the carotid arteries (causing neurological sequelae), the origin of the right coronary artery (causing inferior ischaemia), and finally the aortic valve (causing aortic regurgitation)

If you Clinically Suspect Aortic Dissection What Would You Do?

- Seek a senior input early
- *Never* give thrombolytic therapy, heparin, or antiplatelet therapy
- Obtain a CXR to look for mediastinal widening
- Bedside transthoracic echocardiography (TTE) if available (can visualise intimal flap in acute dissection) N.B. although TOE is an excellent investigation, it must be done by a very senior operator and should be carried out in a cardiothoracic centre with surgeons on standby
- Arrange urgent CT of the chest, abdomen and pelvis – 1st line imaging for definitive diagnosis (nonenhanced CT followed by contrast-enhanced CT angiography)
- Carefully reduce BP with a beta-blocker (e.g. IV labetalol)
- Add a vasodilator (e.g. sodium nitroprusside) if HR and BP are not controlled with a beta-blocker
- Discuss with a cardiothoracic centre urgently

Progress. The patient's ECG now changes at approximately 20 min with 4 mm of convex up-sloping ST elevation in leads II, III and AVF. The diagnosis is an inferior ST elevation MI (STEMI).

WHAT OTHER CONDITIONS CAN CAUSE ST ELEVATION?

- Pericarditis: ST changes are often widespread, involving inferior, as well as anterior leads (Fig. 2.10). ST changes are typically concave with peaked T waves and there is often associated widespread PR depression (a feature specific to pericarditis)
- High ST take-off is seen more commonly in certain racial groups, for example, Afro-Caribbean
- Patients with Brugada syndrome typically get ST elevation in leads V_1–V_3 (with a RBBB)

HOW WOULD YOU NOW MANAGE THIS PATIENT?

All hospitals are expected to have rapid triage for chest pain to ensure that all suspected ACS patients are seen without delay. There should be a multidisciplinary team (MDT) approach with defined guidelines. With all ACS patients:
- Comprehensive ABCDE approach to assessment and management
- Intravenous access should be gained and blood sent for cardiac markers (troponin), biochemistry, lipid profile, FBC and clotting profile
- **Oxygen** only if saturations is <90% on pulse oximetry
- **Aspirin** 300 mg chewed, then 75 to 100 mg daily, should be given
- **Sublingual** glyceryl trinitrate (GTN) 0.3 to 0.6 mg should be given for pain relief, repeated as necessary (provided BP is not compromised). Consider an IV infusion of 1 to 10 mg/h titrated to pain (keep systolic BP >100), if sublingual GTN is ineffective, there is uncontrolled HTN, or evidence of congestive heart failure
- Intravenous **opiates** (e.g. morphine) are used as analgesia
- **Give antiemetic** (e.g. ondansetron or metoclopramide)
- Give any patient who will undergo primary percutaneous coronary intervention (PCI) dual antiplatelet therapy with **a P2Y12 inhibitor** in addition to aspirin based on local protocols, options include prasugrel, ticagrelor or clopidogrel

Note: Proton pump inhibitors, particularly omeprazole, reduce the antiplatelet effect of clopidogrel because they are inhibitors of cytochrome p450 (CYP2C19) but have only a small therapeutic effect
- Urgent **reperfusion** is needed – primary PCI if available within 120 minutes, fibrinolysis if PCI is not available <120 minutes and there are no contraindications (Box 2.3)
- **Anticoagulation** (e.g. unfractionated heparin or enoxaparin) is routinely given during PCI; however, this is normally started by the interventional cardiology team
- Patients with a STEMI ideally should start a **beta-blocker** and an **ACE inhibitor** or angiotensin-II receptor antagonist as soon as they are haemodynamically stable; if there is any doubt, wait until they are stable to avoid the possibility of cardiac shock developing
- All ACS patients should be transferred to a coronary care unit (CCU) for continuous monitoring and further specialist care

Note: IIb/IIIa antagonist infusions have not been proven to be of benefit as medical therapy alone. A GP IIb/IIIa antagonist, for example, eptifibatide, should be given by the interventional cardiology team during PCI to help address a high thrombus burden or no-reflow phenomenon.

BOX 2.3 ■ Contraindications to Thrombolytic Therapy

Absolute Contraindications

- Aortic dissection
- Surgery or procedure within the last month
- Stroke within the last 6 months or coma
- Recent GI haemorrhage or symptoms suggesting active peptic ulcer
- Severe liver disease, oesophageal varices, or acute pancreatitis
- Trauma with risk of haemorrhage
- Haemorrhagic diathesis
- Systolic BP >200 mm Hg

Relative Contraindications

- Pregnancy or active menstruation
- Proliferative diabetic retinopathy
- Known aortic aneurysm or intracardiac thrombus
- Known anticoagulant therapy

GI, gastrointestinal; *BP*, blood pressure

THROMBOLYSIS

Fibrinolysis is recommended unless contraindicated (see Box 2.3) if PCI cannot be delivered within 120 minutes of the time when fibrinolysis could be given. The indications are:

- A history of typical ischaemic chest pain, which started within the last 12 h
- A 12-lead ECG that shows persistent ST-segment elevation in at least two contiguous leads of ≥1 mm in all leads other than leads V2-V3 (where the cut off is 2 mm for men and 1.5 mm for women).

Thrombolytic Therapy

The drug used can vary based on local protocols. A fibrin-specific drug such as **alteplase** ('accelerated' recombinant tissue-type plasminogen activator; rtPA) is commonly used (remember you must give concomitant IV heparin or LMWH for the first 24 h with rtPA).

If a patient has any type of contraindication to thrombolysis, you must discuss the case with a cardiologist immediately.

Progress. This 73-year-old patient with a STEMI received PCI and did not develop any further complications. She was seen by the coronary rehabilitation team.

HOW WOULD YOU CLASSIFY ACUTE CORONARY SYNDROMES?

The term 'acute coronary syndrome' covers the spectrum from unstable angina to STEMI. The definition of a MI has been a rapidly evolving area (Box 2.4). The primary decision to make is:

1. Is this a STEMI or a non-ST elevation MI (NSTEMI)?
2. Or is this unstable angina?

The terms STEMI and NSTEMI are used for patients with clinical characteristics compatible with myocardial ischemia and who demonstrate elevated troponin levels. STEMI refers to such patients with an ECG demonstrating persistent ST-segment elevation in at least two contiguous leads of ≥1 mm in all leads other than leads V2-V3 (where the cut off is 2 mm for men and 1.5 mm for women).

BOX 2.4 ■ Definition of Myocardial Infarction (MI)

Both of the following definitions satisfy the diagnosis of an acute, evolving, or recent MI:
1. Typical rise and gradual fall of troponin with at least one of the following:
   - Ischaemic symptoms (chest pain)
   - ECG changes indicative of ischaemia (e.g. ST depression or elevation, T-wave changes)
   - Development of pathological Q waves on the ECG
   - Following coronary artery intervention, e.g. vangioplasty
2. Pathological findings of an acute MI (usually dead patient)

MI, myocardial infarction

Suspect unstable angina when a patient has symptoms suggestive of myocardial ischaemia with no dynamic troponin rise. It is easy to appreciate from the pathogenesis (Fig. 2.12) how failure to treat unstable angina can allow progression to an MI.

SYMPTOMS SUGGESTIVE OF AN ACS

- Angina occurs at rest, at night or with minimal effort
- The pain might require escalating doses of GTN
- It might be associated with sweating, nausea or breathlessness, especially in an MI
- There might be a background of worsening exertional symptoms prior to the admission episode of pain

CASE HISTORY (2)

You are about to finish your shift when the doctor in the emergency department asks you to look at the ECG of a patient who is about to be sent home. The patient is a 44-year-old male smoker who has had anterior central chest pain on and off at rest for the past 2 days. The first ECG shows some subtle T-wave changes in the anterior leads but his repeat ECG is normal and he is now pain-free following sublingual GTN. The doctor has told him he can go home with a GTN spray and come back to the clinic in 6 weeks. The patient is pleased and is sitting, fully dressed, waiting for his GTN spray, because he is keen to get home to watch the football. Can he go home?

WHAT WOULD YOU DO?

This patient absolutely cannot go home! He needs admission, treatment for unstable angina and risk stratification. This is exactly the type of patient who, if sent home, will go on to have an MI.

Management depends on a fast-track approach: 'time is muscle'. Therapy consists of:
- **Aspirin** 300 mg loading dose (unless significant bleeding risk or known hypersensitivity) then 75 mg daily thereafter
- In addition, give the patient **a P2Y12 inhibitor**, for example, prasugrel, ticagrelor, or clopidogrel (see local guidelines) following input from cardiology
- Analgesia as soon as possible: offer sublingual GTN and IV morphine titrated to effect (with an antiemetic)
- Start him on **anticoagulation** (e.g. fondaparinux 2.5 mg subcutaneously once daily) unless high bleeding risk or immediate coronary angiography planned
- Ensure a **troponin** is sent at the time of admission and at 12 h
- Discuss revascularisation with a cardiologist when the troponin result is known (no dynamic change) and risk assessment is complete. Patients with unstable angina are at significantly

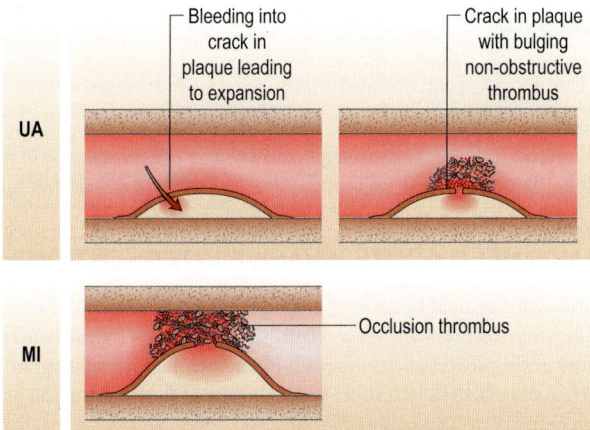

Fig. 2.12 The pathology of unstable angina (UA) versus acute myocardial infarction (MI).

lower risk compared to patients with dynamic troponin changes, suggesting MI. They therefore benefit less from an aggressive invasive approach

■ Start him on a **beta-blocker**, for example, bisoprolol; patients with a sinus tachycardia or HTN will benefit most from this and should be given early beta-blockade

■ Consider an **ACE inhibitor (or an angiotensin-II receptor antagonist)** if the patient has heart failure with reduced LV ejection fraction, diabetes, or chronic kidney disease

■ Assess and correct **risk factors** (smoking, lipids, HTN, diabetes)

REMEMBER

● If the initial ECG is normal, do not discharge the patient. It is possible to have a normal ECG in an ACS
● Repeat the ECG every 20 min for at least 1 h
● Consider other causes of chest
● Further management will depend on risk stratification using the patient's troponin (at 24 h), symptoms and ECG

GLUCOSE AND STATINS

Follow local hyperglycaemia protocols to keep blood glucose levels <11 mmol/L within 48 hours of presentation whilst avoiding hypoglycaemia.

These patients are at very high risk of cardiovascular events, so high-dose statins (e.g. atorvastatin 40-80 mg daily) should be started on admission regardless of low-density lipoprotein cholesterol (LDL-cholesterol) levels. Aim to decrease LDL-cholesterol by >50% from baseline and to achieve LDL-cholesterol <1.4 mmol/L.

Progress. In this patient, the troponins were normal and his symptoms settled. He was admitted under cardiology for further investigation.

CASE HISTORY (3)

A 62-year-old male with type 2 diabetes was admitted to the hospital with a 6-h history of central chest pain radiating to both shoulders and his jaw. The ECG in the emergency department showed 2 mm of ST segment depression in the inferior leads and his initial troponin T was significantly elevated. He was managed as an NSTEMI, his pain settled with medical therapy, and he was referred for PCI.

His angiogram showed a single tight mid-right coronary artery stenosis but no other significant disease. He went on to have a successful angioplasty and a stent, with excellent results.

WHICH PATIENTS NEED ACUTE INVASIVE INTERVENTION?

This is a very rapidly evolving field because of constant advances in techniques and biomechanical engineering, that is, stent technology. As a result, there is a lot of clear evidence from numerous large trials showing improved outcomes with percutaneous intervention in certain groups of patients (FRISC II, Tactics-TIMI 18, GUSTO IV ACS, RITA III – to name just a few). Broadly speaking, these can be put into one of three groups:

1. **STEMI:**
   - Primary intervention: there is clear evidence that PCI is better than thrombolysis for acute STEMI. There is no doubt that given appropriate resources, infrastructure and staff, this is the treatment of choice. In many parts of the world, thrombolysis is still used, although PCI is now more readily available
   - Secondary intervention: patients who are reinfarcting, in whom thrombolysis has failed to resolve the ECG findings and symptoms, have postinfarct angina, or have VT after the first 24 h should be discussed urgently with a cardiologist with a view to urgent PCI
2. **NSTEMI**: stable patients should be risk assessed as per local protocols (e.g. Global Registry of Acute Cardiac Events (GRACE) score) and invasive angiography should be offered within 72 hours of admission to the hospital if the patient is at intermediate or higher risk of future adverse cardiac events
3. **Unstable angina**: patients with ongoing symptoms and evidence of ischaemia, despite medical treatment, should be discussed with a cardiologist for consideration of PCI.

In the long term, the value of revascularisation – whether by surgery or PCI – in relieving persistent symptoms is beyond doubt. Revascularisation should be considered in all outpatients, taking into account their symptoms, lifestyle and investigation results. Generally, bypass surgery is used in left main stem disease, three-vessel disease, diffuse disease with a poor ventricle and diabetics.

Cardiogenic Shock

INFORMATION

Definition

Persistent hypotension (<90 mm Hg systolic) is associated with reduced end-organ perfusion due to low cardiac output. Usually the result of acute MI and manifested by poor peripheral perfusion and low urine output, often associated with clinical/radiological evidence of left ventricular failure (LVF). Mortality approaches 80% with treatment and is much higher without. Predisposing factors include:

- Old age
- Previous MI
- Large anterior MI
- Prior HTN/diabetes
- Inadequate or late thrombolysis

You are called at 2 a.m. to see a 68-year-old female with diabetes who was admitted with a 12-h history of chest pain and ECG changes of an extensive anterior STEMI. She received PCI at 2 p.m. the previous day. She has previously had an inferior NSTEMI. She has remained hypotensive with a poor urine output since admission and is now feeling very unwell. Her current CXR is clear.

HOW COULD YOU MANAGE THIS PATIENT? (SEE FIG. 2.16 LATER)

- Get a repeat ECG to look for evidence of reperfusion or continuing ischaemia
- Check the patient's volume status – consider invasive monitoring, for example, central venous pressure (CVP), pulmonary artery catheter
- Check that there is no structural cause by performing an urgent transthoracic echo:
  - Ventricular septal rupture (murmurs at the left sternal edge – may be inaudible if large); usually occurs after 2 to 3 days
  - Papillary muscle rupture giving severe mitral regurgitation (usually murmur but might be silent)
- Give inotropes IV if there is no response to volume replacement:
  - Dobutamine and/or low-dose dopamine
  - If possible, try to avoid adrenaline (epinephrine) or noradrenaline (norepinephrine) because they will worsen any ischaemia
- Discuss with cardiology immediately for further intervention
- Consider an intraaortic balloon pump (IABP) if available: this is a highly effective way of improving cardiac perfusion and should be used in any patient in whom there is a reasonable prospect of further definitive treatment (e.g. revascula/repair ventricular septal defect). It cannot be used in the presence of significant AR.

Progress. This patient was treated with IV dobutamine with some initial improvement in BP and peripheral perfusion, but 24 h later, she remained anuric and developed acute pulmonary oedema and shock unresponsive to increasing inotropic support. She was too unstable for further coronary invention and died shortly after.

REMEMBER

- In patients on prior beta-blockers, competitive blockade may persist for 24 h or more and will require much higher doses of dobutamine/dopamine
- It is probably simpler in this situation to use milrinone/enoximone, which bypasses the beta-adrenoceptor

INFORMATION

When heart muscle is subjected to acute ischaemia, it might cease to contract but remain viable. This is a potentially reversible cause of haemodynamic problems in acute MI:

- Myocardial stunning – if the blood supply to the relevant area is restored as a result of natural recanalisation of occluded arteries, pharmacological thrombolysis, or angioplasty, the functional capacity might return relatively quickly (over a matter of a few hours)
- Hibernating myocardium – a similar state of affairs might occur on a more chronic basis, usually in severe three-vessel disease. In this case, the cellular ultrastructure might become seriously deranged even though the ischaemic myocytes are still potentially viable. This is known as hibernating myocardium; such myocardium can be restored by revascularisation.

Right Ventricular Infarction

Right ventricular infarction is often associated with volume-dependent hypotension that responds well to fluid replacement.

CASE HISTORY

A 58-year-old male is admitted with an inferior STEMI (Fig. 2.13) and has a successful PCI within 90 minutes of the onset of pain. Although ST elevation and pain largely resolve within 1 h, he remains hypotensive with a systolic BP of 70–80 associated with a low urine output. A further ECG with right-sided chest electrodes (Fig. 2.14) suggests RV infarction with ST elevation in V_3R–V_4R.

HOW DOES RV INFARCTION DIFFER CLINICALLY FROM OTHER AREAS OF INFARCTION?

Right ventricular infarction is:
- Diagnosed readily by elevation of ST segment in V_3R–V_4R on right-sided ECG
- Associated with volume-dependent hypotension

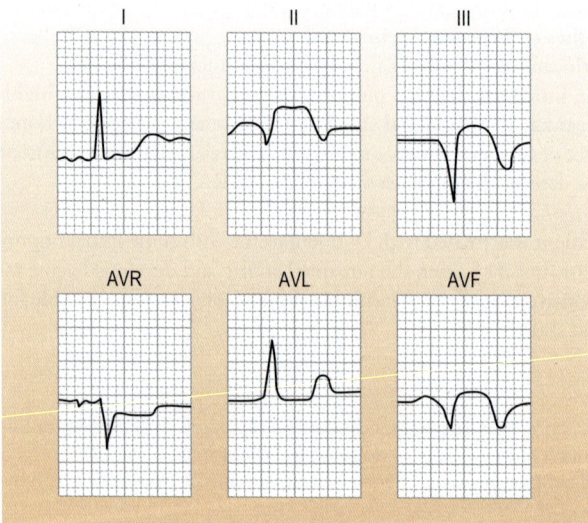

Fig. 2.13 An acute inferior wall myocardial infarction. Note the raised *ST segment and Q waves* in the inferior leads (II, III and AVF).

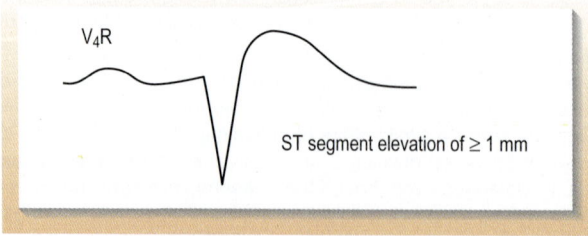

Fig. 2.14 Right ventricular infarct.

- Often associated with elevation of JVP without other evidence of heart failure
- Associated with a higher incidence of all post-MI complications, for example, arrhythmias and cardiac rupture.

Heart failure and cardiogenic shock usually reflect extensive cardiac damage, but cardiac 'stunning' might be present, and active treatment can save lives.

HOW WOULD YOU MANAGE HYPOTENSION IN THIS PATIENT?

Intravenous crystalloid should be given to patients with RV infarction to maintain cardiac output, BPs and coronary artery filling pressures.

Aside from RV infarction, IV fluids should be limited in an acute MI and should only be considered after an appropriate assessment of the patient's filling status (consider invasive measurement in the critical care setting, e.g. CVP or pulmonary artery catheter readings).

Progress. A fluid challenge with 1 L of crystalloid given over 30 minutes restores the BP to 110 systolic with a good urine output. The patient was given medical therapy with aspirin, clopidogrel, beta-blockers and LMWH and was stable after 5 days. He was referred for urgent PCI.

Heart Failure Following Myocardial Infarction

CASE HISTORY

A 63-year-old male has been on the CCU for 5 days following his second MI. He has been managed with PCI and, on this occasion, has had two drug-eluting stents in his left anterior and circumflex arteries. You are asked to see him because he has felt breathless over the last hour.

On examination, he is tachypnoeic with a pulse of 90/min and a BP of 140/80. His venous pressure is raised and he has a gallop rhythm and basal crackles. You suspect **acute heart failure.**

HOW WOULD YOU MANAGE THIS PATIENT?

Initial Treatment

The presence of heart failure, even if transient or only evident on CXR or echo, places the patient with an MI in a far worse prognostic group. Treatment options include:

- An IV nitrate infusion (if no known serious obstructive valvular disease), titrated to BP (keep systolic blood pressure [SBP] >90 mm Hg) and symptoms
- Boluses of IV furosemide 40 to 80 mg, although an infusion is better in severe heart failure
- Invasive monitoring to help guide therapy
- Intravenous inotropes if the patient remains hypotensive despite these measures

After Stabilisation

- Introduce an angiotensin-converting enzyme inhibitors (ACEIs) (or angiotensin receptor antagonist) as soon as possible: ACEIs have been shown to reduce the mortality of this high-risk group by 20% to 30%. Initiate this therapy as soon as the patient is off inotropes and haemodynamically stable with stable renal function. Ramipril (1.25 mg initially) is a good choice, given its simple dosing regimen. A slight deterioration in renal function (up to 30%) might be seen; if this happens, do not increase the dose. If, despite this, renal function continues to worsen, withdraw the ACEI and reconsider at a later date
- Introduce a **beta-blocker** as soon as it is safe: there is a wealth of evidence supporting the use of beta-blockers in heart failure to improve prognosis. Even patients with severe heart

failure benefit from the cautious introduction of beta-blockers (provided the patients are not on IV inotropes or vasodilators), for example, carvedilol, starting at 3.125 mg × 2 daily or bisoprolol, starting at 1.25 mg daily (titrated to response)

- A ldosterone antagonists (e.g. spironolactone 12.5 to 50 mg daily) are recommended in heart failure with a reduced ejection fraction (HFrEF)
- Consider further revascularisation: remember patients will benefit from revascularisation if part of their poor ventricular function is due to viable stunned or hibernating myocardium. All patients with postinfarct cardiac failure should be seen by a cardiologist

Progress. The patient was treated intensely with diuretics, an ACEI and a beta-blocker. He made a very slow recovery but was able to be discharged in 2 weeks and followed up by cardiologists.

Post-Infarction Arrhythmias and Heart Block

CASE HISTORY (1)

A nurse on the CCU calls you at 5 a.m. A 56-year-old male without previous heart disease was admitted with an inferior MI and underwent PCI at 11 p.m. the previous evening. The nurse had been looking at the monitor and noticed that the patient kept having ectopics and has had two short five-beat bursts of nonsustained VT. When you arrive, the patient is lying flat, fast asleep with a HR of 50 (sinus rhythm), and haemodynamically stable. He was given a beta-blocker on admission, and when you look at his results, all his electrolytes (including Mg^{2+} and Ca^{2+}) are normal. You are asked by the nurses whether this patient should be prescribed anything?

WHAT DO YOU DO?

- Additional antiarrhythmics are not indicated. In the CAST trial, postMI patients with asymptomatic ventricular arrhythmias were randomised to antiarrhythmic drugs or placebo; the patients given antiarrhythmics had a worse outcome
- There is no role for giving empirical IV Mg^{2+} to all patients with an acute MI, as shown by the MAGIC trial
- Arrhythmias—atrial and ventricular—are common in the first 24 h after an MI and might be life-threatening. For this reason, all these patients must be in monitored beds on the CCU. Late arrhythmias (after the first 24 h) are of more prognostic significance and will require specialist evaluation

EARLY VENTRICULAR ARRHYTHMIAS

- Ectopics and nonsustained VT are very common, particularly in the 1 to 2 h after thrombolysis ('reperfusion arrhythmias') and usually require no treatment. Check K^+, Mg^{2+} and Ca^{2+}, and correct if needed
- For sustained VT (or after VF), cardioversion/defibrillation is indicated followed by antiarrhythmic medication (options include amiodarone or lidocaine)
- Early use of IV beta-blockers, for example, metoprolol, often reduces the incidence of ventricular arrhythmias

Progress. This patient's arrhythmias settled without the need for anti arrhythmics. He was discharged with an outpatient appointment with the cardiologist.

CASE HISTORY (2)

A 72-year-old female with diabetes was admitted with an anterior MI and received thrombolysis 8 h after the onset of pain. The CXR demonstrated pulmonary venous congestion. The ECG after thrombolysis is shown in Fig. 2.15.

During the night, the nurses observed isolated nonconducted P waves but no action was taken. The next morning, the patient collapsed with an HR of 28 bpm and a complete heart block; she had not passed urine since admission. A wire was passed via the internal jugular route, and she was successfully paced. Despite this, she developed increasing heart failure and died 2 days later.

INFORMATION

Anterior MI and (complete) heart block (CHB) carry a very high in-hospital and 1-year mortality.

HEART BLOCK

Management is usually very different for inferior and anterior MI. In inferior infarcts, a conduction disturbance is common. Provided the patient is not haemodynamically compromised, temporary pacing is usually not required, and the problem resolves within 2 weeks; permanent pacing is rarely required. However, heart block in anterior infarcts invariably represents extensive myocardial damage and nearly always needs pacing (temporary and permanent).

INFORMATION

Indications for Temporary Pacing Post-MI

- Mobitz II heart block with anterior MI
- Third-degree CHB with inferior MI if hypotensive or cardiac failure, *always* with anterior MI
- Bifascicular block (RBBB with left or right axis deviation): usually anterior MI and at risk of CHB
- Trifascicular block (long PR interval and either LBBB or RBBB with axis deviation): usually anterior MI and at risk of CHB
- Alternating LBBB and RBBB: usually extensive myocardial injury and high risk of CHB

Note: Do not use the subclavian route after thrombolysis; instead, choose either the jugular or the femoral route because there is less risk of haemorrhagic complications

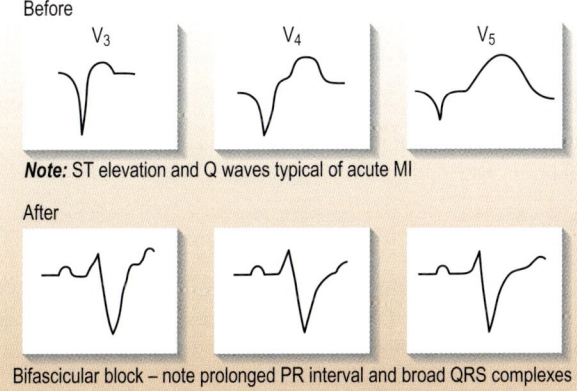

Note: ST elevation and Q waves typical of acute MI

Bifascicular block – note prolonged PR interval and broad QRS complexes

Fig. 2.15   Electrocardiogram following thrombolysis in this patient.

MANAGEMENT OF LATE ARRHYTHMIAS

- Atrial fibrillation/SVT: commonly associated with pericarditis or heart failure. Usually self-limiting or responds to digoxin. Consider cardioversion if this fails or the patient is compromised. Treat pericarditis or cardiac failure actively
- Ventricular tachycardia: as a late event carries a bad prognosis
- Beta-blockers: all patients should be on these unless contraindicated
- Intravenous amiodarone: if there is recurrent VT that has not settled with beta-blockers
- All patients must be referred for early inpatient angiography, appropriate EP investigations, and management as necessary (usually implantation of an internal defibrillator)
- Avoid other antiarrhythmics, especially those that are negatively inotropic, for example, flecainide

REMEMBER

Ventricular 'escape' rhythms are common in bradycardia due to increased vagal tone and usually respond to atropine

Myocardial Infarction – Secondary Prevention

The greatest concern of patients who have recovered from a heart attack is whether they will have another. As well as lifestyle changes, a wide range of drugs is available for secondary prevention, with strong evidence to support their use. The following should be undertaken:

- Smoking cessation
- Strict control of BP
- Diet modification with a view to appropriate weight loss: low fat, low salt, fish oils, high vegetable content
- Exercise
- Drug therapy

DRUG THERAPY

Antiplatelet Therapy

Aspirin
- Dose: 75 mg daily (indefinitely).
- Contraindications: clear history of type 1 allergic reaction (angio-oedema, anaphylaxis). If there is a history suggestive of peptic ulceration disease, give a proton pump inhibitor. *Note:* check later for the presence of *Helicobacter pylori* and eradicate

P2Y12 inhibitor
- Continue the P2Y12 inhibitor used in the acute phase for 12 months
- Follow local protocols – options include prasugrel, ticagrelor and clopidogrel

Beta-blockers

- Should be used in all patients
- Evidence: 20% to 25% mortality reduction; greatest benefit in the high-risk group (prior MI, diabetes, transient heart failure). Likely a class effect but documentary evidence for propranolol, timolol, metoprolol and acebutolol
- Contraindications: reversible airways disease

Calcium-channel Blockers

- Nondihydropyridines (e.g. verapamil): should not be routinely used, and in STEMI, have not been shown to improve mortality (INTERCEPT trial). However, they can be given when beta-blockers are contraindicated and rate control is needed
- Dihydropyridines, for example, nifedipine: have no place in secondary prevention and might be harmful

Angiotensin-converting Enzyme Inhibitors (ACEIs)

Should be given to all patients with post-ACS (HOPE trial); those with reduced ventricular function obtain most benefit. There are many large trials to show this. Although it is probably a class effect, ramipril, lisinopril and enalapril are most commonly given; captopril is less used because it causes more severe first-dose hypotension.

Monitor BP and renal function. If ACEIs are contraindicated or not tolerated due to cough, an angiotensin receptor antagonist such as losartan is given. In the VALIANT trial, it was shown that valsartan is equivalent in efficacy to, but no better than, an ACEI.

Lipid-lowering Drugs

'Statins' should be given to all patients because there is a huge amount of evidence backing their use in primary (WOSCOPS) and secondary prevention (4S trial) in ischaemic heart disease. This is highly likely to be a class effect. Pravastatin has the best side-effect profile, but atorvastatin is more powerful in reducing cholesterol. These should be started on the day of admission (ensure a lipid profile has been sent; see earlier). Occasionally, myalgia/myositis can occur in the first few weeks in some patients. Do not forget to look at and treat low-high-density lipoproteins (HDLs).

Anticoagulation

There is no evidence that this is routinely of any benefit. However, it might be valuable in:

- Patients with proven LV thrombus, those at risk of LV thrombus (large ventricle and LV dysfunction)
- Those with AF

WHICH PATIENTS WOULD BE AT HIGHER RISK FOLLOWING MI?

- Prior ischaemic heart disease, HTN, diabetes mellitus
- Heart failure (even transient)
- Late arrhythmias (>24 h after MI)
- Age >60 years
- Impaired ventricular function
- Inability to perform exercise tolerance tests because of cardiac symptoms

REMEMBER

- All patients should be offered cardiac rehabilitation
- Strict blood sugar control improves prognosis in diabetics; a 3-month regimen of subcutaneous (SC) insulin is often needed
- After MI, the lipid levels might fall for up to 2 months. Ideally, check the lipid profile at this stage, although statin therapy is given (after a random cholesterol has been sent) at presentation
- High-risk patients benefit most!

Heart Failure Recognition and Acute Management

Differentiating heart failure from lung disease as a cause of breathlessness can be difficult because there is often coexisting cardiac and respiratory disease. In the case of smokers, this usually consists of ischaemic heart disease and chronic obstructive pulmonary disease (COPD). There is thus a tendency to give a concoction of therapy to cover both cardiac failure and an exacerbation of COPD, often with antibiotics added in to cover infection, especially in the elderly. This section attempts to provide a diagnostic route to clarify the problem and seek therapeutic solutions.

CASE HISTORY

At 3 a.m., a doctor in the emergency department refers to you an 80-year-old male with a 4-day history of increasing breathlessness, wheeze and nonproductive cough. He lives alone in a first-floor flat and smokes 10 cigarettes a day. The doctor is not sure of the diagnosis but suspects a chest infection.

COULD IT BE HEART FAILURE?

Remember that wheeze and cough occur in heart failure, as well as respiratory disease. Although the onset of breathlessness is often rapid in heart failure, it can also be rapid in respiratory disease. Clinical examination might help you further differentiate the two, but you often need the results of investigations to help distinguish the causes.

- In heart failure, the ECG will most likely be abnormal
- The echo will invariably show depressed systolic function (but beware of a small percentage of patients with diastolic heart failure and normal systolic function)
- The CXR will help, as will respiratory function tests (but remember respiratory function tests may be of no help in the acute phase)
- Serum natriuretic peptides are useful in the diagnosis of heart failure; serum brain natriuretic peptide (BNP) >200
- Assess response to therapy

Progress. The patient gives you a history of sudden onset of breathlessness, preceded by dull chest pain, which started 4 days ago. On examination, he is apyrexial, tachypneic, and sitting up; he has crackles at both his lung bases, a small left-sided pleural effusion, a raised JVP and a BP of 160/95. His ECG showed an old anterior MI.

He clearly has LV failure, the aetiology of which is likely to be ischaemic heart disease with HTN.

WHAT ARE THE COMMON CAUSES OF HEART FAILURE?

Common causes of acute cardiac failure include:

- Ischaemic heart disease
- Hypertension
- Valvular heart disease
- Profound tachy- or bradycardia
- Myocarditis
- Myocardial depression by drugs
- Cardiac tamponade

If you can't identify an aetiology for the cardiac failure and the ECG is normal, reconsider your diagnosis; don't forget the possibility of constrictive pericarditis or diastolic ventricular dysfunction. This latter diagnosis is difficult to make but is more common in elderly hypertensives and can be diagnosed with an echo.

When cardiac failure appears, consider what has precipitated it and treat this, as well as the failure itself. Such precipitating factors include:

- Arrhythmia: tachycardia or bradycardia (e.g. AF, CHB)
- Myocardial infarction
- Excess fluid intake (e.g. postoperative IV fluids)
- Excess fluid retention (e.g. NSAIDs, acute kidney injury)
- Anemia, thyrotoxicosis or any precipitating illness, such as infection in the elderly
- Either precipitating drugs or poor medication compliance in a patient on antifailure drugs

Rule out the above with the appropriate investigations and correct them if possible.

Progress. The patient remained breathless despite an initial bolus of furosemide 80 mg. His CXR confirmed that he had pulmonary oedema.

HOW WOULD YOU FURTHER MANAGE THIS PATIENT? (FIG. 2.16)

He needs rapid therapy to improve his clinical condition, with acute treatment to correct his breathlessness, followed by further therapy to maintain and improve LV function.

The acute phase of therapy can consist of:

- Intravenous **nitrates** (e.g. GTN 10–400 µg/min, start low and titrate to response not <90 mm Hg): these provide excellent and rapid symptomatic relief by offloading the ventricle.
- Continue IV diuretics, initially as boluses (e.g. furosemide 40–80 mg) but this patient might need a furosemide infusion
- Angiotensin-converting enzyme inhibitors or angiotensin receptor antagonist:
    - Start after acute symptoms have settled and the patient is haemodynamically stable

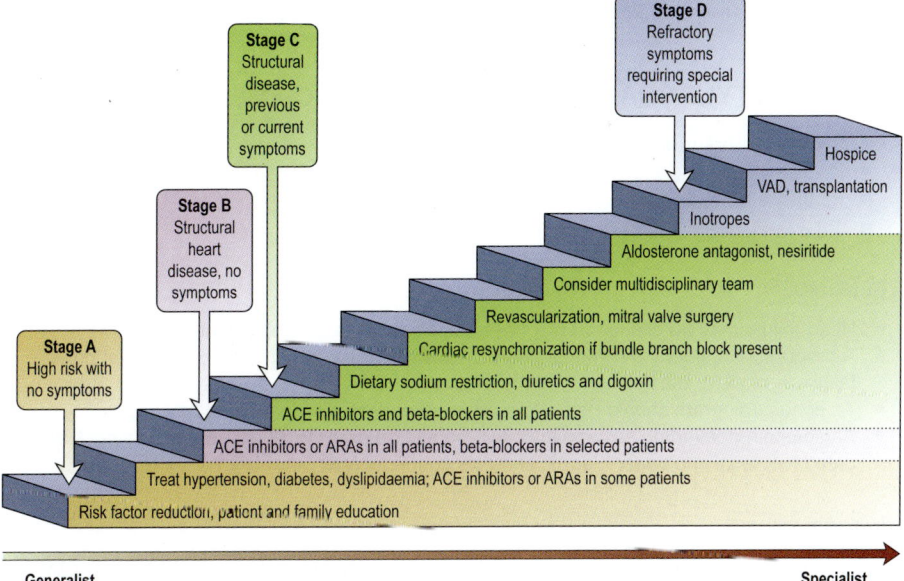

Fig. 2.16 Stages of heart failure and treatment options for systolic heart failure. ACE, angiotensin-converting enzyme; ARA, angiotensin II receptor antagonist; VAD, ventricular assisted device. (From Feather A, Randall D, Waterhouse M, eds. *Kumar and Clark's Clinical Medicine*, 10th edn. Edinburgh: Elsevier; Fig. 30.57.)

- Remember to monitor renal function
- Use an appropriate dose of ACEIs, or they will be ineffective
- **Beta-blockers:**
  - There is excellent evidence to back their use (e.g. CIBIS II, MERIT) and they should be started as soon as the patient is haemodynamically stable and off IV inotropes and IV vasodilators. There is now evidence to support their use even in patients with severe heart failure. Either carvedilol or bisoprolol is the first-line drug (see starting dose, mentioned earlier)
  - Up-titration of the drugs must be very gentle (every 2 weeks). Warn patients that they might initially feel worse. If their symptoms worsen, do not increase the dose; if they continue to worsen, reduce or stop the beta-blockers
- **Spironolactone:** 12.5 to 50 mg daily should be given to all patients with a reduced ejection fraction; check the potassium because of the risk of hyperkalaemia
- **Digoxin:**
  - Valuable in AF
  - Shown to reduce the rate of hospitalisation, not mortality (VA study)
- Noninvasive ventilation (NIV): patients often respond very well to just continuous positive pressure ventilation (CPAP) alone, but they might need bilevel positive airway pressure (BIPAP). You should be aware that positive pressure ventilation might cause hypotension: monitor the patient appropriately

---

INFORMATION

Patients are often left on excessively high doses of diuretics and can easily become dehydrated on discharge, unless their therapy is reduced. However, patients developing heart failure while on diuretics usually require to be discharged on a higher dose than on admission.

The trend would be to increase the dose of the ACEI while reducing the diuretic dose and assessing the response by monitoring symptoms, signs and weight. Ideally, this should be done by a heart failure clinic; these are often nurse-led and are excellent for such patients.

WHAT LIFESTYLE CHANGES WOULD YOU RECOMMEND?

- Reduce alcohol intake
- Reduce weight
- Reduce salt intake
- Take moderate regular exercise

REMEMBER

- Heart failure may be difficult to diagnose, especially with diastolic dysfunction
- A proportion of elderly patients are on diuretics but have no objective evidence of heart failure (systolic or diastolic)
- An echocardiogram should be performed on all patients to identify the aetiology
- Angiotensin-converting enzyme inhibitors should be given to all patients unless contraindicated (i.e. renal impairment, aortic stenosis and renal artery stenosis)

INFORMATION

- Systolic heart failure is associated with a decreased left ventricular ejection fraction (LVEF) (also known as heart failure with reduced ejection fraction [HFrEF]). The heart is enlarged and there is frequently accompanying diastolic heart failure. The cause is often ischaemic heart disease

- In diastolic heart failure (also known as heart failure with preserved ejection fraction [HFpEF]), there is normal LV systolic function with a small heart and impaired LV filling. It often occurs in the elderly in association with HTN.

Progress. This patient was treated according to the algorithm in Fig. 2.16. He made a gradual recovery but was unable to go home. He was placed in a nursing home but was readmitted with a recurrence of pulmonary oedema and died.

Pericardial Disease

Pericarditis is inflammation of the pericardium and typically presents with chest pain. The pericardium consists of an outer layer (fibrous pericardium) and inner layer (serous pericardium), which rub against each other when inflamed. Most cases are idiopathic or caused by viral infection and resolve spontaneously with antiinflammatory medication in <4 weeks. Rarely chronic recurrent pericarditis can develop.

CASE HISTORY (1)

A 41-year-old male presents with a 2-day history of sharp retrosternal chest pain that is worse on inspiration. He also reports having fevers and generalised muscle aches. The chest pain is worse when lying flat but sitting forward relieves it. He is a smoker but otherwise has no other medical problems and takes no regular medication.

On examination, a high-pitched noise is heard on auscultation over the left sternal border on end expiration, but the other heart sounds are normal.

Based on this presentation, you suspect a diagnosis of **pericarditis**.

WHAT ARE THE RISK FACTORS?

Risk factors include:
- Male
- Aged 20 to 50 years old
- Recent cardiac surgery or transmural infarction
- Recent viral or bacterial infection
- Uraemia or ongoing dialysis
- Systemic autoimmune disorders

See Table 2.4 for a full list of potential causes.

WHAT INVESTIGATIONS WOULD YOU REQUEST?

- A 12-lead ECG is required for any patient with suspected acute pericarditis. ECG changes occur in up to 60% of cases and typically include (Fig 2.10):
  - Global 'saddle-shaped' ST elevation with PR depression
  - J-point depression and PR elevation in leads aVR and V1
- Full blood count, urea and electrolytes, liver function tests
- Inflammatory markers (C-reactive protein [CRP] and consider erythrocyte sedimentation rate [ESR])
- Serial troponins if myocardial ischaemia or myocarditis is suspected

TABLE 2.4 ■ **Aetiology of Pericarditis**

Idiopathic	Most Common
Infectious	Bacterial, e.g. *pneumococcal, meningococcal, Haemophilus*, tuberculosis
	Viral, e.g. Epstein-Barr, cytomegalovirus, HIV, influenza
	Fungal, e.g. *Candida*
Inflammatory	Autoimmune disorders, e.g. SLE, rheumatoid arthritis, reactive arthritis, vasculitis
	Secondary inflammatory processes, e.g. post myocardial infarction (Dressler) syndrome, paraneoplastic
Metabolic	Uraemia, myxoedema
Iatrogenic	Drug related, e.g. amiodarone, isoniazid, phenytoin, hydralazine, chemotherapy
	Radiotherapy

SLE, systemic lupus erythematosus

- Echocardiogram: up to 50% will have pericardial effusion
- Consider CXR to assess for evidence of heart failure (can visualise classic 'flask-shaped' heart in large pericardial effusions)

HOW WOULD YOU MANAGE THIS PATIENT?

- Treat potential underlying cause (e.g. bacterial infection) or stop potential causative agent if potentially iatrogenic
- Advise to stop all strenuous exercise for the duration of symptoms
- Non-steroidal anti-inflammatory drugs (NSAIDs), such as aspirin or ibuprofen, are first-line (consider proton pump inhibitor [PPI] cover). These reduce fever, pain and inflammation but do not prevent complications. Aspirin is preferred if there is a history of coronary disease as other NSAIDs impair myocardial healing
- Start colchicine (unless tuberculosis is suspected) if the patient has suspected idiopathic or viral pericarditis and continue for 3 months. This significantly reduces the risk of recurrent pericarditis. Colchicine has a narrow therapeutic window so be wary of drug interactions
- Corticosteroids can be considered if an infectious cause is unlikely and first line treatment is not effective or an autoimmune cause is suspected

Progress. This patient had a normal echocardiogram, his symptoms improved significantly with NSAIDs and he was discharged to outpatient follow-up with a plan to complete 3 months of colchicine.

CASE HISTORY (2)

A 71-year-old female presents to the emergency department with worsening shortness of breath over the last 3 days associated with a sharp chest pain and bilateral ankle oedema. She has a history of nonsmall-cell lung cancer for which she is receiving chemoradiotherapy. She has no previous history of cardiac disease.

On examination, she is anxious and has a respiratory rate of 25 breaths/min, an HR of 115 bpm and a BP of 95/52 mm Hg. Her JVP is significantly elevated, there is pitting oedema to the ankles and her heart sounds are muffled on auscultation.

WHAT ARE THE POTENTIAL COMPLICATIONS OF PERICARDITIS?

- Pericardial effusion with or without cardiac tamponade (in up to 3% of cases)
- Chronic constrictive pericarditis
- Recurrent pericarditis
- Purulent pericarditis

WHAT IS THE MOST LIKELY CAUSE OF THIS PATIENT'S SYMPTOMS?

Diagnosis – cardiac tamponade.

This is a medical emergency and requires prompt treatment. It results from the accumulation of fluid, blood, pus, or air within the pericardial space restricting filling and decreasing cardiac output. Patients commonly present with chest pain and shortness of breath. Most will not present with all of the features of Beck's classic triad:

- Hypotension
- Muffled heart sounds
- Raised JVP

INVESTIGATIONS

- 12-lead ECG is essential: examine rhythm strip for electrical alternans (alternating QRS amplitude), which is rarely seen in the absence of tamponade
- Full blood count, U and Es, CRP (consider ESR) and troponins – may help determine the etiology
- Transthoracic echocardiogram – assesses effusion size, gives rapid haemodynamic data

HOW DO YOU ACUTELY MANAGE CARDIAC TAMPONADE?

- **Pericardiocentesis** – paraxiphoid approach, aspirate and consider exchanging for a pig-tailed catheter to facilitate continuous drainage. Use ultrasound guidance if available. Send fluid for culture and cytology. Do not drain >1 L initially as larger volumes are associated with dilation of the right ventricle
- **Surgical drainage** – consider if history of trauma or high suspicion of haemopericardium, purulent effusion or neoplastic disease

REMEMBER

Carry out a full assessment and risk stratification, including an echocardiogram, before considering discharging a patient with suspected pericarditis.

Valvular Heart Disease

AORTIC STENOSIS

In the UK, the most common cause of aortic stenosis in the elderly is degenerative calcific disease; in younger patients, it is more often due to a congenital bicuspid valve. Although it is now less common, do not forget rheumatic heart disease as a cause.

CASE HISTORY (1)

A 75-year-old male is brought to the hospital after he had blacked out when running for a bus. He had fully recovered when he reached the hospital.

Cardiac examination revealed a normal pulse, with normal rhythm and BP of 160/95. The heart sounds were soft with an ejection systolic murmur heard all over the precordium.

The CXR was normal and the ECG showed LBBB. A clinical diagnosis of aortic stenosis was made.

How Should You Manage This Patient?

- Given the syncopal episode, this patient should be admitted for monitoring and to quantify the severity of his aortic stenosis with an echocardiogram
- Patients with severe aortic stenosis have a very high 1-year mortality
- If he has severe aortic stenosis, he should be referred for consideration of aortic valve replacement as an inpatient

REMEMBER

If in doubt, refer for echo *and* cardiac assessment.

Progress. His echo showed a gradient across the aortic valve of 70 mm Hg with good LV function. He had an aortic valve replacement on that admission without complications and was well at follow-up 18 months later.

INFORMATION

In aortic stenosis, the physical signs can be misleading and do not necessarily correlate with severity:

- Postexercise syncope in someone with a systolic murmur is suggestive of significant aortic stenosis
- A diagnosis of aortic sclerosis should not be made without a full echo assessment
- Soft heart sounds in the context of an aortic murmur often suggest significant stenosis
- Although the pulse might be useful in diagnosing aortic valve lesions (Fig. 2.17), you should note that in elderly patients, the pulse might not be reduced because of loss of arterial tree elasticity
- Severe aortic stenosis with symptoms needs a referral for inpatient surgery
- Elective aortic valve replacement for aortic stenosis either at surgery or via a trans-catheter implantation with a balloon-expandable stent valve (transcatheter aortic valve replacement (TAVR)) is associated with a very low mortality and is excellent curative surgery for symptomatic aortic stenosis with good ventricular function

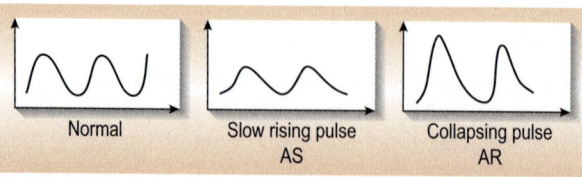

Normal   Slow rising pulse
AS   Collapsing pulse
AR

Fig. 2.17 Pulse *patterns* in aortic valve disease. AR, aortic regurgitation; AS, aortic stenosis.

AORTIC REGURGITATION (AR)

There are many causes of AR, including both valve and aortic root disease. Degenerative disease, rheumatic disease, congenital valvular diseases, and infective endocarditis are some of the more common aetiologies.

> **REMEMBER**
>
> In acute AR (e.g. endocarditis), the murmur might become inaudible and be replaced by a third heart sound. If this happens, the patient needs *urgent* surgical referral.

> **INFORMATION**
>
> In AR, the physical signs do tend to correlate with its severity, that is, the worse the lesion, the more marked the collapsing pulse, the wider the pulse pressure and the longer the murmur:
> - Carry out echo to quantify the severity and LV size, and monitor these parameters on a regular basis thereafter
> - When the ventricle begins to dilate, referral for consideration of surgery is necessary
> - Medical therapy with an ACEI may delay the time until surgery is needed

MITRAL VALVE DISEASE

> **CASE HISTORY (2)**
>
> A 64-year-old male was admitted with heart failure and with signs of mitral regurgitation. He had been in the hospital 6 months earlier with heart failure but had been well since then on maintenance medical therapy. He had cardiomegaly on CXR, but the ECG showed no ischaemic changes. An echocardiogram confirmed papillary muscle dysfunction causing posterior valve leaflet prolapse with resultant severe mitral regurgitation; the LV was dilated and had some impairment of function. Cardiac catheterisation showed normal coronary arteries and confirmed the echo findings. He had an intraoperative TOE and then mitral valve repair and made a good recovery.

In mitral regurgitation (MR), the underlying cause must be adequately treated; this alone can cause a marked improvement in severity. Surgery should be considered in all patients with functional disability (despite adequate medical therapy) and/or worsening LV function documented by echo. The threshold for surgery is constantly dropping with improving technique. Outcome often depends on LV function, so refer early. All patients with MR should be discussed with a cardiologist to arrange appropriate follow-up, investigation and surgical referral.

WHEN SHOULD YOU CONSIDER SURGERY IN VALVULAR DISEASE?

- **Aortic stenosis:** this is usually well compensated but deterioration is rapid once symptoms have developed. Refer for operation if there is dyspnoea, chest pain or syncope. *Note:* do this as an inpatient if stenosis is severe
- **Aortic regurgitation:** refer for operation when the LV starts to dilate (end-systolic dimension >5.5 cm)
- **Mitral stenosis:** refer for an opinion when symptoms are uncontrolled on medical treatment. Remember that percutaneous valvuloplasty may be a first-line option. Generally, when the valve area is <1 cm², intervention is needed
- **Mitral regurgitation:** refer if there are progressive symptoms despite medical therapy and/or LV dilatation

> **REMEMBER**
>
> Age is not a barrier to valvular surgery if LV function is good and no major coronary disease is present

PROSTHETIC VALVE COMPLICATIONS

All of these should be referred urgently to a cardiologist:

- Heart failure: must be assumed to be due to valve malfunction until proved otherwise
- Murmurs: paraprosthetic leaks are common but should be formally assessed by urgent echo followed by TOE
- Infection: blood cultures must be taken for any febrile illness before giving antibiotics. Endocarditis of the prosthetic valve should be referred to a cardiothoracic centre
- Anticoagulants: control is essential (INR 3.5). *Always* take specialist advice before any surgical intervention. *Do not stop a patient's warfarin or reduce the dose until they are fully anticoagulated with IV heparin*

Infective Endocarditis

Infective endocarditis is an endovascular infection of cardiovascular structures, including cardiac valves, atrial and ventricular endocardium, large intrathoracic vessels, and intracardiac foreign bodies, for example, prosthetic valves, pacemaker leads, and surgical conduits. The annual incidence in the UK is 6 to 7 per 100,000, but it is more common in developing countries. Without treatment, the mortality approaches 100%, and even with treatment, there is a significant morbidity and mortality.

Delay in the diagnosis of infective endocarditis might:

- Make medical treatment more prolonged
- Increase the risk of death
- Promote the need for surgery, which might have been avoided had treatment been started earlier

It follows that endocarditis is a diagnosis that needs to be kept in mind when dealing with any pyrexial or constitutional illness in patients with valvular or congenital heart disease.

Diagnosis is made using the modified Duke criteria (Box 2.5).

> **REMEMBER**
>
> The main problem with endocarditis is delay in the diagnosis. *Never* delay empirical antibiotic therapy; take the appropriate cultures and start treatment.

> **CASE HISTORY**
>
> One of your colleagues hands over a patient who has just been admitted. He is a 28-year-old male who presented with a pyrexia and history of feeling unwell for 6 weeks. His doctor had prescribed amoxicillin for a flu-like illness 3 weeks previously. He has a pyrexia of 38.5°C and looks unwell. There is a mid-systolic murmur radiating to the neck and the apex. Careful inspection of the nail beds showed some splinter haemorrhages. Blood cultures were taken on arrival. Your colleague wants you to look these up tomorrow and, depending on the results, start antibiotics.

WHAT DO YOU DO, AND WHAT ELSE DO YOU WANT TO ASK THE PATIENT?

- If you have good clinical grounds for a diagnosis of endocarditis, you must start empirical treatment as soon as you have taken at least three sets of cultures (from different sites). You

> **BOX 2.5** ■ **Modified Duke Criteria for Endocarditis. The Diagnosis of Infective Endocarditis is Definite When: (a) A Microorganism is Demonstrated by Culture of a Specimen from a Vegetation, an Embolism, or an Intracardiac Abscess; (b) Active Endocarditis is Confirmed by Histological Examination of the Vegetation or Intracardiac Abscess; (c) Two Major Clinical Criteria, One Major, and Three Minor Criteria, or Five Minor Criteria are Met**
>
> **Major Criteria**
>
> - A positive blood culture for infective endocarditis, as defined by the recovery of a typical microorganism from two separate blood cultures in the absence of a primary focus (*Viridans streptococci*, *Abiotrophia* species and *Granulicatella* species; *Streptococcus bovis*, HACEK[1] group, or community-acquired *Staphylococcus aureus* or Enterococcus species); *or*
> - Persistently positive blood cultures, defined as the recovery of a microorganism consistent with endocarditis from either blood samples obtained more than 12 h apart or all three or a majority of four or more separate blood samples, with the first and last obtained at least 1 h apart; *or*
> - A positive serological test for Q fever, with an immunofluorescence assay showing phase 1 IgG antibodies at a titre >1:800; *or*
> - Echocardiographic evidence of endocardial involvement:
> - An oscillating intracardiac mass on the valve or supporting structures, in the path of regurgitant jets, or on implanted material in the absence of an alternative anatomical explanation; or
> - An abscess; or
> - New partial dehiscence of prosthetic valve; *or*
> - New valvular regurgitation
>
> **Minor Criteria**
>
> - Predisposition: predisposing heart condition or IV drug use
> - Fever: temperature ≥38°C (100.4°F)
> - Vascular phenomena: major arterial emboli, septic pulmonary infarcts, mycotic aneurysm, intracranial haemorrhage, conjunctival haemorrhages, Janeway lesion
> - Immunological phenomena: glomerulonephritis, Osler nodes, Roth spots, rheumatoid factor
> - Microbiological evidence: a positive blood culture but not meeting a major criterion as noted previously, or serological evidence of active infection with an organism that can cause infective endocarditis[2]
> - Echocardiogram: findings consistent with infective endocarditis but not meeting a major criterion as noted previously
>
> ---
>
> [1]*HACEK, Haemophilus species, Actinobacillus actinomycete mcomitans, Cardiobacterium hominis, Eikenellacorrodens*, and *Kingella kingae*.
> [2]Excluded from this criterion is a single positive blood culture for coagulase-negative *staphylococci* or other organisms that do not cause endocarditis. Serological tests for organisms that cause endocarditis include tests for *Brucella, Coxiellaburnetii, Chlamydia, Legionella*, and *Bartonella species*.

take blood for an FBC and a further blood culture, *now* so that he can have his first dose of antibiotics without delay

- You should ask him if he has had any recent dental work, is an IV drug user or has ever been told he has a murmur (preexisting lesion)
- You should send off baseline U and Es, CRP, ESR, urinalysis and microscopy, and arrange an ECG

Progress. While taking the cultures, you ask him a few questions and he tells you someone mentioned he had a murmur when he was a child but nothing further was done. He also says he had root canal work 8 weeks ago. Follow local guidance and seek advice from a microbiologist;

recommended empirical antibiotic regimens may differ between regions (depending on whether the valve is native, previous antibiotic treatment, local epidemiology and resistance patterns).

All sets of his cultures subsequently show he has *Streptococcus viridans*, and his echo demonstrates a vegetation on a bicuspid aortic valve but no significant gradient (stenosis) or regurgitation.

He makes an uneventful recovery on 2 weeks of slow IV therapy penicillin 1.2 g 4-hourly plus gentamicin 80 mg 12-hourly, followed by oral penicillin for a further 4 weeks.

WHAT ADVICE DO YOU GIVE HIM REGARDING FURTHER DENTAL PROCEDURES?

Antimicrobial prophylaxis is not routinely indicated in healthy patients unless an infective process is already present. Prophylaxis is recommended for patients with cardiac risk factors, including previous endocarditis, prosthetic valves, certain congenital defects and transplant patients with valvulopathy. They may also be indicated for dental procedures in severely immunocompromised patients.

INFORMATION

- Prosthetic valve endocarditis is very difficult to manage and must be referred to a cardiothoracic surgical centre
- Haemodynamic deterioration might precipitate the need for surgery in endocarditis. The difficulty is that operative results are clearly better if the surgeons can wait to allow adequate antibiotic therapy to enable them to operate in a field that is no longer infected. However, in some cases, this might not be possible because fatal haemodynamic deterioration can be prevented only by early surgery
- Transthoracic echocardiography does not always exclude a diagnosis of endocarditis, and TOE will often help; the cardiologist will give appropriate advice
- Development of first-degree AV block strongly suggests an aortic root abscess: hence the need for regular ECGs in all cases
- Always discuss cases that are either not responding or worsening with the surgeons, via the cardiologist
- Right-sided endocarditis is a disease that is characteristic of IV drug users. The condition presents with cardiac signs such as a murmur or evidence of tricuspid regurgitation on the JVP. However, there might be few signs at the outset, and the major abnormality could be on the CXR, with areas of apparent consolidation suggestive of a bronchopneumonia. The condition can present with a 'white-out' of the two lung fields

Pulmonary Hypertension

CASE HISTORY (1)

A 54-year-old female presents with increased breathlessness over 2 weeks. She is a heavy smoker with a chronic productive cough. She recently developed a cold, followed by a cough with purulent sputum and increased breathlessness.

On examination, she is cyanosed and tachypnoeic at rest. Her pulse is 120/min and irregularly irregular (AF). Her JVP is raised by 5 cm. She has a systolic murmur at the left sternal edge with an enlarged pulsatile liver and bilateral leg and ankle oedema.

On examination, of her chest, she had generalised wheezing with bilateral basal crackles.

WHAT IS THE LIKELY DIAGNOSIS?

Cor pulmonale – pulmonary hypertension secondary to COPD.

PULMONARY HYPERTENSION/COR PULMONALE

Pulmonary HTN is a pathophysiological condition defined as an increase in mean pulmonary artery pressure ≥25 mm Hg. Pulmonary HTN can be present for years without causing symptoms.

Cor pulmonale describes impairment of the right ventricle secondary to increased afterload due to chronic hypoxia and subsequent pulmonary vasoconstriction from primary lung disease in patients who have no other cause of ventricular dysfunction. Symptoms include worsening exertional dyspnoea, fatigue and chest pain. On examination, JVP is raised and there is an RV parasternal heave, a loud pulmonary component of the second heart sound, fluid retention and peripheral oedema.

PATHOPHYSIOLOGY OF COR PULMONALE

Pulmonary HTN leads to the elevation of RV pressure and dilatation of both the right ventricle and the right atrium. This produces the physical findings of peripheral oedema, raised JVP, hepatic enlargement (which might be pulsatile because of the tricuspid regurgitation) and ascites. The cause of the fluid retention in cor pulmonale is still debated because there is little evidence that it is truly due to haemodynamic dysfunction of the right ventricle. The most likely explanation is that hypercapnia – an almost invariable feature of cor pulmonale – interferes with the humoral mechanisms controlling sodium and water balance, leading to fluid retention.

In practice, it is relatively common to encounter patients in whom there is evidence of fluid retention, RV hypertrophy and LV problems. Presumably, this occurs because of coexistent primary problems such as ischaemic heart disease and HTN.

HOW WOULD YOU MANAGE A CASE OF COR PULMONALE?

You must treat the underlying disease process, hopefully with the aim of avoiding this final common pathway. Some of these patients are at risk of pulmonary emboli and need anticoagulation: discuss this with the cardiologist. Otherwise, treatment of cor pulmonale is symptomatic with diuretics for fluid retention. There is not yet any direct evidence of benefit from ACEIs for RV dysfunction alone. However, patients will often have coexisting LV disease that benefits from ACEIs.

In COPD, a PaO_2 of <7.3 kPa is an indication for home oxygen treatment. This has been shown to reduce mortality, pulmonary resistance and hypoxia and might produce symptomatic relief.

INVESTIGATIONS

Cor Pulmonale
- Arterial blood gases
- Chest X-ray: showing large pulmonary arteries ± evidence of underlying lung disease
- Electrocardiogram: showing RV strain pattern with right axis deviation and often P-pulmonale
- Echocardiogram: showing large right ventricle and atrium, tricuspid regurgitation and high pulmonary artery pressures
- Computed tomography chest with contrast: to delineate underlying lung disease and pulmonary vasculature further

WHAT IS THE PROGNOSIS?

In COPD, the development of cor pulmonale is always a sinister sign because it invariably represents the final common pathway. The prognosis of cor pulmonale in COPD without treatment is poor (5-year survival is about 30%) compared with treatment (5-year survival of about 60%). Although cor pulmonale is not an invariable feature of COPD, it usually heralds the terminal phase of the illness in those who develop it.

REMEMBER

Patients with long-standing lung disease may develop pulmonary HTN.

Progress. This patient's underlying COPD was treated with bronchodilators, and she was given antibiotics and told to stop smoking. After recovery from the acute episodes, her blood gases showed a PO_2 of 7.1 kPa, and arrangements were made for domiciliary oxygen. She was continued on anticoagulation with warfarin, and her AF was controlled with digoxin. She is being followed by the pulmonary rehabilitation team.

CASE HISTORY (2)

A 21-year-old male presents with an 8-week history of increasing breathlessness; he is now only able to walk less than 20 m, having previously been fit and active. He has no past medical or drug history and has never smoked.

On examination, he is cyanosed, and has a JVP raised to his ears with 'cv' waves, an RV heave, a pansystolic murmur at the right sternal edge and peripheral oedema.

His CXR shows strikingly enlarged pulmonary arteries but clear lung fields. His echo demonstrates an enormous right heart with torrential tricuspid regurgitation but no significant left-sided problems.

WHAT IS THE LIKELY DIAGNOSIS AND PROGNOSIS?

Primary pulmonary artery HTN is the most likely diagnosis. This is an aggressive disease process with a very poor outlook.

Progress. This patient was assessed in the transplantation centre and is awaiting heart–lung transplantation.

Cardiomyopathies

Cardiomyopathy is a primary disease of the heart muscle. Generally, these fall into three functional categories: dilated, hypertrophic and restrictive cardiomyopathies.

> **REMEMBER**
> - Cardiomyopathies are rare in acute medical practice but do not forget them in your differential
> - Echocardiograms are essential in defining the problem

> **CASE HISTORY (1)**
>
> A 42-year-old male is admitted with increasing breathlessness and signs of pulmonary oedema. There is no history of chest pain or palpitations. He had a severe episode of flu 3 months ago and since then has not been able to return to his marathon running. He has never smoked and drinks less than 10 units per week.
>
> **On examination**, he is tachypnoeic. His pulse is 120/min and regular, with BP 100/60. His venous pressure is raised, and he has a gallop rhythm on auscultation. He also has bilateral basal crackles but no peripheral oedema. His CXR confirms cardiomegaly and pulmonary oedema.

WHAT IS THE LIKELY DIAGNOSIS?

Acute heart failure with pulmonary oedema. He is given immediate treatment for this (see 'Heart Failure Recognition and Acute Management'). He has a dilated cardiomyopathy.

DILATED CARDIOMYOPATHY (DCM)

There are a number of causes of DCMs. This case history is suggestive of either a postviral or idiopathic cardiomyopathy. A thorough history, examination and investigations will enable you to rule out many causes of cardiomyopathy, for example, alcohol-induced cardiomyopathy.

Progress. Further investigations show no ischaemia on the ECG and global ventricular systolic dysfunction on his echo. Cardiac MR shows dilatation. Viral titres to enteroviruses are positive.

Treatment is as for acute heart failure. He recovers well and can return to normal activities after 4 months.

MANAGEMENT OF DCMS

- In principle, the treatment is the same as the treatment of heart failure, but you should ask for cardiology input early for advice on specialist investigations and further treatment
- Define an aetiology if possible, as this might identify a reversible/treatable cause, for example, alcohol excess:
  - An echo is essential
  - An endocardial biopsy might be helpful
- It is possible to make a complete recovery from a DCM, especially those of viral aetiology (remember to check viral titres)
- Some acute DCMs run an aggressive course with rapidly worsening ventricular function and cardiac transplantation might be required. Surgically implanted left ventricular assist devices (LVADs) are becoming increasingly common as a bridge to either recovery or transplantation

REMEMBER

Ischaemic heart disease can present as a DCM; it can respond well to treatment with secondary prevention and, where appropriate, revascularisation.

CASE HISTORY (2)

You are a doctor in clinic and see a new and urgent GP referral. She is a 35-year-old female who presented to the emergency department with syncope and palpitations. She was noted to have a soft systolic murmur. She was sent home as her palpitations had settled, and her ECG was thought to be normal. The GP is concerned and has asked you to see her because the patient's sister, age 28, 'dropped dead' while ironing. The patient's ECG shows LV hypertrophy with an S in V_1 of 21 mm plus an R wave in V_6 of >35 mm (see Fig. 2.19 later).

WHAT CONDITION ARE YOU CONCERNED ABOUT?

Hypertrophic cardiomyopathy (HCM).

HYPERTROPHIC CARDIOMYOPATHY

This is an autosomal dominant condition with variable penetrance. There is disorganisation of myocytes and myofibrils, which often results in ventricular hypertrophy that most often affects the septum. The septal hypertrophy can cause LV outflow obstruction, resulting in symptoms such as exercise-induced syncope. The main risk is sudden death.

Some Practice Points for HCM

- On echocardiogram (which all patients must have), cardinal features include asymmetrical septal hypertrophy, systolic anterior motion of the mitral valve, and an outflow gradient
- The degree of outflow obstruction and hypertrophy does not correlate reliably with the risk of sudden death
- Screening of family members and referral to a geneticist are essential because certain HCM mutations are associated with a higher risk of sudden death. Do not forget, HCM can be sporadic as well as hereditary
- Beta-blockers are the mainstay of medical therapy, but amiodarone can be useful. However, certain patients will benefit from an AICD
- Patients with outflow obstruction might benefit from septal reduction by either percutaneous alcohol ablation or surgical myomectomy
- Sometimes, differentiation of HCM from aortic stenosis can be difficult (Fig. 2.18; Table 2.5) – seek specialist advice!

Progress. This patient was treated with beta-blockers but had further episodes of syncope. She has been fitted with an AICD.

Hypertension (HTN)

CASE HISTORY (1)

An anxious 42-year-old female comes to the emergency department with a bad migraine. Her BP has been recorded as 180/120 on a number of occasions while she is waiting to be seen by the medical team.

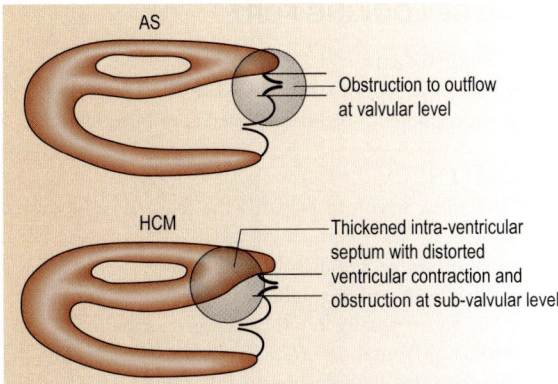

Fig. 2.18 The difference between aortic stenosis (AS) and hypertrophic cardiomyopathy (HCM).

TABLE 2.5 ■ Differentiation of Aortic Stenosis (AS) and Hypertrophic Cardiomyopathy (HCM)

	AS	HCM
Murmur	Ejection systolic	Ejection systolic
		There may be additional MR murmur
Pulse/Additional heart sounds	May be slow-rising	Described as jerky fourth sound possible (associated with double apical pulsation)
ECG	LVH in later stages. May be normal even when AS is severe	LVH (including early stages)
		There may be bizarre changes, including large septal Q waves
CXR	Heart size may be normal even when AS is severe	Heart size may be normal
Echo	Aortic valve thickened Gradient on Doppler across valve LVH if severe	Characteristic:
		Asymmetric septal hypertrophy
		Systolic anterior motion of mitral valve
		Mid-systolic closure of aortic valve

AS, differentiation of the artic stenosis; *HCM*, hypertrophic cardiomyopathy; *CXR*, chest X-ray; *LVH*, left ventricular hypertrophy; *MR*, mitral regurgitation.

HOW WILL YOU ASSESS HER?

First, you need to decide on the significance of the BP reading:

- Relevance of anxiety: a raised BP is a common response to stress, more so in some individuals than in others. Twenty-four-hour ambulatory BP monitors can be of help in these situations
- Prior history of high BP: adds significance to the present reading
- Presence of family history HTN: probably the single most useful determinant in essential HTN
- Relationship to migraine: no direct link between this and HTN has been established
- Relationship to age: BP does rise with age but still carries an adverse cardiovascular risk. The WHO/International Society of HTN classifies HTN as a systolic pressure of >130 mm Hg and a diastolic of >85 mm Hg
- Relationship to lifestyle: high alcohol intake, obesity and lack of exercise are common contributory factors in patients with high BP

WHAT SHOULD YOU BE LOOKING FOR?

- Clinical signs of end-organ damage:
  - Fundoscopy: hypertensive retinopathy grades I to IV
  - Left ventricular hypertrophy: forceful/displaced apex beat, loud A2
  - Proteinuria
- Causes of secondary HTN:
  - Coarctation of the aorta: have you palpated the femoral pulses, especially in the young patient?
  - Renal disease: renal bruits, proteinuria, U and Es
  - Cushing syndrome: obesity, striae; might have low K^+
  - Conn syndrome: no signs; usually low K^+ and high normal Na^+
  - Phaeochromocytoma: presentation often atypical (e.g. acute pulmonary oedema, sweating attacks) rather than textbook flushing/palpitations
- Baseline investigations:
  - Urea and electrolytes, estimated glomerular filtration rate (eGFR) and glucose: look for electrolyte imbalances (e.g. Conn, renal disease and diabetes)
  - Electrocardiogram: a very insensitive detector of LVH but when voltage criteria are present this carries considerable prognostic risk and should not be ignored. Fig. 2.19 shows LVH with S in lead V_2 and R in $V_5 > 35$ mm
  - Chest X-ray: cardiomegaly might be present but rarely adds much to good clinical examination (rib notching exciting, but coarctation should not have been missed clinically!)
  - Echocardiogram: a more sensitive indicator of LVH

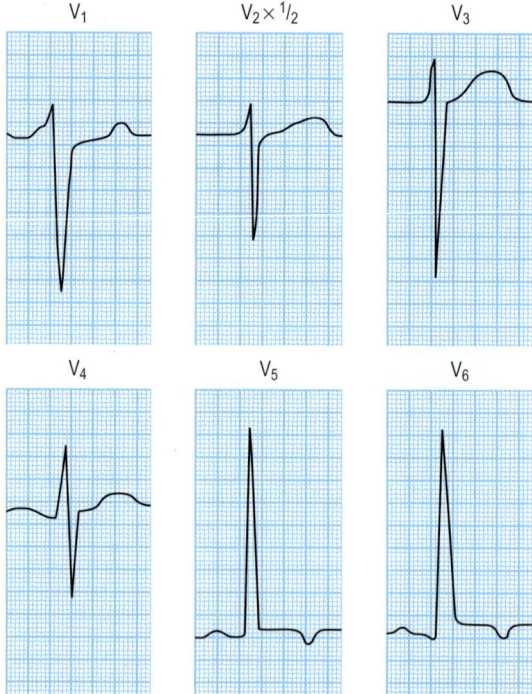

Fig. 2.19   Electrocardiogram showing LV hypertrophy (S in V_2 and R in $V_5 > 35$ mm).

WHAT WOULD RAISE YOUR SUSPICION OF A SECONDARY CAUSE?

- Young patient (under 45) and no family history of HTN
- Those with HTN resistant to treatment.
- Those with accelerated HTN

HOW WOULD YOU FURTHER INVESTIGATE FOR A SECONDARY CAUSE?

Potential investigations include:
- Renal ultrasound: noninvasive, readily available, excludes major renal pathology
- Isotope renogram (+ captopril stress): reasonable screening test for renal artery stenosis but not very sensitive (might miss some)
- Magnetic resonance angiography with contrast: will give a definitive diagnosis in renal artery stenosis. Although renal angiography is the gold standard, this tends to be used only when intervention (renal angioplasty) is considered
- Twenty-four-hour urine collection: catecholamines and cortisol: these require separate bottles! Plasma catecholamines are most accurate for phaeochromocytoma, if available
- Computed tomography/MRI abdomen: when adrenal disease is suspected/confirmed. Perform CT and MRI angiography for reno-vascular disease

REMEMBER

- High BP is a significant risk factor for future cardiac events and should be followed up, especially in diabetics
- Secondary causes, apart from renal disease, are rare – but you will see a few cases

Progress. This patient's hypertension was treated with candesartan 8 mg daily. Her BP fell to 160/100, and therefore bendroflumethiazide 2.5 mg daily and amlodipine 5 mg daily have been added to her treatment. She was also prescribed a statin. Her BP is now controlled at 140/85.

CASE HISTORY (2)

A 50-year-old male is brought to the emergency department by his relatives after behaving oddly. His BP is recorded by the nurses as 220/140 in both arms. This is **accelerated HTN.**

HOW WOULD YOU ASSESS THIS PATIENT?

Clinical assessment:
- Central nervous system: orientation, focal neurological signs (differentiation of hypertensive encephalopathy and a small stroke might be difficult)
- Fundi: haemorrhages/exudates and/or papilloedema indicate accelerated HTN
- Left ventricular hypertrophy: clinical and ECG. Most patients with severe HTN have ECG evidence of LVH
- Urinalysis: to look for renal disease and diabetes
- Remember to look for secondary causes and treat as appropriate

INVESTIGATIONS

- Renal function: renal impairment is likely in severe HT and may be accompanied by electrolyte disturbance
- Computed tomography head scan: if focal signs present to exclude stroke

WHAT ARE THE TREATMENT OPTIONS FOR HTN?

- Oral:
  - Angiotensin-converting enzyme inhibitors (Fig. 2.20)
  - Diuretics, for example, thiazides
  - Calcium-channel blockers, for example, nifedipine, diltiazem
- Intravenous treatment (labetalol, nitroprusside) should be reserved for a real emergency, for example, aortic dissection, when minute-to-minute control is needed. But lower BP *cautiously*
- In this patient, careful titration of IV labetalol would be a suitable choice as the history is suggestive of hypertensive encephalopathy. The initial goal of therapy in hypertensive emergencies is to reduce mean arterial BP by no more than 25%

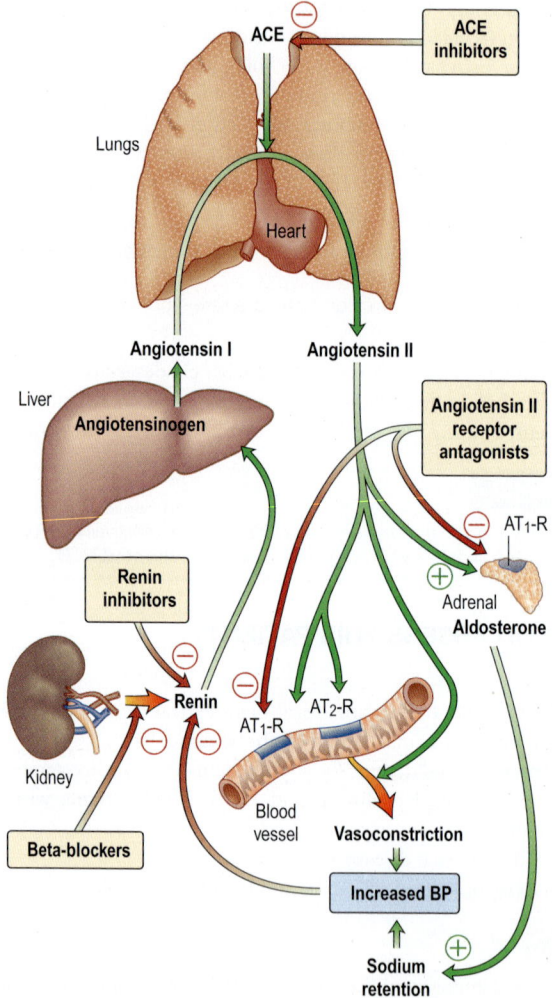

Fig. 2.20 The renin–angiotensin–aldosterone system. ACE, angiotensin-converting enzyme.

LONG-TERM TREATMENT OF HYPERTENSION

Don't forget non-pharmacological measures, including weight loss, diet, smoking cessation and regular exercise; these are often glossed over and can have a significant impact. Current practice includes all major classes of antihypertensive drugs. However, in many patients, an ACEI or ARB would be a sensible first choice (especially for patients under 55 or those with type 2 diabetes). Remember, strict control is of paramount importance in diabetic patients.

SIDE-EFFECTS OF ANTIHYPERTENSIVE MEDICATION

- Beta-blockers:
  - Asthma
  - Symptomatic bradycardia (especially in the elderly)
  - Cardiac failure
  - Masking of hypoglycaemic symptoms
  - Worsening of peripheral vascular disease symptoms
- Diuretics:
  - Gout
  - Hypokalaemia (if severe, i.e. <2.5 mmol/L: consider Conn syndrome)
  - Diabetes (often overlooked)
- Angiotensin-converting enzyme inhibitors:
  - Cough (often overlooked)
  - Hypotension/falls (especially in the elderly)
  - Renal failure (especially in diabetics and claudicants, where renal artery stenosis is more common)
- Calcium-channel blockers:
  - Nondependent ankle oedema (especially nifedipine and amlodipine)
  - Constipation (especially verapamil)

The Swollen/Painful Leg

Common causes of a swollen leg include:
- Deep vein thrombosis (DVT)
- Acute rupture of knee joint/Baker's cyst
- Trauma, for example, rupture of tendon/muscle
- Infection: cellulitis, osteomyelitis

CASE HISTORY (1)

A 36-year-old female on the oral contraceptive pill developed pain in her left calf 3 days ago; it had become increasingly swollen since. Examination revealed oedema of the lower leg without any change in color or prominence of the veins; there was tenderness along the line of the deep veins. You suspect a DVT.

HOW WOULD YOU INVESTIGATE FOR A DVT?

- D-dimer assay:
  - Has a high negative predictive value, that is, if low, a DVT is unlikely
  - Can be used in conjunction with a clinical risk score (e.g. Wells score) to decide if a patient needs treatment and ultrasonographic studies
  - Do not use in pregnancy
- B mode venous compression ultrasound: is generally the first-line investigation of choice It detects clot reliably only in the popliteal/femoral vein, not in calf veins. However, 30% of patients with calf vein clots will have an extension, and anticoagulation is now recommended.
- Venography: although probably the gold standard, can be misleading if there is a past history of venous thrombosis and is no longer used as a first-line investigation

HOW WOULD YOU TREAT THIS PATIENT IF A DVT IS CONFIRMED?

Anticoagulation should be commenced to prevent the propagation of the thrombus in the deep veins, reduce the risk of PE, and reduce the risk of recurrence. The choice of anticoagulant should be decided based on the patient's comorbidities and contraindications (e.g. bleeding risk).

Direct oral anticoagulants (DOACs), such as dabigatran (a direct thrombin inhibitor) or rivaroxaban, or edoxaban (Factor Xa inhibitors), are now commonly used.

If commencing **warfarin**, the patient should be started on subcutaneous LMWH until formal anticoagulation with warfarin is at the target level (INR 2.5).

Consider investigating for malignancy and/or other causes of thrombophilia if there are no obvious provoking factors.

Current recommendations for anticoagulation are:

- Three months minimum
- Consider a longer duration if unprovoked, high risk of recurrence, PE

CASE HISTORY (2)

A 78-year-old male developed sudden pain and weakness in the left hand. The hand was cold and pulseless, indicating **acute limb ischaemia.** He was in sinus rhythm, but a systolic murmur was noted at the apex. Successful embolectomy was performed. Echo showed a mass in the left atrium, which proved at surgery to be an atrial myxoma and was removed.

INFORMATION

- Atrial fibrillation (even when paroxysmal) is the most common cause of embolic events but do not forget rare causes, such as endocarditis, ventricular thrombosis and atrial myxoma
- If you suspect a peripheral embolus, involve a vascular surgeon early because minimising time to embolectomy is as vital as 'door to needle' time in an MI
- In a patient with acute abdominal pain and AF, do not forget mesenteric ischaemia in your differential

---

Progress. This patient's hand recovered following embolectomy. He was left with a mild sensory loss but has had no further problems.

Further Reading

Atrial Fibrillation

Hindricks, G., et al., 2021 Feb 1. 2020 ESC guidelines for the diagnosis and management of atrial fibrillation developed in collaboration with the European Association for Cardio-Thoracic Surgery (EACTS). Eur. Heart J. 42 (5), 373–498.

Link, M.S., 2018. Paradigm shift for treatment of atrial fibrillation in heart failure. N. Engl. J. Med. 378, 468–469.

Marrouche, MF., Brachmann, J., Andresen, D., et al., 2018. Catheter ablation for atrial fibrillation with heart failure. N. Engl. J. Med. 378, 417–427.

NICE, CKS. 2021. Atrial fibrillation: diagnosis and management.

Valvular Heart Disase

NICE, CKS. 2021. Heart valve disease presenting in adults: investigation and management

Otto, C.M., 2019. Informed shared decisions for patients with aortic stenosis. N. Engl. J. Med. 380, 1769–1770.

Otto, C.M., et al., 2021 Feb 2. 2020 ACC/AHA guideline for the management of patients with valvular heart disease: a report of the American College of Cardiology/American Heart Association Joint Committee on clinical practice guidelines. Circulation 143 (5), e72–227.

Infective Endocarditis

Rajani, R., Klein, J.L., 2020. Infective endocarditis: a contemporary update. Clin. Med. 20, 31–35.

Heart Failure

Bozkurt, B., et al., 2021 Apr 1. Universal definition and classification of heart failure: a report of the Heart Failure Society of America, Heart Failure Association of the European Society of Cardiology, Japanese Heart Failure Society and Writing Committee of the Universal Definition of Heart Failure. J. Card. Fail. 27 (4), 387–413.

McDonagh, T.A., Metra, M., Adamo, M., et al., 2021 Sep 21. ESC Scientific Document Group. 2021 ESC guidelines for the diagnosis and treatment of acute and chronic heart failure. Eur. Heart J. 42 (36), 3599–3726.

NICE, CKS. 2018. Chronic heart failure in adults: diagnosis and management

Respiratory Disorders

Acute Breathlessness

You are called by the nurses to see a 63-year-old male who has become breathless. As you walk over to the ward, you consider what the causes could be.

REMEMBER

Respiratory diseases can cause breathlessness within minutes or hours, or slowly over days, weeks or months.

The systems involved would most probably be cardiac or respiratory. You go through the list in Box 3.1 as you walk to the ward.

Despite the long list, the most likely causes for this 63-year-old male are chronic obstructive pulmonary disease (COPD), chest infection, or heart failure; if the onset was sudden, it could also be a pulmonary embolus (PE).

HOW WOULD YOU INITIALLY ASSESS THIS PATIENT?

- What does the patient look like? Is he in shock?
- What is the severity of the problem?
- Tachypnoea?
- Is the patient using his accessory muscles?
- Is there any respiratory distress?
- Colour: is the patient cyanosed?
- Pulse: rate, type, volume?
- Blood pressure (BP)?

Then make a full cardiac and respiratory examination. Is there any evidence of deep vein thrombosis (DVT)?

This vague history shows the vast number of diagnostic possibilities (see Box 3.1), but a shorter differential diagnosis can be made in the context of the age of the patient, the past medical history and the current clinical situation.

Progress. This patient turned out to have acute heart failure. He was treated with furosemide 40 mg daily and, 3 days later, was discharged to be followed up in the outpatient heart failure clinic.

CASE HISTORY (2)

A 29-year-old male had been at a party, where he had consumed a lot of alcohol. He managed to get home with the help of his friend, but he then vomited and fell to the floor. He was holding his throat and had great difficulty in breathing. The friend realised that he was in great distress and called an ambulance.

BOX 3.1 ■ Causes of Breathlessness

Sudden-Onset Breathlessness
- Inhaled foreign body
- Pneumothorax
- Pulmonary embolus

Breathlessness Developing Over a Few Hours
- Asthma/chronic obstructive pulmonary disease (COPD)
- Pneumonia
- Pulmonary oedema
- Respiratory muscle disease, e.g. Guillain–Barré

Intermittent Breathlessness
- Asthma
- Pulmonary oedema
- Pulmonary emboli

Breathlessness Developing Over a Few Days
- Pleural effusion
- Carcinoma of the bronchus
- Pneumonia, including pulmonary tuberculosis

Breathlessness Developing Over Months or Years
- Fibrosis alveolitis
- Chronic obstructive pulmonary disease
- Sarcoidosis
- Chest wall or neuromuscular disease
- Occupational lung disease
- Nonrespiratory causes: anaemia, hyperthyroidism

WHAT IS THE LIKELY DIAGNOSIS?

Upper airways obstruction. *This is an emergency!*

Features include:
- Stridor
- Respiratory distress
- Cyanosis ± shock

Fortunately, the paramedics recognised the problem and tried to clear the airway and gave back blows. There was no improvement, so abdominal thrusts were performed, and a large bone was expelled with immediate relief of the male's respiratory distress. He was taken to the emergency department for assessment but discharged after 2 h of observation.

REMEMBER

Abdominal thrusts can be used to expel an inhaled foreign body:
- Stand behind the patient
- Encircle the upper part of the abdomen, just below the patient's rib cage, with your arms
- Give a sharp, forceful squeeze, forcing the diaphragm sharply into the thorax

This should expel sufficient air from the lungs to force the foreign body out of the trachea. If this fails, urgent assessment by an experienced ear, nose and throat (ENT) clinician is required. Fibre-optic or rigid bronchoscopy will be required if the obstruction is beyond the vocal cords.

TABLE 3.1 ■ Causes of Upper Airways Obstruction (With Management Strategies)

Cause	Action
Anaphylaxis: laryngeal oedema	Adrenaline (epinephrine) 0.5 mg IM
	O_2
Carcinoma of upper airway	Call ENT for laryngoscopy
Tracheal compression, e.g. bleeding postthyroidectomy	Tracheal decompression, e.g. release skin sutures
Inhaled foreign body	Heimlich manoeuvre

ENT; Ear, nose and throat.

Causes of upper airway obstruction are shown in Table 3.1. All of these require emergency management, which is also shown.

Cough

Cough is common and, when persistent, can cause considerable fear and distress. Apart from the immediate discomfort of coughing, paroxysmal cough can interrupt sleep, provoke retching, or vomiting and, if severe, result in rib fractures or syncope. Always enquire about sputum and its colour.

CASE HISTORY

A 67-year-old male was admitted to hospital with a myocardial infarction. Following successful coronary intervention, he was discharged on anti-platelet therapy, atorvastatin and enalapril. When seen again 2 weeks later, he was very well but complained of a persistent hacking cough. This had been keeping him awake at night.

WHAT IS THE LIKELY DIAGNOSIS?

In this case, as the patient has only a cough and is not breathless, the cause is very likely to be the angiotensin-converting enzyme (ACE) inhibitor (enalapril). This should be stopped and an ACE receptor antagonist (e.g. valsartan) started. Unlike ACE inhibitors, angiotensin receptor antagonists do not affect bradykinin metabolism and do not produce a cough.

WHAT ARE THE IMPORTANT CONDITIONS TO CONSIDER WHEN ASSESSING A COUGH?

Cough is provoked by stimulation of mucosal and stretch receptors that are present in the larynx, carina and proximal airways of the lung. Accordingly, it has a number of causes.

Acute Cough

- Inhalation of direct irritants, for example, smoke, chlorine gas, ozone and other air pollutants
- In the asthmatic, inhalation of specific allergen, for example, pollen or nonspecific low-concentration irritants, for example, perfume, tobacco fumes
- Upper and lower respiratory tract infections (yellow/green sputum)

Chronic Cough

- Large airway obstruction, for example, carcinoma of the bronchus or inhaled foreign body (*Note:* peanuts and other inhaled food will not be radio-dense)
- Persistent bronchial inflammation, for example, asthma, bronchiectasis, COPD, smoking
- Persistent infection, for example, tuberculosis (TB), lung abscess
- Interstitial lung disease, for example, pulmonary fibrosis, asbestosis
- Raised left atrial pressure, for example, mitral stenosis, left ventricular failure (LVF)
- Gastro-oesophageal reflux disease (GORD) and bulbar dysfunction. (Laryngopharyngeal reflux disease – cough, hoarse voice, postnasal drip)
- Iatrogenic, for example, ACE inhibitors, radiation pneumonitis

INVESTIGATIONS

All patients with persistent cough should have a chest X-ray (CXR). Other investigations will depend on the likely cause, for example, serial peak flow in asthma, or contrast studies if GORD or aspiration is suspected and sputum culture, including a request for *Mycobacterium tuberculosis* isolation, if the cough is productive.

Breathlessness and Wheeze

Asthma causes breathlessness, cough and wheeze. However, all that wheezes is not asthma.

INFORMATION

- Asthma provocation tests might be required to exclude mild-moderate and variable bronchial irritability
- Bronchoscopy will be required in all chronic cases remaining undiagnosed

The differential diagnosis of wheeze includes:

- Chronic obstructive pulmonary disease:
  - Patient usually >40 years of age
  - Heavy smoker: >20 pack years (*Note:* patients with asthma might also smoke)
  - History of variable wheeze: in patients with asthma, chest wheeze is usually worse at night and may only be episodic
- Upper airway obstruction with stridor:
  - Occurs when there is a mechanical obstruction in the larynx or trachea
  - Is heard during inspiration and expiration, but inspiratory sound when mouth is open is most typical
  - Might be associated with vigorous accessory muscle activity and obvious distress
- Left ventricular failure (LVF):
  - Acute LVF can be difficult to differentiate from asthma
  - Nocturnal symptoms are common to both

Fig. 3.1 shows causes and triggers of asthma.

INFORMATION

Causes of Stridor

- Tumour
- Foreign body
- Bilateral vocal cord palsy
- Laryngeal oedema
- Thyroid goitre

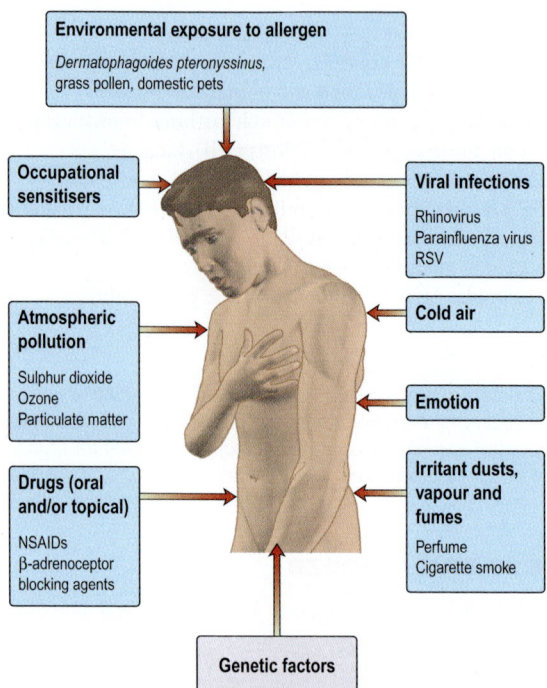

Fig. 3.1   Causes and triggers of asthma. NSAIDs, Nonsteroidal antiinflammatory drugs; RSV, respiratory syncytial virus.

CASE HISTORY

A 24-year-old female was admitted with breathlessness for 6 h. She has had a 'cold' for 2 days. Past history revealed her being 'chesty' as a child. It was noticed that she could not complete sentences easily. Heart rate was 126 beats per minute (bpm) and respiratory rate (RR) was 30/min. There was expiratory wheeze over the lung fields. You diagnose this patient with severe acute asthma.

REMEMBER

Severe Acute Asthma

- Increased breathlessness/cannot complete sentences
- Respiratory rate >25/min
- Heart rate >110 bpm
- Peak expiratory flow rate (PEFR) 30%–50% of best

HOW WOULD YOU INITIALLY MANAGE AND INVESTIGATE THIS PATIENT?

Immediate management should be:

- Reassurance
- Titrate supplemental **oxygen** to maintain SpO_2 >94%

TABLE 3.2 ■ Normal Blood Gas Values (With F$_i$O$_2$ 21%)

Analysis	Normal Range	
	SI Units	Non-SI Units
PaO$_2$	10.6–13.3 kPa	80–100 mmHg
PaCO$_2$	4.5–6.0 kPa	34–45 mmHg
Hydrogen ions	37–45 nmol/L	pH 7.35–7.43
Bicarbonate	24–28 mmol/L	24–28 mEq/L

F$_i$O$_2$, Inspiratory O$_2$ concentration.

To convert kPa to mmHg, multiply by 7.5.

- Nebulised short-acting β$_2$ agonist (SABA), for example, **salbutamol** 5 mg with oxygen (*N.B.* Only 10% of drug reaches the lungs)
- Systemic **corticosteroids**:
  - Prednisolone 40–50 mg daily or
  - Intravenous hydrocortisone 100 mg 6-hourly
- Monitoring of SaO$_2$ by oximetry
- Arterial blood gases (ABGs):
  - Initially if SaO$_2$ <90%
  - Recheck (2-hourly) if PaO$_2$ is <8 kPa or PaCO$_2$ is >5 kPa until PaCO$_2$ is stable and saturation is >90%
- PEFR 4-hourly, Note: performing PEFR might be distressing for patient: do not demand unnecessary repeat testing
- Electrocardiogram
- Chest X-ray

Normal ranges are shown in Table 3.2 later.

Thirty minutes later, there has been no significant improvement in her breathlessness and PEFR.

WHAT WOULD YOU DO NEXT?

- Call for senior help
- Continue with nebulised β$_2$ agonist, now with added ipratropium (500 μg). Repeat every 30 min if necessary
- Consider **magnesium sulphate** 1.2–2 g IV infusion over 20 min with cardiac monitoring
- Intravenous **aminophylline** infusion can be used if patient does not respond to repeated nebulisation with β$_2$ agonist and ipratropium. Loading dose 250–500 mg over 1 h (check local protocols) *Do not use this* if oral aminophylline has been taken

INFORMATION

Life-Threatening Acute Asthma
- Silent chest, feeble respiration, cyanosis
- Bradycardia/hypotension, arrhythmia
- Exhaustion/confusion
- Peak expiratory flow rate <33% of best
- Arterial oxygen saturation <92%

WHAT ARE THE POTENTIAL INDICATIONS FOR HIGH DEPENDENCY UNIT (HDU) OR INTENSIVE CARE?

- Presence of life-threatening features *and*
- PaO_2 <8 kPa on 60% oxygen
- $PaCO_2$ >6 kPa
- Previous history of requiring ventilation

> **REMEMBER**
>
> **Beware of the** *silent chest!*
> If asthma is very severe, air entry will be minimal and breath sounds quiet or absent.

Progress. There is now an improvement in PEFR and breathlessness with the nebulised β_2 agonist and ipratropium.

WHAT TREATMENT SHOULD BE OFFERED TO THE PATIENT NOW?

Continuing management should be:
- Keeping SaO_2 >94% with oxygen supplementation
- Corticosteroids: prednisolone 40–50 mg daily, on a reducing dose
- 2–4-hourly nebulised SABA therapy and tiotropium

WHEN COULD SHE BE DISCHARGED?

The patient can be discharged when:
- Symptoms, particularly nocturnal symptoms, have improved
- Ideally, PEFR is 75% of best and diurnal variation (i.e. 'morning dips') <25%. If the patient is improving and compliance is expected to be good, an earlier discharge is reasonable

Twenty-Four to Forty-Eight Hours Before Discharge

- Add inhaled corticosteroids, for example, beclometasone, to oral steroids
- Replace nebulised bronchodilators with inhalers
- Introduce inhaled long-acting β_2 agonists (LABAs), for example, salmeterol
- Check inhaler technique (? might need spacer)
- Determine the cause of this attack (noncompliance, infection, allergen exposure)

Liaise With Asthma Specialist Nurse

At discharge, the patient should have:
- Oral and inhaled corticosteroids and LABA. Long-acting β_2 agonists should be administered as fixed-dose combinations with corticosteroids (e.g. salmeterol/fluticasone or formoterol/budesonide) in the same inhaler. Short-acting β_2 agonists (SABAs) can be used on an 'as required' basis
- Peak flow meter and diary
- Management plan if condition deteriorates

Progress. This patient was discharged after 7 days on treatment as above. She requires close follow-up because of the severe acute attack.

The discharge letter to her general practitioner (GP) should include:

- Admission and discharge PEFR
- Recommended GP follow-up in 1 week
- Asthma clinic follow-up, preferably within 4 weeks

Hyperventilation

CASE HISTORY

A 15-year-old male is brought by his teacher to the emergency department feeling dizzy and faint. You notice that he is anxious and has erratic ventilation. There are no other physical signs on examination. His teacher volunteered that the patient was anxious about impending examinations.

WHAT SHOULD YOU DO?

- Full systematic physical examination
- Monitor pulse oximetry
- Consider PEFR or spirometry

You suspect that her symptoms are due to hyperventilation. If an ABG is performed, it would demonstrate a respiratory alkalosis with a low $PaCO_2$ and (H^+). Reassure the patient and ask him to focus on controlled breathing exercises: when settled, he can be discharged with further reassurance. *Note:* mild asthma is a common provocative cause and might require further investigation.

HYPERVENTILATION SYNDROME

Hyperventilation syndrome refers to a condition of recurrent attacks of anxiety, sometimes phobic in nature, and provoking profound hyperventilation such as to cause a reduction in arterial pCO_2 and ensuing tetany. Other features include perioral and digital paraesthesia, carpopedal spasm, muscle weakness, dizziness and a sense of impending loss of consciousness or fear.

An attack of hyperventilation can be induced by a strong emotional experience in otherwise normal individuals, for example, witnessing an accident.

In many patients, the label of hyperventilation syndrome is inappropriately given when mild asthma or other conditions, such as heart failure, lie behind the respiratory sensation. Indeed, hypocapnia resulting from hyperventilation might further provoke bronchoconstriction.

Clinically obvious hyperventilation can also result from a metabolic acidosis and will be recognised by ABG analysis: a reduced pH and bicarbonate (HCO_3), contrary to the alkalosis of respiratory hyperventilation.

Tetany: hyperventilation can cause tetany.

Progress. This patient settled quickly. He was reassured that there was nothing seriously wrong with him. He was taken home to his parents with a pamphlet explaining hyperventilation syndrome.

Haemoptysis

CASE HISTORY

A 63-year-old male smoker presents with a 4-month history of cough. Recently, he has been coughing up blood in his sputum. He has also been breathless on exertion.

Coughing up blood is a dramatic symptom and can be frightening for patients and their families.

COLOUR OF BLOOD

This can differ with different causes.

- Pink frothy sputum: pulmonary oedema
- Rusty sputum: pneumonia
- Make sure it is not haematemesis, which would be suggested by:
  - History of retching
  - Altered blood (resembling coffee grounds)
  - Low pH of contents

Enquire about epistaxis, which may cause confusion. Blood-stained saliva suggests bleeding from gums.

WHAT CONDITIONS CAN COMMONLY PRESENT WITH HAEMOPTYSIS?

- Carcinoma of the bronchus:
  - Smoker
  - Age >40 years
  - Usually abnormal CXR
- Pulmonary embolism:
  - Risk factors for DVT
  - Chest X-rays are often negative
  - History of acute breathlessness
  - Pulmonary TB:
  - More common in Africa and Asia, people drinking alcohol in excess, patients with HIV infection
  - Age often <40 years
  - Chest X-ray usually shows patchy opacities in the upper lobes
- Bronchiectasis:
  - History of purulent sputum and/or possibly recurrent haemoptysis over years
  - Cystic lesions on CXR at lung bases in some but not all patients
  - High-resolution CT scan of the lungs is diagnostic, with bronchial dilatation, loss of airway tapering at the periphery, bronchial wall thickening and cysts at the end of the bronchioles
  - Bronchiectasis is also a feature of cystic fibrosis

Less common causes of haemoptysis include:

- Vasculitis (both of the following are antineutrophil cytoplasmic antibody (ANCA)-positive):
  - Granulomatosis with polyangiitis
  - Microscopic vasculitis
- Pulmonary haemorrhage:
  - Goodpasture syndrome
  - Idiopathic pulmonary haemosiderosis
- Chronic venous congestion of lungs:
  - Mitral stenosis
  - Left ventricular failure
- Aspergilloma: seen in association with cavitatory lung disease

REMEMBER

- Chest X-ray might be normal, for example, pulmonary embolism (PE)
- Large opacity: consider malignancy or TB

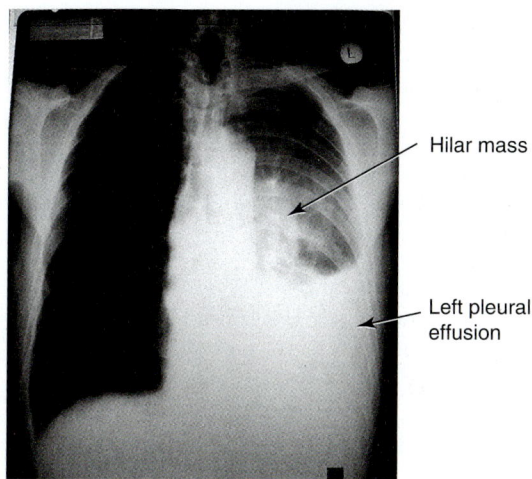

Hilar mass

Left pleural effusion

Fig. 3.2 Chest X-ray showing a left pleural effusion and a hilar mass.

Progress. A CXR was taken (Fig. 3.2 and Information box) and showed a pleural effusion and a hilar mass. The pleural effusion was aspirated and sent for cytology. A pleural biopsy was taken under ultrasound control and showed no evidence of malignancy on histology.

Video-assisted thoracoscopy was then performed, and this allowed visualisation of the pleura. The biopsy showed a squamous cell carcinoma.

The patient was referred to the multidisciplinary team (MDT) for discussion of treatment options.

INFORMATION

Chest X-rays

A standard CXR is taken posteroanteriorly (PA), with the patient facing the X-ray plate; the beam is directed at the patient's back at a standard distance.

An emergency department film is often taken anteroposteriorly (AP), with the patient lying down (supine) on the X-ray plate; the beam is directed at the patient's front; the distance from X-ray source can vary.

In an AP:

- Heart size and mediastinum are magnified
- A pleural effusion that lies along the back of the chest cavity when the patient is supine might be missed
- Film quality may be poor

Do not request an AP 'portable' film unless it would be unsafe for the patient to have a PA film.

HOW WOULD YOU MANAGE MASSIVE HAEMOPTYSIS?

As little as 250 mL can fill the bronchial tree and be life-threatening. This is uncommon but it requires prompt management:

- Monitor pulse oximetry, RR, BP and pulse rate
- Perform mobile CXR if possible

- Send urgent bloods: ABG, full blood count (FBC), U and Es, liver function test (LFT) and full coagulation profile
- Endotracheal intubation and suction might be required
- Urgent bronchoscopy by an experienced doctor is sometimes needed
- A cuffed tube can also be employed to protect the unaffected lung. It is inserted into the bronchus via a bronchoscope.
- Bronchial artery embolisation is highly effective if the bleeding vessel can be identified

INFORMATION

Massive haemoptysis can occur in the following conditions:
- Tuberculosis
- Bronchiectasis
- Aspergilloma
- Carcinoma of the bronchus

REMEMBER

Only a minority of patients have a malignant cause of massive haemoptysis.

Approach to Chest Pain

Diagnosing the cause of a chest pain can be straightforward but is often difficult, taking days to diagnose correctly. A careful history (eliciting site, character and radiation of the pain) is often more useful than tests:
- Exercise-induced central chest pain is usually cardiac in origin
- Rest pain might be cardiac, pleuritic, musculoskeletal, nerve root irritation, oesophageal, mediastinal, or referred pain from the abdomen
- Lung diseases cause pain only if the pleura, mediastinum, intercostal nerves, or bones are involved

IS IT CARDIAC PAIN?

See Chapter 2.

Typically central chest pain that radiates to the arms and neck. There is a dull ache, with a severe, heavy, 'constricting' character. It may be associated with breathlessness.

Typical Angina

Occurs on exercise and is eased by rest.

Acute Coronary Syndrome

Pain at rest or on minimal exertion, sometimes very severe with sweating; pain persists.

Pericarditis

Dull or sharp, central; eased by sitting forwards, may be worse with breathing.

Aortic Dissection

Severe sudden onset might be described as 'tearing' pain in the back or anterior chest; patient often shocked.

IS IT PLEURISY?

Sharp pain in the sides of the chest, which 'catches' with breathing. This is often accompanied by fever, cough with or without sputum or haemoptysis, indicating underlying lung disease.
Think of:
- Pneumonia and pleurisy
- Pulmonary infarction/embolism
- Pneumothorax
- Malignant invasion of pleura

IS IT MUSCULOSKELETAL?

- Trauma:
  - Rib fracture: 'point' tenderness
  - Crushed vertebra: pain often referred around the chest
- Chronic pain:
  - Osteoarthritis (OA): long history with acute episodes; look for spinal deformity
  - Rib or spine disease: might be metastatic cancer; local tenderness and swelling, lumps, history of cancer
- Muscles: Bornholm disease. Follows an upper respiratory tract infection; a low-grade fever can occur. Ache in muscles. Might be tender. Definite cases are rare
- Costochondral junction: Tietze disease; local pain on pressure over costochondral junctions. Responds to NSAIDs

IS IT NERVE ROOT IRRITATION?

- Typically in a dermatome distribution around the chest. Might be unilateral
- Vertebral OA, osteomyelitis, prolapsed disc
- Malignant nerve root compression
- Herpes zoster (shingles): is there a vesicular rash (pain may precede rash)?

IS IT OESOPHAGEAL?

Reflux causes retrosternal burning pain, usually after food. Worse lying flat and eased by antacid. Can be severe and mimic myocardial infarction.

Oesophageal Rupture

Central pain with shock. Might have associated pleural effusion. Occurs after severe vomiting or more commonly endoscopy at which dilatation has been performed for a malignant lesion.

IS IT REFERRED PAIN FROM OUTSIDE THE CHEST?

Diaphragm irritation may cause shoulder tip pain. Localisation might be difficult for the patient. Patients with several abdominal emergencies might have chest pain with or without abdominal pain.

Think of:
- Acute cholecystitis
- Acute duodenal ulceration
- Subphrenic abscess
- Perforated bowel
- Peritonitis
- Pancreatitis

COULD BE FUNCTIONAL?

Exclude organic disease in *all* cases. A tiny minority of patients with chest pain may have functional chest pain. These patients may also have an underlying disease process that could go undiagnosed.

WHAT INVESTIGATIONS WOULD YOU REQUEST FOR A PATIENT PRESENTING WITH CHEST PAIN?

After a good history and examination, do the following (as a minimum):
- Electrocardiogram – repeat if first ECG is normal
- Chest X-ray
- Serum cardiac troponins (if consistent with history)
- Full blood count, U and E, C-reactive protein (CRP)

Many diagnoses will now be obvious but remember:
- A normal ECG does not exclude cardiac pain
- A normal CXR does not exclude PE

If still in doubt:
- Retake the history, reexamine the patient and consider unusual causes
- Arrange further investigations, for example, CT, MRI scan

Bronchiolitis

CASE HISTORY

A 4-month-old female is brought to the emergency department with rhinorrhoea, difficulty breathing, and fevers for the last 24 hours. Her oral intake has been reduced over the last 1 to 2 days, and there have been fewer wet nappies than usual. She was born at term, and the pregnancy and delivery were uncomplicated. There is a maternal history of asthma, and her father smokes within the house.

On examination, her temperature is 38.1°C and her RR is 51 breaths per minute with pulse oximetry showing saturations of 89% on room air. Examination of the chest reveals moderate intercostal and subcostal recession with widespread crackles and expiratory wheeze bilaterally on auscultation.

WHAT IS THE MOST LIKELY DIAGNOSIS?

This presentation is most consistent with **bronchiolitis.** This is an acute viral infection of the lower respiratory tract that predominantly affects infants (generally <12 months, rare over the age of 3 years). Typically, respiratory distress is preceded by several days of upper respiratory tract symptoms, such as rhinitis and cough. Fever is normally low grade (<40°C) and additional systemic symptoms are common (e.g. irritability, malaise, reduced oral intake). Symptoms of lower respiratory tract disease develop later and include retractions, wheezing and scattered crepitations.

INFORMATION

Bronchiolitis is most commonly caused by respiratory syncytial virus (RSV) – responsible for up to 80% of cases. Other possible viruses include:
- Rhinovirus (2nd most common)
- Human bocavirus
- Human metapneumovirus (hMPV)
- Adenovirus
- Influenza and parainfluenza

WHAT WOULD BE YOUR DIFFERENTIAL DIAGNOSES?

Differential diagnoses include:
- Viral-induced wheeze: more common in older children (1–5 years); consider if episodic wheeze, no crepitations on auscultation and/or family history of atopy
- Bacterial pneumonia: far less common, typically higher fever, focal crepitations with minimal wheeze
- Laryngotracheobronchitis (croup): characterised by fever, barking cough and inspiratory stridor (often worse at night)
- Aspiration/foreign body inhalation: sudden onset, history of gagging/choking, no infective symptoms

WHAT ARE THE RISK FACTORS FOR SEVERE BRONCHIOLITIS?

- Prematurity (<37 weeks) and/or low birth weight
- Previous mechanical ventilation
- Age <12 weeks
- Chronic lung disease (e.g. cystic fibrosis, bronchopulmonary dysplasia)
- Congenital heart disease
- Immunocompromise
- Congenital defects of the airways
- Trisomy 21
- Regular exposure to cigarette smoke

HOW WOULD YOU MANAGE THIS PATIENT?

- Give oxygen supplementation if their oxygen saturation is:
  - <90% for children aged 6 weeks and over
  - <92% for babies under 6 weeks or children of any age with underlying health conditions
- Supportive care: give fluids by nasogastric or orogastric tube if they cannot take enough fluid orally. Give IV fluids to those unable to tolerate this or if there is evidence of impending respiratory failure
- High-flow nasal cannula therapy (HFNC) delivers a humidified, heated air and oxygen mixture at high flow and can be used as a rescue therapy for hypoxaemic children who do not respond to standard therapy
- Nasal continuous positive airway pressure (CPAP) can be considered if there is no response to HFNC or if there are signs of impending respiratory failure (e.g. exhaustion, recurrent apnoeic episodes)
- Intubation and mechanical ventilation may be necessary if there is no response to noninvasive ventilation (NIV)

REMEMBER

- In most children with bronchiolitis, no investigations are required
- Investigations (e.g. CXR, blood tests, virological testing) should only be undertaken when the presentation is atypical
- Medications, other than simple analgesia, are not routinely indicated. Do not routinely administer bronchodilators, steroids, antibiotics or antivirals

Respiratory Failure

Respiratory failure (PaO_2 <8 kPa) is a common medical emergency, often presenting with nonspecific symptoms such as mild confusion or agitation. Recognition requires ABG analysis.

Oximeters that estimate SaO_2 from the finger or ear lobe (SpO_2) are useful in assessment or monitoring. Oximeters might, however, be falsely reassuring in the patient breathing oxygen. Importantly, they will not detect alveolar hypoventilation, producing high pCO_2.

Respiratory failure commonly results from either a problem with ventilation or intrinsic lung disease.

REMEMBER

All breathless patients should have oximetry checked at triage in the emergency department.

VENTILATION FAILURE CAUSES A RAISED PACO$_2$

You should think of:
- Severe air-flow limitation, for example, COPD
- Neurological depression, for example, coma, sedatives, overdose
- Chest wall problems, for example, flail chest, pneumothorax
- Neuromuscular disease, for example, Guillain–Barré syndrome, old poliomyelitis

IN INTRINSIC LUNG DISEASE HYPOXAEMIA CAN BE COMBINED WITH A REDUCED PACO$_2$

The hypoxaemia arises primarily from a mismatch of ventilation and perfusion in the pulmonary alveolar bed. Hypoxic stimulation of ventilation, coupled with abnormal respiratory sensation, then leads to a reduced arterial pCO_2 (alveolar hyperventilation). A raised $PaCO_2$ indicates impending respiratory arrest as it suggests a reduction in ventilatory effort.

Consider:
- Infection, for example, pneumonia
- Shock, for example, sepsis, hypovolaemia, acute respiratory distress syndrome (ARDS)
- Cardiac disease, for example, LVF, pulmonary hypertension
- Pulmonary embolism

ARTERIAL BLOOD GAS SAMPLING

Arterial blood gas sampling can be used to:
- Assess severity
- Identify type, that is alveolar hypo- or hyperventilation
- Appreciate the degree of compensation (i.e. the chronicity of the condition)
- Recognise the base excess (BE) value as a coexisting metabolic acidosis commonly causes confusion

> **REMEMBER**
>
> Arterial blood gas sampling is painful, and local anaesthetic should be used. Heparin has a low pH and should be expelled from the syringe. When taking ABG samples, it is essential to note the inspiratory O_2 concentration (F_iO_2).

SUMMARY OF ACID–BASE CHANGES (FIG. 3.3)

In a Respiratory Acidosis

Carbon dioxide clearance is reduced – there is alveolar hypoventilation. The $PaCO_2$ and (H^+) rise. In chronic respiratory acidosis, HCO_3 is also increased due to renal compensation.

Examples include exacerbation of COPD, flail chest injury and Guillain–Barré syndrome.

In a Respiratory Alkalosis

There is alveolar hyperventilation, and both the $PaCO_2$ and (H^+) are decreased. The HCO_3 is slightly decreased.

Examples include acute asthma and anxiety attack.

In a Metabolic Acidosis

There is disturbance of HCO_3 regulation or excessive H^+ production. The HCO_3 is reduced and the $PaCO_2$ falls because of respiratory compensation.

Examples include diabetic ketoacidosis, chronic kidney disease and shock.

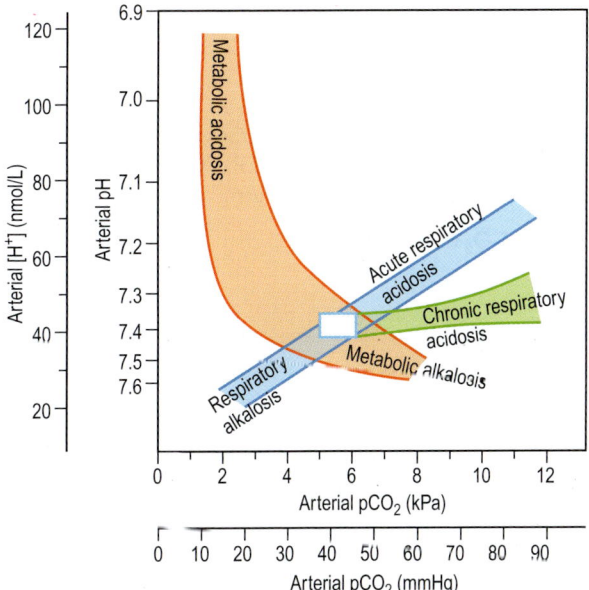

Fig. 3.3 The Flenley acid–base nomogram. The bands show the 95% confidence limits representing the individual varieties of acid–base disturbance. The central white box shows the approximate limits of arterial pH and pCO₂ in normal individuals.

In a Metabolic Alkalosis

The HCO_3 is increased and relative hypoventilation leads to a small compensatory increase in the $PaCO_2$.

Examples include excessive vomiting and profound hypokalaemia.

> **REMEMBER**
>
> The BE value provided by the ABG analyser is the concentration of base required to titrate the blood back to a normal plasma pH at a normal pCO_2 and 37° C.

EXAMPLES OF COMMON ABG ABNORMALITIES

Normal blood gas values are shown in Table 3.2.

Life-Threatening Asthma

- pH: 7.2
- PaO_2: 15.4
- $PaCO_2$: 6.0
- HCO_3: 16.2
- BE: −7.3

Supplemental O_2 is being provided (note the high PaO_2). There is a metabolic acidosis (note the pH and BE) as a result of metabolic demands exceeding O_2 delivery and producing a lactic acidosis. Airflow limitation limits the normal respiratory compensation to this profound acidosis.

Acute or Chronic Respiratory Failure in a Patient With COPD

- pH: 7.3
- PaO_2: 25.8
- $PaCO_2$: 12.6
- HCO_3: 42.1
- BE: +4.3

This is acute or chronic respiratory acidosis exacerbated by a high F_iO_2 using a variable-performance mask (40%–60% O_2) (note high PaO_2 and $PaCO_2$). The high HCO_3 results from renal compensation. The patient was changed to 28% oxygen.

Severe Pneumonia (F_iO_2 60%)

- pH: 7.15
- PaO_2: 4.8
- $PaCO_2$: 3.5
- HCO_3: 12.5
- BE: −9.3

Despite high F_iO_2, this patient is hypoxaemic because of ventilation–perfusion ($\dot{V}/\dot{Q}$) mismatch. The profound hypoxia despite oxygen and the associated metabolic acidosis indicate the need for urgent intubation and intermittent positive pressure ventilation (IPPV) and are a reflection of circulatory failure resulting from septic shock.

MANAGEMENT

Respiratory failure can be difficult to assess or manage. Always review the CXR. Discuss with your consultant or other more senior staff. If you feel that the situation is unstable, do not hesitate to call anaesthetics and intensive care unit (ICU) for support. Semielective intubation is much preferred to a respiratory arrest. It should be performed in the ward before transfer of the patient to the ICU.

WHAT ARE THE POTENTIAL SIGNS OF IMPENDING RESPIRATORY ARREST?

- Tachycardia >120
- Tachypnoea, RR >30
- Hypotension
- Sympathetic activation: pale and sweaty, agitation, confusion
- Progressive increase in $PaCO_2$ or fall in PaO_2
- Rapid desaturation on disconnection from O_2, for example, when drinking or coughing

Evaluation is often at the 'end of the bed'. Is the patient getting tired? Be sensitive to subtle changes or a failure to improve.

TREATING THE CAUSE

- Individual causes will require different actions: for example, an intercostal drain for a tension pneumothorax or large pleural effusion
- In neurological coma, intubation might be necessary for airway protection or to manage raised intracranial pressure by hyperventilation
- Drug-induced respiratory failure can be confirmed by a therapeutic trial with a specific antidote, that is, a bolus injection of naloxone for opiates and flumazenil for benzodiazepines. Infusions will be required if a positive response is obtained, as antidotes have a short half-life
- Oxygen supplementation should be aimed at raising the PaO_2 to beyond the steep part of the oxygen dissociation curve (Fig. 3.4). Very high PaO_2 values are unnecessary but careful controlled O_2 therapy via a fixed-performance mask is necessary in chronic respiratory failure resulting from COPD

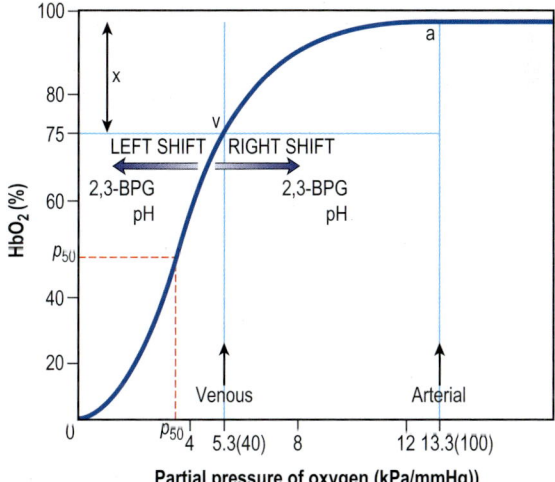

Fig. 3.4 Oxygen dissociation curve. BPG, Bisphosphoglycerate; a, arterial point; v, venous point; x, arterial venous difference; HbO_2, oxygen saturation of haemoglobin.

CASE HISTORY

A 65-year-old male with advanced COPD was admitted with a 1-week history of cough, breathlessness and purulent sputum. In the previous 24 h, he had become mildly confused. He was agitated with an RR of 35 and BP of 170/90 and was sweaty with an oximeter reading on air of 72%. There was widespread wheeze and coarse crackles suggestive of retained secretions. Arterial blood gas analysis revealed pH 7.32, PaO_2 5.8, $PaCO_2$ 8.1 and HCO_3 28.

WHAT DO THESE BLOOD GASES INDICATE?

Hypoxaemia with mild acute respiratory acidosis. There is no evidence of chronic respiratory failure with chronically elevated pCO_2, as HCO_3 is normal, that is, there is no compensation.

The initial treatment in the emergency department was:

- Nebulised bronchodilators (salbutamol 5 mg nebulised + ipratropium bromide 500 μg)
- 28% O_2 by controlled mask
- Antibiotics (in the context of increasingly purulent sputum) as per local guidelines, for example, amoxicillin (doxycycline if patient is penicillin-allergic)
- Intravenous steroids (this is a conventional treatment although there is limited evidence for effectiveness): for example, oral prednisolone 30 mg daily
- Encouragement to clear secretions, including sitting patient up and asking the physiotherapist to attend
- Chest X-ray to exclude pneumothorax or demonstrate associated pneumonia

INFORMATION

Controlled oxygen via a Venturi mask commonly leads to intermittent therapy, as the mask is poorly tolerated by agitated, breathless patients. Oxygen via nasal prongs at 1 or 2 L/min is more effective and continuous but is not 'controlled'.

Progress. Repeat ABGs were requested: pH 7.20, PaO_2 6.5, $PaCO_2$ 12.5, HCO_3 30.

These results show further CO_2 retention and a deteriorating situation. Oxygen should not be removed, as this will precipitate severe hypoxaemia. Alveolar ventilation must be increased. Despite using a nasal airway to stimulate cough and aid suction of respiratory secretions, there was no improvement.

WHAT FURTHER TREATMENT WOULD YOU CONSIDER?

Intubation was considered appropriate but a trial of NIV, bi-level positive airway pressure (BiPAP) with tight-fitting facial mask can be tried first with repeat gases at 1 h. On NIV, the RR slowed and the acute respiratory acidosis resolved.

Noninvasive ventilatory support employs a nose or face mask to provide ventilatory assistance to breathing (this is termed 'spontaneous pressure support') or timed breaths ('pressure-controlled ventilation'). An exhalation valve reduces rebreathing. NIV is successful in approximately 70% of patients with respiratory failure resulting from COPD.

INFORMATION

Contraindications/Cautions to NIV

- Unconscious or uncooperative patient
- Vomiting
- Large amount of respiratory secretions

- Cardiovascular instability (beware of hypotension)
- Recent facial or upper airway surgery
- Recent upper gastrointestinal (GI) tract surgery
- Inability to protect the airway

MECHANICAL VENTILATION

In an unstable situation, it is essential to maintain oxygenation. As intubation of an acutely unwell patient requires experience you should request ICU and anaesthetic support early.

Aims of Intubation and Mechanical Ventilation

- Quick correction of hypoxaemia
- Slower correction of hypercapnia.
- To allow effective suctioning of respiratory secretions

Hypotension After Intubation

This is very common and relates to:

- High airway pressures limiting venous return and causing a fall in cardiac output
- Vasodilatation directly caused by sedatives
- A fall in sympathetic tone

Progress. This patient continued on BiPAP and his blood gases were monitored. These gradually improved on this regimen and antibiotics. He was discharged and advised to see his doctor as soon as he develops a chest infection.

COPD – Acute Exacerbation

Chronic obstructive pulmonary disease (COPD) is used to describe a number of clinical syndromes associated with destruction of the lung and airflow obstruction.

> ### CASE HISTORY (1)
>
> A 63-year-old male ex-smoker has had a chronic productive cough for 20 years. For 10 years, he has had gradually increasing breathlessness on exertion. His usual exercise tolerance is 200 m on the flat. One week previously, he became breathless on walking between rooms and his sputum became purulent. His normal medication is salmeterol, tiotropium and beclometasone inhalers.
>
> **On examination**, his chest expanded poorly and he was wheezy, but there were no localising signs and no evidence of cor pulmonale or heart failure.
>
> His usual forced expiratory volume in 1 s/forced vital capacity (FEV_1/FVC) was 1.9/3.2 (predicted 3.4/4.4), but on arrival was 0.9/2.6. His CXR showed no acute lesion.

WOULD YOU ADMIT THIS PATIENT?

It was decided not to admit this patient to hospital because:

- He was able to cope at home with the aid of his wife
- He was not cyanosed: oximetry showed SaO_2 97%
- His general condition was good and he had a normal level of consciousness

Progress. He was discharged home with:
- Amoxicillin 500 mg × 3 daily for 1 week
- Prednisolone 30 mg daily for 2 weeks
- Advice to use inhaled SABAs in addition to normal medication bronchodilators 4-hourly via a spacer
- A follow-up appointment at the chest clinic for 2 weeks

AMBULATORY MANAGEMENT OF COPD

- The patient did not need admission because:
  - There was no evidence of respiratory failure
  - There was no evidence of cor pulmonale
  - He was able to cope at home
- If antibiotics are indicated, start a broad-spectrum antibiotic and, in particular, cover the majority of *Haemophilus influenzae* and *Streptococcus pneumoniae* organisms (the most common causes of acute exacerbation). Erythromycin was unnecessary because *Mycoplasma* was unlikely
- Oral steroids were used as an adjunct to antibiotics because the patient was already on inhaled steroids and possibly had a degree of steroid responsiveness. This is a conventional treatment, but there is limited evidence to support it
- The patient was given a spacer (and shown how to use it) in order to increase the lung deposition of aerosol
- The salbutamol dose was given 4-hourly because the effect lasts only 4–6 h and is partly dependent on dose
- Follow-up at the chest clinic was arranged because the patient had moderately severe COPD and had never been assessed:
  - Advise pneumococcal and influenza vaccination
  - Consider referral for pulmonary rehabilitation

However, the patient's doctor, when seeing the patient 1 week later, cancelled the outpatient appointment, believing it is unnecessary. He wrote to the chest physician, saying that he was able to manage the patient himself. He had a spirometer in the surgery and, when well, the patient had an FEV_1 of >50% predicated normal. Furthermore, the doctor said that the patient:
- Had a definitive diagnosis
- Had only moderately severe COPD
- Had no cor pulmonale
- Had no respiratory failure and did not need oxygen
- Did not have bullous lung disease
- Did not have a rapidly declining FEV_1

The patient's doctor was arranging to perform bronchodilator tests himself using a spirometer and checking the response to both salbutamol and ipratropium inhalers. He would arrange vaccination.

> **REMEMBER**
>
> Spirometry is required to assess the severity of COPD. Most COPD patients can be satisfactorily managed in the community.

PROGNOSIS OF COPD

Predictors of a poor prognosis are increasing age and worsening of airflow limitation, that is, a fall in FEV_1.

A patient with a BODE index (Table 3.3) of 0 to 2 has a mortality rate of 10%; one with a BODE index of 7 to 0 has a mortality rate of 80% at 4 years.

CASE HISTORY (2)

A 68-year-old female smoker, with a chronic productive cough and 5 years of gradually increasing breathlessness on exertion, had a usual exercise tolerance of 40 m on the flat and was breathless bending and washing. She was virtually housebound and lived alone. She developed a cough with purulent sputum and had been breathless at rest for 2 days. She was sent in to the emergency department.

On examination, the following were noted:
- Signs of respiratory failure: drowsiness and cyanosis, CO_2 flap
- Pulse 130/min, atrial fibrillation, BP 100/60
- Cor pulmonale with tricuspid regurgitation:
  - Jugular venous pressure (JVP) raised up to the level of the ear
  - Mid-systolic murmur at the left sternal edge
  - Enlarged pulsatile liver
  - Bilaterally oedematous legs to knees
- Respiratory rate 30, shallow breaths using accessory muscles of respiration, generalised wheezing and bilateral basal crackles

Investigations showed:
- Arterial blood gases: pH 7.32, PaO_2 5.6, pCO_2 8.2 on air
- Full blood count: Hb 178 g/L, haematocrit (Hct) 54%, white cell count (WCC) 12,300
- Urea 9.0, K^+ 3.5, creatinine 102
- Electrocardiogram 130 (ventricular rate); atrial fibrillation and right heart strain
- Chest X-ray: over-inflated lungs with prominent pulmonary arteries (indicating pulmonary hypertension) and normal-sized heart

---

WHAT ARE THE KEY CONSIDERATIONS FOR THIS PATIENT?

- The patient is in respiratory failure with raised $PaCO_2$: give oxygen via fixed-performance mask 24%, initially increasing to 28% or 35% if no rise in $PaCO_2$
- Cor pulmonale (right heart failure secondary to lung disease) is difficult to improve while the patient remains hypoxic
- Atrial fibrillation may only be secondary to hypoxaemia and might revert to sinus rhythm when PaO_2 improves

TABLE 3.3 ■ **BODE Index**[a]

Variable	Points on BODE Index			
	0	1	2	3
FEV_1 (% of predicted)	≥65	50–64	36–49	≥35
Distance walked in 6 min (m)	≥350	250–349	150–249	≤149
MMRC dyspnoea scale[b]	0–1	2	3	4
Body mass index	>21	≤21	–	–

FEV_1, Forced expiratory volume in 1 s/forced vital; MMRC, modified medical research council.
[a]Body mass index, degree of airflow Obstruction, Dyspnoea and Exercise capacity.
[b]Scores on the modified Medical Research Council (MMRC) dyspnoea scale range from 0 to 4, with a score of 4 indicating that the patient is breathless when dressing.

HOW WOULD YOU MANAGE THEM ACUTELY?

- Oxygen 28% via Venturi mask and repeat ABGs
- Patient to sit upright to help breathing
- Nebulised bronchodilators:
  - Salbutamol 5.0 mg as required and ipratropium 0.5 mg (max 2 mg/day) via nebuliser
  - Air rather than high-flow O_2 is safer for nebulising bronchodilators
- Chest physiotherapy to help sputum expectoration
- Broad spectrum antibiotics as per local guidelines, for example, amoxicillin 500 mg × 3 daily IV until condition improves and then oral switch
- Intravenous hydrocortisone 100 mg every 6 hours until patient improves and then oral prednisolone 20–30 mg daily for 2 weeks
- Monitor oximetry and mental state, RR and pulse until improvement

WHAT SHOULD YOU DO IF THERE IS NO IMPROVEMENT?

This patient did not improve and she was therefore started on non-invasive ventilation (NIV). The best technique is using a tight-fitting facial mask to deliver BiPAP ventilation support.

Progress
- Patient more alert
- PaO_2 8.0, $PaCO_2$ 8.4, pH 7.35 now on 2 L nasal oxygen
- In sinus rhythm

OXYGEN THERAPY IN ACUTE COPD EXACERBATION (FIG. 3.5)

- Management of oxygen is the most helpful and difficult component of treatment
- Although oxygen by Venturi mask, gives a known concentration, it is uncomfortable and claustrophobic. The mask has to be removed to eat, talk and cough, and for nebulised treatment
- Oxygen by nasal spectacles is more comfortable and can be kept on continuously
- Nasal oxygen gives variable F_iO_2, depending on the pattern of breathing and flow rate between 24% and 35%. It worked on this patient, but in many with COPD, 24% oxygen via a mask is preferable when $PaCO_2$ >8.0 kPa
- It takes 30–40 min to equilibrate blood gases with any change in F_iO_2, and blood gases should not be checked earlier
- It is unnecessary to restore the PaO_2 to normal: aim for it to reach the top of the steep slope of the oxygen saturation curve (see Fig. 3.3)
- If PaO_2 is >8 kPa, a small fall in PaO_2 has little effect on O_2 saturation: this is safer
- If PaO_2 is ≤6.5 kPa, a small fall produces a dangerous fall in SaO_2. *Note:* the oxygen dissociation curve is sigmoid in shape (see p. 326)
- Increasing the inspired oxygen may cause a small rise in $PaCO_2$ (mostly because of the relaxation of hypoxic vasoconstriction in relatively poorly ventilated alveoli). A pH change of <0.1 or $PaCO_2$ of <1 kPa is not significant, so do not reduce or remove the oxygen
- On increasing F_iO_2, this patient had not clinically improved and ABGs showed PaO_2 6.8 and $PaCO_2$ 12.0:
  - Action: the patient still needs oxygen but at a more controlled concentration. Increase F_iO_2 to 35%
  - Get help from a senior, preferably from the respiratory team, and discuss transfer to HDU for NIV or to intensive care unit (ICU) for assisted ventilation

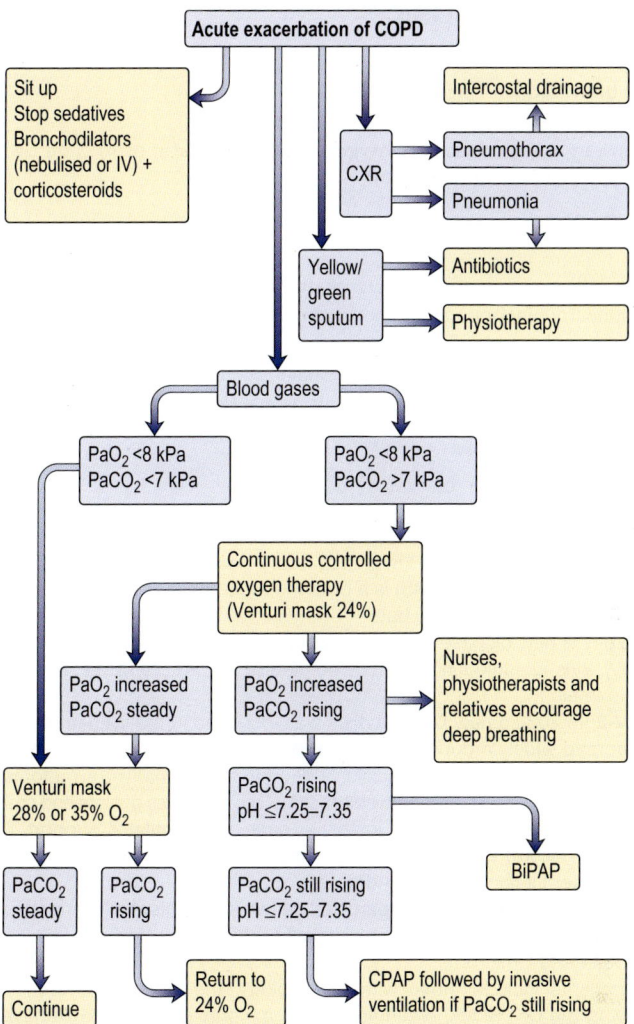

Fig. 3.5 Algorithm for the treatment of respiratory failure in COPD. COPD, chronic obstructive pulmonary disease; BiPAP, bi-level positive airway pressure; CPAP, continuous positive airway pressure; CXR, chest X-ray. (From Kumar, P., Clark, M., eds., 2017. Kumar and Clark's Clinical Medicine, ninth ed. Elsevier, Edinburgh, Fig. 24.24.)

Progress. Before discharge, blood gases were checked on air and showed a PaO_2 of 7.0 and $PaCO_2$ of 6.3. The respiratory nurse was asked to visit to:

- Discuss disease/risk factors, especially to urge smoking cessation and refer to a smoking cessation clinic
- Explain mechanism of action of drugs
- Explain the use of aerosol devices and spacers
- Arrange chest clinic follow-up for 2 weeks

FOLLOW-UP IN CHEST CLINIC

This was arranged to:

- Optimise bronchodilator treatment
- Monitor for polycythaemia and cor pulmonale
- Assess for long-term domiciliary oxygen (indication, PaO_2 of <7.3 on two occasions 3–4 weeks apart when patient is stable)

Pneumonia

Pneumonia is an inflammation of the substance of the lungs. It can be classified by site (e.g. lobar, diffuse, bronchopneumonia) or by aetiological agent (e.g. bacterial, viral, fungal, aspiration, or radiotherapy or allergic mechanisms). Pneumonias can be community-acquired (community-acquired pneumonia (CAP); commonest organism *S. Pneumoniae*), hospital-acquired (often Gram-negative bacteria) or ventilator-associated (multiple organisms, e.g. *Pseudomonas*, *Klebsiella* and *Acinetobacter*).

INFORMATION

Viral Respiratory Epidemics and Pandemics

- **SARS:** In November 2002 a new lower respiratory tract disease occurred in China. Severe acute respiratory syndrome (SARS) is a bronchopneumonia caused by a coronavirus (SARS-CoV), probably spread by bats
- **MERS:** In 2012 a new disease caused by a coronavirus, Middle East respiratory syndrome (MERS-CoV), was identified in patients who died of respiratory failure, the virus being spread via camels
- **SARS-CoV-2:** In 2020 a new **Coronavirus** was identified in the Wuhan district of China. This virus spread widely around the world and was declared a pandemic in March 2020

  People can be asymptomatic, but infective, or develop symptoms. The symptoms include a high temperature, a new continuous cough with shortness of breath, a loss of taste and smell, and fatigue.

  Patients can require admission to intensive care and ventilator support. Complications include multiorgan failure, septic shock and venous thromboembolism. Rarely children can develop a multisystem inflammatory syndrome.

  Spread is via exhaled droplets and particles, as well as contact. Several variants of SARS-CoV-2 have been identified that have sequentially replaced each other (the most significant being Alpha, Delta and Omicron).

  High-risk patients include those with comorbidity, the elderly, the immunosuppressed, and the obese. In the UK, Black, Asian and ethnic minority (BAME) people have had a higher incidence.

  Measures were taken by many countries to ban large gatherings and to enforce social distancing of 2 metres. All nonessential shops and workplaces were required to close during 'lockdowns', with people being encouraged to work at home and online where possible. The social implications were huge and it caused worldwide economic recessions.

  Testing and contact tracing were shown to slow the spread of the virus in many countries. Facial masks were also recommended in many countries for confined spaces, and in some countries, on leaving home.

  Treatment is largely supportive, but dexamethasone and hydrocortisone have been shown to be of benefit in severe cases. Empirical broad-spectrum antibiotics should be started if there is suspicion of a secondary bacterial infection. Antivirals, for example, remdesivir, are also recommended in severe disease. There is also evidence that interleukin-6 inhibitors (e.g. tocilizumab, sarilumab) and JAK inhibitors (e.g. baricitinib) reduce mortality in severe disease.

  Multiple vaccines have been developed that significantly reduce the likelihood of becoming critically ill. Countries developed national vaccination programmes and now offer yearly boosters (based on the current circulating strain) to those most at risk.

CASE HISTORY (1)

A 33-year-old female nonsmoker was admitted to the medical assessment unit with a 2-day history of fever, sweating and cough, productive of yellow, lightly blood-stained sputum. She had pleuritic pain in the right axilla.

PHYSICAL EXAMINATION

- Fever 39°C
- Respiratory rate 28/min
- Blood pressure 100/65 mmHg
- Dullness to percussion right lung base; consolidation
- Bronchial breathing right lung base; consolidation

This is the typical history of CAP

LIKELY INFECTING ORGANISMS

- *S. pneumoniae:* the most likely cause (35%–80% of cases)
- *H. influenzae:* especially in smokers with COPD
- *Mycoplasma* (4-yearly epidemics)
- *Legionella*
- *Staphylococcus aureus.*
- Viral: influenza
- *Chlamydia psittaci*

INVESTIGATIONS

- Chest X-ray
- Arterial blood gases
- Full blood count, WCC + differential
- Urea and electrolytes (U and Es)
- Urinalysis for sugar (is patient diabetic?)
- Blood and sputum culture
- Blood for viral serology and *Legionella/Mycoplasma*
- Serology for pneumococcal antigen (blood, sputum and urine)
- Rapid urine test available for *Legionella*

HOW WOULD YOU ASSESS THE SEVERITY OF THIS PATIENT'S PNEUMONIA?

The CURB-65 criteria (Box 3.2) indicate the severity of CAP.

Progress. This patient was young, previously fit and not breathless or shocked. The CXR (Fig. 3.6) showed a right lower lobe pneumonia. The WCC was raised, normal urea, PaO_2 10.5 kPa.

This pneumonia is not severe on the CURB criteria.

The patient was treated with oral antibiotics and was discharged in 24 h (see antibiotic choices).

CASE HISTORY (2)

A 73-year-old male was brought to the emergency department by his very anxious wife. He had had winter bronchitis for the last 5 years and was currently smoking 20 cigarettes/day. One week ago, he had the 'flu', and this morning became increasingly breathless, sweaty, pale and confused. A diagnosis of angina was made 2 years ago.

Bedside assessment summary:
- Confusion
- Respiratory rate >30/min
- Blood pressure 110/40
- Dehydrated

- Preexisting COPD
- Preexisting angina

That is CURB-65 score of 4+ (no blood tests done yet for urea)

Investigations showed:

- Chest X-ray (Fig. 3.7):
  - Diffuse opacification in both lungs
  - Ring opacities in right lung
- Urea 9 mmol/L
- White cell count 28,000
- Arterial blood gases: PaO_2 9.0 kPa, $PaCO_2$ 5.3 kPa, on FiO_2 40%

BOX 3.2 ■ CURB-65 Criteria for the Diagnosis of Severe Community-Acquired Pneumonia

- *C*onfusion*
- *U*rea >7 mmol/L
- *R*espiratory rate ≥30/min
- *B*lood pressure (systolic <90 or diastolic ≤60 mm Hg
- Age >*65* years

Score 1 point for each feature present:

Score 0–1 – Treat as outpatient

Score 2 – Admit to hospital

Score 3+ – Often require ICU care

Mortality rates increase with increasing score.

Other Markers of Severe Pneumonia

- CXR – more than one lobe involved
- PaO_2 <8 kPa
- Low albumin (<35 g/L)
- WCC (<4 × 10^9/L or high >20 × 10^9/L)
- Blood culture – positive

---

*Confusion is described as new disorientation in person, place or time.

ICU, Intensive care unit; CXR, chest X-ray; WCC, white cell count.

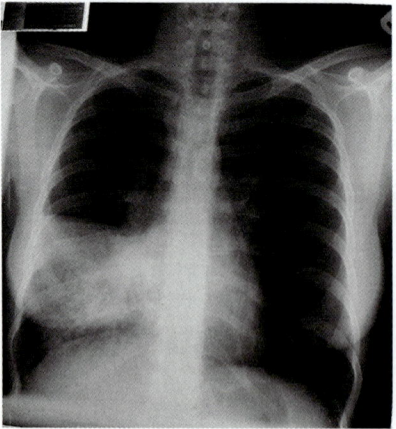

Fig. 3.6   Right lobar pneumonia.

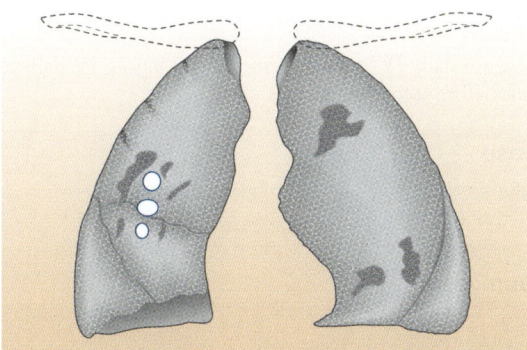

Fig. 3.7   Diagram of chest X-ray showing bilateral diffuse opacities and ring opacities in the right lung.

This is a high-risk case. The patient has influenza and a superinfection with *S. aureus*, causing severe CAP with early abscess formation (ring opacities on the CXR).

HOW WOULD YOU MANAGE THIS PATIENT?

- Rehydration: IV fluid
- Intravenous antibiotics (see antibiotics choices later): severe CAP
- Pulse oximetry: give O_2 to try to keep O_2 saturation >88%
- Nursing: where he can be easily observed or in an HDU (hourly BP, pulse, RR)
- Watching: for respiratory failure, as IPPV might be needed
- Physiotherapy: if he has difficulty coughing up sputum

INFORMATION

Potential Indications for Intensive Care Monitoring and Assisted Respiration

- PaO_2 <8 kPa on 60% O_2
- $PaCO_2$ >6.4 kPa
- Patient exhausted, drowsy or unconscious
- Shock
- Hypotension or circulatory failure

ANTIBIOTIC CHOICES FOR CAP

Always consult your hospital formulary and seek guidance from microbiology when required. Example antibiotic regimes include:

Uncomplicated Mild/Moderate CAP

- Treat for 5 days with oral medication unless patient is not swallowing or not absorbing
- Oral amoxicillin 500 mg × 3 daily + erythromycin 500 mg × 4 daily (or clarithromycin)
- In penicillin-allergic patient with underlying lung disease (*H. influenzae* suspected) give clarithromycin 500 mg × 2 daily

Severe CAP

- Intravenous antibiotics until significant improvement. Coamoxiclav 1.2 g IV × 3 daily and clarithromycin 500 mg IV × 2 daily
- Antibiotics for up to 10 days

Staphylococcal Pneumonia

- Treat for 10–14 days
- Flucloxacillin 2 g × 4 daily IV + gentamicin 3.0–5.0 mg/kg IV daily as single dose (check gentamicin levels before second dose)

Legionnaire Disease

- Treat for 3 weeks
- Clarithromycin 500 mg × 2 daily (for severe cases IV)

Mycoplasma Pneumonia

- Treat for 2 weeks
- Clarithromycin 500 mg × 2 daily IV or oral

Q Fever and Psittacosis

- Tetracycline 250–500 mg up to × 4 daily for 10 days

REMEMBER

- Clarithromycin resistance is a significant problem and it should be used with care.

Progress. This patient made a significant improvement on his IV antibiotics. He was switched to oral antibiotics and made a slow recovery.

CASE HISTORY (3)

A 24-year-old male, recently arrived in the UK from East Africa, presented with breathlessness of 2 weeks' duration, gradually increasing in severity, with a dry cough and sweats. He had a diarrhoeal illness 6 months ago and has recently noticed swollen glands in his neck.
Bedside assessment summary:
- Worried-looking patient
- Respiratory rate 34/min
- Tachycardia 120 bpm
- Temperature 41°C
- No abnormal signs in chest
- Preexisting illness: HIV infection
- Arterial blood gases: PaO_2 9.0 kPa; on F_iO_2 60% $PaCO_2$ 3.2 kPa
- White cell count 23 × 10^9/L
- Normal serum urea
On **investigation**, the CXR had:
- Ground glass appearance of lung fields
- Bilateral and perihilar shadowing

WHAT IS THE LIKELY DIAGNOSIS?

You should investigate whether this patient has HIV with a *Pneumocystis jirovecii* pneumonia because of the history of recent travel, 6-month history of illness, lymphadenopathy, low WCC and appearance on CXR (Fig. 3.8).

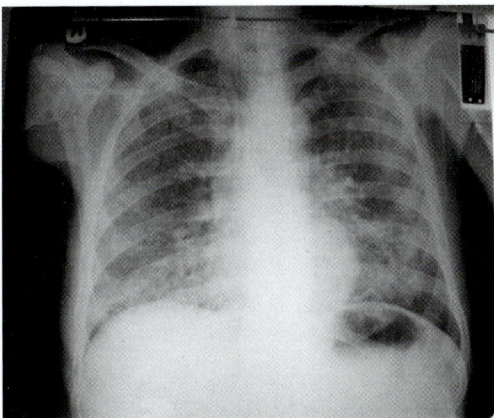

Fig. 3.8   Chest X-ray showing *bilateral perihilar shadowing* in *Pneumocystis jirovecii* pneumonia.

WHAT TREATMENT SHOULD BE STARTED IN THIS PATIENT?

Treatment should start in this patient for *P. jirovecii* infection (follow local guidance):

- Give high-dose IV co-trimoxazole
- Consider IV cefuroxime and erythromycin if in doubt as to the cause of the pneumonia
- Refer to an HIV specialist
- Patient may need high-dose steroids IV if his condition deteriorates
- Titrate O_2 to achieve O_2 saturation 94%–98%
- Arrange for induced sputum collection the next day

Progress. This patient improved on antibiotics, and his care was taken over by the HIV team.

CASE HISTORY (4)

A 68-year-old female smoker was admitted by the surgical team 9 days previously with intestinal obstruction. A laparotomy showed severe diverticulitis with a pelvic mass, and a defunctioning colostomy was performed. She has been very slow to mobilise postoperatively and developed a troublesome cough. Two days ago, she developed a fever and has now become breathless and tachycardic, with right-sided pleuritic chest pain.

Bedside assessment summary:
- Drowsy and diaphoretic
- Respiratory rate 24/min
- Pulse 112 bpm regular
- Temperature 40°C
- Coarse crackles in right lung base, patchy bronchial breathing
- Pleural rub
- No evidence of DVT
- Recent vomiting
- Recent surgery
- The surgeons gave her 5 days of IV amoxicillin postoperatively

Her National Early Warning Score (NEWS) (see Fig. 1.1) has increased to 4.

Investigations revealed:
- Chest X-ray: patchy opacification of right lung base
- Arterial blood gases: PaO_2 7.3, $PaCO_2$ 4.6
- White cell count: $16 \times 10^9/L$
- Urea: 10 mmol/L
- Electrocardiogram: sinus tachycardia

WHAT IS THE DIAGNOSIS?

Severe hospital-acquired pneumonia. However, for all cases, remember that:
- Deep vein thrombosis with pulmonary emboli might coexist
- Inhalation of vomit causes aspiration pneumonia
- Previous antibiotics could have selected out Gram-negative organisms
- The IV cannula may be infected
- There may be preexisting lung disease – smoker

WHAT ARE THE COMMON ORGANISMS IN HOSPITAL-ACQUIRED PNEUMONIA?

There is a wide range of possible organisms:
- Gram-negative bacilli (50%):
  - *Acinetobacter spp.*
  - *Escherichia coli*
  - *Proteus* spp.
  - *Klebsiella* spp.
  - *Pseudomonas* spp.
  - *H. influenzae*
- Gram-positive cocci:
  - *S. aureus*
  - *S. pneumoniae*
- Anaerobes:
  - *Bacteroides* spp.
  - *Clostridia* spp.

HOW WOULD YOU MANAGE THIS PATIENT?

- Titrate O_2 to achieve O_2 saturation 94%–98%
- Rehydrate with IV crystalloid

- Give broad-spectrum IV antibiotics as per local guidelines, for example:
  - **Piperacillin with tazobactam:** 4.5 g three times a day (increased to 4.5 g four times a day if severe infection)
- If improving after 48 h and able to swallow, switch to oral antibiotics such as:
  - Coamoxiclav (500/125) 625 mg × 3 daily + oral metronidazole 400 mg × 3 daily
- Patient is at high risk of PE: check that prophylactic low-molecular-weight heparin (LMWH) is prescribed
- Watch for deterioration
- Arrange chest physiotherapy to encourage effective cough

Progress. She responded slowly to antibiotics and was discharged a week later.

Lung Abscess

This is a severe localized suppuration in the lung. The CXR shows cavity formation, often with the presence of a fluid level (not due to TB).

The causes of lung abscess include aspiration, particularly amongst alcohol users. Lung abscesses also frequently follow the inhalation of a foreign body into a bronchus. They can also occur when the bronchus is obstructed, for example, by a bronchial carcinoma. Chronic or sub-acute lung abscesses can also follow inadequately treated pneumonia.

CASE HISTORY

A 74-year-old male presented with a 1-month history of a productive cough with offensive-tasting sputum, malaise and weight loss. His dentition was very poor. He had just stopped smoking.

On examination, he had a temperature of 39.8°C, a few crackles at the right base but no other respiratory signs. A CXR (Fig. 3.9) showed a cavity.

WHAT ARE THE DIFFERENTIAL DIAGNOSES?

- Lung abscess
- Cavitating lung cancer
- Tuberculosis

Progress. Bronchoscopy showed thick secretions in the right lower lobe. There was no bronchial obstruction and cytology was negative.

Diagnosis – pyogenic abscess. The patient responded to antibiotics (cefuroxime and metronidazole), and the abscess resolved in 6 weeks. It probably resulted from aspiration, with mouth anaerobes contributing to the unpleasant smell and taste of the sputum. Aspiration usually occurs on the right side, as the right bronchus is more vertical.

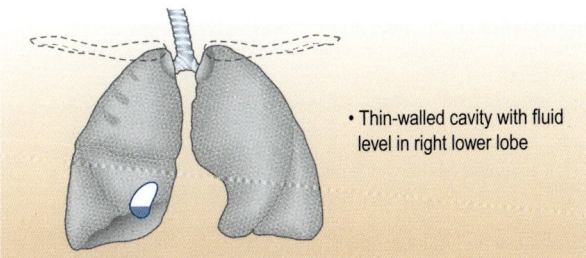

- Thin-walled cavity with fluid level in right lower lobe

Fig. 3.9   Diagram of chest X-ray showing a *cavity* (lung abscess).

Tuberculosis (TB)

CASE HISTORY (1)

An 18-year-old male who came to the UK 2 years ago from the Indian subcontinent presented with general malaise, photophobia, unproductive cough, weight loss and night sweats.

On examination, his temperature was 39.5°C. He looked unwell and appeared rather vague. There was no neck stiffness or any abnormal chest signs.

Investigations revealed Na 120, K 2.6 and urea 2.8, Hb 104 g/L and WCC 6.4; serum alanine aminotransferase (ALT) and alkaline phosphatase were slightly raised. A portable AP chest film appeared.

The patient was admitted with a diagnosis of **pyrexia of unknown origin**. He had blood and urine cultures and Cerebrospinal fluid (CSF) examination. Cerebrospinal fluid showed an increased cell count, mostly lymphocytes, raised protein and low glucose. No organisms were seen but cultures were sent. A departmental PA CXR was performed after 2 days and showed miliary mottling.

WHAT IS THE LIKELY DIAGNOSIS?

This patient has miliary tuberculosis with meningitis (TBM). It carries a high morbidity if not treated early. The hyponatraemia is dilutional secondary to inappropriate secretion of antidiuretic hormone.

WHAT DOES TREATMENT CONSIST OF?

Treatment is with antituberculous drugs such as rifampicin, isoniazid and pyrazinamide. These must commence before cultures are available and are continued for at least 9 months. Ethambutol is avoided where possible because of its ophthalmic complications.

Corticosteroids, for example, prednisolone, are given for the first 3 weeks, as they reduce mortality. Relapses and complications (e.g. seizures, hydrocephalus) are common in TBM. The mortality remains over 60%, even with early treatment.

Progress. This patient was started on antituberculous therapy as described. His mental state improved and temperature settled. He was discharged after 3 weeks with an appointment for 3 weeks later in outpatients.

CASE HISTORY (2)

A 50-year-old male, who was a heavy drinker with no fixed abode, was brought to the emergency department after he 'collapsed'. He had stopped drinking alcohol 1 week previously because he had run out of money. He was confused, hallucinating and coughing.

On examination, he was unkempt, emaciated, confused and jaundiced:
- Temperature: 37.9°C
- Pulse: 100 bpm
- Blood pressure: 100/60

On further examination, right upper chest, bronchial breathing + coarse crackles, trachea deviated to the right. The liver was enlarged 3 cm below the costal margin and there was ascites.

Investigations revealed:
- Haemoglobin 180 g/L, mean corpuscular volume (MCV) 106, WCC 8500
- Urea: 1.3
- K+: 3.5
- Creatinine: 60, estimated glomerular filtration rate (eGFR) 98 mL/min
- Na: 126
- Bilirubin: 40
- Alkaline phosphatase and ALT: raised
- Chest X-ray: Fig. 3.10

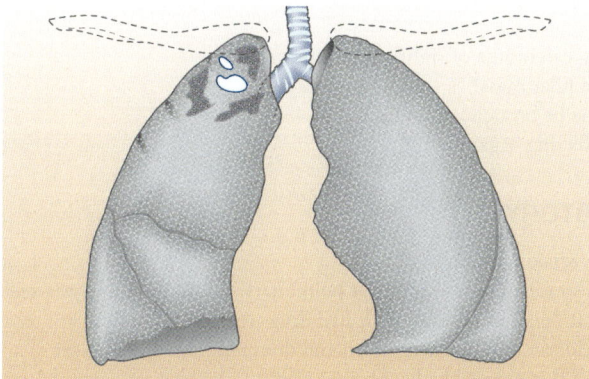

Fig. 3.10　Diagram of chest X-ray – *patchy opacification* with *cavitation* in *right* upper lobe and trachea deviated to the right in tuberculosis.

A provisional differential diagnosis was made of:
- Delirium tremens
- Pulmonary TB
- Alcoholic liver disease

Urgent sputum was sent for staining with auramine–phenol fluorescent test plus culture and sensitivities for AFB (if no organisms are found, send at least three more good sputum specimens). TB bacilli were found in the third sputum specimen (smear-positive).

WHAT ARE THE RISK FACTORS FOR DEVELOPING TB REACTIVATION?

- Heavy alcohol or other drug use
- Diabetes mellitus
- Malnutrition
- Immunosuppression (any cause, including steroid therapy)

HOW WOULD YOU MANAGE THIS PATIENT?

- Isolate patient as smear-positive
- Treat delirium tremens. *Note:* always give thiamine too
- Start anti-TB therapy as soon as possible
- Notify infection control about the patient and ask the TB health visitor to do contact tracing

Progress. The patient was started on anti-TB therapy and treatment for his delirium tremens. He needed directly observed treatment (DOT) because he was unlikely to comply with treatment otherwise. He was also referred to both the respiratory and gastroenterological teams.

CASE HISTORY (3)

A 64-year-old male smoker was treated by his doctor with antibiotics for bronchitis 3 months ago. As his cough had not resolved, he was admitted to hospital 1 week ago. Initial assessment showed a right upper lobe pneumonia, and he was treated with oral amoxicillin and clarithromycin. Blood and sputum cultures were negative. He had a persistent low-grade fever and the CXR still showed patchy right upper lobe consolidation. You have been called to see him because he has just developed haemoptysis.

WHY IS THIS PNEUMONIA SLOW TO RESOLVE?

Consider:
- Obstructing carcinoma of right upper lobe bronchus:
  - Is there a hilar mass?
  - Should he be bronchoscoped?
- Unusual infecting organism

FURTHER HISTORY

It is always worth retaking the history:
- The patient's mother was treated for pulmonary TB in 1941. He was seen in a chest clinic as a child but does not think that he had drug treatment. He does not recall having Bacillus Calmette-Guerin (BCG) vaccination and does not have a BCG scar
- Pulmonary TB is a possible diagnosis
- Look carefully at a new PA CXR (Fig. 3.11)

WHAT WOULD YOU DO NEXT?

This is TB until proved otherwise.
- Send urgent sputum for auramine staining and TB culture
- Send at least three sputum specimens
- Check blood count, liver biochemistry and renal function

RESULTS

The microbiologist calls you urgently:
- The patient has AFB seen on sputum smear
- Sputum is being cultured for TB
- Culture results will be available in 6–8 weeks
- Sensitivities perhaps may not be available for 12 weeks

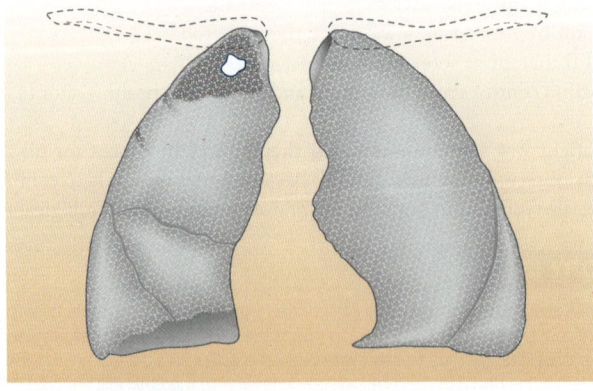

Fig. 3.11 Diagram of chest X-ray – right upper lobe consolidation with small apical cavity. This was probably obscured by the clavicle on the previous chest X-ray.

Progress

- This patient was isolated in a side room (smear-positive)
- Treatment for TB was given
- Tuberculosis is a notifiable disease in the UK and allows contact tracing to be initiated

---

CASE HISTORY (4)

A 34-year-old female who had travelled from Uganda recently presented to the emergency department with high fever, diarrhoea and weight loss. She did not inform the staff that she had been found to be HIV-positive 6 months previously (with a CD count of 250) and had declined further investigation or treatment at that time.

On examination, she appeared unwell and cachectic and was coughing continuously.
Investigations revealed:

- Chest X-ray: right lower lobe shadowing and possible right hilar lymphadenopathy
- Haemoglobin 75 g/L, WCC 4.2, lymphocytes 0.8, platelets 156
- Na^+ 128, K^+ 2.5, urea 11.8, albumin 18

Blood, stool, sputum and urine cultures were taken, and she was admitted and commenced on amoxicillin and erythromycin. She failed to improve, and after 3 days, the antibiotics were changed to ciprofloxacin, although sputum culture was unhelpful. On day 5, the microbiologist was consulted: examination of sputum for AFB was positive, and *M. tuberculosis* was subsequently isolated from blood and stool.

REMEMBER

- Many patients do not volunteer their HIV status
- You must indicate that *M. tuberculosis* is a possibility when requesting sputum examination
- Atypical radiological changes are common in TB in the immunocompromised
- Both *Mycobacterium intracellulare avium* and *M. tuberculosis* can be isolated from stool and blood
- A patient from a country where TB is prevalent who presents with pneumonia should be admitted to a side room until TB has been excluded
- The risk of TB developing in those infected (i.e. disease reactivation) in HIV increases when CD count is <200

Progress. This patient was started on antituberculous therapy. She was taken over by the HIV team and had continued care from the respiratory team for follow-up and contact tracing.

HOW IS TB TREATED?

- Rifampicin: if body weight is <50 kg, 450 mg daily; if body weight is ≥50 kg, 600 mg daily
- Isoniazid: 300 mg daily
- Pyrazinamide: if body weight <50 kg, 1.5 g daily; if body weight ≥ 50 kg, 2 g daily
- Ethambutol: 15 mg/kg (test visual acuity before treatment)
- Give all drugs together once daily with breakfast
- All four drugs for 2 months followed by rifampicin and isoniazid for 4 months (having checked the sensitivities)
- Tuberculous meningitis: recommended duration 12 months:
  - Four drugs for 3 months; rifampicin + isoniazid for 9 months
  - Corticosteroids are indicated in tuberculous meningitis, pericarditis and spinal TB with neurological compression

N.B. This patient may have multiresistant TB (MRTB).

Monitor Therapy

- Liver biochemistry
- Patient compliance with medication

Pleural Effusion

This is an excessive accumulation of fluid in the pleural space. It can be detected on X-ray when ≥300 mL of fluid is present, and clinically when ≥500 mL or more is present. The CXR appearances range from obliteration of the costophrenic angle to dense homogeneous shadows occupying part or all of the hemithorax. Fluid below the lung (a subpulmonary effusion) can simulate a raised hemidiaphragm. Fluid in the fissures may resemble an intrapulmonary mass.

CASE HISTORY (1)

A 63-year-old male presented with a 2-month history of increasing breathlessness and could only walk at a slow pace on the level.

On examination, he showed:
- Reduced chest movement on the left
- Reduced tactile vocal fremitus
- Stony dullness to percussion
- Reduced breath sounds
- Apex beat in anterior axillary line (see Fig. 3.2)

WHAT OTHER CLINICAL SIGNS WOULD YOU LOOK FOR?

- Clubbing: suggests malignancy
- Glands in neck
- Wasting
- Enlarged liver

WHAT WOULD YOU DO NEXT?

The patient was admitted to the medical assessment unit. A diagnostic aspiration was performed after the procedure was explained to the patient and consent obtained. A syringe with a 21 G needle was inserted under ultrasound guidance and 20 mL of fluid was obtained. This was sent to the laboratory for:

- Protein/ lactate dehydrogenase (LDH)
- Cell count
- Culture, including TB
- Cytology for malignant cells

Results

- Fluid is blood-stained
- Fluid protein is >30 g/L, which indicates an exudate
- Few white cells and mesothelial cells
- Cultures sterile
- Malignant cells: probably squamous origin

WHAT IS THE DIAGNOSIS?

Malignant pleural effusion. There is an underlying squamous cell carcinoma of the bronchus.

If the diagnosis had not been obtained on the aspirate, a pleural biopsy and a larger volume of pleural fluid with cytological examination of the spun cellular debris could have been performed. If there is still no diagnosis, refer to a respiratory physician.

WHAT NEXT?

- Treatment should be discussed at an MDT meeting, concentrating on relieving symptoms and possible chemotherapy
- Drain the effusion (following explanation and consent) with an intercostal drain, ideally placed over the top of the diaphragm:
  - Use ultrasound to guide placement
  - A small-bore (10–14 F) intercostal drain should be the initial choice
  - Clamp intermittently and limit flow to 1 L in the first hour to reduce the risk of reexpansion pulmonary oedema or discomfort from mediastinal shift. Reexpansion pulmonary oedema occurs much more commonly following reexpansion of the collapsed lung associated with a pneumothorax. It relates to endothelial dysfunction and is therefore not hydrostatic. Diuretics are not helpful and may exacerbate any tendency to hypovolaemic hypotension

Progress. This patient's breathlessness improved after drainage of the effusion and he was discharged oncology follow-up.

> ### CASE HISTORY (2)
>
> A 43-year-old female developed increasing breathlessness and malaise after being treated for pneumonia with oral cefalexin 2 weeks previously. She was febrile with a temperature of 39°C, flushed and anorexic with signs of a **left pleural effusion**. A pleural tap produced cloudy, infected fluid (an empyema). A diagram of the CXR appearances is shown in Fig. 3.12.

WHAT SHOULD YOU DO?

- Drain the fluid by placing an intercostal drain
- Start antibiotics (after taking blood and fluid cultures) based on local guidelines. This should cover both aerobic and anaerobic organisms; for example, cefuroxime 1 g IV 6-hourly and metronidazole 500 mg IV 8-hourly
- Consult a chest physician/surgeon early if drainage is incomplete. Decortication of the lung or a rib resection and wide-bore drain might be needed
- Bronchoscopy should be performed to exclude bronchial obstruction
- Computed tomography scanning is helpful to assess the presence of an underlying lung abscess

WHAT ARE THE POTENTIAL CAUSES OF PLEURAL EFFUSIONS?

Exudates (protein >30 g/L in patients with a normal serum protein level):
- Malignancy
- Mesothelioma
- Metastatic cancer: breast, bowel
- Lymphoma
- Pneumonia
- Tuberculosis

Transudates (protein <30 g/L in patients with a normal serum protein level):
- Heart failure

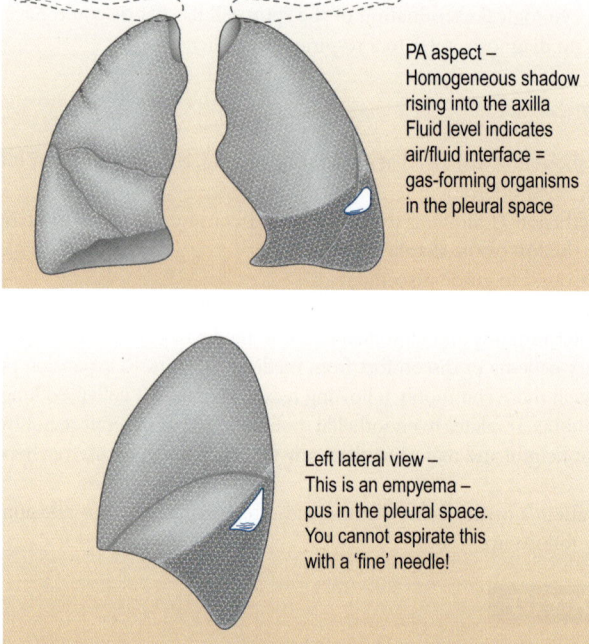

PA aspect –
Homogeneous shadow
rising into the axilla
Fluid level indicates
air/fluid interface =
gas-forming organisms
in the pleural space

Left lateral view –
This is an empyema –
pus in the pleural space.
You cannot aspirate this
with a 'fine' needle!

Fig. 3.12   Diagram of chest X-ray (posteroanterior [PA] and left lateral) of an empyema.

- Nephrotic syndrome
- Liver cirrhosis

Progress. This patient had an **empyema**. She was in hospital for 10 days, as her recovery was slow. She required two further drainages of her empyema but surgery was not necessary. When seen 4 weeks later, she was well.

Pulmonary Embolism (and Deep Vein Thrombosis)

Pulmonary embolism (PE) is due to thrombus formed in the systemic veins (rarely, the right side of the heart), which breaks off and embolises in the pulmonary artery. The clinical scenarios depend on whether the emboli block small/medium arteries or the pulmonary artery itself, causing right ventricular obstruction.

The diagnosis of pulmonary embolism can be difficult for a number of reasons:
- Presumptive treatment is not without risk
- Proving the diagnosis can be difficult

CASE HISTORY (1)

A 24-year-old female had been getting breathless for 3 months when referred. Asthma seemed unlikely (peak flow from the referring doctor was 460 L/min) and the CXR was normal. A short pulmonary early diastolic murmur was noted, and a cardiology opinion sought. Spirometry was normal, but CO gas transfer was reduced (TL_{CO} 60% predicted). The echocardiographic appearances were normal.

About 2 weeks later, she was admitted in shock. The ECG (Fig. 3.13) showed acute right heart strain (S1, Q3, T3 with dominant R waves in V_1–V_3), and the pulmonary artery diastolic pressure with the right atrial pressure was calculated to be 25 cmH_2O (by Doppler echocardiography of the tricuspid regurgitant wave), which is very high.

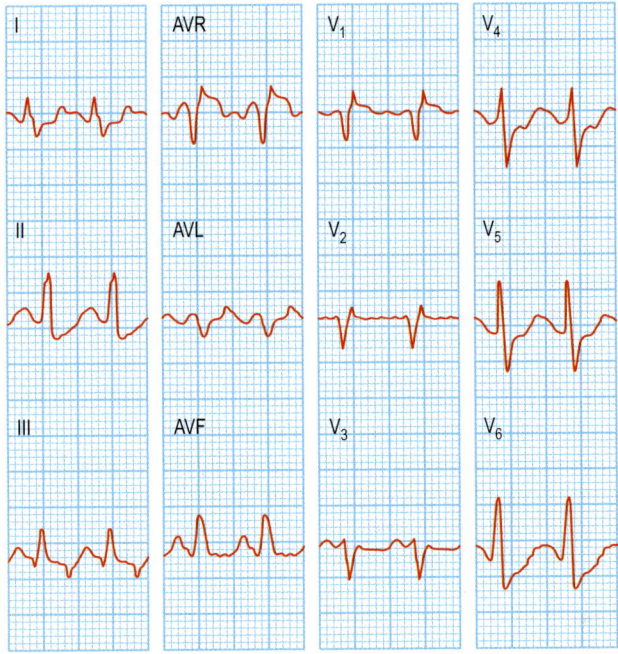

Fig. 3.13   Acute pulmonary embolism shown on a 12-lead ECG. (From Feather, A., Randall, D., Waterhouse, M., eds., 2020. Kumar and Clark's Clinical Medicine, tenth ed. Elsevier, Edinburgh, Fig. 29.1.)

WHAT IS THE DIAGNOSIS?

This is a massive pulmonary embolism.

Progress. She was managed on the cardiac care unit (CCU) and received thrombolysis with alteplase. Doppler echocardiogram was used to monitor response. She was subsequently anti-coagulated with low-molecular-weight heparin (LMWH) and warfarin. She responded well to treatment and was returned to the ward.

A subsequent $\dot{V} / \dot{Q}$ scan revealed the typical multiple patchy perfusion abnormalities of recurrent minor PE, which explains her 3-month history of breathlessness. The scan has remained abnormal and she has continued to be breathless. Leiden factor V deficiency was discovered and the oral contraceptive stopped. She has been advised to remain on long-term warfarin, although the benefits are disputed.

HOW ELSE CAN PULMONARY EMBOLISM PRESENT?

- Acute minor pulmonary infarction producing pleuritic chest pain and possibly haemoptysis
- Episodic nonspecific symptoms in the postoperative patient (such as palpitations and anxiety attacks), possibly followed by a cardiac arrest
- Chronic minor thromboembolism leading to established pulmonary hypertension

WHAT SIMPLE INVESTIGATIONS CAN HELP DIAGNOSE A PE?

These are only helpful if the clinical presentation is suggestive:

- Plasma D-dimers in combination with risk scoring (e.g. Wells' criteria); if the patient has a low pretest probability and the D-dimer is negative it can rule out PE
- Electrocardiogram and/or CXR might reveal evidence of alternative causes such as myocardial infarction, pneumothorax or aortic dissection

REMEMBER

An undetectable plasma D-dimer level (reflecting fibrin activation) essentially excludes significant thromboembolism but a raised value is nonspecific.

WHAT FURTHER INVESTIGATIONS COULD YOU REQUEST FOR A SUSPECTED PE?

CT

Contrast-enhanced, multidetector CT pulmonary angiograms (CTPAs) have a sensitivity of 83% and specificity of 96%, with a positive predictive value of 92% (higher with 64-multislice scanners).

Radionuclide ventilation/perfusion scanning ($\dot{V}/\dot{Q}$ scan)

This is a good test after measurement of D-dimers. It demonstrates ventilation/perfusion defects, that is areas of ventilated lung with perfusion defects. Pulmonary [99m]technetium scintigraphy demonstrates the under-perfused areas, while a scintigram, performed after inhalation of radioactive xenon, shows no ventilatory defect. A matched defect may, however, arise with a PE that causes an infarct, or with emphysematous bullae. This test is therefore conventionally reported as a probability (low, medium or high) of PE and should be interpreted in the context of the history, examination and other investigations.

MRI

This gives similar results to CT and is used if CTA is contraindicated.

Echo

The echocardiogram can be very useful in the diagnosis of massive PEs but is of limited value otherwise:

- It might show RV dilatation with paradoxical septal wall movement; pulmonary artery pressure may also be estimated

- It might exclude or confirm an alternative diagnosis, for example, cardiac tamponade, LVF
- RV clot is occasionally imaged and is an adverse prognostic sign, with 10% mortality risk

Ultrasonography for DVT

Doppler ultrasound and B-mode venous compression ultrasonography of the legs have largely replaced contrast venography, having sensitivities of 90% and 70%, respectively, for proximal thrombus. They can detect clots in the pelvic or ilio-femoral veins.

HOW WOULD YOU TREAT A PATIENT WITH A CONFIRMED PE?

- Supportive therapy with oxygen, IV fluids and analgesia should be given
- Low-molecular-weight is licensed for use in DVT and PE (use unfractionated heparin if rapid reversal is required) and should be started as soon as possible (to prevent further clot formation)
- If using warfarin, then overlap with heparin and discontinue heparin once the INR is therapeutic (INR 2–3)
- Direct oral anticoagulants (DOACs) such as antithrombin agents (e.g. dabigatran) or Factor Xa inhibitors (e.g. rivaroxaban, apixaban, edoxaban) are increasingly being used in place of heparin and warfarin:
    - If using rivaroxaban or apixaban, these can be started without the need for lead in therapy with LMWH
    - If ongoing anticoagulation will be with edoxaban or dabigatran, at least 5 days of lead-in therapy with LMWH is required first. Stop LMWH before starting dabigatran or edoxaban
- Anticoagulation can be stopped after 3 months (or 3–6 months for people with active cancer) if the PE was provoked (if the risk factor is no longer present). Anticoagulation is continued for longer if the PE was unprovoked
- Thrombolytic therapy is used for clot lysis in major PE. Although good evidence of reduced mortality is lacking, there is faster and more complete resolution of echocardiographic abnormalities or $\dot{V}/\dot{Q}$ defects
- Emergency embolectomy is rarely a possibility – it can be performed only in cardiothoracic centres
- Transvenous placement of venocaval filters is used for *recurrent* PE, even though the patient is adequately anticoagulated

REMEMBER

Thrombolysis should be used in all patients with cardiogenic shock due to massive PE. You should discuss this with your senior before treating.

Pneumothorax

CASE HISTORY (1)

A 23-year-old male presented to the emergency department with a sudden onset of right-sided chest pain, worse on deep inspiration and associated with acute breathlessness. This started at rest and was not associated with cough. There were no preexisting medical problems and no other symptoms.
On examination, he was a healthy young male:
- Afebrile, not cyanosed, no signs of DVT
- Pulse rate 100 bpm, RR 30/min
- Trachea central
- Chest movement red right side
- Percussion note hyperresonant right side
- Breath sounds reduced right side
- Key investigation: CXR (Fig. 3.14), which demonstrated pneumothorax = 1/2 hemithorax.
Diagnosis – right-sided spontaneous pneumothorax

> **REMEMBER**
>
> Common causes of pleuritic chest pain and dyspnoea are pneumothorax, PE and pneumonia with pleurisy.

HOW WOULD YOU MANAGE THIS PATIENT?

- If <2 cm, discharge and review next day
- If there is shortness of breath ± >2 cm rim on CXR, aspirate
- If still unsuccessful, insert intercostal drain

This male was symptomatic and had a moderate-sized pneumothorax. Aspiration is the first choice. Explain and obtain consent:

Technique for simple aspiration

- Infiltrate with local anaesthetic down to pleura in second intercostal space in mid-clavicular line using 16 FG cannula (or less) at least 3 cm long
- Once in pleural space, remove needle
- Connect cannula via three-way tap to chest, 50 mL syringe
- Stop aspirating when resistance felt, or patient coughs or complains of discomfort, or when 2.5 L aspirated

Progress. The patient was X-rayed again, and the lung was seen to have partially re-expanded.

HOW WOULD YOU MANAGE THIS PATIENT AFTER ASPIRATION?

The patient was:

- Discharged home after observation and some resolution on CXR, taking his discharge X-ray with him
- Instructed not to fly for 6 weeks or go diving
- Given a follow-up appointment in the chest clinic for 1 week
- Instructed to reattend (bringing the X-ray) if he became breathless

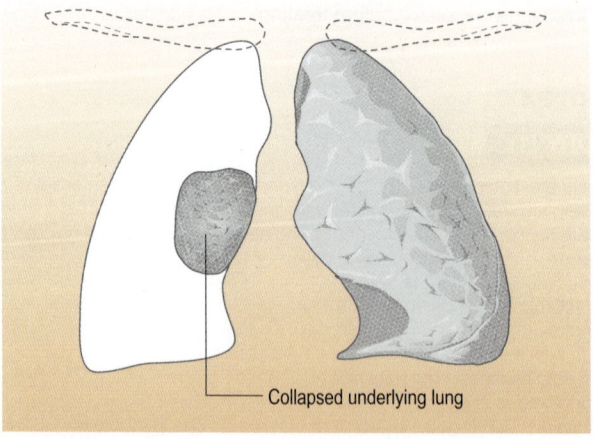

Collapsed underlying lung

Fig. 3.14 Diagram of chest X-ray showing collapsed *right* lung (pneumothorax).

Progress. This male's follow-up X-ray was normal and he has had no further problems.

CASE HISTORY (2)

A 69-year-old male with long-standing COPD and an exercise tolerance of 100 m on the flat became acutely breathless at rest.
On examination, he was distressed and cyanosed:
- Using accessory muscles of respiration
- Respiratory rate 40/min
- Pulse 120, BP 100/60
- Barrel-shaped chest with poor expansion
- Hyperresonant chest on the left with almost inaudible breath sounds, trachea deviated to right

WHAT ARE YOUR MAIN DIFFERENTIAL DIAGNOSES?

- Acute exacerbation of COPD but no obvious infection and symptoms very acute
- Pulmonary embolism
- Pneumothorax
- Acute myocardial infarction with LVF

WHAT IS THE MOST LIKELY DIAGNOSIS?

Life-threatening **tension pneumothorax**: emphysematous lungs with mediastinal shift to the right and complete left pneumothorax.

HOW WOULD YOU MANAGE THIS PATIENT?

- Controlled oxygen as per blood gases
- Urgent needle decompression via insertion of cannula
- Insertion of intercostal tube

INFORMATION

Management of Intercostal Tube

Insertion of Tube

- Explain and reassure patient throughout, obtain consent
- Double-check site of pneumothorax
- Site: 4th–6th intercostal space in anterior axillary line (check site with ultrasound if available) – mark with pen and position patient supine with head at 30 degree and arm abducted to 90 degree
- Wear sterile gloves
- Drain 10–14 FG (adult). Check assembly and tight connection, and make sure that under-water seal is ready
- Local anaesthetic:
  - Intradermal bleb in appropriate intercostal space
  - Infiltrate deeper with blue then green needle to parietal pleura at upper surface of rib; N.B. neurovascular bundle runs along lower surface
  - Use 5–10 mL 1% lidocaine
  - Check intermittently if in pleural space (air aspirated into syringe)

Insertion of Drain

- Make 1–2 cm incision in skin and subcutaneous fat
- Insert two horizontal sutures across incision (leave loose for subsequent sealing of wound on drain site)

- Make wide tract through intercostal muscles down to and through pleura by blunt dissection with forceps (not sharp trocar)
- Insert tube using Seldinger technique and drain assembly without force
- Withdraw metal needle 5 cm and advance tube in apical direction
- Remove metal needle and connect tube to underwater seal
- Secure tube firmly with one or two sutures (one loop through skin and four times round tube); purse string suturing no longer advised as it leaves unsightly scarring
- Loop tube and secure to skin with plaster (*Note:* no kinks)
- Prescribe adequate analgesia.

Removal of Tube

- Leave tube draining until no further bubbling and then X-ray again (X-ray earlier if in doubt about site or efficacy of tube). *Note:* if level is not swinging, tube is blocked. Clear or replace if lung is not reexpanded
- Some patients need premedication for tube removal
- Remove holding suture and withdraw while patient breath-holds in expiration
- Seal wound with one of original sutures
- Observe overnight and if no recurrence of pneumothorax (clinical and X-ray), discharge with chest clinic appointment in 7–10 days

Progress. A CXR at the chest clinic at 10 days showed full expansion of the lungs. The patient was asymptomatic but apprehensive about having a recurrence. He was reassured that this was unlikely.

Carcinoma of the Bronchus

CASE HISTORY

A 53-year-old male presents with a history of coughing up blood a few hours ago. He has been smoking 20 cigarettes a day for the past 30 years.

On examination, there are diminished breath sounds at the right upper chest anteriorly.

WHAT IS THE MOST LIKELY DIAGNOSIS AND WHY?

Carcinoma of the bronchus:

- Cigarette smoking is the most common risk factor
- It is a common cause of haemoptysis in smokers >40 years of age
- Physical sign of diminished breath sounds suggests bronchial obstruction

INFORMATION

Carcinoma of the Bronchus

- Most common form of cancer in both sexes
- Nonsmall cell:
  - Squamous cell carcinoma (39%)
  - Large cell carcinoma (10%–15%)
  - Adenocarcinoma (25%)
  - Alveolar cell carcinoma (2%)
- Small-cell (20%–30%)

WHAT ARE THE DIAGNOSTIC INVESTIGATIONS?

- Chest Xray
- Sputum cytology
- Bronchoscopy for histological diagnosis
- Computed tomography

If histological diagnosis is not made on bronchoscopy, CT-guided percutaneous needle biopsy should be performed.

RADIOLOGICAL MANIFESTATIONS OF LUNG CANCER

Chest X-ray is the first diagnostic screening investigation for lung cancer. Evidence on CXR depends on:

- Location of the tumour
- Its effect on neighbouring tissues:
    - Central lung shadow: about 70% of cancers, mostly small-cell and squamous cell, arise centrally and present as a shadow in the hilar region and/or in the mediastinum due to involvement of lymph nodes (Fig. 3.15)
    - Peripheral lung shadow: some tumours, especially adenocarcinoma, appear as a rounded shadow in the periphery
    - Collapse of lung parenchyma: centrally located tumours often result in collapse of a lobe by obstruction of the bronchus (Figs. 3.16 and 3.17)
    - Collapsed whole left lung (Fig. 3.18). *Note:* Collapse of whole lung is also seen postoperatively due to retained sputum
    - Pleural effusion: a large pleural effusion is almost always due to invasion of pleura by malignant cells and its presence is a contraindication to surgical resection. A small pleural effusion might occur without invasion of malignant cells and hence surgical resection may still be considered
    - Rib erosion: the classic presentation is erosion of the first rib seen with an apical neoplasm (Pancoast tumour), often associated with Horner syndrome. Rib erosion itself is not a contraindication to surgical resection

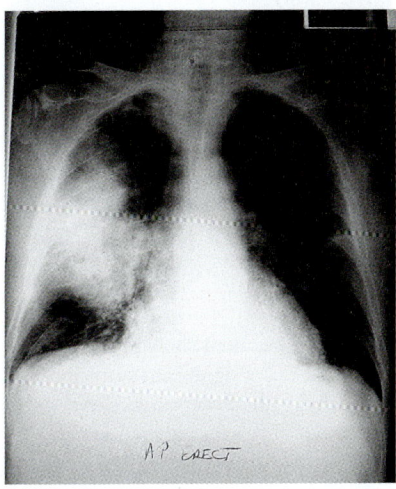

Fig. 3.15 Chest X-ray showing a *shadow* in the *right mid-zone* (note the area of consolidation with *irregular margins*).

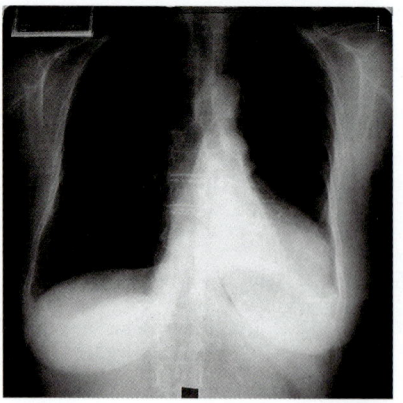

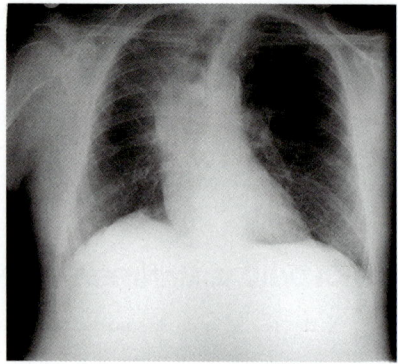

Fig. 3.17 X-ray showing *right upper lobe* collapse.

Fig. 3.16 Chest X-ray showing a *left lower* lobe collapse.

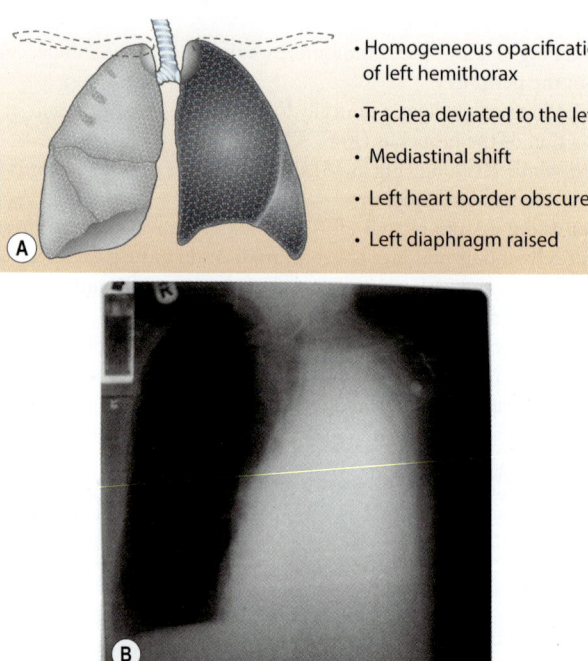

- Homogeneous opacificati
  of left hemithorax
- Trachea deviated to the le
- Mediastinal shift
- Left heart border obscure
- Left diaphragm raised

Fig. 3.18 Diagram (A) and chest X-ray (B) showing a complete collapse of the *left* lung. Note that the mediastinum has been shifted to the *left*.

Contrast-enhanced CT screening has been shown to reduce mortality. Any new abnormality on CXR, or any presentation that raises significant suspicion for lung cancer (despite normal CXR), should have a CT that includes the lower neck, chest, and upper abdomen. These views help define the primary tumour and evaluate for regional spread.

WHAT ARE THE POTENTIAL DIFFERENTIAL DIAGNOSES?

Pneumonia

The possibility of lung cancer should be considered in a smoker with shadow on CXR diagnosed as due to pneumonia:

- Presence of lobar collapse on CXR
- Irregular margins of the lung shadow representing consolidation
- Absence of constitutional symptoms associated with pneumonia
- Symptoms such as haemoptysis and weight loss prior to the development of pneumonia, especially in a middle-aged or elderly smoker

The patient should be investigated for lung cancer if:

- He/she does not respond to treatment, especially if there are risk factors such as smoking and susceptible age group
- Satisfactory radiological resolution has not occurred 6 weeks following treatment for pneumonia resulting in clinical response

Tuberculosis

- Tuberculosis is more often seen in a younger age group
- Constitutional symptoms such as low-grade pyrexia and night sweats are often present in TB
- Cavitation is uncommon in lung cancer but may occur in the squamous cell type. The wall of the cavity is thick and irregular in lung cancer

WHAT ARE THE MAJOR COMPLICATIONS OF BRONCHIAL CARCINOMA AND HOW ARE THEY MANAGED?

Hypercalcaemia

- Intravenous fluids: 3–4 L
- Consider adding a diuretic: furosemide 40 mg IV (ensure adequately rehydrated)
- Intravenous pamidronate: treatment of choice

Weakness of Legs

This suggests spinal cord compression and is a medical emergency, especially with bladder or bowel dysfunction:

- Start corticosteroids as soon as possible e.g. dexamethasone
- Magnetic resonance imaging (MRI) scan of the spine and referral for radiotherapy/surgery

Stridor

This is due to obstruction above the level of the carina (demonstrated in a flow volume loop):

- Start dexamethasone
- Urgent bronchoscopy followed by CT scan of the chest/neck
- Intraluminal growth: referral for laser therapy/stenting
- Extrinsic compression: referral for radiotherapy/stenting

Superior Venocaval Obstruction

- Start on dexamethasone
- Refer for radiotherapy
- Consider heparin or thrombolysis

HOW ARE BRONCHIAL CARCINOMAS CATEGORISED?

For practical purposes, carcinoma of the bronchus can be divided into:
- Small-cell lung cancer (SCLC): this is rarely operable
- Nonsmall-cell lung cancer (NSCLC)

All patients should be referred to an MDT for discussion of management, which is then discussed fully with the patient before decisions are made.

Progress. This patient was found to have nonsmall cell carcinoma of the bronchus, squamous cell type. The MDT consensus was that surgery was not an option. He was given radiotherapy followed by chemotherapy. Follow-up at 6 months showed significant deterioration of his condition, and he was referred to the palliative care team.

SMALL-CELL LUNG CANCER

Prognostic Factors

The staging of SCLC is divided into limited and extensive disease. Systemic therapy is the primary therapeutic modality because of the usually disseminated nature of the disease.

INFORMATION

- Small-cell lung cancer Limited disease: tumour confined to one hemithorax and ipsilateral supraclavicular node
- Extensive disease: involvement of any site outside the hemithorax

---

Treatment

Limited disease is present in approximately 30% of patients. It is best treated with concurrent chemo- and radiotherapy using a combination of cisplatin and etoposide or irinotecan, which increases the survival at 5 years from 15% to 25% compared with radiotherapy alone. A similar degree of improvement can also be achieved with hyperfractionated radiotherapy. Prophylactic whole-brain radiation to prevent cerebral metastases can reduce symptomatic CNS disease and improve overall survival by 5%.

Extensive disease can be palliated with the combination of carboplatin and etoposide or irinotecan; when compared with best supportive care, this can increase median survival from 6 months to 9 to 13 months and 2-year survival to 20%.

Potential complications include:
- Severe pain: potent analgesics, for example, opiates, including fentanyl.
- Bone pain:
  - NSAIDs
  - Local radiotherapy
- Nerve root pain:
  - Amitriptyline
  - Carbamazepine

MANAGEMENT OF PATIENTS WITH NEUTROPENIA FOLLOWING CHEMOTHERAPY

INVESTIGATIONS

- Blood cultures (preferably two samples from two different sites) and urine cultures
- Chest X-ray
- Culture from any suspected site of infection, for example, cannula exit site, sputum

---

What are the Indications for Antibiotic Therapy?

- Absolute neutrophil count <1.0/total WCC <2.5
- Pyrexia

What are the Recommended Antibiotic Regimens?

Broad-spectrum cover is required, follow local guidelines. Examples include:
- Intravenous gentamicin 3–5 mg/kg IV once a day (monitor trough levels) and a ureidopenicillin (piperacillin with tazobactam 4.5 g every 6 h)
- In the presence of severe renal insufficiency, replace gentamicin with IV ceftazidime 1–2 g × 3 daily or ciprofloxacin 400 mg × 2 daily
- Continue antibiotics for 5 days or until WCCs are in normal range and symptoms have remitted

What Would You Do If There Is No Improvement After 48 to 72 h of Antibiotic Therapy?

- Repeat blood and urine cultures and CXR
- Consider the following infections:
  - Fungus: blood and urine cultures. Start fluconazole and/or amphotericin
  - Protozoa: bronchoalveolar lavage
  - Virus: viral serology
  - Resistant staphylococcus: more common with central venous catheter; treat with vancomycin

What Are the Indications for Filgrastim (Recombinant Human Granulocyte-Colony Stimulating Factor, rhG-CSF)?

This is for specialist use only:
- Absolute neutrophil count: 0.2
- Persistent neutropenia (<1.0 for >48 h)
- Stop therapy when absolute neutrophil count is ≥1.5

Sarcoidosis

Sarcoidosis is a multisystem granulomatous disorder of unknown aetiology. It commonly presents with bilateral lymphadenopathy, pulmonary infiltration, and skin and eye lesions.

CASE HISTORY (1)

You are phoned by a primary care physician who has a 28-year-old female in the clinic with tender, bluish lumps on the front of her legs. She also complains of stiffness of the ankles and a temperature. The doctor thinks that this is erythema nodosum (EN) but would like another opinion.

IS THIS EN?

From the description, this sounds very likely and you ask the doctor to send the patient up to outpatients, where you will arrange for a CXR to be performed (Fig. 3.19).

Erythema nodosum with lymphadenopathy on CXR is a characteristic presentation of **sarcoidosis**. When it presents along with arthritis and fever, it is called Löfgren syndrome.

In outpatients, the patient poses several questions on hearing her diagnosis.

WHAT IS SARCOIDOSIS?

You explain that this is a well-recognised disorder for which no cause is known. You emphasise, however, that in her case the skin rash (EN) will subside within 2 months, but the CXR might take up to a year to revert to normal. No treatment is required other than pain relief. The chances of further trouble are negligible.

WHAT ARE THE EXTRAPULMONARY MANIFESTATIONS OF SARCOIDOSIS?

You discuss this case later with your consultant, who reminds you of the extrapulmonary manifestations that can be troublesome (**skin and ocular lesions** are most common):

- **Skin lesions:** 10% of cases. Apart from EN, a chilblain-like lesion (lupus pernio) and nodules are seen
- **Eye involvement:** 5% of cases. Anterior uveitis (misting of vision, pain, red eye) is common. Posterior uveitis may present with a progressive loss of vision. Conjunctivitis and retinal lesions are seen. Asymptomatic uveitis may be found in 25% of patients
- **Metabolic hypercalcaemia:** found in 10% but rarely severe
- Central nervous system **involvement:** rare (2%) but can lead to severe neurological disease
- **Bone and joint involvement:** arthralgia without EN is seen in 5% of cases
- **Cardiac involvement:** rare (3%) clinically, although seen in 20% of postmortems. Ventricular arrhythmias, conduction defects and cardiomyopathy with congestive cardiac failure are seen. The serum ACE is insensitive in cardiac sarcoid and echocardiography should be performed in chronic sarcoidosis.

Progress. The patient made a good recovery and her EN settled after 2 weeks. A follow-up CXR at 6 months was normal.

CASE HISTORY (2)

You are contacted by the ENT registrar because he has seen a 48-year-old patient with nasal stuffiness and a blocked nose. He had also noted some blood-stained nasal discharge. An X-ray of the patient's sinuses shows destruction of the nasal bones. He wants you to see the patient because he found out that this man has had long-standing **pulmonary sarcoidosis**. As you walk to the ENT ward, you go

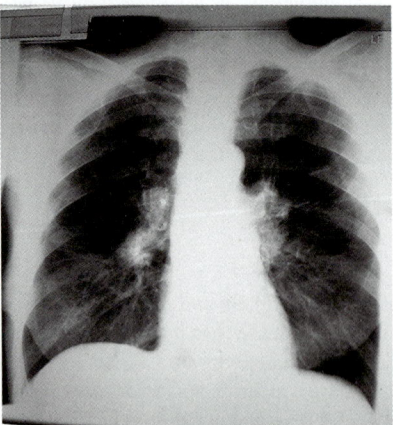

Fig. 3.19 Bilateral hilar lymph node enlargement in sarcoidosis.

over your knowledge of sarcoidosis, remembering that patients with upper respiratory tract involvement usually have pulmonary disease.

On arrival on the wards, you retake the history: the patient has been breathless for years and tells you that all his numerous CXRs show that his lungs are 'full of sarcoid'. He has not been on steroids because of their lack of efficacy and side effects, which have made him noncompliant.

On examination, he is noticeably breathless and cyanosed. Chest examination shows widespread crackles.

You arrange to give the patient oxygen by ordinary face mask (4 L/min).

Investigations are as follows:
- Chest X-ray
- Full blood count:
  - A mild normochromic normocytic anaemia
  - Low lymphocyte count ± low neutrophils
  - Thrombocytopenia
- Blood gases: PO_2 6.8 kPa, pCO_2 4.3 kPa

The next morning, you return with your consultant, having obtained the patient's old notes.

You note multiple CXRs showing widespread pulmonary infiltration with no hilar lymphadenopathy. The latest CXR also shows a rounded opacity in the right apex – thought to be an aspergilloma.

Fibre-optic bronchoscopy with transbronchial biopsies was performed 10 years ago. This showed epithelial and giant cell granulomas (this test has a 90% sensitivity with pulmonary infiltration).

Lung function tests showed:
- Reduced total lung capacity (restrictive ventilatory capacity)
- Impaired gas transfer (TLCO)
- Low compliance
- Raised serum ACE level: done a few years ago

Review of his past treatment shows that he has been given steroids on many occasions and azathioprine and methotrexate as steroid-sparing agents.

Your consultant congratulates you on your review of the notes, which is crucial for the future management of this case. In a patient with such severe disease, he suggests you start high-dose steroids and then a trial of azathioprine and infliximab, for which there is some evidence of efficiency.

Progressive respiratory failure is well recognised in sarcoidosis. Unfortunately, recurrence in the transplanted lung (as well as limited availability of organs) has led many centres not to consider transplantation for end-stage pulmonary fibrosis. Lung transplantation may be indicated if this patient fails to improve.

Progress. This male's chest condition remained static, despite a further trial of steroids and azathioprine. He continues to be breathless but is coping, for the moment. He has been referred to the transplant team for assessment in view of his young age.

Further Reading

Breathlessness and Wheeze

British Thoracic Society/Scottish Intercollegiate Guidelines Network, 2019. British guideline on the management of asthma. Available from: https://www.brit-thoracic.org.uk/quality-improvement/guidelines/.
NICE, CKS, 2021. Asthma: diagnosis, monitoring and chronic asthma management. NICE, London.

Respiratory Failure

British Thoracic Society British Thoracic Society/Intensive Care Society, 2016. Guidelines for the respiratory management of acute hypercapnic respiratory failure in adults. Available from: https://www.brit-thoracic.org.uk/quality-improvement/guidelines/.

Roberts, C.M., Brown, J.L., Reinhardt, A.K., et al., 2008. Non-invasive ventilation in COPD: management of acute type 2 respiratory failure. Clin. Med. 8 (5), 517–521.

COPD – Acute Exacerbation

British Thoracic Society British Thoracic Society/NICE, 2019. Guideline – COPD in over-16s. Available from: https://www.brit-thoracic.org.uk/quality-improvement/guidelines/copd/.
Global Initiative for Chronic Obstructive Lung Disease, 2023. Global strategy for the diagnosis, management, and prevention of chronic obstructive pulmonary disease: 2023 report.

Tuberculosis

Bloom, B.R., 2018. A neglected epidemic. N. Engl. J. Med. 378 (3), 291–293.
Bracchi, M., et al., 2019. British HIV association guidelines for the management of tuberculosis in adults living with HIV 2019. HIV Med. 20 (Suppl 6), s2–s83.
WHO, WHO Global tuberculosis report 2019. Available from: https://www.who.int/tb/publications/global_report/en/.

Pleural Effusion

British Thoracic Society Pleural Disease Guideline Group, 2010. British Thoracic Society Pleural Disease Guideline Group. BTS Pleural Disease Guideline 2010. Thorax 65 (Suppl II). Available from: https://thorax.bmj.com/content/65/Suppl_2#BTSPleuralDiseaseGuideline2010.
Feller-Kopman, D., Light, R., 2018. Pleural disease. N. Engl. J. Med. 378 (8), 740–751.

Pulmonary Embolism (and Deep Vein Thrombosis)

Stevens, S.M., et al., 2021. Executive summary: antithrombotic therapy for VTE disease: second update of the CHEST guideline and expert panel report. Chest 160 (6), 2247–2259.
NICE, CKS, 2023. Venous thromboembolic diseases: diagnosis, management and thrombophilia testing. NICE.

Pneumothorax

MacDuff, A., Arnold, A., Harvey, J., 2010. Management of spontaneous pneumothorax: British Thoracic Society Pleural Disease Guideline 2010. Thorax 65 (2), ii18–ii31. Available from: https://thorax.bmj.com/content/65/Suppl_2#BTSPleuralDiseaseGuideline2010.

Carcinoma of the Bronchus

British Thoracic Society, Guidelines. Available from: www.brit-thoracic.org.uk/guidelines.
Goldstraw, P., Ball, D., Jett, J.R., et al., Non-small-cell lung cancer. Lancet 378 (9804), 1727–1740.
NICE, CKS, 2023. Lung cancer: diagnosis and management. NICE.
Royal College of Radiologists. Royal College of Radiologists: guidelines on the non-surgical management of lung cancer. Available from: www.rcr.ac.uk.
Van Meerbeeck, J.P., Fennell, D.A., De Ruysscher, D.K., 2011. Small-cell lung cancer. Lancet 378 (9804), 1741–1755.

CHAPTER 4

Gastroenterology

Vomiting

Vomiting centres are located on the lateral reticular formation of the medulla. They are stimulated by chemoreceptor trigger zones on the floor of the 4th ventricle and also by vagal afferents from the gastrointestinal (GI) tract.

Causes of vomiting are shown in Box 4.1.

CASE HISTORY

A 70-year-old male was admitted with a 2-week history of repeated vomiting. He had lost more than 6 kg in weight. He had recently developed colicky abdominal pain and constipation without the passage of wind.

On examination, his abdomen was distended, and he was tender in the epigastrium.

You call for surgical advice. The surgeon, in addition to your findings, notes that there are increased bowel sounds. The patient's hernial orifices and rectal examination show no abnormality.

REMEMBER

Non-GI causes are possible; a full examination is therefore necessary. *Note:* look at the fundi for papilloedema.

INVESTIGATIONS

Haematological:

- Full blood count (FBC), erythrocyte sedimentation rate (ESR), C-reactive protein (CRP)

Biochemical:

- Electrolytes
- Urea/creatinine/estimated glomerular filtration rate (eGFR)
- Liver biochemistry
- Calcium
- Amylase

Radiological:

- Abdominal X-ray (AXR)
- Chest X-ray (CXR)

Abdominal X-ray:

- **Normal.** With a history of this length, a normal X-ray would suggest that large or small bowel obstruction is unlikely. High obstruction in the GI tract, that is in the oesophagus or stomach, is possible. Investigate for non-GI causes (metabolic, neurological – exclude brainstem lesion), occasionally severe depression.
- **Abnormal.** Might show evidence of small or large bowel obstruction or gastric distension.
- In this patient, the AXR showed small bowel obstruction (Fig. 4.1). The **differential diagnosis** is shown in the Information box.

Chest X-ray:

- **Normal.** Look for evidence of air under the diaphragm (perforation), signs of pneumonia and hilar mass (tumour).

BOX 4.1 ■ Causes of Vomiting

- Any GI disease
- Infections:
  - Viruses (influenza, norovirus)
  - Bacterial (pertussis, urinary infection)
- CNS disease:
  - Raised intracranial pressure
  - Vestibular disturbance
  - Migraine
- Metabolic:
  - Uraemia
  - Hypercalcaemia
- Diabetic ketoacidosis
- Drugs:
  - Antibiotics

- Chemotherapy
- Digoxin
- Immunotherapy
- Incretins
- Levodopa
- Opiates
- Reflex:
  - Myocardial infarction
  - Biliary colic
- Psychogenic
- Pregnancy
- Alcohol excess

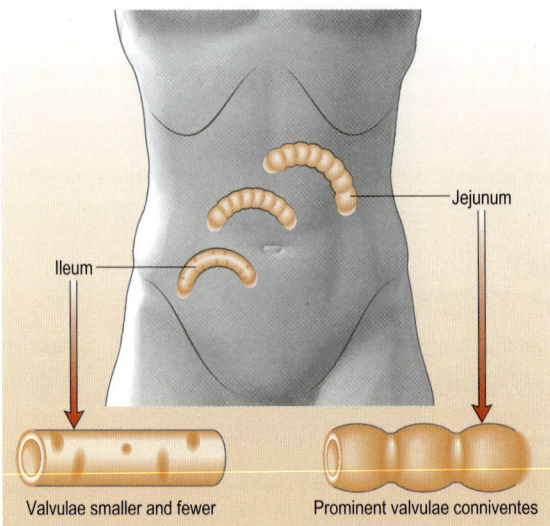

Fig. 4.1   Small bowel obstruction, showing dilated loops of small bowel.

INFORMATION

Small Intestinal Obstruction: Differential Diagnosis

- Adhesions (80% in adults)
- Hernia
- Crohn disease
- Intussusception
- Obstruction due to extrinsic involvement by cancer

Management

The definitive treatment for this patient is to relieve the obstruction. In the interim:

- Infuse glucose/saline to maintain electrolyte balance (with additional K⁺ 20 mmol/L depending on electrolyte results)

- Insert nasogastric tube (on continuous drainage)
- Contact surgeons, await instruction as to further investigations (such as CT scan to localise obstructive lesion)

Progress. At operation, a carcinoma of the ascending colon was found and resected.

Hiccups

Hiccups are due to involuntary diaphragmatic contractions with closure of the glottis. They are very common and usually not sinister, even if persistent.

> **CASE HISTORY**
>
> You are called by the surgical registrar because he is concerned that a 70-year-old male has had continuous hiccups for 48 h, along with a fever, malaise and right hypochondrial pain. Ten days ago, he had been admitted with intestinal obstruction (see case earlier), and a laparotomy for a carcinoma of the ascending colon had been performed. This is a classic situation for a **subphrenic abscess** occurring post surgery in an elderly person.

HOW WOULD YOU INVESTIGATE?

Check haemoglobin (Hb), white cell count (WCC) and liver biochemistry. An urgent ultrasound was performed and confirmed the diagnosis of a subphrenic abscess. Blood cultures were taken, as the patient was febrile.

TREATMENT AND PROGNOSIS OF THE ABSCESS

He had drainage under ultrasound and antibiotics were started. The bacteria causing abscesses are usually *Bacteroides* spp. and/or *Escherichia coli* and he was therefore treated with ciprofloxacin and metronidazole. His hiccups were controlled with chlorpromazine 50 mg as necessary.

OTHER CAUSES OF HICCUPS

- Metabolic, for example uraemia
- Neurological, for example a brainstem tumour
- Other abdominal pathology
- No pathological cause

Weight Loss

Weight loss is often a perceived symptom by patients that needs to be verified. It is a general symptom, which can reflect disease in any part of the body.

Always make sure that the patient has a sufficient calorie intake for his/her requirements, bearing in mind the amount of exercise taken. In a young female, think of anorexia nervosa.

Reduced calorie intake can be caused by intentional dieting but can also be a symptom of generalised disease due to anorexia.

> **CASE HISTORY**
>
> A 40-year-old male has been admitted with a fever, tremor and 10 kg weight loss. He has previously been counselled for alcohol misuse.

WHAT SHOULD YOU DO?

You need to consider a number of diagnoses and this might be helped by additional history and examination:

- Hyperthyroidism: check for symptoms and signs of hyperthyroidism (see Endocrinology & Diabetes chapter)
- Alcoholic liver disease
- Malnutrition: check by asking the patient's family. Perhaps there is a psychiatric history?
- Underlying cancer, particularly lung, bowel and pancreas
- Biochemical investigations: should help determine underlying metabolic or renal disease
- Malabsorption: often causes anorexia, contributing to weight loss

This patient had no signs of chronic liver disease but did admit to recurrent episodes of upper abdominal pain radiating through to his back. These tended to occur on Monday, following his weekend binges. This suggests **pancreatic disease** resulting from his heavy alcohol intake.

WHAT INITIAL INVESTIGATIONS ARE APPROPRIATE?

- Full blood count, urea and electrolytes (U and Es), liver biochemistry, amylase or lipase, calcium, blood alcohol
- Abdominal ultrasound to assess the pancreas for cysts and potential masses

This patient was admitted in a malnourished, hyperdynamic state due to **acute alcohol withdrawal** (see p. 67). Treat this initially and investigate the pancreas later.

FURTHER INVESTIGATIONS

- Computed tomography (CT) scan of the pancreas
- Magnetic resonance cholangiopancreatography (MRCP): this is noninvasive and of value in assessment of the pancreas and biliary tree
- Endoscopic retrograde cholangiopancreatography (ERCP) to delineate the biliary and pancreatic ducts (if MRCP is unavailable)
- Endoscopic ultrasound: can help define pancreatic cysts and masses

Progress. This patient was treated initially with benzodiazepine and IV thiamine (p. 67) and made a good recovery from his acute withdrawal state. Further investigations showed chronic pancreatitis; he was referred to the liver clinic.

Dysphagia

Dysphagia is difficulty in swallowing. It is an immediate, obstructive sensation during the passage of liquid or solid through the pharynx or oesophagus.

CASE HISTORY

A 55-year-old patient has been referred urgently because of acute dysphagia. She gave a history of reflux for years and increasing dysphagia for 6 months. She had been eating an orange, which became lodged in her gullet and all efforts to dislodge it were unsuccessful. The underlying diagnosis is likely to be **food bolus obstruction** on an already present oesophageal stricture.

WHAT SHOULD YOU DO?

Refer the patient for an urgent endoscopy. The endoscopy findings were of a stricture in the mid-oesophagus with no obvious malignant lesion. Biopsies were taken, and the stricture dilated.

> **REMEMBER**
>
> Submucosal cancer can look like a benign lesion.
>
> Unfortunately, this patient developed severe chest pain immediately after the dilatation and surgical emphysema could be felt in her neck. Clinically, an oesophageal tear is suspected.
>
> A CT of the chest and abdomen confirms an oesophageal rupture.

Diagnosis

The underlying cause is more likely to be **oesophageal cancer** because careful dilatation of benign lesions rarely causes a tear.

Initial Management

- Nil by mouth
- Intravenous access for fluids
- Antibiotic prophylaxis
- Surgical referral

Small tears in a peptic stricture can resolve in a few days with conservative management. Large tears generally need surgery in a dedicated thoracic unit. Endoscopic stenting is used initially for tears in malignant lesions but, again, surgery may be required.

Biopsies later confirmed a **squamous carcinoma**.

Management will include assessment for surgery with:

- Blood count, U and Es, liver biochemistry
- Chest X-ray
- Electrocardiography
- Respiratory function tests
- Abdominal ultrasound, CT scan to assess operability
- Endoscopic ultrasound: an accurate way of staging lesion and any local lymph nodes
- Positron emission tomography (PET) scan: to look for distant metastases

Discussion should take place with a multidisciplinary team (MDT) to decide on the patient's treatment.

As investigations showed no distant metastases, surgery with neo-adjuvant (preoperative) and adjuvant (postoperative) chemoradiation treatment was given.

Constipation

Defined by less frequent bowel movements (fewer than three times per week), constipation is characterized by straining and the passage of hard stools.

> **CASE HISTORY**
>
> A trainee doctor inquires about the appropriate prescription for an elderly male who has not had a bowel movement in 5 days. The patient, previously healthy and active, was admitted with a chest infection a week ago. A rectal examination indicated a loaded colon without any localized abnormality.

SHOULD THIS PATIENT BE INVESTIGATED?

Immediate investigation may not be necessary as the constipation is likely due to reduced mobility. However, if there is no improvement with initial treatment, further colonic evaluation may be required.

TREATMENT

Initiate with a laxative to stimulate bowel movements. Glycerol suppositories can be beneficial.

- Consider oral magnesium sulphate, an osmotic laxative, which is cost-effective and typically well-tolerated
- Avoid stimulant laxatives as a first-line treatment
- Discontinue any medications that may contribute to constipation where possible
- For faecal impaction, digital extraction may be needed, followed by the administration of small-volume phosphate enemas
- Educate the patient on the benefits of a high-fibre diet and adequate fluid intake to prevent recurrence

INFORMATION

Causes of Constipation

- Simple/idiopathic constipation without an identifiable organic cause
- Intestinal obstruction or colonic diseases, such as carcinoma
- Anal conditions causing pain which may deter the normal defecation reflex
- Side effects of certain drugs, including codeine, iron supplements, verapamil, tricyclic antidepressants, and opiates
- Endocrine disorders, such as hypothyroidism and metabolic issues like hypercalcaemia
- Psychological factors, particularly depression
- Reduced physical activity and prolonged immobility

Diarrhoea

Increased frequency of defecation, even in a previously fit patient, can produce dehydration and *severe* electrolyte depletion. Diarrhoea can also be a recurrent problem in patients with established GI disease.

WHAT SHOULD YOU DO IN A CASE OF DIARRHOEA PRESENTING IN ACCIDENT AND EMERGENCY?

- Obtain a thorough history, including recent food consumption, travel history and medication use, particularly antibiotics
- Inquire about accompanying symptoms, such as abdominal pain and weight loss
- It is crucial to establish the onset history, determine the frequency, consistency and content of stool, and assess for the presence of blood
- Evaluate the patient's hydration status and electrolyte balance
- Send stool samples for culture, parasites (ova, cysts), and *Clostridium* difficile toxin assay, especially if there is a history of hospitalization or antibiotic use
- Conduct a rectal examination; refer for sigmoidoscopy to the gastroenterology team if bloody diarrhoea is present
- Take blood cultures in severe cases accompanied by fever
- Consider an AXR to rule out complications
- Isolate the patient and take full contact precautions in line with local infection control guidelines

INFORMATION

Likely Pathogens Causing Diarrhoeal

Bacteria (50%):

- *E. coli*

- *Campylobacter* spp.
- *Salmonella* spp.
- *Shigella* spp.

Viruses (1% but seldom produce severe diarrhoea in adults):

- Rotavirus
- Norovirus

Protozoa:

- *Giardia intestinalis*
- *Entamoeba histolytica*
- *Cryptosporidium*

Helminths (e.g. *Strongyloides*)

In some cases, no pathogens or multiple pathogens are found (20%–50% of cases)

Management

- Most diarrhoeal illnesses are self-limiting. Identification of the pathogen will guide specific therapy
- Rehydration is key, with oral rehydration solutions recommended. IV fluids may be necessary in cases of severe dehydration
- Antiemetic medication, such as metoclopramide, may be used if vomiting is present

CASE HISTORY (1)

A 24-year-old returned from travelling for 3 months, during which he passed through several countries. He was fairly well when he came home but after 3 days developed severe diarrhoea, which has now been present for 2 weeks.

On admission to the medical assessment unit (MAU), he is dehydrated and has lost over 5 kg in weight.

WHAT IMMEDIATE ACTION WOULD YOU TAKE?

- Conduct basic blood tests, including FBC, U and Es, and liver function tests
- Rehydrate the patient, prioritizing oral solutions when possible
- Send stool samples for ova, cysts, and culture
- Vomiting might need to be treated with an antiemetic (such as metoclopramide 10 mg × 3 daily)

DIAGNOSIS

This is most likely not acute diarrhoea with a viral/bacterial cause as the patient did not have diarrhoea when he returned to the UK. Viral/bacterial diarrhoea usually starts in the country where the infection occurred and generally clears up within 7 days. Possible causes are shown in the Information box.

INFORMATION

Causes of Nonacute Diarrhoea in a Returning Traveller

- Giardiasis
- Cryptosporidiosis
- Amoebiasis
- Tropical sprue (SE Asia, Caribbean)
- Schistosomiasis
- Strongyloidiasis

Stool samples showed no abnormal findings

Progress. Giardiasis is very likely in this patient. Treatment with metronidazole 2 g a day for 3 successive days was given, with dramatic improvement.

CASE HISTORY (2)

A 30-year-old female patient presented with a 2-week history of passing 6 to 10 motions a day. The stools were loose and contained blood. She felt tired and had lost about 5 kg in weight.
On admission to the MAU, she was not dehydrated but had a fever and was very lethargic.

WHAT IS THE DIFFERENTIAL DIAGNOSIS?

- Infective diarrhoea. Send specimens for microbiological testing
- First presentation of inflammatory bowel disease (IBD) (most likely for this patient)

Inflammatory Bowel Disease (IBD)

In any case of persistent diarrhoea, IBD is a possible cause. A previous history of intermittent diarrhoea or recurrent abdominal pain is often present. In lower/mid-income countries, infective causes are more likely and must be excluded.

WHAT GENERAL MEASURES SHOULD YOU TAKE?

- Acute diarrhoea (for more than 2 weeks) is usually not infective
- Take blood for FBC, ESR, CRP, U and Es, liver biochemistry
- Consider a plain AXR for the presence of stool, mucosal oedema, bowel dilatation or perforation
- Sigmoidoscopy: the presence of an inflamed, friable mucosa with loss of vascular pattern or patchy inflammation indicates IBD. Take a rectal biopsy
- Stool cultures (*N.B.* Infective gastroenteritis must always be ruled out). *Clostridioides difficile* (*C. diff*) toxin assay – four stool specimens (90% sensitivity)

In this patient, you have ruled out infective gastroenteritis, as three stool cultures were negative. Taking into account the history and the sigmoidoscopic finding, you presume this must be IBD. Her Hb was 100 g/L and CRP 84 mg/L.

Acute colitis is associated with diarrhoea, abdominal pain, fever and systemic disturbance. There is blood in the stools in ulcerative colitis but Crohn disease patients only have bloody diarrhoea with Crohn colitis. To assess severity, check the factors shown in Table 4.1.

TABLE 4.1 ■ **Findings in a Severe Attack of Ulcerative Colitis**

Findings	↓/↑	Results
Hb	↓	<100 g/L
Albumin	↓	<30 g/L
Fever	↑	>37.5°C
Stool frequency	↑	>6/day
ESR	↑	>30 mm/h
Pulse rate	↑	>90 bpm
Platelets	↑	–
WCC	↑	–

Hb, Haemoglobin; ESR, erythrocyte sedimentation rate; WCC, white cell count.

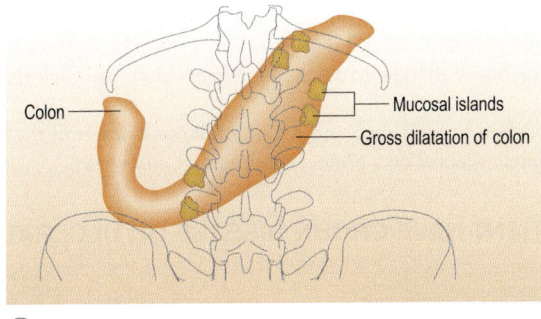

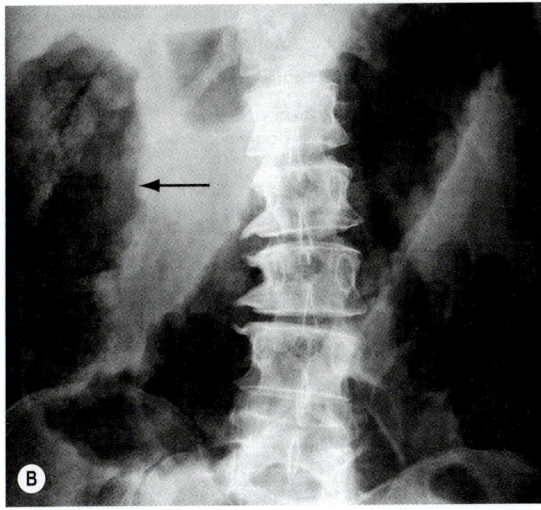

Fig. 4.2 (A) Schematic diagram showing toxic dilatation of the colon; (B) plain abdominal X-ray showing toxic dilatation in ulcerative colitis. *Arrow* shows mucosal island.

Always look for the presence of:

- Toxic dilatation: colon >5 cm in diameter and mucosal islands on plain AXR (Fig. 4.2)
- Perforation (on AXR)

HOW WOULD YOU MANAGE THIS ACUTE SITUATION?

- Intravenous fluids with glucose/saline
- Intravenous therapy with steroids (IV hydrocortisone 100 mg × 4 daily for example), followed by oral therapy (prednisolone 40 mg per day for example) if the patient improves
- Intravenous antibiotics (such as metronidazole/cephalosporin)
- Further management: refer to gastroenterologists; consult GI surgeons

REMEMBER

In acute severe ulcerative colitis, at 3 days post treatment, a CRP >45 mg/L or stool frequency >8/day has an 85% chance of needing a colectomy.

Progress and Management

There was no response to treatment at 3 days (see Information box). The patient was started on infliximab 5 mg/kg as 'rescue therapy' to avoid immediate colectomy. Ciclosporin 2 mg/kg/day is an alternative.

This patient responded to infliximab and is being followed closely in the colitis clinic. She is continuing on infliximab therapy on a protocol, lasting up to 46 weeks.

DOES THIS PATIENT HAVE CROHN DISEASE OR ULCERATIVE COLITIS?

Both can produce acute colitis. The differentiation is by colonoscopy and histological appearance (Table 4.2).

INFORMATION

Crohn Disease

- Affects any part of the GI tract, from mouth to anus
- Seventy percent of cases affect the terminal ileum
- Can be controlled but not cured

Ulcerative Colitis

- Confined to colon
- Cured by colectomy
- Can affect the rectum alone (proctitis); sigmoid and descending colon (left-sided colitis); or the whole colon (extensive colitis)

Both

- Extra-GI manifestations, for example, pyoderma gangrenosum (Fig. 4.3 and Box 4.2)

Abdominal Pain

Most diseases of the GI tract are associated with abdominal pain but pain can also be referred to the chest or back. The characteristics of the pain can help in the diagnosis.

CASE HISTORY

A 40-year-old male presents with epigastric and central abdominal cramping pain. For 48 h the pain has been continuous, severe and associated with vomiting. The pain does not radiate but is getting worse by the hour. **On examination**, he has a temperature of 38°C and a pulse rate of 98 beats per minute (bpm). He has tenderness across the upper abdomen but no other signs. His bowel sounds are normal. He has no alteration of bowel habit and reports no weight loss.

TABLE 4.2 ■ Differentiating Between Crohn Disease and Ulcerative Colitis

Histological Findings	Crohn Disease	Ulcerative Colitis
Inflammation	Deep (transmural), patchy	Superficial (mucosal) continuous
Granulomas	++	Rare
Goblet cells	Present	Depleted
Crypt abscesses	+	++

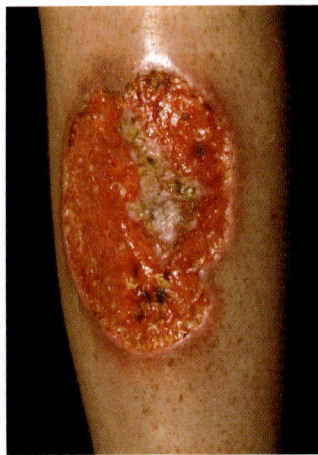

Fig. 4.3 Pyodermagangrenosum. (From James G. Marks, Jeffrey J. Miller, L. Claire Hollins. *Lookingbill & Marks' Principles of Dermatology*, 7e, Fig 19.5, New Delhi, Elsevier INC, 2025.)

BOX 4.2 ■ Extragastrointestinal Manifestations of Inflammatory Bowel Disease

- Eyes:
  - Uveitis
  - Episcleritis, conjunctivitis
- Joints:
  - Type I (pauci-articular) arthropathy
  - Type II (polyarticular) arthropathy
  - Arthralgia
  - Axial spondyloarthritis
  - Inflammatory back pain
- Skin:
  - Pyodermagangrenosum (see Fig. 4.3)
- Liver and biliary tree:
  - Sclerosing cholangitis
  - Fatty liver
  - Chronic hepatitis
  - Cirrhosis
  - Gallstones
  - Nephrolithiasis
  - Venous thrombosis

Immediate Investigations

- Haematological: Hb, WCC, ESR
- Biochemical: U and Es, liver biochemistry, amylase or lipase, CRP
- Radiological: consider AXR for obstruction; CXR in acute pain to assess for intestinal perforation

Management

Develop the management plan to include:

- Symptomatic relief
- Information for patient and relatives
- Further investigations (endoscopy, ultrasound, CT and MRI as necessary to exclude perforation, obstruction, stones, calcification, cancer and ascites)
- Consultation with surgical colleagues

In this case, abdominal pain situated in the epigastrium and central abdomen, and of the severity described, is almost always due to organic disease. Your differential diagnosis should include the following:

- An acute surgical cause:
  Aortic aneurysm dissection
  Appendicitis (even occasionally with upper abdominal pain)

Perforation

Intestinal obstruction.

■ Acute pancreatitis:

Severe pain

Often associated with heavy alcohol use, gallstones, viral infection (e.g. mumps)

↑Serum amylase or lipase

Gastric retention and vomiting

Ultrasonographic changes and contrast-enhanced dynamic CT (best investigation) show pancreatic swelling, necrosis and peripancreatic fluid collection

---

REMEMBER

Acute Pancreatitis: Assessment of Severity and Poor Prognosis (First 48 h): (Glasgow Prognostic Criteria)

- Age >55 years
- Blood glucose >10 mmol/L
- Serum urea >16 mmol/L
- Serum calcium <2 mmol/L
- Serum lactate dehydrogenase (LDH) >600 U/L
- Partial pressure of oxygen <8 kPa
- White cell count >15 × 10^9/L
- Serum albumin <30 g/L
- Serum aspartate aminotransferase (AST) >200 U/L

Note: More than 3 positive factors during the first 48 h suggest **severe acute pancreatitis** and a poorer prognosis.

SYMPTOM RELIEF

Symptom relief depends on diagnosis. Use antispasmodics (hyoscine butylbromide 20 mg × 4 daily) and minor analgesics (such as paracetamol). Opiates like morphine or codeine should be prescribed with caution due to potential side effects like constipation and sphincter of Oddi spasm. Antiemetics such as ondansetron or metoclopramide may be necessary for managing vomiting.

PATIENT INFORMATION

This depends on diagnosis but should be delivered to both patients and relatives sensitively and with an understanding of underlying pathology.

DIAGNOSIS AND PROGRESS

In this case, the 40-year-old patient turned out to have **acute pancreatitis**, with a serum amylase of 1000 units. He quickly settled by being kept nil by mouth and having IV fluids. The aetiology was never established but was thought perhaps to have been viral.

Gastro-Oesophageal Reflux Disease (GORD)

Gastro-oesophageal reflux occurs normally. Gastro-oesophageal reflux disease occurs when the antireflux mechanism fails, allowing acidic gastric contents to make prolonged contact with the oesophageal mucosa.

CASE HISTORY

A 48-year-old male was admitted with severe epigastric pain radiating up into his chest. He thought he had had a heart attack.

WHAT INVESTIGATIONS WOULD YOU DO ON ADMISSION?

It is critical to exclude life-threatening conditions, such as myocardial infarction, pulmonary embolism and pneumothorax, before labelling such pain as due to reflux.

INVESTIGATIONS

- Full blood count, U and Es, liver biochemistry, serum amylase
- Electrocardiogram, repeated after 1 h
- Chest X-ray
- Cardiac markers, such as serum troponins

In this patient, two ECGs, CXR and cardiac markers were normal. Additional features in the history included:
- Long history of reflux (GORD)
- Burning nature of the pain
- Flatulence
- A relationship of the present pain to previous similar pain
- A food-related element
- Exacerbation of pain with drinking hot liquids

Features of gastro-oesophageal reflux
- Burning pain produced by bending, stooping or lying down
- Pain seldom radiates to the arms
- Pain precipitated by drinking hot liquids or alcohol
- Pain relieved by antacids

Features of myocardial ischaemia
- Gripping or crushing pain
- Pain radiates into the neck, shoulders and both arms
- Pain produced by exercise
- Pain accompanied by breathlessness

A diagnosis of **GORD** was made in this patient from the history

Progress and Management

The patient was given a liquid antacid (e.g. Gaviscon or Peptac) and a proton pump inhibitor (PPI, e.g. omeprazole or lansoprazole) to control the symptoms. Endoscopy will need to be performed in this man in view of his age.

REMEMBER

- Reflux can be difficult to diagnose, and although it is often associated with a hiatus hernia, more formal investigation might be necessary, for example, endoscopy followed by oesophageal pH, impedance and pressure monitoring if necessary
- At endoscopy, assess the degree of oesophagitis and check for Barrett oesophagus (including biopsies)

Barrett Oesophagus

This occurs as a result of long-standing reflux. It consists of columnar epithelium with intestinal metaplasia extending upwards into the lower oesophagus and replacing normal squamous epithelium. Barrett oesophagus (even a short segment <3 cm) is premalignant for **adenocarcinoma**. Risk factors for progression are male sex, age >45 years, length of segment >8 cm, early age of onset and duration of symptoms of GORD, the presence of ulceration and stricture and a family history. Dysplasia is patchy and biopsies from all four quadrants (every 2 cm) of the Barrett segment must be performed. There is no evidence that treatment with PPIs or surgery leads to Barrett's regression. Patients without dysplasia do not require **surveillance**. Low-grade dysplasia requires regular endoscopic surveillance. High-grade dysplasia is treated with radiofrequency ablation using the HALO system, but endoscopic ablation therapy or laser is also used.

Peptic Ulcer Disease

CASE HISTORY (1)

In the clinic, you see a 40-year-old male with epigastric pain that has been present on and off for a number of years. The doctor's letter indicates that the patient has been a regular attender and has received antacids, H_2 receptor antagonists and a PPI at some time over the last 5 years. Recently, the patient was found to have *Helicobacter pylori* antibodies in his serum and was given eradication therapy.

WHAT SHOULD YOU DO?

The history of intermittent epigastric pain is highly suggestive of peptic ulcer disease and you note there are no alarm features in the history. The patient has been given *H. pylori* eradication therapy but the general practitioner (GP) has not indicated the drugs that were used. The patient remembers taking two different tablets for 1 week. You ask about smoking (which delays ulcer healing) and also take a drug history. There is no history of NSAID or aspirin use.

REMEMBER

Alarm Features

- Weight loss
- Anorexia
- Dysphagia
- Protracted vomiting
- Haematemesis or melaena

In the absence of alarm features, it is reasonable to try a PPI if the history is suggestive of reflux, for example, heartburn worse on bending.

WHAT WOULD YOU DO NEXT?

You would need to establish whether the patient has had successful *H. pylori* eradication.

Tests for *H. pylori*

- Stool antigen test (current infection)
- Antral biopsy: either for histology or for *Campylobacter*-like organism (CLO, urease) testing (for current infections)

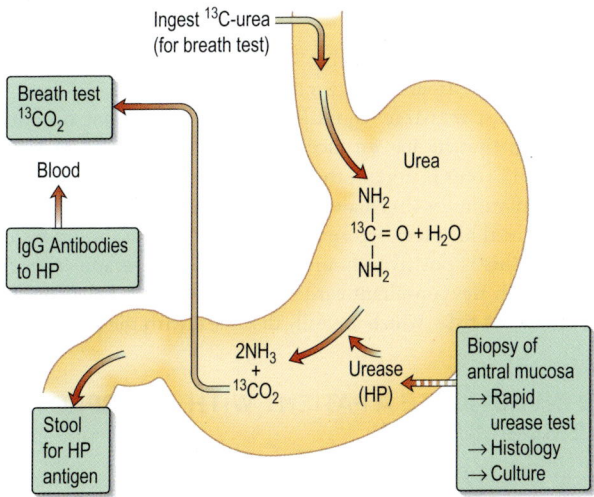

Fig. 4.4 Metabolism of urea by *Helicobacter pylori* (HP), showing the different tests that are available for the detection of *H. pylori*.

- Urea breath tests (for current infections) measuring $^{13}CO_2$ (Fig. 4.4)
- Serological IgG antibodies (useful in the community but testing does not distinguish between past and current infections)

This patient's urea breath test is positive, indicating continuing *H. pylori* infection.

TREATMENT OF *H. PYLORI* INFECTION

Patients with peptic ulcer disease who are *H. pylori*-positive should be given combination eradication therapy, for example:

- Clarithromycin 500 mg × 2 for 1 week
- Amoxicillin 1 g × 2 daily for 1 week
- Omeprazole 20 mg × 2 daily for 2 weeks

With increasing resistance to clarithromycin, quadruple therapy is now being used, as in this patient. He was given lansoprazole 30 mg × 2, tri-potassium di-citratobismuthate 120 mg × 4, tetracycline 500 mg × 4 and metronidazole 500 mg × 3 – all daily for 2 weeks.

Progress. This patient has had no further problems since his therapy and a stool antigen test was negative for *H. pylori*.

CASE HISTORY (2)

You are asked by the cardiologists to see a male patient with epigastric pain. He has been admitted for urgent percutaneous coronary intervention (PCI). He is already on aspirin 75 mg daily. He has had many similar episodes of pain over the years. Approximately 10 years ago, he had an endoscopy and was told that he had an ulcer and given omeprazole. He points with one finger to his epigastrium as the site of his pain.

This is a classic history of duodenal ulcer disease.

WHAT SHOULD YOU DO?

As the PCI is tomorrow, you recommend that he be given a PPI, for example, omeprazole 20 mg × 2 daily, and referred to gastroenterology outpatients.

The cardiology specialist registrar would like to put the patient on antiplatelet therapy post PCI and is worried that he has an ulcer. This is a problem of balancing the risks. As placement of the coronary stent is urgent, they will have to go ahead with antiplatelet therapy with a PPI. The ideal situation for this male would be to perform endoscopy prior to PCI, and if an ulcer is present, to heal his ulcer before the intervention. He should have a stool *H. pylori* antigen checked and, if this is positive, should receive *H. pylori* eradication therapy.

After reassessment with the consultant cardiologist, it is decided that the PCI is still urgent and will go ahead, despite its risks, which are fully discussed with the patient.

HOW DO YOU INVESTIGATE A PATIENT WITH A SUSPECTED ULCER IN THE COMMUNITY?

- Under 45 years of age: *H. pylori* serology. If positive, give eradication therapy. If negative, treat symptomatically
- Over 45 years: patients with new dyspepsia and those with alarm symptoms (e.g. anorexia, weight loss) should be referred for endoscopy (cost-effective)

REMEMBER

- *H. pylori* serology can remain positive, even after successful eradication of *H. pylori*
- Current *H. pylori* infection can be detected by the urea breath test (see Fig. 4.4), endoscopy (urease test, histology or culture) and detection of stool antigen (cost-effective)

CASE HISTORY

A 40-year-old female patient was seen in the emergency department with a sprained ankle. She was sent home with a strapped ankle and given diclofenac to take for the pain. There was no history of indigestion. Ten days later she is brought in by ambulance, having vomited blood. The bleeding was thought to be related to the NSAID therapy.

On examination, she was not shocked, and there are no signs of chronic liver disease. She had stopped bleeding and an endoscopy was performed in the next 24 h.

A bleeding ulcer, with a fresh adherent clot, was seen on endoscopy; it was injected with adrenaline (epinephrine) 1: 10,000 and a heater probe was also used. A biopsy was taken for *H. pylori*.

A bleeding ulcer might have certain stigmata that suggest that rebleeding is likely to recur (see Remember box).

Gastric cancer does not usually cause an acute GI bleed; it is more likely to produce anaemia from chronic blood loss.

REMEMBER

Stigmata of a Recent Bleed From an Ulcer on Endoscopy

- Spurting vessel
- Prominent vessel
- Fresh adherent clot

Progress. The *H. pylori* test was positive, indicating chronic peptic ulcer disease. The haematemesis was precipitated by the NSAIDs.

DISCHARGE POLICY

The patient's age, diagnosis on endoscopy, comorbidity and the presence or absence of shock should be taken into consideration. In general, patients under the age of 60, as well as older patients who are haemodynamically stable and have no stigmata of recent haemorrhage on endoscopy, can be discharged within 24 h.

Note: All shocked patients need careful observation in hospital. Check your own hospital's guidelines.

Iron Deficiency Anaemia

CASE HISTORY

A 40-year-old female patient was found at routine screening to have an Hb of 80 g/L with an iron-deficient appearance on the film.

She admitted to some ankle swelling and increased breathlessness of recent onset. Examination was unhelpful.

Full blood count, film and low serum ferritin confirmed **iron deficiency**.

WHAT DO YOU DO?

- Exclude all obvious causes of bleeding:
  Heavy periods
  Rectal bleeding
  Recurrent nose bleeds
- If there is no obvious menorrhagia it is likely to be secondary to GI disease (always consider malabsorption - coeliac disease is still very underdiagnosed)
- The patient travels abroad a lot and could have a bowel infestation. Remember that hookworm is the most common cause of iron deficiency anaemia worldwide
- Occult bleeding from the GI tract is common and can be confirmed by haemoccult testing

INFORMATION

Faecal Occult Bloods

- Of no use in males or postmenopausal females with iron deficiency anaemia and no other cause for bleeding
- Useful for screening populations for colonic cancer

WHAT ADDITIONAL INVESTIGATIONS ARE APPROPRIATE?

- Rectal examination is mandatory to exclude rectal cancer, and a proctoscopy to exclude piles
- Gastroscopy: peptic ulcer, gastric cancer and GORD can certainly occur in this age group
  Also, do a duodenal biopsy for coeliac disease (Fig. 4.5)

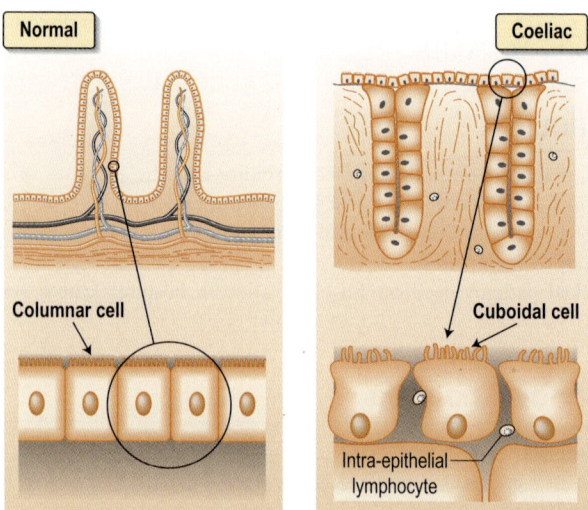

Fig. 4.5 Small intestinal mucosa showing normal villi with normal columnar cells, compared to coeliac mucosa showing subtotal villus atrophy, crypt hyperplasia, lamina propria inflammation and an increase in intra-epithelial lymphocytes.

REMEMBER

Coeliac Disease

- This is increasingly recognised worldwide and has an incidence of <1:100 in many countries. Certain areas of the world are said to have a higher incidence, for example, Ireland and Italy
- HLA-DQ2 and HLA-DQ8 are present in 90%–95% of coeliac patients
- Malabsorption of iron, as well as increased iron loss, can occur. There might be other deficiencies as well, for example, calcium and folic acid
- A history of steatorrhoea can be missed, unless a detailed stool history is taken (*Note:* many patients do not have steatorrhoea or any GI symptoms)
- Coeliac serology with antiendomysial and antitissue transglutaminase (the target antigen for the endomysial antibody) antibodies should be checked. A serum IgA must be performed, as these are IgA in vitro tests. Deaminated gluten peptide (DGP) testing is now available. These tests have a high sensitivity and specificity
- Diagnosis is confirmed by biopsy of duodenal/jejunal mucosa
- Treatment is with a gluten-free diet
- Follow-up: Regular dietary adherence checks, annual reviews for symptoms and nutritional status, and appropriate vaccinations

If gastroscopy is unhelpful, a full colonic assessment is necessary. The best investigation is colonoscopy, which will allow full assessment of the colon; biopsy, polypectomy and laser treatment of angiodysplasia can be performed as appropriate.

If the above investigations are negative, you have a problem. A small minority of patients fall into this category and the host of further investigations, performed with advice from the GI unit, will include:

- Small bowel MRI
- Capsule endoscopy

- Enteroscopy
- Meckel scan
- Angiography: preferably performed when a patient is bleeding, and in this patient, unlikely to be helpful
- Laparotomy with possibly simultaneous on-table endoscopy

Progress. This patient turned out to have menorrhagia due to fibroids.

> **REMEMBER**
>
> - If there is iron deficiency anaemia in a postmenopausal female or any male with no obvious cause of blood loss, there likely be a GI cause
> - Few patients have an inadequate iron intake in developed countries

Rectal Bleeding

Rectal bleeding is characterised by the passage of fresh blood rectally, as opposed to either occult loss, when blood can be detected only by laboratory testing, or melaena.

> **CASE HISTORY**
>
> An 80-year-old female was admitted in a shocked state after having passed 'a great deal' of fresh blood from her rectum. She gave no other history, and prior to the incident, had just returned on her bicycle from doing the shopping. Abdominal examination was normal.

HOW WOULD YOU MANAGE THE PATIENT INITIALLY?

- Establish IV access and give warmed crystalloids
- Check Hb and U and Es
- Group and cross-match blood urgently
- Consider invasive blood pressure monitoring and central venous access

The patient stabilised and had no further bleeding.

ADDITIONAL EXAMINATION

Additional investigations must include a rectal examination, proctoscopy and rigid sigmoidoscopy.

Proctoscopy

This will allow the diagnosis of haemorrhoids and anal fissure. These are the most common causes of rectal bleeding, but rarely – if ever – cause torrential blood loss. Features of bleeding from an anorectal lesion are:

- Passage of blood after a motion, and not mixed with it
- Blood dripping into the pan
- Blood just on the paper
- Anal pain, particularly with an anal fissure

Flexi-Sigmoidoscopy

This will determine the presence of colitis and might show a lesion, for example, carcinoma. If local anorectal disease is excluded, other causes include:

- Cancer
- Diverticular disease
- Colitis
- Angiodysplasia
- Polyps
- Ischaemia

Progress. In this patient sigmoidoscopy showed that the blood was coming from above the limit of the scope. Colonoscopy showed a bleeding polyp; this was excised.

REMEMBER

Even in the presence of severe diverticular disease, a polyp and carcinoma can be the cause of the bleeding and must be excluded by colonoscopy.

Family History of Colon Cancer

CASE HISTORY

A doctor phoned to discuss a possible referral to the gastroenterology clinic. He has just seen an anxious, 32-year-old female patient whose mother has recently died of colonic cancer. The patient has just discovered that her maternal aunt died of a similar complaint. The doctor emphasises that the patient herself has no GI symptoms.

WHAT SHOULD YOU ADVISE?

The patient needs to be seen by a gastroenterologist with a view to a full discussion of the pros and cons of having a colonoscopy.

Family cancer syndromes include:

- **Familial adenomatous polyposis:** multiple polyps are found throughout the colon and upper small bowel. All patients should be screened after age 12 years because *all* will develop colon cancer unless the colon is removed.
- **Hereditary** nonpolyposis cancer of the colon (HNPCC) (Box 4.3): this accounts for 5%–10% of colon cancers; the average age of diagnosis is 45 years. Cancers are mainly in the right-hand side of the colon.

A flexible sigmoidoscope can only reach 60 to 70 cm up the colon, where approximately 60% of cancers occur (Fig. 4.6).

The gastroenterologist advises a colonoscopy for this patient, which she agrees to have after full discussion.

REMEMBER

Risks for Developing Colon Cancer

- Normal: 1:50
- With a first-degree relative: 1:17
- With an elderly first-degree relative: 1:30

MSI-H, microsatellite instability – high

Modified Amsterdam Criteria

- One individual diagnosed with colorectal cancer (or extra-colonic HNPCC-associated tumours) before age 50 years
- Two affected generations
- Three affected relatives, one a first-degree relative of the other two
- Familial adenomatous polyposis should be excluded
- Tumours should be verified by pathological examination

Bethesda Guidelines

- Colorectal cancer diagnosed in patient who is younger than 50 years
- Presence of synchronous, metachronous colorectal, or other HNPCC-associated tumours, irrespective of age
- Colorectal cancer with the MSI-H histology diagnosed in a patient who is younger than 60 years
- Colorectal cancer diagnosed in one or more first-degree relatives with an HNPCC-related tumour, with one of the cancers being diagnosed under age 50 years
- Colorectal cancer diagnosed in two or more first- or second-degree relatives with HNPCC-related tumours, irrespective of age

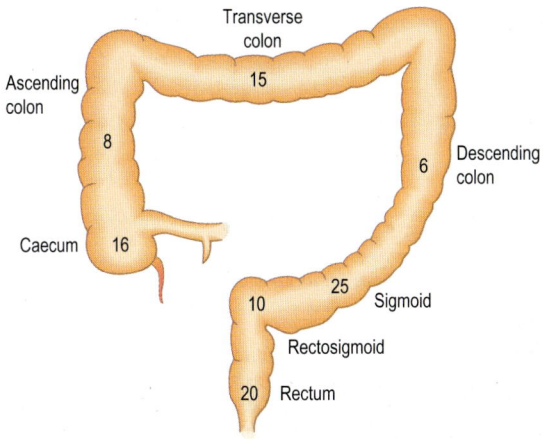

Fig. 4.6 Distribution of colorectal cancer (%).

Progress. This patient's colonoscopy showed a 2 cm polyp, which was fully excised. Histologically, it was a tubular adenoma. She was asked to return for a surveillance colonoscopy in 3 years' time and was told that she would need continuous follow-up in view of the family history.

Functional Bowel Disease

CASE HISTORY

A 30-year-old patient is in the emergency department with severe lower abdominal pain. She is otherwise well and the surgical registrar has found no evidence of serious disease. She has already examined her fully and investigated her with routine blood tests and a CT of her abdomen, all of which are normal.

WHAT DO YOU DO?

- Retake the history
- Reexamine the abdomen: think again of all the causes of an acute abdomen (see Information box)
- Review the investigations

The history supports a diagnosis of IBS but it is important to make sure all other potential causes are excluded. Remember that the pain can be very severe and distressing to the patient.

Management

This can be very difficult, particularly because relatives often feel unable to cope. The situation needs to be calmed down with strong reassurance and pain relief (e.g. simple analgesics and antispasmodics). Refer the patient to gastroenterology outpatients.

INFORMATION

Acute Abdominal Pain of Sudden Onset

- Perforation, for example, duodenal ulcer
- Rupture, for example, aneurysm
- Torsion, for example, ovarian cyst

Acute Abdominal Pain of Gradual Onset

- Inflammatory conditions, for example, appendicitis, back pain

Think of

- Pancreatitis
- Ruptured aortic aneurysm
- Renal tract disease

Pseudomembranous Colitis

This is the condition caused by *Clostridium difficile*; a pseudomembrane is seen on sigmoidoscopy.

CASE HISTORY

A 40-year-old male, who had been on the intensive care unit for 3 weeks with a head injury following a road traffic accident, developed severe diarrhoea. He was on a ventilator and currently was finishing a course of a third-generation parenteral cephalosporin for hospital-acquired pneumonia. According to the nurses, one other patient on the ICU also has diarrhoea.

WHAT OTHER QUESTIONS DO YOU WANT TO ASK?

You would want to know:

- What is the diarrhoea like? Are the stools liquid or bloody?
- How long has the patient been on broad-spectrum antibiotics?
- Does any other patient/member of the staff have diarrhoea? (One of the ICU nurses informs you that another patient did have loose stools, and you need to ascertain if this is really the case and if there were any obvious reasons for this)

WHAT IS YOUR DIFFERENTIAL DIAGNOSIS?

This would include:

- Antibiotic-associated diarrhoea, particularly pseudomembranous colitis
- Diarrhoea due to enteral feeding

- Other bacterial causes, for example, *Salmonella* spp., *Shigella* spp., *Campylobacter* spp. and *E. coli* 0157; these are less likely because the patient has not been eating, but could occur as a result of cross-infection
- Viral gastroenteritis

WHAT INVESTIGATIONS WOULD YOU PERFORM?

You would need to send a stool from the patient to the microbiology laboratory (and also from any other patient/staff member with diarrhoea) for microscopy, culture and sensitivity. If several patients/members of staff are affected, stools should also be sent to the virology department to look for a viral aetiology, for example, small round viruses. In addition, you would specifically need to request an examination for *C. difficile* (toxin) – the organism responsible for the toxin of pseudomembranous colitis. Do a sigmoidoscopy to look for the typical pseudomembrane seen in pseudomembranous colitis and exclude IBD by rectal biopsy.

The patient was thought, on clinical grounds, to have pseudomembranous colitis. This was later confirmed by the microbiology department, which found the stool to be positive for *C. difficile* toxin.

> **REMEMBER**
>
> Culture of *C. difficile* itself in a stool is insufficient evidence that a patient has pseudomembranous colitis; only toxin-producing strains cause this.

HOW WOULD YOU MANAGE THE PATIENT?

The patient should be isolated in a side room, if possible, to prevent cross-infection. You need to ensure that the patient is adequately hydrated. In patients with antibiotic-associated diarrhoea, any broad-spectrum antibiotics that the patient is taking should be stopped if it is at all possible. If it is not feasible to do this, try to change to a narrow-spectrum agent (discuss with microbiology). Specific first-line therapy for pseudomembranous colitis varies depending on region but can include oral metronidazole 400 mg × 3 for 7 to 10 days or oral vancomycin 125 mg four times daily for 7 to 10 days (check local guidance). Fidaxomicin is also effective.

Note: you do not need to check vancomycin levels in patients receiving oral vancomycin because it is not systemically absorbed.

In some parts of the world, enterococcal vancomycin resistance is becoming a major problem. Installing a faecal transplant from a healthy donor can restore normal flora and eradicates *C. difficile* infections.

Progress. This patient initially responded to metronidazole but after 8 days, his diarrhoea returned (up to 30% of cases relapse); he was switched to vancomycin, to which he responded.

He was eventually weaned from the ventilator and made a good physical recovery but with impaired cognitive function.

> **REMEMBER**
>
> **Prevention**
>
> Infection control relies on:
> - Responsible use of antibiotics
> - Hygiene, which should involve all health workers, as well as patients and relatives
> - Washing hands thoroughly using soap and water, which is essential as alcohol disinfectants do not kill *C. difficile* spores

- Hospital cleaning of surfaces, which should be performed regularly to try to reduce transmission from fomites
- Isolation of patients with *C. difficile*

Food Poisoning: *E. coli* O157

Enterohaemorrhagic *Escherichia coli* (EHEC)

Enterohaemorrhagic *Escherichia coli* (usually serotype O157:H7, and also known as verotoxin-producing *E. coli*, or VTEC) is a well-recognised cause of gastroenteritis in humans. It is a zoonosis usually associated with cattle; the organism being found in the intestines of herbivores. There have been a number of major outbreaks (notably in Scotland and Japan) associated with contaminated food. Run-off water from where cattle have been grazing is used in irrigation and therefore salads and vegetables are a source of infection, as well as milk and underdone beef, for example, hamburgers.

Enterohaemorrhagic *E. coli* secretes a toxin (Shiga-like toxin 1), which affects vascular endothelial cells in the gut and in the kidney. After an incubation period of 12 to 48 h, it causes diarrhoea (frequently bloody), associated with abdominal pain and nausea. Some days after the onset of symptoms, the patient may develop thrombotic thrombocytopenic purpura or haemolytic uraemic syndrome (HUS). This is more common in children and may lead to permanent renal damage or death. Treatment is mainly supportive: there is evidence that antibiotic therapy for gastroenteritis might precipitate HUS by causing increased toxin release.

CASE HISTORY

A 15-year-old female patient is admitted to the hospital with bloody diarrhoea; her parents and her three siblings are well. They have apparently all eaten the same food during the last week, except on a single occasion when the patient ate a beefburger cooked at a local party. The mother remembers that it looked rather raw inside. The female had eaten chicken at least three times during the previous week. She looked slightly dehydrated and had a temperature of 37.8°C. Her abdomen was soft but generally tender, and bowel sounds were increased.

WHAT IS THE DIFFERENTIAL DIAGNOSIS IN THIS PATIENT?

Infectious gastroenteritis with bloody diarrhoea due to:
- *Campylobacter* spp. (chicken is the likely source)
- *E. coli* O157 (beef is the likely source)
- *Shigella* spp.
- *Salmonella* spp.
- Onset of IBD

INVESTIGATIONS

Should include:
- Full blood count, including platelets
- U and Es (*E. coli* O157 can cause HUS)
- Blood culture
- Stools for microscopy, culture and sensitivity
Full clinical details should be put on the form accompanying the stool

WHAT WOULD YOUR INITIAL MANAGEMENT BE?

The patient should be admitted to the MAU and put into excretion–secretion isolation (assuming a probable infective aetiology). Ensure adequate hydration. Oral/IV antibiotics can have a place in treating severe infections due to *Salmonella* spp., *Campylobacter* spp. and *Shigella* spp.; they should not be used in infections caused by *E. coli* O157. The disease should be notified to the Health Protection Team/CCDC both by telephone immediately and in writing when the diagnosis has been made. Rapid notification is required if the patient works in the food industry or with the very young, the elderly or the immunosuppressed.

Progress. This patient had *E. coli* O157 and did not develop HUS. She made an uneventful recovery.

INFORMATION

Features of Haemolytic Uraemic Syndrome (HUS)

- Intravascular haemolysis with red cell fragmentation (microangiopathic haemolysis)
- Thrombocytopenia
- Acute kidney injury

Mortality is high in the elderly; treatment is by plasma exchange, with some patients requiring haemofiltration dialysis.

Typhoid

This is the typical form of enteric fever and is caused by *Salmonella typhi*. Enteric fever is an acute systemic illness with fever, headache and abdominal discomfort.

CASE HISTORY

A 35-year-old male presents with a 1-week history of fever, headache, a dry cough and constipation. He is resident in the UK and has just returned from a 6-week holiday in Bangladesh, where he was visiting relatives. He works as a chef in a local restaurant. While he was away, one of the relatives he was staying with had a high fever and severe diarrhoea.

On examination, the patient had a fever of 39.5°C with a pulse rate of only 85/min. Examination of the cardiovascular, respiratory and central nervous systems was unremarkable.

The abdomen was slightly tender.

INVESTIGATIONS

- Full blood count, routine chemistry, CXR and blood cultures taken
- Full blood count shows a slight leucopenia
- Gram-negative rods are seen in a film of the blood cultures taken after 24-h incubation

WHAT IS THE MOST LIKELY DIAGNOSIS?

S. typhi (this was later confirmed as being the definitive diagnosis).

HOW WOULD YOU MANAGE THIS PATIENT?

The patient should be nursed in a side room with excretion–secretion precautions used (consult your local infection control manual). The control of infection officer should be alerted, as should your local CCDC, as soon as a definite diagnosis is made. Your CCDC should be alerted immediately by telephone and also via the formal notification book, which should be available on every ward. This is particularly important because this patient is a food handler. If the patient subsequently develops diarrhoea, adequate fluids are required to avoid dehydration. Pending antibiotic sensitivity testing, the patient should be commenced on antibiotics (e.g. ciprofloxacin 500 mg × 2 daily for 10 days).

> **REMEMBER**
>
> Ciprofloxacin is extremely well absorbed and so can be given by the oral route 500 mg 12-hourly as long as the patient is not vomiting. After starting ciprofloxacin, the patient began to feel better very quickly but it took 3 to 6 days for the temperature to settle.

Progress. The patient was discharged after 6 days, feeling well and with no fever. He needed a follow-up appointment to ensure that he does not become a carrier of *S. typhi*. He must remain away from his job as a food handler until he is known to have negative stool cultures for *S. typhi*.

Further Reading

Constipation

NICE, CKS, 2023. Constipation. NICE.

Diarrhoea

Friedman, S., 2017. Tofacitinib for ulcerative colitis – a promising new step forward. N. Engl. J. Med. 376 (18), 1792–1793.

Lamb, C.A., Kennedy, N.A., Raine, T., et al., 2019. BSG consensus guidelines on management of inflammatory bowel disease in adults. Gut 68 (Suppl 3), s1–s106.

NICE, CKS, 2023. Diarrhoea – adult's assessment. NICE.

Abdominal Pain

Forsmark, C.E., Vege, S.S., Wilcox, C.M., 2016. Acute pancreatitis. N. Engl. J. Med. 375 (20), 1972–1981.

NICE, CKS, 2023. Acute pancreatitis. NICE.

Peptic Ulcer Disease

Cook, D., Guyatt, G., 2018. Prophylaxis against upper gastrointestinal bleeding in hospitalized patients. N. Engl. J. Med. 378 (26), 2506–2516.

Laine, L., 2016. Upper gastrointestinal bleeding due to a peptic ulcer. N. Engl. J. Med. 374 (24), 2367–2376.

Iron Deficiency Anaemia

Goddard, A.F., James, M.W., McIntyre, A.S., et al., 2011. Guidelines for the management of iron deficiency anaemia. Gut 60 (10), 1309–1316.

NICE, CKS, 2023. Coeliac disease. NICE.

Family History of Colon Cancer

Sinicrole, F.A., 2018. Lynch syndrome – associated colorectal cancer. N. Engl. J. Med. 379 (8), 764–773.

CHAPTER 5

Liver and Biliary Tract Disorders

Abnormal Liver Biochemistry

'Liver function tests (LFTs)' are routinely requested.

Serum bilirubin, aminotransferases, alkaline phosphatase, γ-glutamyl transpeptidase (γ-GT) and total proteins are measured. These are, in fact, tests of liver damage (hence the term 'liver biochemistry') rather than actual liver function. Liver function is assessed by serum albumin and the prothrombin time.

> **CASE HISTORY**
>
> A doctor phones you to ask whether a hospital referral is necessary for her patient. The doctor has recently seen a 55-year-old patient for a medical insurance examination. She had found no problems with the patient at the time of the examination, but the liver biochemistry results have come back abnormal. The tests showed:
> - Serum bilirubin: 14 μmol/L
> - Serum alkaline phosphatase: 134 IU/L
> - Aspartate aminotransferase (AST): 70 IU/L
> - Alanine aminotransferase (ALT): 90 IU/L

WHAT ADVICE DO YOU GIVE?

These tests suggest intrahepatic disease and you ask about the patient's alcohol history. The answer is that only occasional alcohol is taken. You suggest that the doctor could arrange the following tests while waiting for an outpatient appointment:

- Repeat liver biochemistry
- Viral markers
- Serum autoantibodies
- Serum ferritin

These tests will yield a diagnosis in most cases.

THE DOCTOR ASKS WHETHER AN ULTRASOUND WOULD BE HELPFUL

This is unlikely to help as the LFTs are not consistent with biliary or pancreatic disease.

You arrange to see the patient with your consultant in outpatients. At outpatients, the history is again unhelpful. There is no history of:

- Blood transfusions
- Previous hepatitis
- Intravenous drug use
- Sexual promiscuity

On examination, you notice a few spider naevi. The liver is not palpable.

The results of the tests performed by the doctor are now available (Table 5.1). Hepatitis C virus (HCV) antibodies indicate **HCV infection** (chronic hepatitis) and the patient will require HCV RNA, liver biopsy and treatment with antiviral therapy.

TABLE 5.1 ■ Further Investigations into the Cause of Abnormal Liver Biochemistry

Test	Result	Implication
Repeat liver biochemistry	Similar to earlier	–
Hepatitis A	IgG-positive	Patient has been infected with HAV in the past or immunised
	IgM-negative	This virus does *not* cause chronic liver disease
HBsAg	Negative	See Table 5.2
HCV antibodies	Positive	
Autoantibody screen	Negative	Positive titres usually found in autoimmune hepatitis
Serum ferritin	110 µg/L	This excludes hereditary haemochromatosis

HbsAg, Hepatitis B surface antigen; HCV, hepatitis C virus; HAV, hepatitis A virus.

TABLE 5.2 ■ Significance of Viral Markers in Hepatitis B

Markers	Significance
Antigens	
HbsAg	Acute or chronic infection
HbeAg	Acute hepatitis B
	Persistence implies:
	Continuous infectious state
	Development of chronicity
HBV DNA	Implies viral replication
	Found in serum and liver
	Levels indicate response to antiviral treatment
Antibodies	
Anti-HBc	Immunity to HBV; previous exposure; vaccination
Anti-HBc	Seroconversion
Anti-HBc	–
IgM	Acute hepatitis B (high titre)
	Chronic hepatitis B (low titre)
IgG	Past exposure to hepatitis B (HBsAg-negative)

HbsAg, Hepatitis B surface antigen; HbeAg, hepatitis B e-antigen; HBc, hepatitis B core antigen.
From Feather, A., Randall, D., Waterhouse, M., eds., 2020. Kumar and Clark's Clinical Medicine, tenth ed. Elsevier, Edinburgh, Box 34.9.

Armed with the HCV result, you discuss IV drug use with your patient, who then admits to the very occasional use of IV drugs in her twenties.

Although this patient did not have HBV, you need to know the significance of HBV markers (Table 5.2).

Progress. This patient was referred to the liver clinic. Her HCV RNA showed 45,000 IU/mL viral load with genotype I infection. Direct-acting antiviral agents are now the standard of care in the treatment of chronic HCV infection. She was treated with glecaprevir–pibrentasvir once daily for 8 weeks, and her liver biopsy showing no evidence of cirrhosis. She had a sustained virological response and continues to be followed up in the liver clinic.

Jaundice

Jaundice is detected clinically when the serum bilirubin is greater than 50 μmol/L (3 mg/dL).

CASE HISTORY (1)

A 45-year-old female patient has been admitted to the Medical Assessment Unit (MAU) presenting with pronounced jaundice. She reports experiencing two severe episodes of abdominal pain, each lasting approximately 30 minutes. Additionally, she notes a significant loss of appetite and subsequent weight loss.

Upon **abdominal examination,** no chronic liver disease signs were present. However, her blood tests revealed elevated serum bilirubin levels, ALT at 50 U/L, and markedly high alkaline phosphatase at 410 IU/L. Based on these findings, and considering her symptomatic history suggestive of biliary colic, an ultrasound of the liver and biliary system is warranted to investigate the possibility of gallstone disease (Fig. 5.1).

INVESTIGATIONS

- Complete blood count and liver biochemistry to assess overall liver function, including international normalised ratio (INR) and albumin levels
- Abdominal ultrasound to visualize the liver and biliary tree structures
- Viral serology to rule out hepatitis as a cause of intrahepatic cholestasis

Ultrasound in extrahepatic obstruction can show:
- Dilatation of the intrahepatic biliary tree
- Dilatation of the common bile duct
- Gallstones in the gallbladder
- Gallstones in the biliary tree
- A pancreatic mass
- Metastatic liver disease

In this patient, the ultrasound showed gallstones in the gall bladder and a dilated common bile duct. Provided this patient's clotting is satisfactory, the next procedure should be an endoscopic

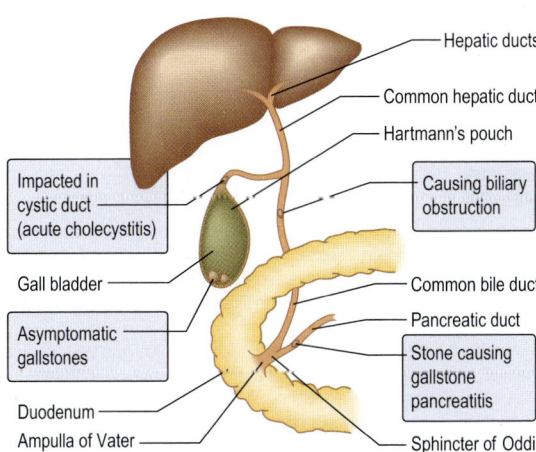

Fig. 5.1 Clinical presentation of gallstones.

retrograde cholangiopancreatography (ERCP). This would enable better visualisation of the system and would allow a gallstone that is causing the obstruction in the common bile duct to be removed. A sphincterotomy would need to be performed beforehand and the stone could be removed with a basket or a balloon. If the stone is very large, it can be crushed and the debris removed. In an elderly patient, stent insertion to maintain drainage is an option.

Progress. In this patient, the stones were cleared from the common bile duct at ERCP and this was followed by a laparoscopic cholecystectomy to prevent recurrence.

REMEMBER

- Cholangitis, an infection of the bile ducts, often occurs with gallstones. Immediate drainage of the biliary tree is crucial, and antibiotic therapy should be administered
- Any remaining stones should be removed endoscopically once the patient has stabilized from the acute episode

CASE HISTORY (2)

A 78-year-old male patient is admitted with marked jaundice. He was previously fit and well but the ultrasound arranged by his doctor showed a dilated biliary system with the probability of a pancreatic mass.

An endoscopic ultrasound and/or CT scan should be performed to assess the possibility of operability, although this is rare.

An ERCP with the placement of a stent through the stricture enables drainage and is the usual treatment. This makes the patient feel a lot better, as well as relieving the jaundice. This was performed in this male.

Jaundice without pain is quite common with carcinoma of the pancreas, but with gallstones, there is usually a history of biliary pain accompanying the jaundice.

A similar obstruction could equally well be related to an obstruction higher up in the duct system, perhaps due to a cholangiocarcinoma. This could arise in preexisting sclerosing cholangitis, although this would usually occur at a younger age.

Complications of ERCP Sphincterotomy (Complication Rate 8%–12%)

- Bleeding (severe in 2%)
- Perforation
- Acute pancreatitis (5%)
- Cholangitis

CASE HISTORY (3)

A 20-year-old female patient is admitted in a confused state and deeply jaundiced. She has recently returned from India, where she had been trekking; she had had a major argument with her boyfriend. A subconjunctival haemorrhage was noticed on examination.

This patient is critically ill with fulminant hepatic failure and it is essential to stabilise her as soon as possible.

A central venous line was inserted, and as her haemoglobin (Hb) was very low, she was given 2 units of red blood cells. The clotting studies give an indication of the degree of damage to her liver and will be useful for daily follow-up. It is also necessary to make sure that the patient's potassium and blood sugar are satisfactory, and whether replacements are necessary.

This female's investigation showed a bilirubin of 130 μmol/L, ALT 900 IU/L, AST 785 IU/L, alkaline phosphatase 109 IU/L, albumin 34 g/L, INR 2.2, indicating **severe hepatocellular damage**.

Further Management

This patient is liable to infection and intravenous antibiotics are required after blood cultures have been taken.

REMEMBER

Hepatic encephalopathy should be treated with a low-protein diet and rifaximin.

It is essential to try to establish the cause of this patient's jaundice. This might be hepatitis A (HAV) or hepatitis E – both are endemic causes of hepatitis in India and often follow an initial respiratory type of illness; they can occasionally cause fulminant liver damage. A paracetamol overdose is also a possibility, as her boyfriend said that she was very upset when they returned to the UK.

Further Investigation

- Viral markers for the above causes
- Paracetamol levels

These must be obtained urgently. Other investigations would include the following if no cause has been found:

- Autoantibodies
- Copper studies
- Alpha-1 antitrypsin levels

In this case, the patient's relatives arrive and say they have found empty containers labelled 'paracetamol 500 mg tablets' in her bedroom.

The patient might well stabilise at this stage, but a close eye will need to be kept on her for potential infections, particularly with opportunistic organisms. It is reasonable to give acetylcysteine in the initial management of such comatosed patients, whether or not the paracetamol blood level is high.

This patient's clinical condition deteriorated, with an early warning score (NEWS) of 5. She became increasingly drowsy and confused and developed a flapping tremor and fetor hepaticus. Her investigations now showed a serum bilirubin of 320 μmol/L, ALT of 3800 U/L, AST of 4200 U/L and serum albumin of 32 g/L, with an INR of 3.62. Urgent advice was sought from the nearest liver unit.

INFORMATION

Indicators for Transfer to a Specialised Unit

- International normalized ratio >3.0 at 48 hrs (or >4,5 at any time)
- Presence of hepatic encephalopathy (grade 3 or 4)
- Hypotension after resuscitation with fluid (BP < 80 mm Hg)
- Oliguria or serum creatinine >200 μmol/L
- Metabolic acidosis (pH <7.3 after resuscitation)

Persistent hypoglycaemia

Severe thrombocytopaenia

You arrange for transfer. In specialised units, 70% of patients with paracetamol overdose and grade IV encephalopathy survive. Factors that indicate a poor prognosis with paracetamol overdose (without transplantation) are:

- Arterial pH <7.3 *or*
- Serum creatinine >300 μmol/L
- Prothrombin time >100 s
- Grade III to IV encephalopathy

Progress. This female was seriously ill with acute hepatic failure. She survived with supportive therapy, and transplantation was not necessary.

Acute Liver Disease

CASE HISTORY

A medical student turns up in the emergency department with jaundice. He is very worried that he has gallstones and might need surgery. He has never seen jaundice outside a surgical ward.

HOW DO YOU APPROACH THIS SITUATION?

First, you point out that gallstones are rare in a young person and that viral hepatitis is, by far and away, the most likely diagnosis. You quickly ascertain that he has been previously immunised against hepatitis B and only drinks beer after rugby. He denies IV drug use. You suspect infection with hepatis A virus (HAV). There is no clue as to how he could have acquired this from the history:

- No contact with jaundice
- No prodromal features
- No travel abroad

On examination, apart from jaundice, there are no other abnormal signs.

Take blood for:

- Liver biochemistry
- Hepatitis serology including hepatitis A virus IgM (to indicate acute HAV infection).

You tell him to go back to his student flat, be careful with his personal hygiene and return in 2 days for his results (Table 5.3).

HAV IgM-negative! You realise that although HAV is very, very common in such a situation, there are other causes. You had omitted to take a careful drug history from someone you knew.

Progress. This student turned out to have glandular fever (Epstein–Barr virus infection), which can occasionally present with jaundice.

TABLE 5.3 ■ **Test Results in Acute Liver Disease**

Test	Result	Implication
Serum bilirubin	70 μmol/L	–
AST	300 IU/L	Compatible with acute hepatitis
ALT	280 IU/L	
Alkaline phosphatase	140 IU/L	
HAV IgM	Negative	

AST, aspartate aminotransferase; ALT, alanine aminotransferase; HAV, hepatitis A virus.

Ascites

Ascitis is fluid within the peritoneal cavity due to sodium and water retention, for example, cirrhosis or heart failure, or secondary to malignant deposits.

CASE HISTORY (1)

A 45-year-old female patient presents with ascites gradually increasing over 2 weeks.

Examination shows no abnormality outside the abdomen.

Determining the cause of the ascites is essential to developing a management plan and she is admitted to the MAU.

INVESTIGATIONS

- Liver biochemistry
- Full blood count (FBC)
- International normalized ratio and serum albumin
- Ascitic tap – for white cell count (WCC), culture, protein, malignant cells

INFORMATION

Paracentesis (Ascitic Tap)

- Obtain the patient's consent after explaining the procedure
- Use ultrasound (if available) to assess the location of ascites and the optimal needle insertion point (if no ultrasound this can be assessed via percussion of the right or left lower quadrant)
- Clean the skin and inject local anaesthetic (1% lidocaine) into the skin using an orange needle
- Insert a 21-gauge needle (green) on a 20 mL syringe into the fluid
- Withdraw approximately 20 mL
- Withdraw the needle and apply a dressing

Ascitic Fluid

The ascitic protein concentration, as well as the serum:ascites albumin gradient (SAG), helps differentiate a transudate (<5 g/L or SAG >11 g/L) from an exudate (>25 g/L or SAG >11 g/L).

In this case, a high ascitic protein (>25 g/L) suggests a tumour or infection.

Malignant cells were present; further imaging with ultrasound and abdominal and pelvic CT was performed to determine the tumour site.

DIAGNOSIS

In this patient, the age and sex suggested an **ovarian malignancy** and this was confirmed.

Progress. She was referred to the gynaecology department for further management.

CASE HISTORY (2)

A 45-year-old male patient has attended his doctor on many occasions with alcohol-related problems. He is sent to the emergency department with a swollen abdomen. He admits to drinking 60 to 80 units per week for 20 years.

On examination, he is not jaundiced, but he does have spider naevi, liver palms, Dupuytren contractures and testicular atrophy, as well as gross ascites and pitting ankle oedema.

WHAT SHOULD YOU DO?

An ascitic tap is necessary to rule out infection and malignancy, even though he has **chronic liver disease**.

Ascitic fluid showed 25 cells/mm^3 and protein content of 23 g/L, with a SAG of <9 g/L, suggesting a transudate.

- A transudate (<25 g/L) suggests cirrhosis without any complication
- In a patient with known liver disease, a high WCC and high protein levels suggest infection (spontaneous bacterial peritonitis)

Ultrasound of the liver and spleen is now performed. It shows splenomegaly (portal hypertension) and an irregular liver with fat, indicative of cirrhosis.

Immediate Management

- Salt restriction
- Daily weights and U and Es
- Start diuretics – spironolactone 100 mg/day (increasing gradually to 400 mg/day) to obtain a weight loss of 500 g/day
- If there is an inadequate response to these measures, introduce furosemide 40–120 mg/day
- Give thiamine 25–50 mg daily

The patient *must* stop drinking.

Subsequent Management

It may be necessary to perform a liver biopsy to confirm the cause of cirrhosis but only after the ascites is removed. If it is impossible to do a percutaneous liver biopsy (due to ascites and prolonged clotting), then a biopsy can be undertaken through the jugular vein under X-ray control.

Progress. This patient was referred to the Alcohol Dependency Unit after resolution of his ankle swelling and ascites. He may require liver transplantation and should be referred to a Liver unit for assessment. He continues to abstain from alcohol but, at present, does not fit the criteria for transplantation (Model for End-stage Liver Disease [MELD] – Score 7).

Haematemesis and Melaena

Haematemesis is vomiting blood. Melaena is the passage of black, tarry stools, usually from a lesion proximal to the right colon.

CASE HISTORY

A 70-year-old male was admitted, having vomited blood this morning. His stools have been loose and black (melaena).

On initial assessment, he looked pale and was shocked, with a tachycardia of 110 beats per minute (bpm) and a BP of 80/60 mmHg.

An IV cannula was immediately inserted, blood taken for Hb, U and Es, clotting, and grouping and cross-matching for four units. He was initially given fluid replacement and transferred to the intensive care unit (ICU).

Resuscitation

- Intravenous access (wide-bore)
- Consider invasive arterial blood pressure monitoring and central venous access (with central venous pressure monitoring)
- Fluid replacement
- Blood transfusion
- O_2 if hypoxic

REMEMBER

Haemoglobin <100 g/L, urea ↑, postural hypotension present, pulse rate 110 bpm. This patient is severely compromised and needs urgent treatment.

The gastroenterologists and surgical teams were informed. He was admitted to the high-dependency unit and a CVP line was inserted.

Many hospitals have multidisciplinary teams (MDTs) and protocols. Keep the patient nil by mouth until the bleeding has stopped. Causes of upper gastrointestinal (GI) bleeding are shown in Fig. 5.2.

A further history of this male revealed that he had had a high alcohol intake of 70 units/week for many years. He had no history of long-term dyspepsia and did not take NSAIDs, including aspirin.

On examination, he had signs of chronic liver disease with spider naevi. His liver was 4 cm palpable and he had splenomegaly.

REMEMBER

Shock
- Pallor
- Cold peripheries
- ↓ Systolic BP

Common Causes of a GI Bleed

- Peptic ulcer
- Gastric erosions
- Oesophageal varices

Management

The patient's Hb was returned as 90 g/L and the urea was raised at 10 mmol/L. A blood transfusion was started to resuscitate him (Fig. 5.3). On improvement, he had an endoscopy, which

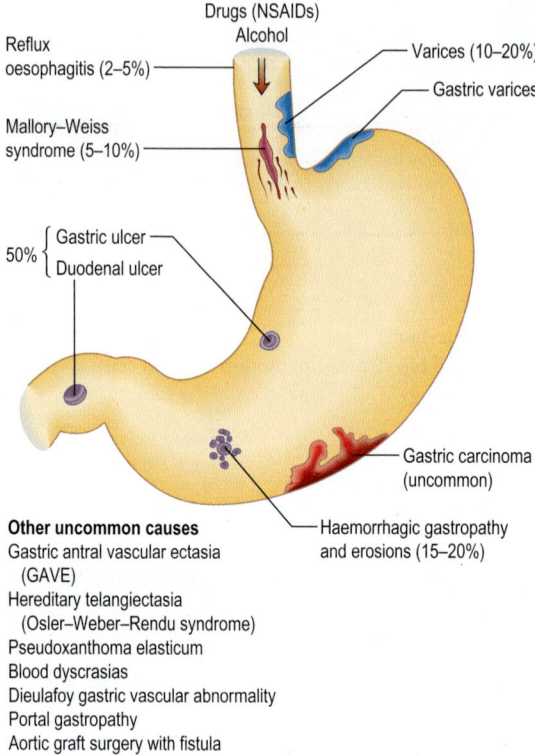

Fig. 5.2 Causes of upper gastrointestinal bleeding.

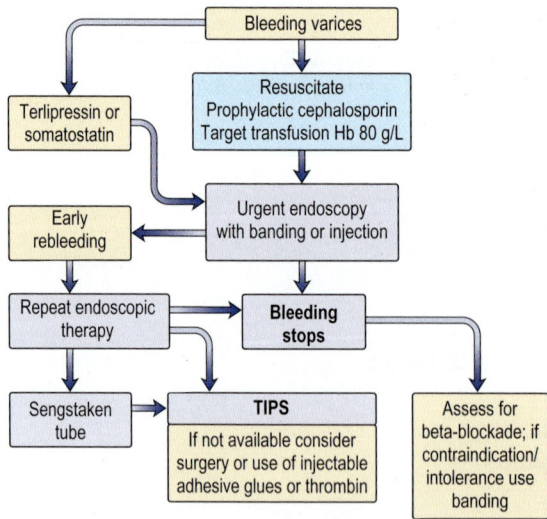

Fig. 5.3 Management of gastrointestinal haemorrhage due to oesophageal varices. TIPS: Transjugular intra-hepatic portosystemic shunt.

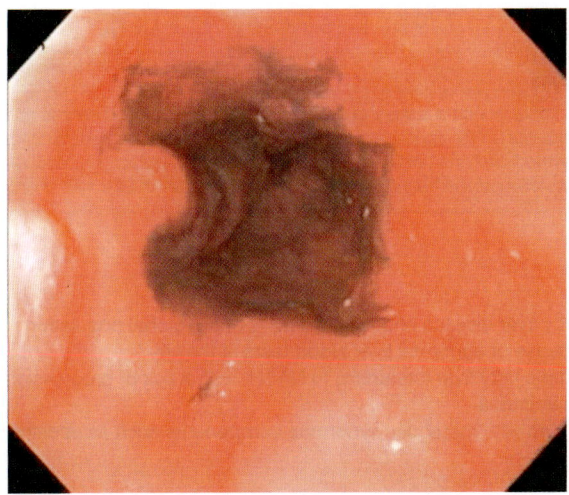

Fig. 5.4 (A) Oesophageal varices; (B) with band in place. (From Akiyama, T., Abe, Y., Iida, H., et al. 2010. Endoscopic therapy using an endoscopic variceal ligation for minute cancer of the esophagogastric junction complicated with esophageal varices: a case report. Journal of Medical Case Reports 4, 149.)

showed oesophageal varices, and these were banded (Fig. 5.4). On return to the ward, he had a further haematemesis 4 h later. Vasoconstrictor therapy was given.

Vasoconstrictor Therapy

The main use of this is for emergency control of bleeding while waiting for endoscopy and in combination with endoscopic techniques. The aim of vasoconstrictor agents is to restrict portal inflow by splanchnic arterial constriction.

- **Terlipressin.** This is the only vasoconstrictor shown to reduce mortality. It should not be given to patients with ischaemic heart disease. The patient is likely to complain of abdominal colic, will defecate and have facial pallor owing to the generalised vasoconstriction
- **Somatostatin.** This drug has few side effects and appears to reduce bleeding but has no effect on mortality. It should be used if there are contraindications to terlipressin

Balloon tamponade with a Sengstaken–Blakemore tube can be used if the bleeding continues. Use the gastric balloon only initially, but if the bleeding is not controlled, inflate the oesophageal balloon, remembering that continuous inflation leads to oesophageal damage. It has serious complications and should be left in situ for only 24 h.

If these measures fail, a transjugular intrahepatic portosystemic shunt (TIPS) might be required; this is often used as the treatment of choice for gastric varices.

Progress. Unfortunately, this patient continued to bleed, despite a repeat endoscopy with injection of the varices. A Sengstaken–Blakemore tube was put in place, and he was therefore referred urgently to a liver unit for TIPS insertion.

REMEMBER

Erosions can bleed profusely and be very difficult to control.

Nonalcoholic Fatty Liver Disease (NAFLD)

CASE HISTORY

A 58-year-old male presents with a history of type 2 diabetes mellitus and central obesity. He reports fatigue and a dull sensation in his right upper quadrant. He does not consume alcohol. His LFTs have been persistently elevated over the past 4 months, with ALT levels notably higher than AST levels. An ultrasound scan indicates increased hepatic echogenicity suggestive of fatty liver changes.

INFORMATION

- Nonalcoholic fatty liver disease affects up to 25% of the global population
- Most common cause of abnormal liver blood tests in the UK
- Ranges from simple fatty liver (steatosis) to NASH, with a risk of progression to cirrhosis or hepatocellular carcinoma
- Strongly associated with metabolic syndrome components such as obesity, diabetes, and dyslipidaemia

WHY IS CARDIOVASCULAR RISK ASSESSMENT IMPORTANT IN NAFLD PATIENTS?

Patients with NAFLD have an increased risk of cardiovascular disease, which is the most common cause of death in this population. Regular cardiovascular risk assessments are crucial for early detection and management of potential complications. Weight loss, particularly a reduction of 5% to 10% of body weight, can significantly improve liver steatosis, inflammation, and fibrosis. It is one of the most effective management strategies for NAFLD.

INVESTIGATION

- Persistently elevated ALT levels for more than 3 months, exceeding AST levels
- Ultrasound findings indicating steatosis
- Use noninvasive tools like the NAFLD Fibrosis Score or Fibrosis-4 Score to assess fibrosis risk

Management

Advise gradual and sustained weight loss, targeting a 5% to 10% reduction over 6 months.

Implement a Mediterranean diet and encourage water over sugar-sweetened beverages.

Promote physical activity, aiming for at least 150 minutes of moderate-intensity exercise per week.

Optimize control of comorbidities such as diabetes, hypertension and dyslipidaemia.

REMEMBER

Nonalcoholic fatty liver disease should not be ruled out based on normal LFTs or liver ultrasound alone. Cardiovascular disease, not liver-related complications, is the leading cause of death in NAFLD. Lifestyle modifications remain the cornerstone of NAFLD management.

Progress. Upon follow-up, the patient has managed to lose 5% of his body weight through dietary changes and increased physical activity. His LFTs show a modest improvement, and he reports a reduction in fatigue. The decision is made to reassess his condition annually for metabolic risk factors and every 3 years for advanced liver fibrosis.

Liver Failure

CASE HISTORY

A 60-year-old female has been a known user of alcohol for the past 20 years. She is admitted because of a deterioration in her health, with confusion and the development of ascites.

Further history indicates that she stopped drinking some 2 months ago and suffered no withdrawal symptoms.

On examination, you wonder whether she has liver failure.

WHAT SIGNS INDICATE LIVER FAILURE?

- Jaundice
- Ascites/portal hypertension (splenomegaly)
- Hepatic encephalopathy:
  - Hepatic flap
  - Fetor hepaticus
  - Constructional apraxia
  - Signs of chronic liver disease, for example,
  - Spider naevi
  - Gynaecomastia
  - Dupuytren's contracture
  - Liver palms

If there is no risk of bleeding, concentrate on determining the level of encephalopathy:

- Grade 1: disorientated
- Grade 2: confused
- Grade 3: comatose
- Grade 4: unconscious

Early signs can be demonstrated by asking the patient to copy a five-pointed star.

INFORMATION

Portosystemic encephalopathy (PSE) is a neuropsychiatric syndrome that occurs in cirrhosis. The blood bypasses the liver via collaterals, allowing 'toxic' metabolites to pass directly to the brain. The nature of these 'toxins' is unclear but they appear to be related to ammonia. Treatment is aimed at reduction of protein breakdown in the gut and rifaximin therapy.

Immediate Management

- Measure full blood count, U and Es, blood sugar, liver function and liver biochemistry
- Perform an ascitic tap to rule out infection
- Institute a low-protein and low-salt diet
- Give parenteral thiamine
- Monitor blood glucose levels and treatment hypoglycaemia with intravenous glucos infusion
- Start diuretic therapy (see Ascites)
- Use purgatives: lactulose 10–20 mL × 3/day to produce 2–3 stools a day
- Determine the presence of infection both in ascites (ascitic tap) and systemically (blood culture), and treat.

Further Management

Monitor daily:
- Weight
- Conscious level (Glasgow coma score (GCS) score)
- Liver biochemistry and coagulation
- Electrolytes and blood sugar

Progress. This patient's condition improved dramatically, and she was ready for discharge from hospital after 10 days. She was referred to the alcohol dependency unit and regular follow-up was arranged at the liver clinic.

Excess Alcohol Use

CASE HISTORY

A 45-year-old male presents with a history of excessive alcohol intake for 10 years since his marriage failed. He has sought help from counselling services but has been unable to remain sober. His presenting symptoms were collapses in the street and home – the most recent collapse was witnessed and reported as epileptic.

Neurological examination shows that he is conscious and aware of his surroundings but confused (GCS 13). He has nystagmus and ataxia when asked to walk. **Examination of his legs** shows diminished sensation to light touch, pinprick and vibration below the knees. Ankle jerks are absent.

This male has two features of excess alcohol consumption.
1. **Central findings:** Wernicke–Korsakoff syndrome. This is sometimes reversible with parenteral thiamine therapy.
2. **Peripheral neuropathy:** usually not reversible on alcohol abstinence or vitamin therapy.

Management

Initiate intravenous vitamin therapy without delay, prioritizing parenteral administration of B and C vitamins over the initial 3-day period. Due to the risk of serious allergic reactions, administer injections slowly and be prepared to manage anaphylaxis. Concurrently, administer oral thiamine throughout the hospital stay.

INFORMATION

Seizures occurs in 3% to 10% of patients who have alcohol dependence associated with:
- Alcohol intoxication
- Alcohol withdrawal
- Hypoglycaemia

A full history and examination must be undertaken to exclude:
- Neurological damage (central, peripheral)
- Hepatic damage/signs of liver failure
- Concurrent use of other drugs

Further Treatment

- Enforce complete alcohol withdrawal
- Provide sedation through adequate benzodiazepine dosing, while closely monitoring for respiratory depression
- Maintain close supervision and avoid combining sedatives

- Gradually taper benzodiazepines over the following 5 days, monitoring for the resolution of withdrawal symptoms such as:
  - Perspiration
  - Tremors
  - Nausea and vomiting
  - Restlessness
  - Hallucinations
- Refrain from using antiepileptic drugs

Further Management

Refer patient to specialized agencies for alcohol and drug use for comprehensive assessment and management. Lesser degrees of damage than in the case described can occur in excess alcohol use and must always be assessed in all patients attending hospital. These findings are commonly hidden and should be sought using a nonjudgemental interviewing style.

Additional laboratory investigations, including mean corpuscular volume (MCV), triglycerides, uric acid, and gamma-glutamyl transferase (γ-GT), can provide insights into the extent of physical damage resulting from chronic alcohol use.

REMEMBER

Excessive alcohol consumption can originate from various precipitating factors and cause multifaceted damage encompassing financial, social, psychological and physical domains. A holistic approach addressing all these areas is crucial for effective intervention and recovery.

Progress. This patient was discharged from hospital with regular attendance at the alcohol dependence unit. His attendance became erratic and he started drinking again.

Cholecystitis

CASE HISTORY

A 28-year-old male presents to the emergency department with right hypochondrial pain. This has been persistent, increasing in severity over the last 3 days.

On examination, there is right hypochondrial tenderness. In view of his age and general good health, he is sent home after surgical review, given paracetamol and told to see his doctor for follow-up.

Two days later, a rather concerned doctor phones to say that the patient's pain has persisted and the tenderness is marked. You ask him to send him back to the emergency department. **On examination**, you confirm the doctor's findings of marked tenderness in the right hypochondrium. He has a temperature of 37.8°C.

WHAT SHOULD YOU DO NOW?

Given the ongoing pain and the secondary referral, the patient should be admitted. Conduct the following blood tests as indicated in the investigations box:

INVESTIGATIONS

- Full Blood Count
- Urea and Electrolytes
- Liver Biochemistry
- Serum Amylase
- Blood Culture (considering the presence of fever)

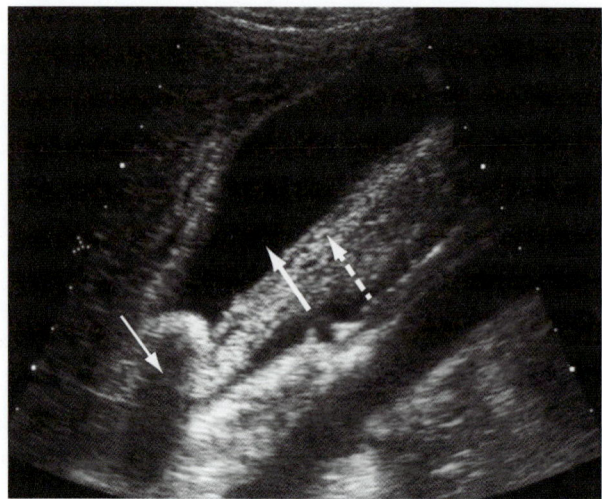

Fig. 5.5   Ultrasound scan in a patient with acute cholecystitis. There is a stone (casting an acoustic shadow – *thin arrow*) impacted in the gall bladder neck, with a distended gall bladder (*thick arrow*), and thickening and oedema of the gall bladder wall (*dashed arrow*). (From Kumar, P., Clark, M., 2017. Kumar and Clark's Clinical Medicine, ninth ed. Biliary tract and pancreatic disease, Edinburgh, Elsevier Ltd, Fig. 15.4.)

Shortly after, a report reveals a raised WCC of 19,000, indicating an infection. Promptly arrange for an urgent ultrasound while informing the surgical registrar of the findings. The patient, previously discharged by the same registrar, is now under review again. The ultrasound scan (Fig. 5.5) shows:

- Presence of gallstones in the gallbladder
- Positive sonographic Murphy's sign
- Thickening of the gallbladder wall
- Pericholecystic fluid

DIAGNOSIS

> **REMEMBER**
>
> - Acute appendicitis is a differential diagnosis, although the pain location is slightly higher than typical
> - Acute cholecystitis is confirmed despite the patient's age and gender; gallstones are not exclusive to any specific demographic
> - Consider other serious conditions like localized perforation, but rely on imaging for accurate diagnosis

The diagnosis of **acute cholecystitis** is made. The surgical specialist registrar initiates treatment with antibiotics (for instance, cefuroxime), places the patient on nil-by-mouth status, and starts IV fluids. A laparoscopic cholecystectomy is scheduled.

> **REMEMBER**
>
> Gallstones can occur at any age. Always think of appendicitis in a young patient with acute pain. Ultrasound/CT scans are invaluable in making the diagnosis.

Progress.   A successful laparoscopic cholecystectomy was performed with no complications.

Acute Cholangitis

CASE HISTORY

A 45-year-old female, with a past medical history of gallstones, presents to the emergency department with a 48-hour history of severe right upper quadrant pain, fever and jaundice. She appears acutely ill and reports chills and changes in stool colour. Her vital signs reveal tachycardia and fever. Laboratory findings demonstrate elevated white blood cell count, abnormal liver enzymes, and direct hyperbilirubinemia. An abdominal ultrasound shows dilated intrahepatic bile ducts and a common bile duct stone.

INFORMATION

Acute cholangitis is a bacterial infection of the bile duct usually secondary to obstruction. Risk factors include gallstones, biliary strictures and previous biliary surgery. Mortality can be high if not treated promptly, but outcomes are excellent with timely antibiotic therapy and biliary decompression.

WHAT IS THE SIGNIFICANCE OF HYPOTENSION AND ALTERED MENTAL STATUS IN ACUTE CHOLANGITIS?

Charcot triad consists of right upper quadrant pain, fever and jaundice. It is commonly used to diagnose acute cholangitis, indicating bile duct obstruction and infection. Hypotension and altered mental status, in addition to Charcot triad, constitute Reynold pentad, which suggests acute suppurative cholangitis, a more severe form that can lead to sepsis and requires urgent intervention.

INVESTIGATIONS

- Elevated liver enzymes, particularly alkaline phosphatase and gamma-glutamyl transferase (GGT)
- Direct hyperbilirubinemia and elevated bilirubin levels
- Ultrasound or CT scan showing biliary dilation and potential causes of obstruction

Management

- Initiate empirical broad-spectrum antibiotics after obtaining blood cultures
- Provide supportive care with fluids and electrolyte management
- Perform biliary drainage using ERCP or percutaneous transhepatic cholangiography (PTC) when ERCP is not available or feasible
- Plan for cholecystectomy after the resolution of cholangitis to prevent recurrence

REMEMBER

Early recognition and prompt antibiotic therapy are key to managing acute cholangitis. Consider acute cholangitis as a potential cause of sepsis in patients with known biliary disease. Monitor for signs of systemic inflammatory response syndrome (SIRS) and sepsis, which can occur in severe cases.

Progress. Following admission, she receives intravenous fluids, broad-spectrum antibiotics and urgent ERCP to remove the obstructing stone. Her symptoms and laboratory abnormalities improve significantly postprocedure. She is scheduled for an elective cholecystectomy to prevent future episodes.

Further Reading

Abnormal Liver Biochemistry

Zeuzem, S., Foster, G.R., Wang, S., et al., 2018. Glecaprevir-pibrentasvir for 8 or 12 weeks in HCV genotype 1 or 3 infection. N. Engl. J. Med. 378 (4), 354–369.

Jaundice

Kindler, H.L., 2018. A glimmer of hope for pancreatic cancer. N. Engl. J. Med. 379 (25), 2463–2464.
NICE, CKS, 2023. Jaundice in adults. NICE.

Excess Alcohol Use

NICE, CKS, 2023. Alcohol – problem drinking. NICE.

Nonalcoholic Fatty Liver Disease

NICE, CKS, 2023. Non-alcoholic fatty liver disease. NICE.

Ascites

Lucey, M.R., 2014. Liver transplantation for alcoholic liver disease. Nat. Rev. Gastroenterol. Hepatol. 11 (5), 300–307.
Moore, K.P., Wong, F., Gines, P., et al., 2003. Management of ascites in cirrhosis. Report on the consensus conference of the International Ascites Club. Hepatology 38 (1), 258–266.

Haematemesis and Melaena

BSG (British Society for Gastroenterology), 2022. UK guidelines for the management of variceal haemorrhage in cirrhotic patients. Available from: www.bsg.org.uk/clinical-resource/uk-guidelines-for-the-management-of-variceal-haemorrhage-in-cirrhotic-patients/.
Jalan, R., Hayes, P.C., 2000. UK guidelines on the management of variceal haemorrhage in cirrhotic patients. Gut 46 (Suppl 3–4), III1–IIII5.

Cholecystitis

NICE, CKS, 2023. Cholecystitis – acute. NICE.

CHAPTER 6

Kidney and Urinary Tract Disease

Presentation of Kidney and Urinary Tract Disease

HOW DO PATIENTS COMMONLY PRESENT WITH KIDNEY AND URINARY TRACT DISEASE?

- Presenting complaints directly related to the urinary tract or urine output, for example, frequency, dysuria, burning micturition, urgency, colic, polyuria, nocturia, haematuria, oliguria and anuria
- Discovery of abnormal laboratory findings during routine investigations, for example, proteinuria, haematuria, elevated plasma creatinine, electrolyte and acid–base disturbances
- Symptoms and signs of renal disease (e.g. uraemia, anaemia, anuria, hypertension and oedema) in the absence of prior renal disease
- Discovery of renal and urinary tract disease as part of involvement in systemic disease, for example,
  - Metabolic disease (e.g. diabetes mellitus): the most common cause of end-stage renal disease (ESRD) in developed nations
  - Autoimmune rheumatic diseases (e.g. systemic lupus erythematosus (SLE), vasculitis, systemic sclerosis, rheumatoid arthritis)
  - Infectious diseases (e.g. Gram-negative sepsis, infective endocarditis, mycobacterial, protozoal, viral)
  - Cardiovascular diseases (e.g. hypertension, heart failure)
  - Blood dyscrasia (e.g. multiple myeloma, amyloidosis, lymphoma, haemolytic uraemic syndrome/thrombotic thrombocytopenic purpura [HUS/TTP])

REMEMBER

- Decline in glomerular filtration rate (GFR): is this due to prerenal, postrenal or intrarenal disease?
- Intrinsic renal disease: divides into glomerular or nonglomerular disorders (e.g. tubular, interstitial or vascular)
- Differentiate between primary renal diseases and renal disorders secondary to systemic disease
- Identify preventable or reversible diseases

Fluid Balance and Electrolytes: Assessing Fluid Status

CLINICAL ASSESSMENT

Take a quick history, particularly of fluid and electrolyte intake (oral or IV) and output (renal, gastrointestinal [GI] tract or skin), and then examine the patient (Fig. 6.1, Table 6.1).

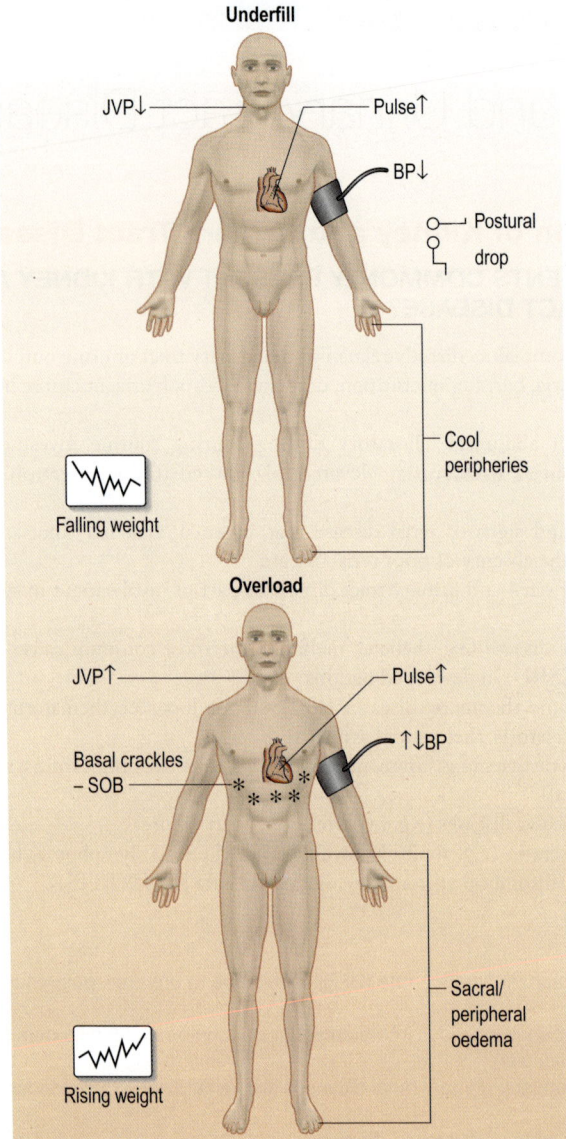

Fig. 6.1   Examining the patient: underfill and overload. SOB, shortness of breath.

CASE HISTORY (1)

A 43-year-old male is brought to the emergency department with a 4-day history of severe abdominal pain and watery diarrhoea up to 10 times daily. He has felt so bad that he has hardly drunk or eaten anything over the last few days. He has lost 5 kg in weight.

He is normally fit and well, and he wonders whether he has some form of severe gastroenteritis.

On examination, he is dehydrated with dry tongue. Abdominal examination reveals some generalised tenderness.

Fig. 6.1A shows the other signs of hypovolaemia.

TABLE 6.1 ▪ **Tools to Assess Fluid Status**

Useful	Not So Useful
Clinical examinations	
BP (especially postural or postexercise drop)	Skin turgor
Oedema	Eye turgor
JVP	Mucous membranes
Peripheral perfusion	
Pulse	
Basal crackles	
Charts	
Serial weight (on same machine)	Fluid balance (input/output)
Additional tools	
CVP line – use dynamically	CVP – absolute
CXR	Urine Na$^+$
Pulmonary artery flow catheter	Osmolality

BP, Blood pressure; CXR, chest X-ray; JVP, jugular venous pressure.

INVESTIGATIONS

- Serum Na 123 mmol/L
- Serum K 2.1 mmol/L
- Chloride 86 mmol/L
- Urea 35 mmol/L
- Creatinine 120 µmol/L
- Haemoglobin (Hb) 154 g/L
- Packed cell volume (PCV) 0.58

WHAT IS THE MOST LIKELY DIAGNOSIS?

Prerenal failure due to dehydration secondary to GI fluid loss.

HOW SHOULD THIS PATIENT BE MANAGED?

Volume replacement can often be achieved with oral rehydration solutions, but because of hypotension, this male was given IV 0.9% saline initially over 1 h, followed by 1 L of 0.9% saline plus 20 mmol K$^+$ 4-hourly for 24 h.

He quickly improved and clinically appeared euvolaemic (normal venous pressure, pulse and BP) by the next day. Stool cultures grew *Campylobacter*, which is a common cause of severe gastroenteritis.

REMEMBER

- Examine the patient again!
- Then again later (today)!!
- And again (tomorrow)!!!
Laboratory tests are no substitute for clinical assessment.

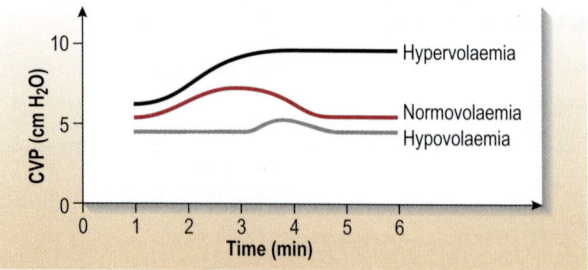

Fig. 6.2   Fluid challenge.

CASE HISTORY (2)

A 24-year-old male was involved in an road traffic accident (RTA), receiving injuries to his chest and abdomen.

On admission to the trauma unit, he is shocked, with a tachycardia of 120 beats per minute (bpm), BP 90/55, and cold clammy peripheries. His Glasgow Coma Scale (GCS) score is 12.

Examination of his chest reveals a right haemothorax. Abdominal examination shows a tender, rigid abdomen with no bowel sounds, suggestive of peritonitis.

HOW SHOULD THIS PATIENT BE MANAGED?

- A comprehensive and systematic ABCDE approach to assessment and management should be taken
- Large-bore intravenous cannulas were inserted and resuscitation with IV crystalloid commenced. A urinary catheter was inserted to monitor urine output
- Arterial and central venous pressure (CVP) lines were inserted to assist with haemodynamic monitoring (Fig. 6.2), facilitate repeat blood sampling and improve venous access. The patient responded both clinically and haemodynamically to the fluid challenge suggesting hypovolaemia. Rapid blood transfusion was started with repeated checks on his fluid status
- An emergency CT scan confirmed the haemothorax and an intercostal tube drain was inserted
- Abdominal CT confirmed free fluid in the abdomen and an abnormal small intestine, suggestive of ischaemia. The liver, spleen and other organs seemed normal
- The patient proceeded to laparotomy

Progress. Postoperatively, his vital signs were stable but he had not passed urine despite fluid replacement. His urea and creatinine had risen significantly on his postoperative bloods indicating acute kidney injury (AKI) due to acute tubular necrosis. Further management was provided by the intensive care unit with the aim of controlling fluid and electrolyte balance whilst treating sepsis until the kidneys spontaneously recover. After 10 days' management, including haemofiltration (necessary for uncontrolled hyperkalaemia), he started to pass urine and eventually made a good recovery.

Fluid Balance and Electrolytes: Sodium

WHAT ARE YOU ACTUALLY ASSESSING WHEN YOU MEASURE SERUM SODIUM?

Serum sodium concentration is effectively a ratio of:
- Extracellular Na^+ in mmol
- Extracellular water in litres

TABLE 6.2 ▪ **Hyponatraemia and Hypernatraemia**

Ratio (Na⁺: Water)	Extracellular Water
Hyponatraemia	
Water ↑	→ or ↓
Water ↑ >Na⁺ ↑	↓↓
Na⁺ ↓	↓
Hypernatraemia	
Water ↓	→ or ↓
Water ↓ >Na⁺ ↓	↓↓
Na⁺ ↑	↑

Using this concept, you can describe how serum Na⁺ becomes abnormally low (hyponatraemia) or high (hypernatraemia) (Table 6.2).

Hyponatraemia is defined as a sodium concentration <135 mmol/L.

Hypernatraemia is defined as a sodium concentration >145 mmol/L.

The key is to determine the extracellular water – examine the patient carefully (see Fig. 6.1).

CASE HISTORY (1)

The gynaecology team is worried about a 53-year-old female who had a trans-abdominal hysterectomy 3 days ago. Her serum Na⁺ has fallen to 123 mmol/L. On examination, there are no features of fluid depletion. The gynaecology trainee asks whether the female should be given IV saline. The polite answer is 'No'!

REMEMBER

Wherever sodium goes, water is sure to follow, and vice versa.

HOW WOULD YOU ASSESS THIS PATIENT?

- Fluid assessment
- Examine fluid charts

You then discover that she had been receiving 5% glucose by IV infusion since surgery 3 days ago. This is a potential cause of hyponatraemia in a surgical patient. Other causes are listed in Box 6.1.

HOW WOULD YOU MANAGE THIS PATIENT?

Stop IV fluids, restrict oral fluids to 1 L daily and allow food as requested by the patient.

Progress. Forty-eight hours later, her serum sodium is 132 mmol/L and she is discharged.

CASE HISTORY (2)

A 47-year-old male is in the neurosurgical unit having had a pituitary tumour removed by transsphenoidal surgery. He has made a normal postoperative recovery, but on review, prior to discharge, he complains of excess thirst and nocturia.

Review of the fluid balance charts show that he is drinking nearly 5 L a day, with a urinary output of 3.5 L.

Recent blood tests show a serum Na⁺ of 153 mmol/L.

You diagnose cranial diabetes insipidus, which you know occurs transiently for a few days or weeks after pituitary surgery.

BOX 6.1 ▪ Other Causes of Hyponatraemia

- Diuretic therapy: loop diuretics, in particular, cause large renal losses of salt and water and metabolic alkalosis
- Severe heart failure, advanced liver cirrhosis or nephrotic syndrome: hyponatraemia with increased total body sodium and even greater excess of water, resulting in ascites and oedema. Plasma osmolality is low. Increased water orally continues in the face of salt restriction, diuretic therapy or both and will aggravate the ascites and oedema
- Syndrome of inappropriate antidiuretic hormone (SIADH) production
- Pseudohyponatraemia: e.g. hyperlipidaemic states where sodium is confined to the aqueous phase or monoclonal gammopathies, hyperglycaemia (10 mmol rise reduces sodium by approximately 2 mmol)

WHAT ARE THE OTHER CAUSES OF HYPERNATRAEMIA?

- Iatrogenic: IV infusion of hypertonic sodium bicarbonate ($NaHCO_3$), hyperalimentation by IV route or nasogastric tube, sodium chloride tablets, sea water drowning or mineralocorticoid excess; total body sodium is elevated in these conditions. Signs are of hypervolaemia
- Impaired thirst/unconscious patient: total body sodium is low because of both sodium and water deficit, but water losses are greater than the losses of sodium. Signs are of hypovolaemia
- Osmotic diuresis, for example, diabetic ketoacidosis, radiocontrast, mannitol: total body sodium is low because of both sodium and water deficit, but water losses are greater than sodium losses. Urine is not maximally concentrated despite the hyperosmolar state, in contrast to GI losses of sodium and water where urine is maximally concentrated. Signs are of hypovolaemia
- Water loss, for example, diabetes insipidus: normal total body sodium. Signs are of euvolaemia

---

REMEMBER

True Na^+ overload is invariably iatrogenic and gives a clinical picture of fluid overload.

HOW WOULD YOU MANAGE THIS PATIENT?

- The goal of treatment is to:
  - Treat any underlying disorder
  - Correct hypovolaemia if present with electrolytes and free water
  - Correct dehydration by replacing free water losses
- Fluid requirement can be estimated by calculating water deficit using the formula:

$$\text{Water deficit (L)} = TBW \times ([\text{serum}[Na^+][\text{mmol/L}] / 145] - 1)$$

TBW = total body water and is estimated by multiplying the lean body weight (in kg) by 0.6 for children and adult males, 0.5 for adult females and elderly males, and 0.45 for elderly females.

- Avoid rapid correction – serum Na^+ should not fall by >1 mmol every 2 h, that is 10 mmol/24 h (Fig. 6.3)
- Give hypotonic fluids (e.g. IV 0.45% saline, 5% dextrose, oral water) with frequent monitoring of volume status and serum Na^+ level
- If shocked, give isotonic fluid (e.g. 0.9% saline) to restore volume
- If poor renal function or severe hyponatraemia (e.g. >170 mmol/L), consider haemofiltration
- Correct any other electrolyte abnormalities, for example, hypokalaemia

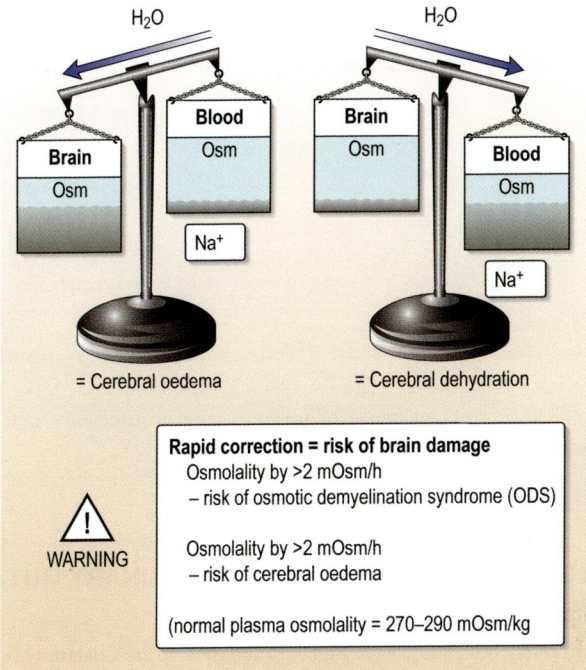

Fig. 6.3 Effect of changes in sodium concentration on the brain.

Low Urine Output

WHAT SHOULD YOU DO?

- Take a detailed history of the type of surgical procedure
- Ask about GI bleeding, dehydration or other fluid losses, nephrotoxic drugs, drugs associated with hypersensitivity reaction causing tubulo-interstitial nephritis (e.g. penicillins,

TABLE 6.3 ▪ Shock – Failure of Organ Perfusion

	BP	Peripheral Perfusion	CVP	Brief Action
Hypovolaemia	↓	↓	↓	Look for overt/covert loss and replace with appropriate fluid, e.g. saline or blood
Cardiogenic	↓	↓	→↑	Myocardial infarction might need inotropes
Sepsis	↓	→↓	→↓	Look for source, give antimicrobials ± inotropes if hypotensive

CVP, Central venous pressure.

NSAIDs, cephalosporins), evidence of previous renal insufficiency, and any radiological procedure with contrast enhancement
- Anuria usually means obstructive uropathy or vasculitides rather than acute tubulo-nephritis (ATN); evidence of these conditions should be sought

WHAT ARE THE COMMON CAUSES OF LOW URINARY OUTPUT?

- Urine retention: always catheterise
- Dehydration: assess fluid status (see Fig. 6.1) and look at fluid balance charts
- Shock: Table 6.3
- Drugs: look at medicines chart

Progress. There is no urine draining from this patient's catheter, and he is hypovolaemic on clinical assessment. His fluid chart is incorrectly filled in, but the patient seems to have received 2 L of fluid (IV and oral) over the last 48 h.

HOW WOULD YOU INITIALLY MANAGE THIS PATIENT?

This male is fluid-depleted and needs fluid replacement (Table 6.4):
- Commence IV crystalloid, for example, Hartmann solution or 0.9% saline. Add 20 mmol/K^+ to maintain 1 mmol/kg/day potassium unless hyperkalaemic
- Write up initial regimen: modulate according to patient age/size and severity of fluid depletion
- Reassess fluid status regularly
- Check U and Es regularly
- Stop potentially nephrotoxic drugs
- Stop antihypertensive drugs
- Ask nurses to record daily weights and to make careful notes of fluid intake and urine output on the fluid chart

WHAT WOULD YOU DO IF THE PATIENT STILL DOES NOT PASS URINE?

- Recheck fluid status
- Check that the urine catheter is not blocked or misplaced
- The patient might now have established AKI – refer to a nephrologist

TABLE 6.4 ▪ **Fluid Replacement**

IV Fluid	Na+ (mmol/L)	K+ (mmol/L)	HCO₃ or Equivalent (mmol/L)	Cl⁻ (mmol/L)	Ca²⁺ (mmol/L)	Indication (See Below)
Normal plasma values	**142**	**4.5**	**26**	**103**	**2.5**	–
1. Sodium chloride 0.9%	150	–	–	150	–	1
2. Sodium chloride 0.18% + glucose 4%	30	–	–	30	–	2
3. Glucose 5% + potassium chloride 0.3%	–	40	–	40	–	3
4. Sodium bicarbonate 1.26%	150	–	150	–	–	4
5. Compound sodium lactate (Hartmann's)	131	5	29	111	2	5
6. Plasma-Lyte 148	140	5	–	98	–	–

1. Volume expansion in hypovolaemic patients. Rarely to maintain fluid balance when there are large losses of sodium. The sodium (150 mmol) is greater than plasma and hypernatraemia can result. It is often necessary to add KCl 20–40 mmol/L.
2. Maintenance of fluid balance in normovolaemic, normonatraemic patients.
3. To replace water. Can be given with or without potassium chloride. May be alternated with 0.9% saline as an alternative to (2).
4. For volume expansion in hypovolaemic, acidotic patients alternating with (1). Occasionally for maintenance of fluid balance combined with (2) in salt-wasting, acidotic patients.
5. Used for maintenance of fluid balance after surgery. The potassium content may be dangerous in renal failure but occasionally useful in the diuretic phase of acute tubular necrosis where hypokalaemia occurs.
6. (6) For fluid replacement with glucose and electrolytes. Used for head injury, intra-operative fluid replacement, fracture and infection.

From Kumar, P., Clark, M., eds., 2017. Kumar and Clark's Clinical Medicine, ninth ed. Elsevier, Edinburgh.

Progress. Fortunately, this male responded to fluid replacement and produced urine, initially 50 mL/h.

REMEMBER

- Do not miss urine retention
- Recognise shock
- Assess fluid status regularly
- Most cases will need fluid replacement, and failure to achieve this can result in established renal failure

Acute Heart Failure

Acute heart failure (AHF) occurs when cardiac function falls, causing elevated cardiac filling pressure. This causes severe breathlessness with fluid accumulating in the interstitial and alveolar spaces of the lung (pulmonary oedema).

CASE HISTORY

A 65-year-old 50 kg female who smokes 20 cigarettes per day, and has a history of intermittent claudication, presented to the emergency department with acute shortness of breath (SOB).

On examination, she was centrally cyanosed and peripherally cold and clammy. She had a raised jugular venous pressure (JVP), and on auscultation, she had a gallop rhythm and bilateral coarse crackles up to both mid-zones. She had absent foot pulses and bilateral femoral bruits. Her BP at presentation was 195/98.

Her ECG showed hypertensive changes (with left ventricular hypertrophy), and a CXR showed bilateral perihilar shadowing. Initially, her biochemistry was:

- Na: 142 mmol/L
- K: 3.1 mmol/L
- Urea: 12 mmol/L
- Creatinine: 115 μmol/L, estimated glomerular filtration rate (eGFR) 44 mL/min/1.73 m^2

WHAT IS THE LIKELY DIAGNOSIS?

Flash pulmonary oedema

Progress. She responded well to oxygen, IV morphine, and IV furosemide but 4 days later her biochemistry was:

- Na: 142 mmol/L
- K: 6.0 mmol/L
- Urea: 54 mmol/L
- Creatinine: 500 μmol/L (Fig. 6.4), eGFR 8 mL/min/1.73 m^2

WHAT DO THESE RESULTS SUGGEST?

It is very likely that she has developed acute kidney injury (AKI) due to underlying renovascular disease.

WHAT CLINICAL FEATURES ARE CONSISTENT WITH RENOVASCULAR DISEASE?

- Most patients will have disseminated atheroma with missing pulses and/or bruits and a history of smoking
- Abdominal/renal bruits are rare (although they have a very strong association with renal artery stenosis [RAS])

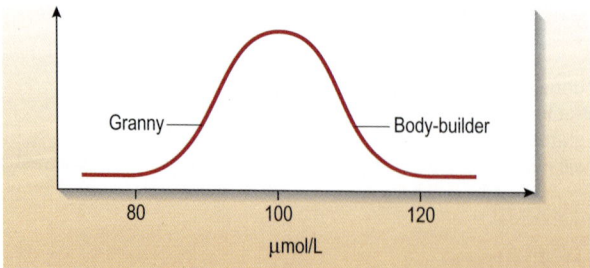

Fig. 6.4 Interpreting serum creatinine. The serum creatinine in the healthy population is normally distributed according to muscle bulk. Only large, well-muscled males will usually have a creatinine >110 if their renal function is normal. Therefore, for small people, creatinine does not enter the 'abnormal' range until half their renal function has been lost.

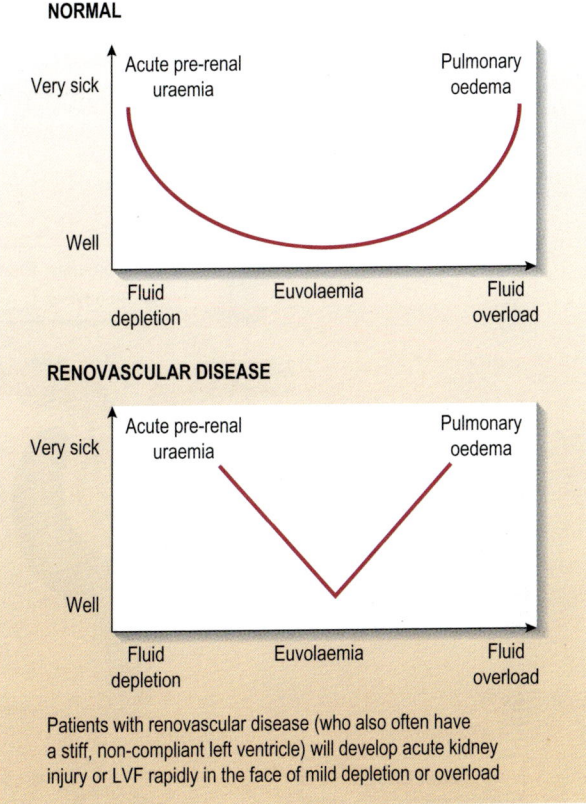

Fig. 6.5 Fluid status in normal and renovascular disease. LVF, Left ventricular failure.

- 'Flash pulmonary oedema' (without an obvious precipitant) is a good predictor of renovascular disease
- There is a brittle response to volume loading or off-loading (Fig. 6.5)

Note: this patient's renal function was abnormal at presentation, but angiotensin-converting enzyme (ACE) inhibitors can cause acute kidney injury in patients with renovascular disease (Fig. 6.6).

HOW SHOULD PATIENTS LIKE THIS BE MANAGED?

The key to successful management is very careful fluid control.

Managing Acute Heart Failure (AHF) in the Presence of Suspected Renovascular Disease

- Treat the pulmonary oedema with IV diuretics, for example, furosemide: it is a dangerous and very distressing condition
- Avoid ACE inhibitors (ACEIs)/A II blockers: use other vasodilators
- Avoid rapid volume off-loading: titrate the diuretic dose against renal function
- Examine (and weigh) the patient regularly

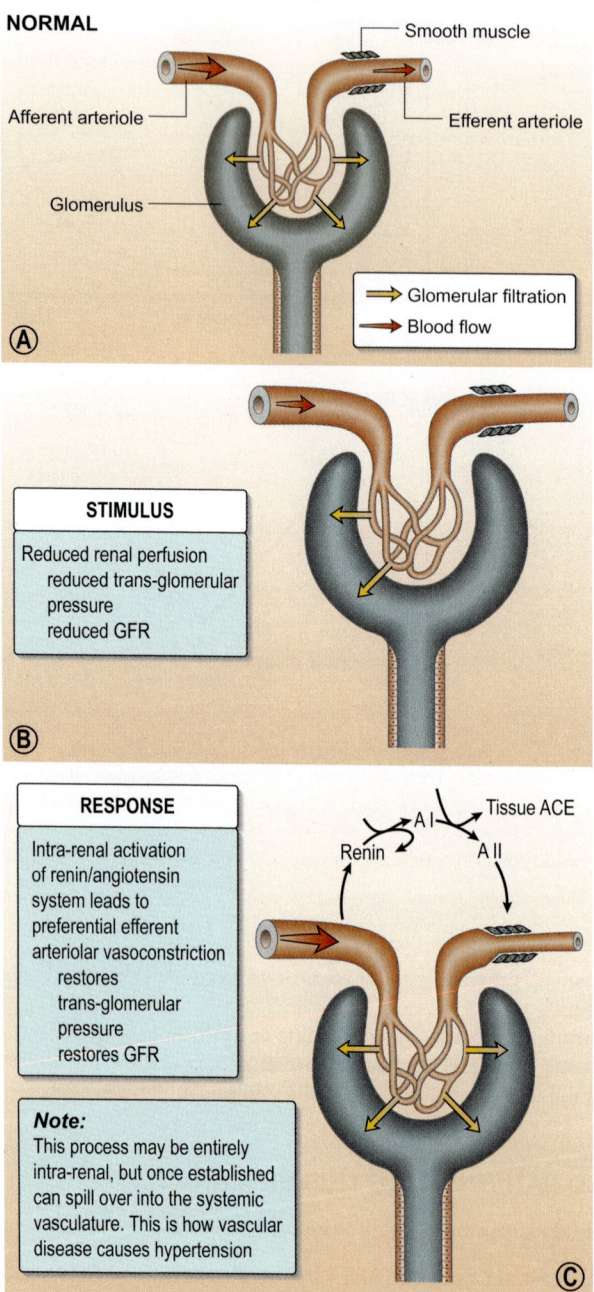

NORMAL

Smooth muscle

Afferent arteriole

Efferent arteriole

Glomerulus

⟹ Glomerular filtration
⟹ Blood flow

Ⓐ

STIMULUS

Reduced renal perfusion
reduced trans-glomerular
pressure
reduced GFR

Ⓑ

RESPONSE

Intra-renal activation
of renin/angiotensin
system leads to
preferential efferent
arteriolar vasoconstriction
restores
trans-glomerular
pressure
restores GFR

Tissue ACE
A I
Renin   A II

Note:
This process may be entirely
intra-renal, but once established
can spill over into the systemic
vasculature. This is how vascular
disease causes hypertension

Ⓒ

Fig. 6.6   (A–D) Effect of angiotensin-converting enzyme (ACE) inhibitors/blockers. A I/A II, angiotensin I/II.

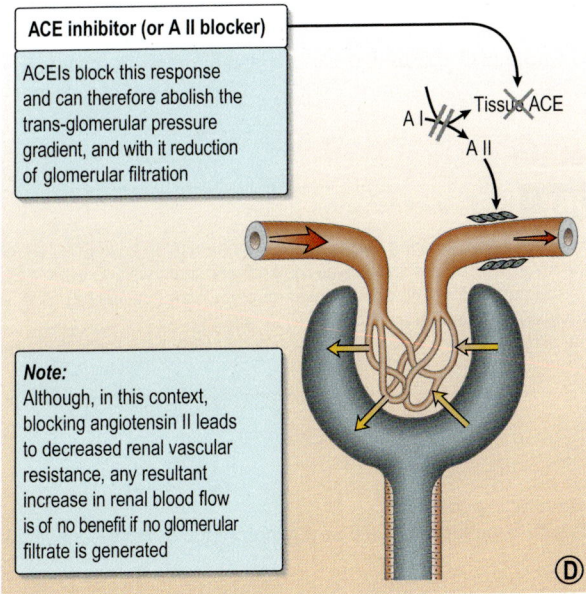

ACE inhibitor (or A II blocker)

ACEIs block this response and can therefore abolish the trans-glomerular pressure gradient, and with it reduction of glomerular filtration

Note:
Although, in this context, blocking angiotensin II leads to decreased renal vascular resistance, any resultant increase in renal blood flow is of no benefit if no glomerular filtrate is generated

Fig. 6.6—cont'd

Renal Imaging Investigations

- Ultrasound: unequal renal size (>2 cm difference) is a good predictor of renovascular disease, but its absence does not exclude RAS. Duplex ultrasound is used to demonstrate renal artery perfusion
- Isotope renography: unequal function, slow transit and altered dynamics with captopril are all suggestive of renovascular disease. In experienced hands and with good renal function, its sensitivity and specificity are 70% (creatinine <150 μmol/L); however, in inpatients with severe renal impairment, its sensitivity falls below 30%
- Magnetic resonance (MR) angiography is increasingly used to visualise the renal arteries
- Intraarterial angiography: rarely undertaken but is the gold standard – should be carried out by experienced radiologists with minimal contrast load

Progress. This patient responded to treatment of her AHF, her pulmonary oedema resolved and her renal function returned to normal.

She was then investigated for RAS, with MR angiography showing a narrowing of the right renal artery, thought to be due to atherosclerosis.

She was continued on diuretics and amlodipine, with good control of her BP. She is under regular review.

NATURAL HISTORY OF ATHEROMATOUS RENOVASCULAR DISEASE

- ACE inhibitors/A II blockers will cause AKI only if both kidneys are affected by RAS or if only one functioning kidney is present. However, the atheroma is diffuse and progressive. Complete renal artery occlusion with total loss of renal function on one side is usually clinically silent

- Anatomical renovascular disease is very common and much of it is not physiologically significant (but you cannot tell which is which until it is too late)
- Small vessel (intrarenal) disease behaves identically to main renal artery disease (but you cannot treat it)

Hyperkalaemia

CASE HISTORY

A 70-year-old female has been admitted by vascular surgeons with an acutely ischaemic lower limb. The right leg, below the knee, was cold, the skin was mottled, and there was no pulse palpable. The patient was in agony with the pain in the limb and she was given IV morphine 10 mg. She is on an ACEI and diuretic for hypertension and also on an NSAID.

It is 2 a.m. The surgical trainee calls you because her K^+ has come back at 7.2 mmol/L and wants your help.

REMEMBER

- This is a life-threatening condition
- Most patients with hyperkalaemia will be asymptomatic or have nonspecific symptoms only

WHAT WOULD YOU DO NEXT?

- 12-lead ECG
- Immediate **cardioprotection**:
  - 30 mL of 10% Ca gluconate (or 10 mL 10% calcium chloride) over 10 min
  - *Note:* action is relatively short-lived but dose can be replaced every 15 min
- **Get K^+ inside cells** (Fig. 6.7): 50 mL of 50% glucose with (or followed by) 10 U insulin (consider also administering nebulised salbutamol)
- Consider IV 50 mL $NaHCO_3$ 8.4% over 1 h for severe acidosis
- Consider emergency haemofiltration in the presence of end-stage renal failure or if the potassium is rising rapidly and/or is not responding to medical management
- *Note:* if the patient has a nasogastric tube, then put it on free suction because it will remove acid and potassium, causing systemic alkalosis and encouraging the influx of potassium intracellularly (Fig. 6.7)
- Alongside this, administer an oral cation-exchange resin, such as sodium zirconium cyclosilicate (Lokelma), to rapidly increase potassium excretion

Now you have time to stop and think. Find and treat the cause of the hyperkalaemia.

REMEMBER

1 mL of 8.4% $NaHCO_3$ = 1 mmol Na^+. Do not harm your patient with sodium overload (see Fig. 6.1).

WHAT ARE THE COMMON REVERSIBLE CAUSES OF HYPERKALAEMIA?

- Tissue hypoxia/damage
- Acidosis
- K^+-sparing diuretics
- Angiotensin-converting enzyme inhibitors

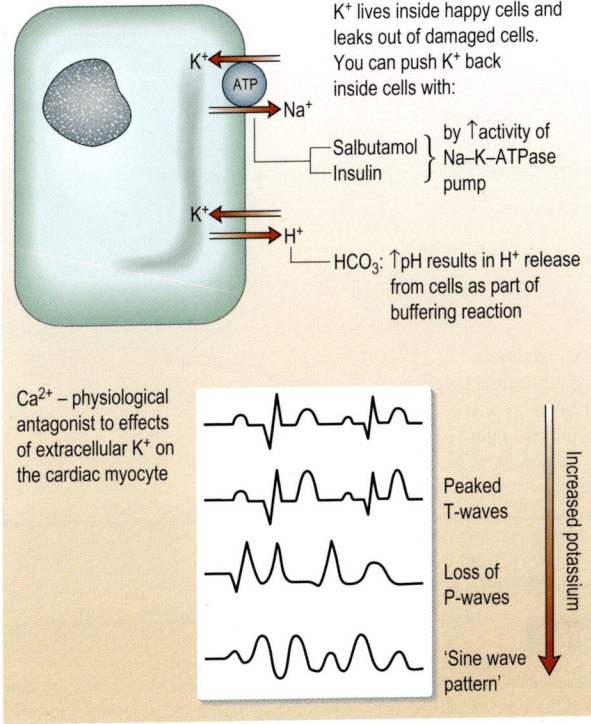

Fig. 6.7   Potassium: some facts.

- Blood transfusion
- Acute kidney injury

Less common causes of hyperkalaemia are listed in Box 6.2.

WHAT QUICK AND SIMPLE INTERVENTIONS CAN IMPROVE HYPERKALAEMIA?

- Establish a diuresis
- Stop ACEIs/NSAIDs
- Stop blood transfusion
- Successfully treat sepsis

REMEMBER

If K^+ is not responding, your patient might need dialysis. If the patient's early U and Es suggest acute or chronic kidney disease (CKD), make arrangements to move him/her to a dialysis unit after initial resuscitative measures. Do not sit too long on such patients – dialysis could be the only option.

Progress. An urgent angiogram was performed, which showed a thrombosis in the right femoral artery near the junction of the popliteal artery.

Thrombolysis was initially used, as the surgeons felt removal of the thrombus would not be feasible. The patient did not respond and gangrene occurred, so that a below-knee amputation then became necessary.

BOX 6.2 ▪ Less Common Causes of Hyperkalaemia

Endocrine

- Addison disease
- Isolated hypoaldosteronism
- C-21 hydroxylase deficiency
- Congenital adrenal syndromes, e.g. 3-β hydroxy dehydrogenase deficiency

Additional Drugs

- Ciclosporin
- Succinylcholine
- NSAIDs

Others

- Tumour lysis syndrome
- Periodic hyperkalaemia paralysis
- Malignant hyperthermia
- Familial hyperkalaemia acidosis

NSAIDs, Nonsteroidal antiinflammatory drugs.

The Acidotic Patient

CASE HISTORY

A 50-year-old female with CKD developed laryngeal oedema as an idiosyncratic reaction to a phenothiazine. She became hypotensive and oliguric. On admission, her blood gases showed:

- pH: 6.9 (Fig. 6.8)
- PO_2: 6.0
- PCO_2: 8.2
- Bicarbonate (HCO_3): 15

Following intubation, ventilation and fluid resuscitation, her BP rose to 145/70. Her blood gases returned to normal over the next 12 h.

REMEMBER

Only <5% of patients admitted with pH 7.0 or less survive to discharge from hospital. This is because severe acidosis is usually a reflection of serious underlying problems.

HOW WOULD YOU MANAGE A SEVERELY ACIDOTIC PATIENT?

First, assess:

- Airway
- Breathing
- Circulation

Problems with any of these will contribute to acidosis and must be corrected.

Then identify and treat the underlying problem. Tissue damage/hypoxia is by far the most common cause of metabolic acidosis due to lactic acidosis. Examples include:

- Sepsis:
    - Hypotensive patient with warm peripheries
    - Often apyrexial and/or normal WCC on presentation, especially if very sick or elderly
    - Sometimes develop low PO_4

- Remember pH is a log scale. A pH of <7.15 means that the $[H^+]$ (hydrogen ion concentration) has doubled.
- Before pH falls significantly, extensive buffering capacity must be consumed. Once this has happened, patients are highly unstable.

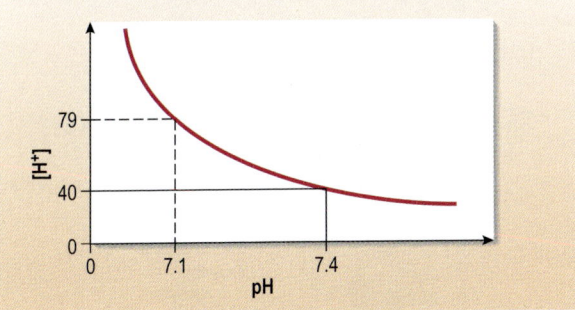

Fig. 6.8 pH: some facts.

- Rhabdomyolysis:
  - Areas of muscle necrosis not always clinically evident
  - $PO_4 \uparrow, K^+ \uparrow$
  - Might have a biphasic Ca^{2+} pattern (initially $\downarrow$ due to binding to damaged muscle, then $\uparrow$)
- Bowel ischaemia:
  - Severe acidosis
  - $PO_4 \uparrow, K^+ \uparrow$
  - Often have evidence of peripheral vascular disease
- Heart failure:
  - Pump failure leading to tissue hypoperfusion
  - Often accompanied by renal hypoperfusion and impaired renal function
- Overproduction of acid or inability to excrete acid. Examples include:
  - Diabetic ketoacidosis
  - Kidney injury
  - Alcoholic ketoacidosis
  - Salicylate intoxication
  - Methanol poisoning
  - Ethylene glycol ingestion

Note: all the above can result in metabolic acidosis with high anionic gap.

Examples of normal anionic gap acidosis (hyperchloraemic acidosis):

- Diarrhoea
- Renal tubular acidosis
- Dehydration
- Interstitial renal disease
- Ureterosigmoidostomy
- Carbonic anhydrase inhibitors (acetazolamide)
- Arginine hydrochloride ingestion
- Ammonium chloride ingestion

REMEMBER

Find and treat the underlying cause.

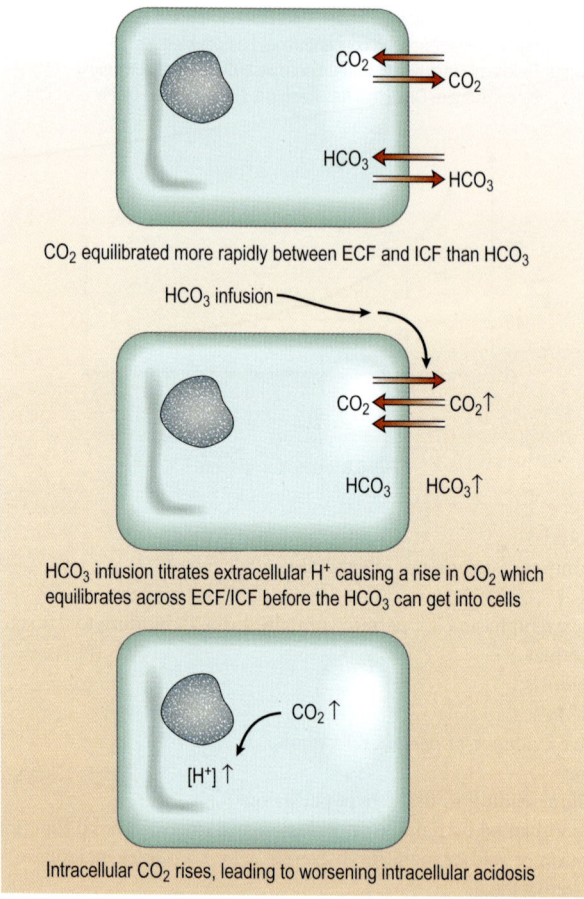

Fig. 6.9 Theoretical reasons for adverse effect of HCO_3 in small rodent models of lactic acidosis. Conclusions: if you are called to accident and emergency (A and E) to see a rat with lactic acidosis, do not under any circumstances give it IV $NaHCO_3$. ECF, Extracellular fluid; ICF, intracellular fluid.

WOULD YOU GIVE IV HCO₃ TO THIS PATIENT?

- The role of IV HCO_3 is not clear (Fig. 6.9)!
- Remember, 8.4% HCO_3 = 1 mmol/mL Na^+. It is very easy to precipitate volume overload
- HCO_3 might be indicated if pH is <7.25 in an attempt to reduce the depression of myocardial function produced by severe acidosis

REMEMBER

Bicarbonate will not save your patient if you do not correct the underlying cause of acidosis (but it might help keep them alive until you do)

Acute Kidney Injury

Acute kidney injury is an abrupt deterioration of renal function over the course of a few days or weeks. It is usually (but not always) reversible.

TABLE 6.5 ▪ **KDIGO Classification of Acute Kidney Injury**

Stage	Serum Creatinine Concentration (SCr)	Urine Output Criteria
1	SCr 1.5–1.9 times baseline OR ≥26.5 µmol/L (0.3 mg/dL) increase	<0.5 mL/kg per h for 6–12 h
2	SCr 2–2.9 times baseline	<0.5 mL/kg per h for 6–12 h
3	SCr 3 times baseline OR Initiation of renal replacement therapy OR In patients <18 years, decrease in eGFR to <35 mL/min/1.73 m²	Anuria for ≥12 h

eGFR, Estimated glomerular filtration rate; KDIGO, Kidney Disease: Improving Global Outcomes; SCr, serum creatinine.

CASE HISTORY

A 75-year-old male has a 5-day history of anorexia, nausea, vomiting and lethargy. His doctor has noted the following findings:
- Haemoglobin: 100 g/L
- Urea: 48 mmol/L
- Creatinine: 820 µmol/L; eGFR 6 mL/min/1.73 m²
- K⁺ 6.1 mmol/L

His previous medical history includes mild hypertension and osteoarthritis.

WHAT ARE THE DIAGNOSTIC CRITERIA FOR AKI?

The definition of AKI used in clinical and epidemiological studies is based on specific criteria that have been sequentially developed. The Kidney Disease: Improving Global Outcomes (KDIGO) definition and staging system is the most recent and preferred (Table 6.5). Others include the (risk, injury, failure, loss of kidney function and end-stage kidney disease (RIFLE) criteria; Table 6.6), and a subsequent modification proposed by the Acute Kidney Injury Network (AKIN) and others.

The KDIGO criteria differ from the RIFLE classification in that the former utilise only changes in serum creatinine and urine output for staging, not changes in GFR; the exception is made for children under the age of 18 years, for whom an acute decrease in eGFR to <35 mL/min/1.73m² is included in the criteria for stage 3 AKI.

WHAT ARE YOUR TREATMENT PRIORITIES?

- Treat the hyperkalaemia (see p. 224)
- Fluid assessment (see Fig. 6.1):
  - Hypovolaemic: treat with fluids
  - Hypervolaemic: treat with fluid restriction

In this case, the patient has a K⁺ of 6.1 mmol/L and he is euvolaemic. At this stage, review/stop any drug therapy. Now, you have to consider:
- Why does this patient have an AKI?
- Is it reversible?

TABLE 6.6 ▪ **RIFLE Criteria for Acute Kidney Injury[a]**

Grade	GFR Criteria	UO Criteria
Risk	SCr × 1.5 or GFR decrease >25% (within 48 h)	<0.5 mL/kg per h × 6 h
Injury	SCr × 2 or GFR decrease >50%	<0.5 mL/kg per h × 12 h
Failure	SCr × 3, GFR decrease >75%, SCr >350 µmol/L with an acute rise >40 µmol/L	<0.3 mL/kg per h × 24 h
Loss	Persistent AKI >4 weeks	
ESKD	Persistent ESKD >3 months	

ESKD, end-stage kidney disease; GFR, Glomerular filtration rate; RIFLE, risk, injury, failure, loss of kidney function and end-stage kidney disease; SCr, serum creatinine; UO, urinary output.
[a]There is a consensus definition that merges RIFLE criteria and the Acute Kidney Injury Network definition (Kidney Disease: Improving Global Outcomes [KDIGO] group 2012).
From Bellomo, R., Ronco, C., Kellum, J.A. et al. 2004. Acute renal failure – definition, outcome measures, animal models, fluid therapy and information technology needs: the Second International Consensus Conference of the Acute Dialysis Quality Initiative (ADQI) Group. Crit Care 8, R204. https://doi.org/10.1186/cc2872.

- Do you need to refer to a renal unit?
- What further investigations would you request?

Urinalysis

Blood and protein suggest active glomerular disease in the absence of infection. Some hospitals provide a facility for urinary red blood cell (RBC) morphology on fresh urine by polarising microscopy. Predominant dysmorphic RBCs are highly suggestive of glomerular pathology.

INVESTIGATIONS

- Ultrasound
- Immunological markers: antinuclear antibodies (ANA), extractable nuclear antigen (ENA), antineutrophil cytoplasmic antibody (ANCA), antiglomerular basement membrane (GBM) antibodies, cryoglobulins, complements, antistreptolysin O titre (ASOT)
- Serum protein electrophoresis
- Twenty-four-hour urinary protein loss

Renal Tract Imaging (Box 6.3)

In this case, the renal ultrasound is normal. This tells you:
- There is a low probability of obstruction
- There is potentially a reversible component

Renal Unit Referral

- Do not delay! The most common concern expressed by renal units is that referring teams wait too long to transfer cases and patients are in a critical condition when they arrive at the unit
- Be ready to provide further information

WHEN WOULD DIALYSIS BE INDICATED?

There is no magic level of urea or creatinine. Dialysis is indicated:
- In uncontrolled hyperkalaemia and/or uraemia

BOX 6.3 ▪ **Renal Tract Imaging**

Ultrasound

- Noninvasive
- Independent of renal function
- Can measure size (renal length and cortical thickening)
- Limited or no view of ureters
- Low detection rate of renal calculi
- Operator-dependent

CT

- Has largely replaced IVU
- First-line investigation for cases of ureteric colic

Intravenous Urogram (IVU)

- Good visualisation of pelvico-calyceal system and ureters
- Gives some functional information

- In unresponsive pulmonary oedema
- When patient symptoms demand

Progress. In this case, the patient turned out to be taking a therapeutic excess of NSAIDs. He required haemodialysis for uncontrolled vomiting and subsequently had a renal biopsy. This showed tubulo-interstitial nephritis secondary to NSAIDs. He responded well to a short course of steroids.

WHAT QUESTIONS WILL YOU BE ASKED WHEN REFERRING TO A RENAL UNIT?

- Is the patient passing urine?
- What is the patient's fluid status?
- Have you done a renal ultrasound (Box 9.4)?
- What are the urinalysis results?
- Any nephrotoxic drugs?
- Hepatitis status?
- Any information on the patient's prior renal function?

Chronic Kidney Disease

Chronic kidney disease (CKD) is used to describe long-standing, usually progressive, impairment in renal function.

CASE HISTORY

A 35-year-old female registers with a new doctor and is found to be hypertensive (180/105), with blood and protein in her urine. She has no specific symptoms.

On examination, there is pallor, BP 180/105, grade II hypertension, retinopathy. On renal ultrasound, a small, nonobstructed kidney is seen.

INVESTIGATIONS

- Haemoglobin: 85 g/L
- Urea: 18.0 mmol/L
- Creatinine: 310 μmol/L; eGFR: 20 mL/min/1.73 m^2 (Box 6.4)

BOX 6.4 ▪ **Equations Used to Estimate Glomerular Filtration Rate (GFR) in Clinical Practice**

Modification of Diet in Renal Disease (MDRD) Equation

- Calculates GFR from 4 to 6 variables (age, sex, race, serum creatinine concentration ± urea, albumin)
- It is not valid for use in patients with malnutrition or those who have had a limb amputation. Interpret it with caution at extremes of body weight
- The four-variable MDRD equation is the most widely used eGFR measurement in clinical practice

Cockcroft–Gault Equation

- Well validated but the formula requires an accurate weight

―――――――

eGFR: estimated glomerular filtration rate.

Clinical features seen in CKD are shown in Fig. 6.10 and classification in Table 6.7.

This female has irreversible CKD and subsequent follow-up showed a progressive rise in creatinine. *Note:* Not all patients with CKD have small, shrunken kidneys. Normal or larger-than-normal kidneys can be seen in diabetic nephropathy, amyloidosis, polycystic kidneys and hydronephrosis (here, cortical thinning is the sign of irreversibility).

HOW DO YOU MANAGE THIS PATIENT?

REMEMBER

Control of hypertension is the single most useful factor in CKD.

The approach should be multidisciplinary (Fig. 6.11).

Preparing the Patient

- Educate: a specialist counsellor should be consulted.
- Renoprotection (Box 6.5).

SPECIFIC CONDITIONS

Hyperparathyroidism

- Measure parathyroid hormone (PTH): X-rays become diagnostic only in advanced cases
- Control phosphate:
  - Dietitian
  - Phosphate-binding drugs, for example, calcium carbonate, calcium acetate, Sevelamer and aluminium hydroxide (in selected cases)
- Vitamin D analogues (e.g. alfacalcidol)
- Monitor Ca^{2+}, phosphate, PTH and alkaline phosphatase levels

Anaemia

- Correct iron deficiency (if present)
- Erythropoietin: can only be given IV or by subcutaneous (SC) injection × 1–3 weekly. Epoetin alfa can only be given by IV route because of increased risk of pure red cell aplasia (PRCA)
- Target Hb 115–130 g/L
- Monitor BP

Progress. This patient with CKD had well-controlled BP, but her renal function gradually deteriorated. She eventually agreed to have haemodialysis and possible transplantation in the future.

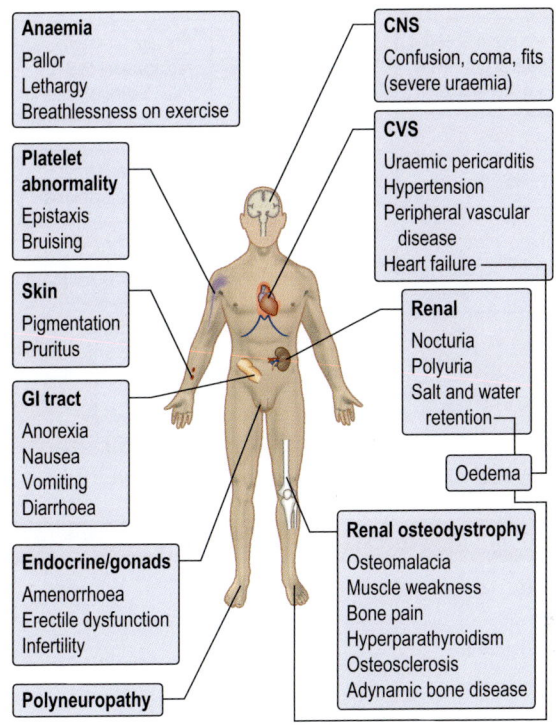

Fig. 6.10 Symptoms and signs of chronic kidney disease. (From Kumar, P., Clark, M., eds., 2017. Kumar and Clark's Clinical Medicine, ninth ed. Elsevier, Edinburgh.)

TABLE 6.7 ▪ Classification of CKD

Stage	GFR (mL/min per 1.73 m²)	Description
1	≥90	Normal or increased GFR with other evidence of kidney damage
2	60–89	Slight decrease in GFR with other evidence of kidney damage
3A	45–59	Moderate decrease in GFR with or without other evidence of
3B	30–44	kidney damage
4	15–29	Severe decrease in GFR with or without other evidence of kidney damage
5	<15	Established renal failure

CKD, Chronic kidney disease; GFR, glomerular filtration rate.

Note: The suffix 'P' can be applied to the stage of CKD if the patient has significant proteinuria, defined as urinary albumin:creatinine ratio >65 mg/mmol or protein: creatinine ratio >100 mg/mmol,

From Kidney Disease: Improving Global Outcomes (KDIGO) CKD Work Group, 2013. KDIGO 2012 clinical practice guideline for the evaluation and management of chronic kidney disease, Kidney Int. 3 (1), 1–150.

REMEMBER

- Chronic kidney disease is an insidious condition with no specific symptoms. In some cases, patients do not present until they have reached the stage when dialysis is required
- Preparing the patient for dialysis is a specialist task: refer!
- Chronic kidney disease is a major cardiovascular risk factor: the average dialysis patient is at an approximately 20 times higher risk

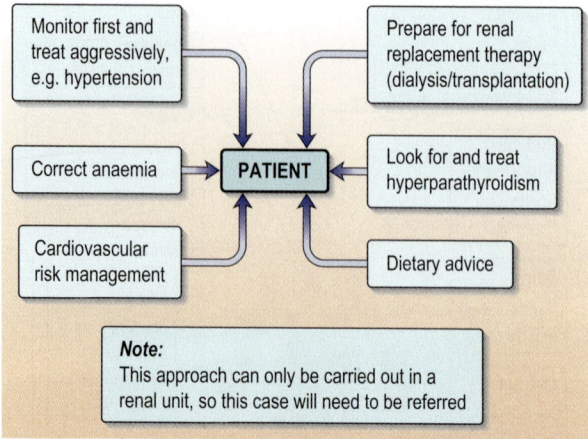

Fig. 6.11 Multidisciplinary approach to chronic kidney disease.

BOX 6.5 ▪ Renoprotection

Goals of Treatment

- BP <120/80
- Proteinuria <0.3 g/24 h

Treatment

Patients with CKD and proteinuria >1 g/24 h:

- ACE inhibitor increasing to a maximum dose
- Add angiotensin receptor antagonist if goals are not achieved
- Add diuretic to prevent hyperkalaemia and to help control BP
- Add calcium-channel blocker (verapamil or diltiazem) if goals are not achieved

Additional Measures

- Statins to lower cholesterol to <4.5 mmol/L
- Smoking cessation (threefold higher rate of deterioration in CKD, if a smoker)
- Treat diabetes (HbA_{1c} <7%/53 mmol/moL)
- Normal protein diet (0.8–1 g/kg body weight)
- Decide on the mode of therapy: haemodialysis vs. peritoneal dialysis versus pre-emptive renal transplantation if a live-related or spousal kidney donor is willing to donate
- Plan access surgery: an arteriovenous fistula requires at least 6 weeks before it can be used
- In type 2 diabetes, start with angiotensin receptor antagonist

ACE: Angiotensin-converting enzyme, CKD: chronic kidney disease, HbA_{1c}: glycated haemoglobin.

Multisystem Vasculitis/Acute Glomerulonephritis

CASE HISTORY

A 54-year-old male with a 1-month history of cough and SOB, which has not responded to two courses of antibiotics from his doctor (amoxicillin, then clarithromycin and coamoxiclav), represented to his doctor complaining of fatigue, muscle aches and pains.

A week later, he then presented to the emergency department complaining of acute SOB. His CXR showed fluffy bilateral patchy alveolar shadowing, and his serum creatinine was 350 µmol/L. On further investigation, he was found to be c-ANCA-positive. Renal biopsy showed focal necrotising glomerulonephritis. He responded well to immunosuppression with corticosteroids and cyclophosphamide.

INFLAMMATORY AUTOIMMUNE VASCULITIS: MICROSCOPIC POLYANGIITIS/GRANULOMATOSIS WITH POLYANGIITIS

Presentation is very nonspecific: typically, vague arthralgia and myalgia with fatigue, anorexia and malaise. At a later stage, patients might develop:

- Vasculitic rash
- Mononeuritis multiplex
- Arthritis
- Ear/nose/throat symptoms, such as epistaxis or deafness

At this point, the diagnosis is more obvious, but these diseases respond well to treatment if diagnosed early.

HOW TO DIAGNOSE MULTISYSTEM VASCULITIS

If you find microscopic haematuria in a patient with nonspecific malaise/myalgia:

- Enquire specifically for suggestive symptoms:
  - Nasal congestion/nose bleeds with polyangiitis (granulomatosis with polyangiitis)
  - Rash
  - Neurological symptoms
- Examine carefully for:
  - Splinter haemorrhages
  - Nail-fold infarcts
  - Mouth ulcers
  - Rash
  - Neuropathy
- Do not assume that microscopic haematuria is due to a urinary tract infection (UTI): send mid-stream urine (MSU)
- If there are suggestive symptoms or signs: discuss with a nephrologist
- If there are no suggestive symptoms or signs but MSU is negative for a UTI: check renal function. If it is abnormal, discuss with a nephrologist

Antineutrophil Cytoplasmic Antibody (Fig. 6.12)

- False-positives occur in situations of polyclonal B-cell activation (usually on immunohistology but not against specific target antigens)
- Antineutrophil cytoplasmic antibody-negative small-vessel vasculitis can be clinically and pathologically identical to ANCA-positive vasculitis
- Changes in antibody titre might be unrelated to, lag behind or precede changes in disease activity in different patients

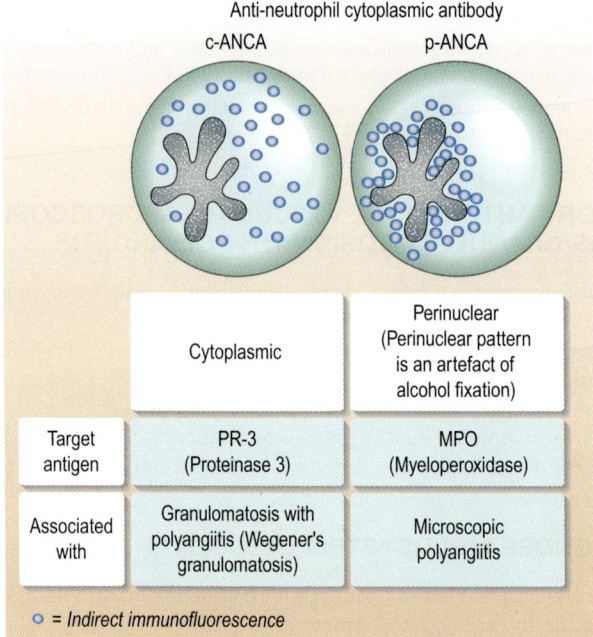

Fig. 6.12 Antineutrophil cytoplasmic antibody.

Other Markers of Disease Activity

↑ Erythrocyte sedimentation rate (ESR), ↑ C-reactive protein (CRP), thrombocytosis

OTHER RAPIDLY PROGRESSIVE GLOMERULONEPHRITIDES

- Goodpasture disease is rare: it is classically described as a 'one-hit' disease and is less likely to be preceded by a nonspecific prodrome than ANCA-positive vasculitis
- Immunoglobin A (IgA) nephropathy, mesangiocapillary glomerulonephritis due to cryo-globulins, and diffuse proliferative glomerulonephritis in SLE can all present with a rapidly progressive, crescentic nephritis

> **REMEMBER**
>
> If diagnosed late, these diseases have difficult and life-threatening complications.

PULMONARY HAEMORRHAGE

- Most common disease-related cause of death in ANCA-positive vasculitis and anti-GBM disease (Goodpasture syndrome)
- Chest X-ray appearances are very variable but there is usually patchy alveolar shadowing (can mimic, or be accompanied by, pulmonary oedema or chest infection)
- Often precipitated by pulmonary oedema/infection/smoking
- Subclinical haemorrhage can be diagnosed noninvasively by finding increased carbon monoxide transfer factor (KCO); transfer factor (carbon monoxide [CO]) binds to blood and gives falsely elevated KCO

Management

The patient requires an urgent nephrology and ICU referral. These individuals can become very sick very quickly and may need ventilation and plasma exchange.

Intercurrent Illness in Dialysis and Transplant Patients

CASE HISTORY (1)

A 72-year-old patient with type 2 diabetic haemodialysis was brought in by urgent ambulance to the emergency department complaining of chest pain and SOB. He was due to be dialysed later that day at the nearest renal unit (5 miles away).

On admission, he had signs of mild biventricular heart failure with a tachycardia, raised venous pressure, gallop rhythm, basal crackles and peripheral oedema. His ECG showed lateral ischaemia and his Hb was 58 g/L.

He was given IV nitrates and 2 units of blood under cover of 40 mg furosemide. As the second unit of blood ran through, he complained of acute SOB and then suffered a cardiorespiratory arrest, from which he could not be resuscitated.

REMEMBER

- Do not give blood transfusion in a dialysis patient unless a nephrologist tells you to. You could precipitate lethal hyperkalaemia and volume overload (and the normal methods of treating these complaints will be ineffective)
- Also, even if your patient survives, you might sensitise them to HLA antigens in the blood, thereby removing the chance of a renal transplant
- As a general rule, dialysis patients should not be transfused while on dialysis

WHAT ELSE REQUIRES CAREFUL CONSIDERATION IN DIALYSIS PATIENTS?

Access Preservation

Dialysis access is essential for life-preserving treatment; potential sites for it are limited and easily damaged irretrievably (Fig. 6.13).

Use veins in hands or feet or the antecubital fossa. For central access use the internal jugular vein.

Fluids

Caution is advised to prevent volume overload. Dialysis patients do *not* routinely need 2 L/day of IV fluid or furosemide postoperatively.

Other Things to Watch Out for in Dialysis Patients

- Vascular disease: ischaemic heart disease is very common in dialysis patients – even young ones. It is often unmasked by anaemia
- Infection: dialysis patients are significantly immunosuppressed functionally. They cope poorly with sepsis and rapidly become systemically unwell. Infections in access sites (lines, fistulae, peritoneal dialysis catheters) are common and might not be clinically evident, for example, subacute infective endocarditis and osteomyelitis – always think of these complications
- Electrolytes: haemodialysis patients are often chronically hyperkalaemic predialysis (and invariably hypokalaemic immediately postdialysis). They will often present with hypercalcaemia (too much vitamin D or Ca^{2+}-based PO_4-binders) or hypocalcaemia (too little)

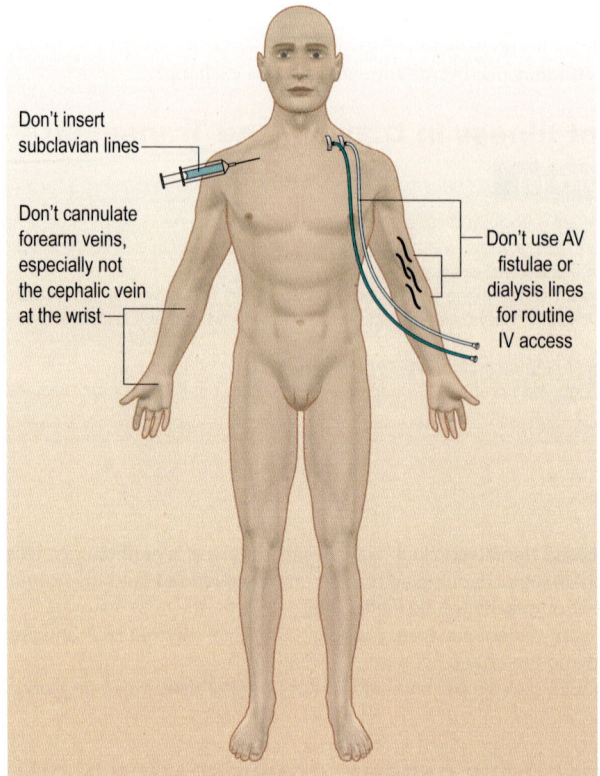

Don't insert subclavian lines

Don't cannulate forearm veins, especially not the cephalic vein at the wrist

Don't use AV fistulae or dialysis lines for routine IV access

Fig. 6.13   Things not to do in dialysis patients. AV, Arteriovenous.

■ Poorly compliant patients are routinely hyperphosphataemic; if they then start taking their 'prescribed' doses of vitamin D (1-α calcidol) and Ca^{2+}-based phosphate binders, their $Ca^{2+} \times PO_4$ product might exceed 7 mmol/L precipitating ectopic calcification

---

CASE HISTORY (2)

A 23-year-old renal transplant recipient (due to reflux nephropathy), on standard triple-therapy immuno-suppression (prednisolone, azathioprine, ciclosporin), presented with a hot, swollen, exquisitely painful right ankle.

    The joint was aspirated. The fluid contained 5000 WCC/mm³ with negative birefringent needle-shaped crystals seen on microscopy.

WHAT IS THE LIKELY DIAGNOSIS?

Gout. Their symptoms responded to colchicine 500 μg × 2 daily and allopurinol was started (300 mg × 1 daily) after 4 weeks.

    Three weeks later, the patient presented shocked with pancytopenia and then developed multiorgan failure.

BEWARE DRUG INTERACTIONS IN TRANSPLANTATION!

Allopurinol and Azathioprine

Azathioprine is metabolised to 6-Mercaptopurine, which is metabolised by xanthine oxidase. Allopurinol inhibits xanthine oxidase and effectively trebles or quadruples the functional dose of azathioprine, leading to significant bone-marrow depression.

This was the cause of the male's pancytopenia and multiorgan failure.

Ciclosporin (CyA)

These drugs increase CyA levels:
- Macrolides, for example, erythromycin
- Calcium-channel blockers
- Triazoles

These reduce CyA levels:
- Rifampicin
- Antiepileptics

WHAT OTHER COMPLICATIONS ARE TRANSPLANT PATIENTS AT RISK FROM?

Infections

The level of immunosuppression is high initially, then reduced. A wide range of opportunistic infections can occur (Box 6.6).

Vascular Disease

This remains very common after transplantation. Death (with a functioning graft) from ischaemic heart disease is the cause of death in 50% of patients.

Nephrotic Syndrome

Nephrotic syndrome is not a diagnosis but a set of signs and symptoms:
- Peripheral oedema
- Proteinuria: usually >3 g per day
- Hypoalbuminaemia

BOX 6.6 ■ **Opportunistic Infections That Can Occur in Renal Transplant Patients**

Viral
- Cytomegalovirus
- Epstein–Barr virus
- Herpes simplex virus
- Varicella zoster virus

Bacterial
- Tuberculosis
- *Listeria*
- *Nocardia*
- *Salmonella*

Protozoal
- *Toxoplasma*

Fungal
- *Pneumocystis*
- *Candida*
- *Aspergillus*

- Hypercholesterolaemia: a secondary phenomenon due to increased liver synthesis associated with increased protein synthesis:
  - It can be very resistant to lipid-lowering drugs
  - Treat the primary condition
- Hypertension, which accompanies the fluid overload
- Thrombophilia: nephrotic syndrome is associated with an increased clotting tendency and risk of thromboembolic disease. It is also a secondary condition. However, while the patient is nephrotic, anticoagulation is indicated, especially in membranous nephropathy.

REMEMBER

In nephrotic syndrome, there is a reduction in *relative* circulating volume in the presence of oedema.

CASE HISTORY

An 18-year-old female presents with a 2-week history of swollen ankles and mild breathlessness on exertion.

On examination, she had dependent oedema of the lower limbs to the knee with some facial oedema. Her pulse was normal, BP 150/90. She had bilateral pleural effusions.

INVESTIGATIONS

- Serum albumin 19 g/L
- Twenty-four-hour urine protein 5.6 g per day confirming the nephrotic syndrome
- Fasting cholesterol 8.7 mmol/L
- Urine analysis: proteinuria, no blood or red cell casts ('bland' urine sediments)

MANAGEMENT

The aim in all such cases is to find the cause.

How?

Although various noninvasive tests might hint at the diagnosis, in most adult cases, a renal biopsy is required.

Renal Biopsy Results

Do not panic – you do not need to know about renal histopathology!

Table 6.8 lists some of the common diagnoses and therapeutic strategies. This patient turns out to have a 'minimal change' disease. She slowly responds to oral steroids (60 mg/m^2 daily) with a significant reduction in urinary protein, but only after 12 weeks of high-dose therapy.

Remember HIV-associated nephropathy (HIVAN) in high-risk patients as a cause of unexplained renal impairment. HIV patients can also develop drug nephrotoxicity and HUS. Modern antiretroviral therapies have resulted in good renal outcomes in patients with nephrotic syndrome due to HIVAN.

REMEMBER

The use of IV albumin is controversial but declining. However, where severe reduction in circulating volume threatens renal function, it might help prevent acute kidney disease.

TABLE 6.8 ▪ **Some Common Diagnoses and Therapeutic Strategies**

Diagnosis	Treatment
Minimal change disease	Steroids (first line)
	Cyclophosphamide
Membranous nephropathy	None
	or ACEIs to reduce proteinuria
	or Steroids
	Alkaloids (cyclophosphamide or chlorambucil)
	Rituximab
Lupus nephritis	Prednisolone + cyclophosphamide/mycophenolate
Diabetic nephropathy	ACEIs or A II receptor antagonist
	Control hypertension: aim for BP <120/80
	Improve glycaemic control
Vasculitis	Prednisolone ± azathioprine
Amyloid	Treat underlying condition
HIVAN (collapsing FSGS)	Antiretroviral therapy

ACEI, Angiotensin-converting enzyme inhibitor; A II, angiotensin II; FSGS, focal segmental glomerulosclerosis; HIVAN, HIV-associated nephropathy.

Future progress. This patient's steroids were reduced, but she subsequently relapsed and was therefore given prednisolone 15 mg daily with cyclophosphamide 2 mg/kg daily for 12 weeks. She is presently in remission.

Haematuria Without Albuminuria

INFORMATION

- Macroscopic haematuria (red colour urine): can be confused with bile pigments, porphyrins, Hb and myoglobin. Confirm haematuria by microscopy
- Microscopic haematuria: >3–5 RBCs per high-power field on microscopy

REMEMBER

Haematuria very rarely causes anaemia. If anaemic, always look for another cause, for example, tuberculosis (TB), neoplasms and blood dyscrasias

WHAT CONDITIONS CAN CAUSE HAEMATURIA?

- Systemic: fever, anticoagulant therapy, sickle-cell trait or disease, strenuous exercise or coagulopathies
- Renal: glomerulonephritis (IgA nephropathy, Alport syndrome, thin basement nephropathy), interstitial tubulonephritis, renal infarcts, TB, polycystic disease, papillary necrosis, neoplasm, trauma, vascular malformations
- Urinary tract: calculi, foreign bodies, neoplasms, endometriosis, trauma, infections

WHAT WOULD YOU ASK IN THE HISTORY?

- Menstrual history to exclude vaginal cause of blood in urine

- Frequency, urgency, dysuria or urethral discharge suggests bladder or urethral involvement
- Pain or colic might be seen with stones, obstruction, infarction, polycystic kidney disease (PCKD)
- Bleeding at the beginning of micturition suggests urethral cause, whereas terminal bleeding is associated with prostate or bladder pathology
- Rectal or perineal pain suggests prostatitis
- Weight loss might suggest a neoplasm
- History of blood dyscrasia or anticoagulant therapy: anticoagulant therapy usage and haematuria should be investigated further for underlying lesions of the urinary tract
- Family history of PCKD, sickle-cell disease or glomerulonephritis (Alport or thin basement nephropathy)
- Upper respiratory tract infection or gastroenteritis suggests exacerbations of IgA nephropathy
- History of easy bruising or vasculitic rash, arthralgia and abdominal pain suggest Henoch–Schönlein purpura. Occasionally, anti-GBM disease, SLE or vasculitis can present as isolated haematuria

WHAT WOULD YOU LOOK FOR ON PHYSICAL EXAMINATION?

- Look for elevated BP or oedema (usually implies renal cause)
- Bilaterally palpable kidneys (PCKD)
- Unilateral mass (neoplasm, cystic or hydronephrotic kidney)
- Fever and tenderness over renal angle (pyelonephritis)
- Tender prostate (prostatitis)
- Presence of atrial fibrillation or valvular heart disease can suggest embolism or renal infarction
- Presence of petechiae, ecchymosis, lymphadenopathy or splenomegaly may signal blood dyscrasia or clotting disorder

INVESTIGATIONS

- Complete urinalysis: polarised microscopy may reveal dysmorphic RBCs (glomerular origin) or isomorphic RBCs (urothelial origin). Pyuria and haematuria with bacterial growth suggest UTI. No bacteriological growth triggers search for TB
- Consider nephritic screen, for example, serum immunoglobulins (IgG, IgA, IgM), serum and urine protein electrophoresis (exclude myeloma), serum complement, autoantibodies (ANA, antidouble stranded DNA, ANCA, antiglomerular basement membrane antibodies), antistreptolysin O titre (ASOT), HBsAg and anti-HCV
- Imaging:
  - Ultrasound scan of kidneys and bladder with residual bladder volume assessment
  - IVU/CT KUB (CT of kidney, ureter and bladder): stones and urinary tract lesions can be missed on ultrasound scan alone
  - Cystoscopy

Urinary Tract Infection (UTI)

CASE HISTORY

You are called to see a 19-year-old female who is complaining of a 2-day history of frequency, dysuria, urgency and right loin pain. She has a temperature of 39.8°C and a heart rate of 118 beats/min. Yesterday she had a rigor. You suspect a UTI and likely acute pyelonephritis in view of her high fever and right loin tenderness. She tells you that this is her first episode of a UTI. She has recently started to have frequent sexual intercourse with a new partner. She has no vaginal discharge and has never had a history of sexually transmitted infections. A complete physical examination shows no abnormality, apart from right loin tenderness. There is no urinary bladder distension or suprapubic tenderness.

- **Frequency** is defined as voiding every 2 h or more than seven times per day. A variety of factors can affect voiding intervals, including fluid intake, drugs (diuretics), alcohol and caffeine. Patients with polyuria from any cause complain of frequency with an increased urine flow. By contrast, bladder inflammation can cause frequency without an increase in urine flow
- **Urgency** is described as a powerful sensation to void, regardless of bladder volume. Typically, voided volumes of these patients are small – much less than the patient's normal maximum bladder capacity. Urgency is often caused by bladder inflammation but prostatic enlargement and external compression of the bladder by masses (as in pregnancy) can also generate a feeling of urgency
- **Dysuria** (painful micturition) suggests irritation or inflammation in the bladder neck or urethra, usually because of bacterial inflammation

- Urinary dipstick – presence of nitrite and/or leucocytes can be suggestive of bacterial infection (do not use for patients with indwelling catheters)
- Urine microscopy: pyuria, bacteriuria and leucocyte casts are consistent with UTI, send MSU specimens for culture and sensitivity
- Full blood count, serum U and Es, CRP and blood cultures
- Imaging: ultrasound is first line and should be performed when pyelonephritis is suspected to rule out calculi obstruction and incomplete emptying

HOW WOULD YOU MANAGE THIS PATIENT?

- Admit patients with acute pyelonephritis if it is severe or they have any signs or symptoms that suggest a more serious illness or condition, for example, sepsis (this patient's heart rate in this context would be concerning for sepsis)
- Provide analgesia and IV crystalloid if evidence of shock
- The most common bacterial cause of a UTI is *Escherichia coli*. Given this patient has suspected pyelonephritis, administer an appropriate broad-spectrum IV antibiotic (as per local guidelines) while waiting for the culture report. Consider previous urine culture and susceptibility results, as well as previous antibiotic use (which may have led to resistant bacteria). For example, in the UK, the National Institute for Health and Care Excellence (NICE) recommends the following intravenous antibiotics first-line for males and nonpregnant females:
  - Amoxicillin/clavulanate
  - Cefuroxime
  - Ciprofloxacin
  - Gentamicin (if severe/signs of sepsis, caution if renal function reduced)
- Advise prophylactic measures to prevent further UTIs:
  - A 2 L daily fluid intake
  - Voiding at 2- to 3-h intervals with double micturition if reflux is present
  - Voiding before bedtime and after intercourse
  - Avoidance of constipation, which may impair bladder emptying

Renal and Ureteric Colic

A 36-year-old male presented to his local emergency department with excruciating colicky right flank pain and vomiting. Physical examination is usually unremarkable, except for the presence of flank tenderness.

WHAT IS THE MOST LIKELY DIAGNOSIS?

Renal colic (often unilateral) is typically characterised by excruciating intermittent pain originating in the flank or kidney area and radiating across the abdomen towards the suprapubic region. The pain of ureteric colic has similar characteristics but typically radiates along the course of the ureter, frequently into the region of the genitalia and inner thigh.

AETIOLOGY

- Renal colic is usually caused by stretching of the renal capsule due to acute inflammation or bleeding within the kidney. Acute pyelonephritis, an expanding cyst or an acute expansion of the renal pelvis due to pelvi-ureteric obstruction by calculus or blood clot are the usual causes
- Ureteric colic is often caused by the passage of a calculus, sloughed papilla or blood clot
- Renal stones are usually calcium oxalate or calcium phosphate and are caused by hypercalciuric or hyperoxaluric states. Other types of stones are struvite (magnesium ammonium phosphate) stones, which are caused by urea-splitting organisms, cystine stones (the result of an inherited disorder of cystinuria) and urate stones (idiopathic or hyperuricosuric state)

WHAT WOULD YOU ASK ABOUT IN THE HISTORY?

- Pain: this is usually associated with GI symptoms (nausea, vomiting, abdominal distension)
- Chills, fevers and increased frequency: common
- Age at which symptoms of stones were first noted
- Family history of nephrolithiasis
- History of fractures or prolonged immobilisation
- Previous urinary infections or recent instrumentation

HOW WOULD YOU INVESTIGATE THIS PATIENT?

- Urinalysis: the urine might be normal despite multiple calculi. Macroscopic or microscopic haematuria is common. Pyuria with or without bacteria may be seen
- Computed tomography of the kidneys, ureters and bladder (CT-KUB) is carried out during the episode of pain. The CT-KUB appearances in a patient with acute left ureteric obstruction are shown in Fig. 6.14

HOW WOULD YOU MANAGE THIS PATIENT?

Give adequate hydration and analgesia. NSAIDs (unless contraindicated) are first line, for example, diclofenac IM/PR. Titrate opioids if required.

Progress. This patient passed a small stone later in the day; it was found to be a calcium oxalate stone. He was referred to the renal physician to investigate the cause of his stone formation. He was advised to take a high fluid intake and to restrict dietary oxalate (refer to a dietitian).

HOW CAN YOU FURTHER INVESTIGATE STONE FORMATION?

- Urinary excretion of calcium, phosphate, oxalate, urate and cystine can be performed on at least two separate occasions
- Morphological and biochemical analyses of passed stones can be performed

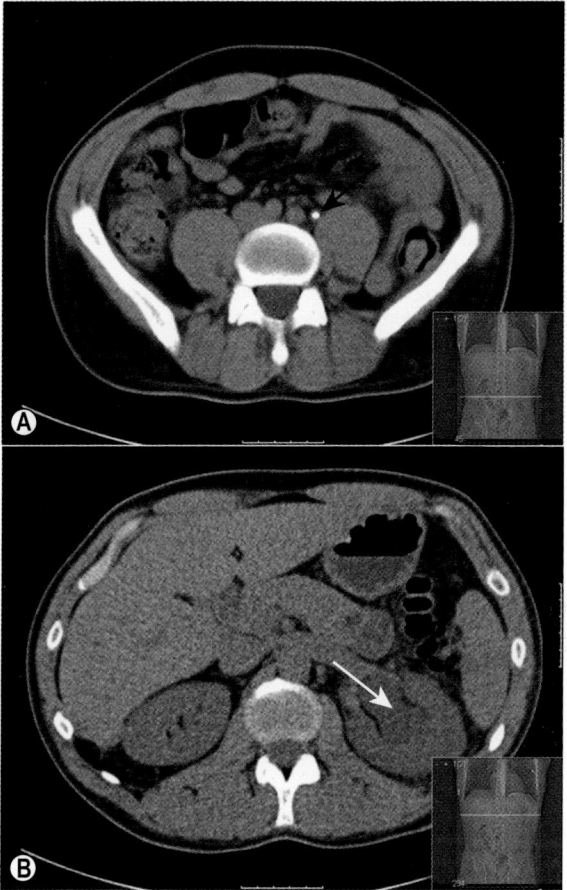

Fig. 6.14 (A) Left ureteric calculus. (B) A dilated renal pelvis (*arrow*) proximal to the ureteric stone in (A).

Further Reading

Fluid Balance and Electrolytes: Sodium Problems

Sterns, R.H., 2015. Disorders of plasma sodium – causes, consequences and correction. N. Engl. J. Med. 372 (1), 55–65.

The acidotic patient

Berend, K., 2018. Diagnostic use of base excess in acid–base disorders. N. Engl. J. Med. 378 (15), 1419–1428.

Chronic Kidney Disease

Ashby, D., et al., 2019. Renal association clinical practice guideline on haemodialysis. BMC Nephrol. 20 (1), 379.

Kalantar-Zadeh, K., Jafar, T.H., Nitsch, D., Neuen, B.L., Perkovic, V., 2021. Chronic kidney disease. Lancet 398 (10302), 786–802.

NICE, CKS, 2021. Chronic kidney disease: assessment and management. NICE.

Multisystem Vasculitis/Acute Glomerulonephritis

Berden, A.E., Ferrario, F., Hagen, E.C., et al., 2010. Histopathological classification of ANCA-associated glomerulonephritis. J. Am. Soc. Nephrol. 21 (10), 1628–1636.

Sethi, S., De Vriese, A.S., Fervenza, F.C., 2022. Acute glomerulonephritis. Lancet 399 (10335), 1646–1663.

Nephrotic Syndrome

Tervaert, T.W.C., Moovaart, A.L., Amann, K., et al., 2010. Pathological classification of diabetic nephropathy. J. Am. Soc. Nephrol. 21 (4), 556–563.

Urinary Tract Infection

Hooton, T.M., 2012. Uncomplicated urinary tract infection. N. Engl. J. Med. 366 (11), 1028–1037.
NICE, CKS, 2018. Urinary tract infection (lower): antimicrobial prescribing. NICE.

Renal and Ureteric Colic

British Association of Urological Surgeons, 2018. Guidelines for the management of acute ureteric colic. British Association of Urological Surgeons.
NICE, CKS, 2019. Renal and ureteric stones: assessment and management. NICE.
Worcester, E.M., Coe, F.L., 2010. Calcium kidney stones. N. Engl. J. Med. 363 (10), 954–963.

CHAPTER 7

Neurologia

Diplopia

Diplopia (double vision) occurs when there is an acquired defect of movement of an eye (paralytic squint). It is maximal in the direction of action of the weak muscle.

CASE HISTORY (1)

A 70-year-old male with type 2 diabetes presents with a 12-hour history of double vision. He is taking metformin and glibenclamide for his diabetes.

On examination, there is ptosis in the left eye, which is deviated downwards and laterally (down and out) and fails to elevate or move medially (Fig. 7.1). The pupils both react normally. He is otherwise well. Random blood glucose is 11.5 mmol/L. Glycated haemoglobin (HbA1c) is 8% (64 mmol/moL).

You suspect a diagnosis of **mononeuritis** (usually a pupil-sparing IIIrd nerve palsy), a complication of diabetes mellitus.

WHAT IMMEDIATE ACTION WOULD YOU TAKE?

- Achieve better diabetic control
- Put a patch over the eye
- Reassure the patient that recovery is likely (but not definite) over weeks

If recovery does not occur, refer the patient to a neurologist for an MRI scan and investigation of causes of mononeuritis multiplex.

INFORMATION

- A **painless IIIrd nerve palsy with preserved pupil reactions** commonly occurs in the setting of diabetes due to nerve infarction
- If a headache, especially of sudden onset, is present, a posterior communicating artery aneurysm compressing the IIIrd nerve in front of the midbrain is a likely cause. Such a lesion also commonly involves the parasympathetic pupillary constricting fibres so that the pupil is fixed and dilated. Magnetic resonance (MR) angiography is indicated in this situation (Fig. 7.2)

Progress. This male's diplopia improved over the next 2 months.

CASE HISTORY (2)

A 35-year-old female presents with 3 months of intermittent double vision.

On examination, there is mild restriction of upgaze and lateral gaze of the left eye, as well as mild restriction of upgaze of the right eye. There is mild bilateral ptosis. Further examination reveals fatigability of the ptosis and the eye movements.

A clinical diagnosis of myasthenia gravis was made.

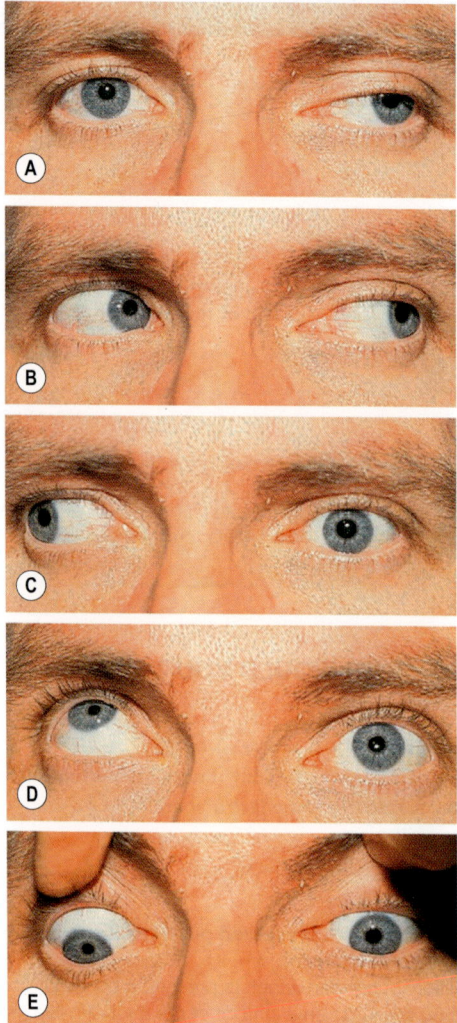

Fig. 7.1   Partial left IIIrd nerve palsy with mild ptosis in a male *without diabetes*. (A) Large left pupil; (B) normal left gaze; (C) no adduction of left eye on right gaze; (D) poor elevation; (E) poor depression.

WHAT ACTION WOULD YOU TAKE?

Confirm the diagnosis of myasthenia by:

- Measurement of serum acetylcholine receptor (Ach-R) antibodies (present in 40% of cases with eye involvement only with 100% specificity)
- Serum muscle-specific tyrosine kinase (MuSK) antibody testing for all patients negative for ACh-R antibodies
- Electromyography studies
- Magnetic resonance imaging of mediastinum to exclude thymoma

This patient was diagnosed as having myasthenia gravis and was referred urgently to a neurologist. Myasthenia gravis is sometimes restricted to the ocular system and can present as a variable

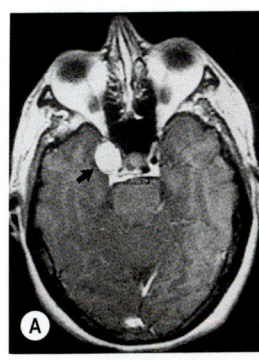 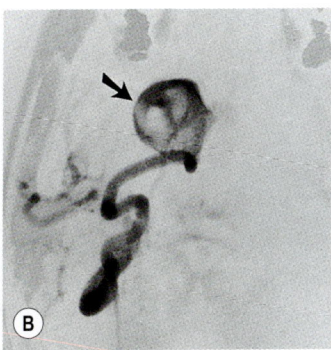

Fig. 7.2 (A) Magnetic resonance imaging showing left cavernous carotid aneurysm (*arrow*); (B) Magnetic resonance angiogram showing an aneurysm (*arrow*). (From Albert, D., Miller, J., Azar, D., et al., 2008. Albert and Jakobiec's Principles and Practice of Ophthalmology, third ed. Philadelphia, PA, Saunders/Elsevier, with permission.)

BOX 7.1 ■ Causes of Diplopia

Muscle/Obstructive
- Orbital masses
- Orbital pseudotumour (ocular myositis)
- Myasthenia
- Latent squint (visible when tired)

Cranial Nerves
- Mass lesion in path of IIIrd, IVth or VIth nerves
- Mononeuritis multiplex
- False localising due to raised intracranial pressure

Central
- Brainstem inflammation
- Demyelination
- Brainstem mass lesion
- Infarction
- Haemorrhage

---

gaze palsy that is difficult to interpret in terms of individual muscles or cranial nerves. There is not always a history of fatigability. Some of the many causes of diplopia are listed in Box 7.1.

HOW WOULD YOU TREAT THIS PATIENT?

Treatment of myasthenia gravis includes oral anticholinesterases, for example, neostigmine or pyridostigmine (dosage gradually increased), steroids, immunosuppression and plasmapheresis. Restricted ocular myasthenia carries a better prognosis, as swallowing and the respiratory muscles may be permanently spared.

Thymectomy may be necessary, even in patients without a thymoma.

Progress. This patient remains well on pyridostigmine at regular intervals through the day, but in view of the high doses required (>360 mg), she was put on immunosuppressive therapy

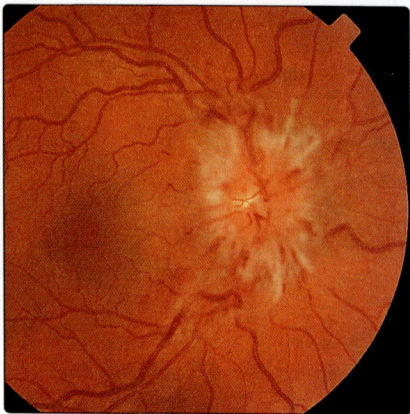

Fig. 7.3   Papilloedema.

(azathioprine and steroids). She experienced side-effects of abdominal colic from the pyridostigmine and this was helped by oral propantheline.

CASE HISTORY (3)

A 30-year-old, 27-week pregnant female patient complains of 4 weeks of headache, nausea, brief 1-second episodes of visual loss, and horizontal double vision that is worse on distance gaze.

On examination, she is found to have bilateral papilloedema (Fig. 7.3) and bilateral restriction of lateral gaze consistent with VIth nerve palsy.

WHAT ACTION WOULD YOU TAKE?

Magnetic Resonance Imaging or CT Scan of Head

In this case the ventricles were normal, and therefore it was safe to proceed to a lumbar puncture. The opening pressure was recorded at 30 cm (normal pressure <25 cm). A volume of cerebrospinal fluid (CSF) (usually around 20 mL) should be removed, so as approximately to halve the opening pressure.

WHAT IS THE DIAGNOSIS AND WHAT ARE THE COMMON PRECIPITATING FACTORS?

This patient has **idiopathic intracranial hypertension (IIH)**. This is most common in overweight female patients.

Precipitating Factors

- Pregnancy
- Weight gain
- Polycystic ovaries
- Tetracyclines
- Vitamin A excess (including retinoids)
- Steroids

WHAT IS THE MANAGEMENT?

Repeated lumbar puncture and removal of CSF, for example, every 1 to 2 weeks, has been widely used but is probably not helpful. Weight reduction is effective in improving symptoms. Drugs such as acetazolamide can be of assistance. Treatment is directed primarily at preventing visual loss due to uncorrected papilloedema and secondly at relief of headache/diplopia. The visual fields must be checked formally at intervals by screen perimetry to monitor any enlargement of the blind spots. If repeat puncture is unsuccessful in this usually self-limiting condition, optic nerve fenestration or even ventriculoperitoneal shunting may be necessary.

> **REMEMBER**
>
> - There are a number of secondary causes of raised intracranial pressure (ICP) without dilated ventricles or other space-occupying lesion, for example, venous sinus thrombosis and meningeal disease
> - Magnetic resonance imaging/MR venography and examination of CSF constituents are therefore mandatory

Progress. This patient's condition improved postpartum.

Acute Loss of Vision

CASE HISTORY (1)

A 64-year-old male presents to the emergency department with a 3-hour history of visual loss in the right eye. He had a previous episode several months earlier. He describes the loss as a horizontal screen descending over his vision. You are called by the triage nurse to give an opinion. When you arrive, the visual loss has recovered.

WHAT IS THE MOST LIKELY DIAGNOSIS?

Temporary monocular visual loss with a horizontal defect in this age group is very likely to be **amaurosis fugax**. This is often caused by thromboembolism in the ophthalmic artery and is a symptom of carotid stenosis.

WHAT IS THE DIFFERENTIAL DIAGNOSIS?

Transient ischaemic attacks (TIAs) are usually diagnosed clinically. Other causes of visual loss are shown in Box 7.2.

Remember giant cell arteritis, which causes acute visual loss. It responds to steroids.

Abrupt and progressive visual loss over days is also seen in elderly hypertensives. There is often disc swelling and later disc pallor. This is due to an arteriopathy of the posterior ciliary artery resulting in ischaemia of the optic disc and causing an anterior ischaemic optic neuropathy.

HOW WOULD YOU INVESTIGATE AND MANAGE THIS PATIENT?

See pp. 226 and 227.

BOX 7.2 ■ Causes of Acute or Transient Visual Disturbance

Ophthalmological

- Glaucoma
- Amaurosis fugax
- Giant cell (temporal) arteritis
- Anterior ischaemic optic neuropathy
- Central retinal vessel occlusion
- Vitreous haemorrhage
- Retinal detachment
- Uveitis, keratitis

Neurological

- Optic neuritis/demyelination
- Compressive lesion of the optic nerve, chiasm, tract
- Transient ischaemic attack/stroke of posterior cerebral circulation
- Migraine
- Occipital, temporal, parietal haemorrhage
- Occipital, temporal, parietal space-occupying lesion
- Temporal lobe epilepsy
- Raised intracranial pressure

Progress. This patient's carotid Doppler showed a 70% stenosis in the carotid artery and an internal carotid endarterectomy was performed. He has had no further episodes.

CASE HISTORY (2)

A 24-year-old female complains of several attacks of loss of vision, lasting up to 1 hour, in the right eye, accompanied by a left-sided pounding headache. Closer questioning reveals that the defect is, in fact, in the right visual field of both eyes.

WHAT IS THE LIKELY DIAGNOSIS?

Visual hemifield disturbance, sometimes with shimmering or jagged line scotomata, is a relatively common aura experienced by patients with **migraine**. Occasionally, there is no headache.

If the symptoms are dramatic or atypical, or especially if there are any fixed symptoms or signs, an MRI scan should be performed to check for an underlying vascular lesion, such as an arteriovenous malformation or underlying epileptogenic lesion, including occipital tumour.

HOW WOULD YOU MANAGE THIS PATIENT?

- Paracetamol 1 g, aspirin 900 mg (dispersible formulation) or another NSAID, for example, ibuprofen 400–600 mg or naproxen 500 mg, is given, as early as possible during an attack. Gastric emptying is reduced during the attack, and so dispersible formulations are preferred
- Antiemetics (e.g. metoclopramide 10 mg or domperidone 10 mg) can also be given
- If these measures are ineffective, use a 5-hydroxytryptamine $(5HT)_{1B}/_{1D}$ serotonin receptor agonist (triptan). These drugs relieve both the pain and the nausea. Triptans should be avoided in patients with vascular disease or uncontrolled/severe hypertension. They should

be given at the onset of the headache (e.g. during the aura phase). There are several triptans available with a spectrum of efficacy, for example,

- Sumatriptan 25–100 mg by mouth at onset of headache; repeat if necessary, after at least 2 h, maximum 300 mg in 24 h; subcutaneous (SC) 6 mg sumatriptan has the highest efficacy and produces the most rapid response
- Zolmitriptan 2.5 mg by mouth at onset; repeat if there is only a partial response after 2 h; 5 mg also available
- Rizatriptan 10 mg at onset; repeat after 2 h if there is only a partial response
- Oro-dispersible formulations exist for some triptans but absorption is slower
- If there is no response to an initial dose, do not persist with subsequent doses during the same attack. However, the drug may be effective in subsequent attacks

Progress. This patient's headache improved with paracetamol and sumatriptan. With subsequent episodes of migraine, she was able to self-administer sumatriptan, an antiemetic and paracetamol at the onset of her headaches. In this regimen, her migraine has been manageable.

Gradual Loss of Vision

Gradual loss of vision can be caused by a multitude of conditions. It can be very concerning for some patients, but in others, it can be so subtle, it is only picked up on routine screening.

CASE HISTORY

A 53-year-old male with a 20-year history of type 2 diabetes mellitus presents with worsening vision in his left eye. He has a history of poor glycaemic control and is poorly compliant with his metformin and gliclazide. His HbA1c is 78 mmol/moL.

On examination, his visual acuity is 20/100 in the left eye and examination of the retina demonstrates hard exudates, microaneurysms and macula thickening.

WHAT IS THE LIKELY DIAGNOSIS?

Diabetic retinopathy (DR). This is the chronic retinal manifestation of diabetic microvascular damage and is potentially sight-threatening. There are two stages:
- Nonproliferative: early stage, can cause moderate visual loss
- Proliferative: late stage, severe visual loss

The characteristic features include micro-aneurysms, hard exudates (deposition of proteins leaking from retinal vessels), haemorrhages and cotton wool spots (axonal debris secondary to ischaemia) in nonproliferative DR (Fig. 7.4). Proliferative DR is characterised by neovascularisation.

WHAT ARE THE OTHER IMPORTANT CAUSES OF GRADUAL VISUAL LOSS?

Painless:
- Age-related macular degeneration: progressive chronic disease of the central retina, typically causes visual distortion and loss of central vision (scotoma)
- Primary open-angle glaucoma: characterised by raised intraocular pressure with an open iridocorneal angle that causes progressive peripheral vision loss
- Cataracts: opacification of the lens that typically causes glare and vision loss
- Optic nerve compression: rare, consider if associated with headaches or associated neurological abnormalities

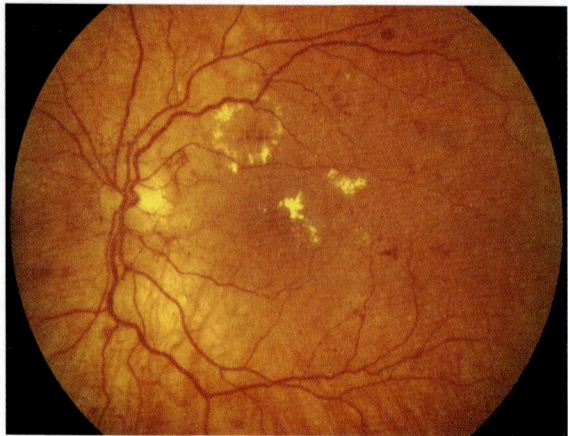

Fig. 7.4 Background diabetic retinopathy. Exudates, microaneurysms and small haemorrhages can be seen in the posterior pole. (From Goldman, L., Cooney, K.A., 2024. Goldman-Cecil Medicine, Twenty-seventh ed. Diseases of the Visual System, Fig. 391.22, Philadelphia, PA, Elsevier INC.)

- Drugs/toxins: amiodarone, ethambutol, isoniazid, sildenafil, isotretinoin
- Nutritional deficiency: vitamin A deficiency

Painful (much rarer)

- Optic nerve lesions: examples include optic neuritis or granulomas
- Neoplastic: choroidal melanoma
- Intracranial pathology
- Sarcoidosis

WHAT ARE THE MANAGEMENT OPTIONS FOR THIS PATIENT?

The main goals of treatment are to optimise glycaemic, lipid and blood pressure control, as well as stopping any disease before visual loss occurs.

Target an HbA1c below 50 mmol/moL, aim for a systolic blood pressure less than 130 mm Hg and commence lipid-lowering therapy.

Ophthalmic interventions include laser treatment aimed at causing regression of new vessels and reducing macular thickening. Other options include intravitreal steroids and antivascular endothelial growth factor treatment (e.g. aflibercept).

Red Eye

Red eye is a very common presentation and is mostly caused by benign self-limiting conditions. It can prove a diagnostic challenge to identify the small proportion of patients with serious conditions that require urgent treatment.

CASE HISTORY

A 46-year-old male presents to his local emergency department with severe pain in his right eye associated with blurred vision, tearing and photophobia. The eye is red with a small irregular pupil and purulent discharge is noted. On examination with a slit lamp, the assessing doctor notes injection around the corneal limbus and cells in the anterior chamber.

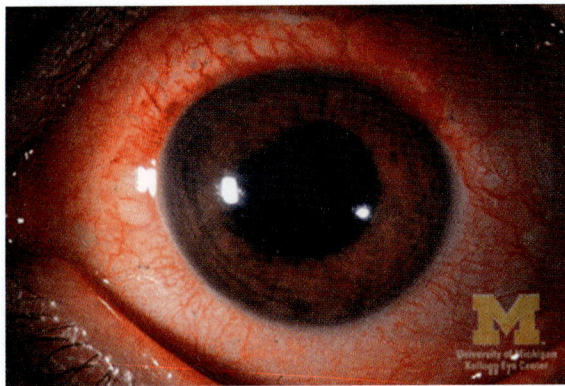

Fig. 7.5 Anterior uveitis (Red eye). (Courtesy University of Michigan, Kellogg Eye Center.)

WHAT IS THE DIAGNOSIS?

Anterior uveitis (iritis). Uveitis is a broad term for inflammation of the uvea which is the vascular area between the retina and sclera of the eye. Anterior uveitis is the inflammation of the iris and ciliary body, and it can be acute, recurrent or chronic. It typically presents with unilateral eye pain and redness with photophobia. It can cause a constricted, abnormally shaped and/or nonreactive pupil. Characteristic signs on slit lamp examination include circumlimbal injection and the presence of cells in the aqueous humour (Fig. 7.5).

WHAT ARE THE DIFFERENTIAL DIAGNOSES?

Other causes of a painful red eye include:
- Acute angle closure glaucoma: raised intraocular pressure due to obstructed anterior chamber angle
- Episcleritis
- Scleritis
- Endophthalmitis: severe inflammation of the anterior and/or posterior chambers of the eye (usually due to bacterial or fungal infection)
- Trauma/foreign body/abrasion
- Keratitis: inflammation of the cornea typically due to infection

WHAT ARE THE POTENTIAL CAUSES OF THIS CONDITION?

- Idiopathic (up to 70% of cases)
- Infectious: herpes simplex virus (*HSV*), varicella-zoster virus, cytomegalovirus, HIV, Lyme disease, tuberculosis (TB), syphilis
- Noninfectious: autoimmune disorders, inflammatory bowel disorder, seronegative arthropathies, sarcoidosis, multiple sclerosis (MS)

WHAT IS THE MANAGEMENT OF THIS CONDITION?

All patients require urgent review by an ophthalmologist. If caused by an underlying condition (see previous discussion), then the management of this should be optimised.

Corticosteroids can be started to rapidly control the inflammation, for example, prednisolone or dexamethasone eye drops. Periocular or intraocular corticosteroids can also be considered. Oral steroids can be used in severe cases or if patients cannot tolerate injections.

Cycloplegics (e.g. ophthalmic atropine or cyclopentolate) can be considered to relieve pain and prevent adhesions.

Bell's Palsy

CASE HISTORY

You are called to see a 45-year-old male who woke up this morning with a 'numb' left face, a droopy left eyelid and drooling from the left side of his mouth.

On examination, it is apparent that his 'numbness' represents left facial weakness in the upper and lower distributions. There is no sensory loss and there are no lesions of the skin around or inside the ear (Ramsay Hunt syndrome).

WHAT IS THE LIKELY DIAGNOSIS?

An acute VIIth nerve lesion, **Bell's palsy** (Fig. 7.6), is usually due to a viral infection (often herpes simplex). It involves the VIIth (facial) nerve (motor only), occasionally with a loss of taste on the tongue and hyperacusis. There should be no sensory loss or other cranial nerve involvement.

HOW WOULD YOU MANAGE THIS PATIENT?

- Treatment is with steroids (60 mg prednisolone for a week, tailing down over the subsequent 1–2 weeks)
- An antiviral, for example, valaciclovir 1000 mg × 3 daily also for 1 week, is recommended by some for severe paralysis (randomized trials are inconclusive)
- The patient should be reassured and the cornea protected if exposed
- Sometimes recovery is incomplete and faulty reinnervation of the facial muscles or of the lacrimal gland may occur. Relapses are seen.
- Bilateral or recurrent Bell palsy, or one that shows no recovery after several weeks, should be investigated with an MRI scan, possibly CSF analysis, and investigations for causes of **mononeuritis multiplex**.

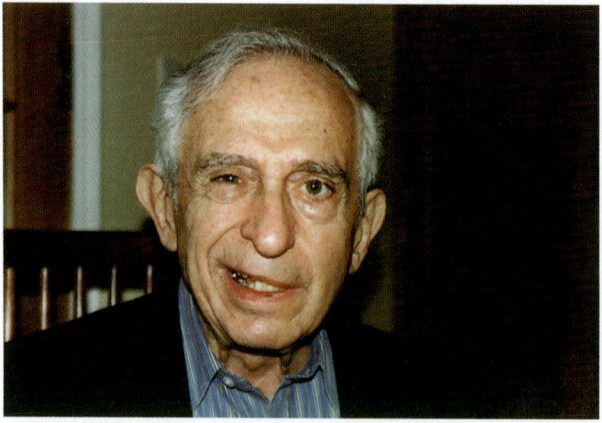

Fig. 7.6 Bell palsy.

INVESTIGATIONS

Mononeuritis Multiplex

- Full blood count (FBC)
- Urea and electrolytes (U and Es)
- Blood glucose
- Serum auto-antibodies
- Serum anticardiolipin antibodies
- Serum antineutrophil cytoplasmic antibody (ANCA)
- Treponemal serology
- *Borrelia* serology
- Serum and CSF angiotensin-converting enzyme (ACE)
- Serum electrophoresis and Bence Jones protein
- Chest X-ray

REMEMBER

- Sarcoidosis should be suspected in cases of bilateral Bell palsy
- Melkersson–Rosenthal syndrome is a rare condition causing bilateral Bell palsy and tongue swelling with other features
- Progressive multiple cranial nerve palsies should lead to suspicion of malignant meningitis, or lymphomatous or carcinomatous infiltration

Progress. This patient was treated with steroids and aciclovir, and the palsy resolved over a few weeks. He has had no further recurrences.

Vertigo

Vertigo, the definite illusion of movement of the subject or surroundings, typically rotatory, indicates a disturbance of the vestibular nerve, brainstem or, very rarely, cortical function. Deafness and tinnitus accompanying vertigo indicate involvement of the ear or cochlear nerve.

CASE HISTORY (1)

An 85-year-old female presented to the emergency department with a history of severe nausea, vomiting and dizziness, which started on waking one morning 2 weeks previously. She was confused and dehydrated. On rehydration, she was able to give a clear history of true vertigo (the sensation of the environment spinning or rotating about her). The symptoms were precipitated by head movement, especially when she turned her head in bed.

On examination, she has normal eye movement. The rotational nystagmus in both eyes was brought on by sudden head movements (Hallpike manoeuvre).

WHAT IS THE LIKELY DIAGNOSIS?

This history is typical of **vestibular neuronitis**, the aetiology of which is uncertain. It occurs at any age. Recovery generally takes place over 2 to 3 weeks, although complete recovery might take several months. Cinnarizine and other vestibular suppressants give symptomatic relief but are best avoided in the long term.

Peripheral vestibular lesions are characterised by positional vertigo, which is influenced – often in a stereotyped way – by head movement. This is manifest in the Hallpike test (see Information box and Fig. 7.7), which characteristically reveals a rotational nystagmus.

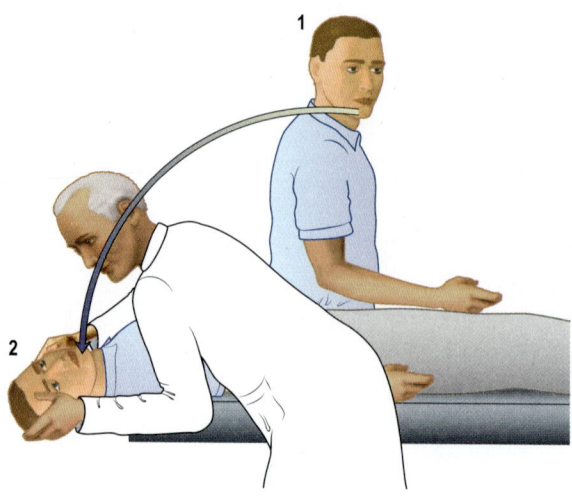

Fig. 7.7   Hallpike manoeuvre for diagnosis of benign paroxysmal positional vertigo.

INFORMATION

Hallpike Test

The patient is sat on a couch with the eyes open and facing the side of the lesion. The examiner swings the patient backwards so that he/she is supine and the head is below the horizontal. Nystagmus following a latent interval of a few seconds is commonly noted if the test is positive.

A **central vestibular lesion** is sometimes also positional but generally fails to habituate (i.e. on Hallpike testing, continued repetition of the same movement results in no reduction in the unpleasantness or in the nystagmus).

Caloric tests are the definitive investigation to differentiate the two sites and to lateralise the lesion.

REMEMBER

- If there is suspicion of a central lesion, an MRI scan should be performed
- Always check for associated deafness, tinnitus, cranial nerve lesions or cerebellar disturbance for early identification of a cerebellopontine angle lesion, most commonly, an VIIIth nerve schwannoma ('acoustic neuroma')

WHAT ARE THE POTENTIAL CAUSES OF VERTIGO?

Peripheral

- Vestibular neuronitis
- Benign paroxysmal positional vertigo (BPPV)
- Ménière syndrome
- Lesion of the VIIIth nerve, for example, schwannoma
- Inner ear infections, infiltrations

Central

- Brainstem infarction, inflammation or demyelination
- Brainstem space-occupying lesion
- Posterior circulation TIA
- Migraine
- Complex partial seizures

Progress. This patient's vertigo settled after 5 days and has not recurred.

CASE HISTORY (2)

A 65-year-old female presents to the emergency department with occasional, very brief, blackouts and a long history of dizziness in crowds or when walking past fast-moving traffic. She prefers to avoid any sudden head movements, especially in certain directions and when turning in bed. Hallpike test is positive.

WHAT IS THE LIKELY DIAGNOSIS?

Benign paroxysmal positional vertigo (BPPV). This is a relatively common disorder presenting with true vertigo, particularly on head movement. There are often vague 'vestibular hypersensitivity' symptoms, especially precipitated when there are conflicting visual inputs such as being stationary in a fast-moving visual field. Occasionally, the vertigo may be so sudden and dramatic as to present as a blackout. Diagnosis is largely clinical, although caloric testing may reveal mild dysfunction and MRI helps to exclude other conditions.

WHAT ARE THE MANAGEMENT OPTIONS?

Vestibular physiotherapy is given in the form of Cawthorne–Cooksey exercises (repetitive eye and head movements) and vestibular suppressants (e.g. β-histine). In some cases the cause is said to relate to fragments of calcification in the semicircular canals; some specialists perform the Epley manoeuvre. This gentle manipulation and rotation of the head attempt to dislodge these fragments away from the receptors. Some severe cases may be successfully treated by surgical section of the nerve to the ampulla of the posterior semicircular canal.

Progress. The patient has vestibular physiotherapy and was taught to continue the exercises at home. She continues to have dizziness in crowds but is better.

CASE HISTORY (3)

A 70-year-old male presents with sudden onset of vertigo, vomiting, gait unsteadiness and left facial numbness.
  On examination, there is coarse unidirectional nystagmus, a reduced left corneal reflex, a left Horner syndrome, mild dysphagia and palatal deviation to the right, left-sided ataxia and impaired pinprick on the right arm and leg.

WHAT IS THE LIKELY DIAGNOSIS?

This is a **partial left lateral medullary syndrome** due to a stroke in the territory of branches of the posterior or anterior inferior cerebellar arteries. The vertigo is usually not positional. Nystagmus of brainstem origin is often coarse, may be in any direction, and is frequently unidirectional and sometimes monocular.

WHAT IS THE MANAGEMENT?

As for stroke – see next section.

Stroke

This is the sudden onset of focal neurological symptoms caused by interruption of the vascular supply to a region of the brain (ischaemic stroke) or intracerebral haemorrhage (haemorrhagic stroke). It is a common cause of mortality and physical disability.

PATHOPHYSIOLOGY

Ischaemic stroke (infarction of central nervous tissue) results from cerebral infarction secondary to either arterial thromboembolism or emboli arising from the heart (e.g. in atrial fibrillation, mural thrombus after acute myocardial infarction, or rarely from vegetations in infective endocarditis).

Cerebral haemorrhage is often caused by microaneurysm rupture in small penetrating arteries in hypertensive patients. It can also occur because of rupture of an aneurysm or arteriovenous malformation or because of amyloid angiopathy in older patients. It accounts for around 15% of strokes.

Other causes of stroke in younger patients include arterial dissection, venous sinus thrombosis, thrombophilia, vasculitis and paradoxical embolisation through a patent foramen ovale.

CASE HISTORY (1)

A 70-year-old male presents with a 2.5-hour history of right-sided arm, leg and face weakness and loss of speech. He has no headache but is mildly confused. He has a history of ischaemic heart disease.

On examination, he had a global dysphasia, full visual fields, upper motor neurone (UMN) distribution right facial weakness, and dense weakness (UMN distribution) of the right side with absent reflexes and an upgoing plantar response on that side. His pulse was regular.

A clinical diagnosis of left middle cerebral artery stroke is made.

INFORMATION

Stroke Diagnosis

Simple history and examination – FAST:

- *Face* – sudden weakness of the face
- *Arm* – sudden weakness of one or both arms
- *Speech* – difficulty speaking, slurred speech
- *Time* – the sooner treatment can be started, the better

WHAT IMMEDIATE ACTION WOULD YOU TAKE IN THIS CASE (I.E. CEREBRAL INFARCT)?

- Is thrombolysis to be considered? **Yes**
- Computed tomography will distinguish haemorrhage, but infarction cannot be seen early on (see Fig. 7.8A). An early CT scan is also useful in stroke to check for subarachnoid or

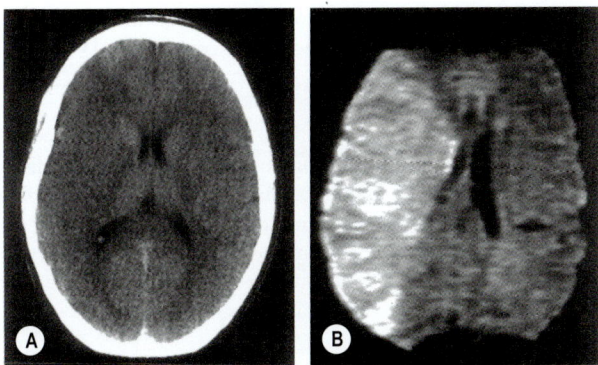

Fig. 7.8 (A) Computed tomography of a middle cerebral infarct performed in the early stages, showing subtle changes in the right middle cerebral artery territory; (B) Magnetic resonance imaging of same region done at the same time as the CT, showing the full extent of the damage. (Courtesy Dr Paul Jarmon.)

intracerebral haemorrhage and to help exclude other conditions that may masquerade as stroke, such as tumour, cerebral abscess and cerebral venous sinus thrombosis.

- Consider diffuse weighted MRI with stroke-specific sequences if the diagnosis remains uncertain after CT (see Fig. 7.8B)
- **In this patient** the CT showed no evidence of haemorrhage; therefore **cerebral infarction** was likely
- He was given **alteplase** (IV tissue plasminogen activator [tPA]) after ruling out contraindications and obtaining patient consent as soon as possible (*minutes count*): total dose 0.9 mg/kg; maximum 90 mg. Give 10% of the total dose over 1 min and the remainder over 60 min by infusion

(If there had been a contraindication to the therapy or if thrombolysis was not available, he would have been given 300 mg aspirin.)

> **REMEMBER**
>
> - If cerebral haemorrhage is shown on CT, *do not* give any therapy that might interfere with clotting, for example, aspirin or heparin
> - If it is a posterior fossa haemorrhage, refer to the neurosurgeons for possible emergency clot evacuation

WHAT ELSE WOULD YOU DO FOR THIS PATIENT?

Acute Management

- Electrocardiogram – exclude arrhythmia, for example, atrial fibrillation
- Blood tests – FBC, U and Es, glucose, lipid profile, HbA1c
- Direct admission to stroke unit
- Check:
  - Blood pressure: do not overcorrect systemic hypertension in acute phase
  - Swallowing: nil by mouth and IV fluids in any major stroke; assess properly by speech therapist (Speech and Language Therapy [SALT] team)
  - Asymptomatic aspiration: common, and therefore early referral to physiotherapy and other support services should be arranged

- Any concurrent infection, other illness or electrolyte disturbance: check for and treat
- If there is evidence of cerebral oedema and risk of coning, give IV mannitol or hypertonic saline

Thrombolysis

This significantly increases the chances of having no disability or minimal disability after stroke by reducing infarct size. Recombinant tissue plasminogen activator (rt-PA; alteplase) should be given as soon as possible within 4.5 hours of symptom onset. It is also being considered up to 9 hours after symptom onset if there is evidence of the potential to salvage brain tissue on CT or MRI perfusion studies.

Thrombectomy

Thrombectomy should usually only be considered in patients with:

- A prestroke functional status of less than three on the modified Rankin scale; and
- A score of more than five on the National Institutes of Health Stroke Scale (NIHSS)

Thrombectomy should be offered within 6 hours of symptom onset to patients with confirmed ischaemic stroke secondary to occlusion of the proximal anterior circulation.

If perfusion imaging shows potentially salvageable brain tissue, these patients can also be considered for thrombectomy between 6 and 24 hours after symptom onset.

Thrombectomy should also be considered for patients with confirmed ischaemic stroke occluding the proximal posterior circulation if there is potential to salvage brain tissue.

Further Management

- Start aspirin 75 mg daily following a 300 mg loading dose (usually 24 h after if tPA has been given)
- Dual antiplatelet therapy (add either clopidogrel or ticagrelor) for patients presenting within 24 h of minor stroke with a low risk of bleeding
- Anticoagulants if in atrial fibrillation
- Serum cholesterol: if fasting is >3.5 mmol/L (not in acute situation), start atorvastatin

Progress. This patient did not make an early clinical improvement, as can occur after thrombolytic therapy (37%), but by 3 months he was ambulant, with a minor neurological deficit, and had improved speech.

CASE HISTORY (2)

A 56-year-old male presents with weakness of the left hand and face lasting 3 hours and resolving gradually. He had a similar episode 3 months earlier and made a complete recovery. He is a type 2 diabetic and a smoker. A Doppler ultrasound reveals that he has a 90% stenosis at the origin of the right internal carotid artery.

WHAT IS THE LIKELY DIAGNOSIS?

Diagnosis: Transient Ischaemic Attack (TIA)

A TIA is a transient episode of neurological dysfunction caused by focal brain, spinal cord or retinal ischaemia without acute infarction. The previous definition, with its arbitrary 24-hour timescale, is no longer used as the end point is now tissue injury.

Examples include:

- Anterior circulation – sudden transient loss of vision in one eye (amaurosis fugax), aphasia, hemiparesis; *or*

- Posterior circulation – diplopia, ataxia, hemisensory loss, dysarthria, transient global amnesia

Transient ischaemic attacks may herald the onset of stroke (one-quarter of patients developing stroke have had a TIA, usually within the previous week):

- If patients are at a high risk or have had two recent TIAs, especially within the same vascular territory, they should be admitted for investigation and treatment
- *All* patients should be referred to a TIA clinic and ideally seen within 24 h. Investigation and treatment should be regarded as *urgent* and should be *completed* within 7 days

INVESTIGATIONS

- Full blood count, U and Es, fasting lipids and glucose, HbA1c
- Electrocardiogram – assess for arrhythmia (e.g. atrial fibrillation) or ischaemia
- Look for the source of the embolus – carotids (Doppler) and cardiac (echo)
- Computed tomography brain
- Further investigation with MRI of the brain and vascular system is often required

HOW WOULD YOU TREAT THIS PATIENT?

- Antiplatelet therapy as for stroke
- Modification of vascular risk factors – smoking, hypertension; give statins as discussed earlier
- Early endarterectomy for symptomatic 70%–99% carotid artery stenosis (within 1 week if possible)
- Anticoagulation for atrial fibrillation

Progress. In this patient an endarterectomy was performed. He has made lifestyle changes and has been well over the last 2 years.

CASE HISTORY (3)

A 40-year-old male presents with a 1-week history of headache followed by loss of speech and a right hemiparesis. His weakness worsens over the next 24 hours and he becomes confused. A CT scan is normal at this time. A subsequent MRI scan reveals an infarct in the left frontal lobe with small haemorrhages elsewhere in the hemispheres. His erythrocyte sedimentation rate (ESR) and auto-antibodies are normal. CSF analysis reveals 35 lymphocytes/mm^3 but is otherwise normal. A right frontal brain biopsy reveals **primary cerebral granulomatous angiitis** (a rare necrotising inflammation with granulomatous vasculitis of the brain and meningeal vessels). He is treated with high-dose steroids and cyclophosphamide.

WHAT ARE THE CAUSES OF STROKES IN THIS YOUNG AGE GROUP?

In the younger age group, there are other causes of stroke, such as vasculitis or structural cardiac lesions. In many of these conditions, specific treatment is indicated. Cerebral vasculitis is difficult to diagnose because systemic inflammatory markers may be normal. The CSF and intraarterial angiography are sometimes also normal. Even a cerebral/meningeal biopsy may miss involved vessels because the condition is often patchy.

INVESTIGATIONS

Additional Investigations in the Younger Age Group
- Magnetic resonance imaging head
- Auto-antibodies, including anticardiolipin, ANCA
- Lupus anticoagulant
- Serum electrophoresis
- Serum lactate/pyruvate
- Urine for protein and casts
- Urine homocysteine
- Echocardiogram
- Twenty-four-h ECG
- Consider CSF analysis

Progress. This patient was initially treated with high-dose steroids and cyclophosphamide. The steroids were reduced gradually and oral cyclophosphamide continued for 6 months.

Subdural Haemorrhage

This is caused by venous bleeding in the subdural space from rupture of a vein, often following a head injury.

CASE HISTORY

A 77-year-old female was admitted as she was unable to manage at home alone. There had been a 2-year history of cognitive decline that seemed to have accelerated to precipitate the admission.
    On examination, she was confused and disorientated, unable to repeat a five-digit number, and had an upgoing left plantar response. Her Glasgow Coma Scale score (GCS) was 12.
    A CT scan revealed **bilateral subdural haematomas** (Fig. 7.9).

WHAT RISK FACTORS ARE ASSOCIATED WITH THIS CONDITION?

Subdural haemorrhage can present rather acutely following a fall, with sudden onset of headache and diminished consciousness. The diagnostic challenge lies in identifying other cases that present vaguely without focal signs and with no history of trauma. A number of factors are associated with increased risk of apparently spontaneous subdural haemorrhage:
- Old age
- Cerebral atrophy, dementia
- Alcohol excess, general debility
- Bleeding diathesis/anticoagulant therapy
- Intracranial lesions such as tumour
- Brain surgery, especially ventricular shunt insertion for normal pressure hydrocephalus

WHAT ARE THE MANAGEMENT OPTIONS?

The management of subdural haematomas depends on their size and the severity of symptoms. Small ones may simply be managed conservatively with follow-up CT scanning. Larger or more acutely symptomatic subdurals should be surgically evacuated.

Progress. This patient had an acute subdural haemorrhage that precipitated her deterioration. This was managed surgically with overall improvement in her cognitive state.

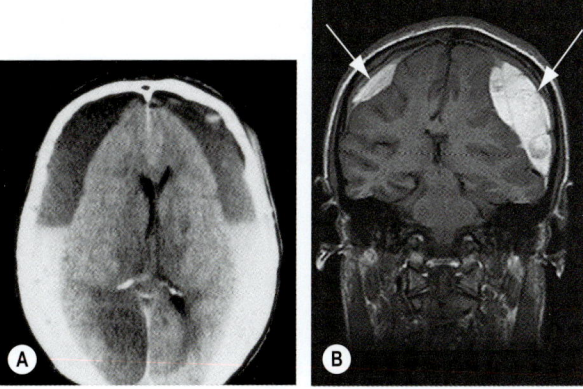

Fig. 7.9 Bilateral subdural haematomas (*arrows*). (A) CT scan; (B) MR (T1) image.

Encephalitis

This is an inflammation of the brain parenchyma, which is often due to a virus.

> **CASE HISTORY (1)**
>
> A 45-year-old male presents with a 1-week history of malaise, followed by increasing confusion, headache, meningism and a seizure.
>
> **On examination**, he was confused, with a GCS of 10. He had fever, neck stiffness and hyperreflexia of the left arm and leg.
>
> A tentative diagnosis of encephalitis was made.

WHAT ACTION WOULD YOU TAKE?

- Supportive care: including respiratory support if necessary
- Treatment of any seizures: ictal and postictal states are a reversible element of changes in conscious level
- Computed tomography (CT) scan: showed no space-occupying lesion
- Lumbar puncture: there was a lymphocytosis
- Serology and polymerase chain reaction (PCR): for likely aetiological agents (see later)
- *If there is even a remote possibility that the cause is HSV1), start aciclovir immediately, IV 10 mg/ kg × 3 daily.* Herpes simplex virus is treatable; most other causes are not (Box 7.3). Patients have been known to relapse and respond to further treatment

> **REMEMBER**
>
> - Most cases of viral encephalitis present in the same way, the symptoms being milder than those for a bacterial meningitis. In many cases the viral cause can be worked out from the epidemiological pattern, for example, from the geographical area where the disease was contracted and the season of the year
> - The term 'encephalitis' encompasses any acute febrile illness, perhaps with some meningeal involvement, that is accompanied by acute generalised or focal cerebral disturbance. Thus there is considerable overlap with meningitis

---

BOX 7.3 ■ Causes of Encephalitis/Meningoencephalitis

Viral

- Herpes simplex (HSV 1 and 2)
- Measles
- Rubella
- Epstein–Barr virus
- Varicella zoster virus
- Echo
- Coxsackie
- Cytomegalovirus
- Human immunodeficiency virus
- Japanese B (most common worldwide)
- West Nile encephalitis
- Tick-borne encephalitis
- Postviral: acute disseminated encephalomyelitis (ADEM)

Bacterial

- Legionnaire
- *Mycoplasma*
- *Listeria*
- Tuberculosis

In immunocompromised people, think of unusual organisms, for example, fungal.

INVESTIGATIONS

Further Investigations

- An MRI scan showed temporal oedema
- An electroencephalography (EEG) excluded generalised or complex partial status epilepticus
- If there is a possibility of immunosuppression (as a result of AIDS, lymphoproliferative disorders or iatrogenic), this should be investigated

Progress. The MRI was highly suggestive of an **HSV1 encephalitis** and this was confirmed by serology and PCR. The patient was treated with IV aciclovir. Although he survived, he was left with a significant residual deficit. He was sent for rehabilitation but had problems with his memory, which is particularly common following HSV1 encephalitis.

REMEMBER

- All cases of encephalitis should be given aciclovir.
- Herpes simplex virus is treatable; most other causes are not

---

CASE HISTORY (2)

A 25-year-old female has an upper respiratory tract infection. Following recovery, she becomes drowsy over a period of 48 hours.

On examination, she is apyrexial with a GCS of 9. She has abnormal eye movements and gaze-evoked nystagmus. There is marked spasticity in the limbs.

Investigations: CT shows effacement of cerebral sulci, but it is deemed safe to do a lumbar puncture. Lumbar puncture reveals 40 lymphocytes/mm³. The patient requires intubation to protect the airway.

A provisional diagnosis of HSV1 encephalitis is made.
Follow-on: a subsequent MRI scan reveals diffuse and confluent T2 hyperintensities in the periventricular white matter and brainstem, as well as within the cerebral grey matter.

WHAT IS THE DIAGNOSIS?

Acute disseminated encephalomyelitis (ADEM). This is considered to be a postviral (sometimes post *Mycoplasma*) inflammatory condition, mainly affecting the white matter, although the distinction from a direct viral encephalitis may be blurred. At the other end of the scale, the distinction from a severe initial attack of MS might also be unclear, although the latter attack is usually milder, more likely to be associated with CSF oligoclonal bands, and characterised in retrospect by repeated attacks. However, treatment of both ADEM and MS attacks is similar, namely, with high doses of steroids. Because of the nature of presentation of ADEM, antivirals are usually also given.

Progress. This patient was treated with IV methylprednisolone, followed by a course of oral steroids, and made a good recovery after several weeks, with some residual pyramidal gait difficulty.

Meningococcal Meningitis and Septicaemia

CASE HISTORY

An 18-year-old female is brought into the emergency department after collapsing. The previous day, she had apparently been well, apart from symptoms of a minor upper respiratory tract infection. She woke up feeling very unwell with a severe headache and asked her flatmate to call the emergency doctor. The flatmate noted that her friend had a couple of spots on her chest but by the time the doctor arrived, she was developing a more widespread petechial rash. The emergency doctor transferred her immediately to hospital after giving her a single dose of benzylpenicillin.
The patient was febrile with a temperature of 38°C
A petechial rash was present
The patient was hypotensive and shocked.

WHAT IS THE MOST LIKELY DIAGNOSIS?

This young female has **fulminant meningococcaemia**, which has a worse prognosis than meningococcal meningitis and usually follows an extremely rapid downhill course.

WHAT IS THE ACUTE MANAGEMENT?

Take blood and throat cultures, and then start antibiotics immediately (following local protocols), common regimes include:
- Intravenous benzylpenicillin, initially 2.4 g 4-hourly or
- Intravenous cefotaxime 2 g × 6-hourly or
- Intravenous ceftriaxone 2 g × 2 daily

REMEMBER

The first doctor to see a patient suspected of having meningococcal sepsis or meningitis should immediately give benzylpenicillin IM injection before immediate transfer to hospital.

WHAT INVESTIGATIONS SHOULD BE PERFORMED?

Relevant investigations are shown in the box. Other causes of meningitis/septicaemia should be excluded.

INVESTIGATIONS

- Full blood count and differential: leucocytosis common (but can be normal)
- U and Es, calcium, phosphate, magnesium: derangement common
- Liver biochemistry
- Coagulation profile: can cause disseminated intravascular coagulation
- C-reactive protein (CRP) (or procalcitonin)
- Blood cultures: always before starting antibiotics
- Throat swab to look for meningococcal carriage
- Computed tomography brain if signs of raised ICP, for example, focal neurology, papilloedema, seizures
- Consider lumbar puncture only once patient is stable and if raised ICP is ruled out

---

WHO SHOULD BE INFORMED AND WHAT FURTHER ACTION SHOULD BE TAKEN?

Microbiology and the relevant public health authority must be informed if a clinical diagnosis of meningococcal disease is made. Formal notification should then be given in writing. Chemoprophylaxis can then be arranged for any close contacts, ideally within 24 hours of identification of the index case.

Contacts (irrespective of vaccine status), who should receive prophylaxis?

- People who live in the same household as the case or who have lived there in the previous week
- Sexual partners
- Work fellows sharing a small office, that is an office for two
- The patient herself at the end of her parenteral therapy
- School contacts if more than one case in a school
- Healthcare providers having unprotected contact with patients' respiratory secretions

Once the public health authority has been informed, they will usually arrange chemoprophylaxis but might ask the hospital doctor to do this for the patient's relatives.

Ciprofloxacin and rifampicin are both recommended but ciprofloxacin is normally used as 1st line treatment.

Progress. This patient was treated with intravenous ceftriaxone 2 g IV × 2 daily in the intensive care unit (ICU). After a stormy course, she made a full recovery. There were no secondary cases.

Meningitis

CASE HISTORY (1)

A 55-year-old male, a heavy alcohol user, is brought to the emergency department with headache, confusion and a high fever.

On examination, he is found to be photophobic and to have neck stiffness. He is thought by the emergency department staff to have meningitis and is immediately given IV ceftriaxone because they were unclear about the most likely organism. You are called urgently to review him.

WHAT WOULD YOU DO?

You quickly check the neurological signs and agree this is meningitis. You also note that there is no purpuric rash of meningococcal septicaemia. You try to see the patient's fundi but are unsure whether papilloedema is present. You are worried about doing a lumbar puncture because he is semiconscious and you are concerned about the possibility of 'coning'. You arrange an immediate CT scan, which is normal. You proceed with a lumbar puncture, and the CSF, which is turbid, is sent urgently to the microbiologists.

INFORMATION

Lumbar Puncture

This should be performed with sterile measures. Check there are no signs of raised ICP.

- Obtain patient consent
- Place patient in lateral decubitus position
- Identify L4 to 5 interspace (intersection of imaginary line between iliac crests and spine)
- Clean area with antiseptic, for example, chlorhexidine
- Local anaesthetic (2% lidocaine) into skin and subcutaneous tissue
- Insert lumbar puncture spinal needle (bevel upwards) into skin over L4 to 5 interspace horizontally and slightly towards the head
- When needle penetrates the dura mater (a slight decrease in resistance is felt), withdraw stylet and allow a few drops of CSF to escape
- Measure CSF pressure by connecting manometer to a needle; it rises and falls with respiration and heartbeat
- Collect CSF in three sterile tubes (2 mL per tube)
- Send to laboratory. Note if clear, cloudy, yellow (xanthochromic) or red
- Remove needle and apply sterile dressing
- Patient should lie horizontal for 4 h to avoid headache, analgesics might be required

Indications and contraindications are shown in Box 7.4.

BOX 7.4 ■ Indications for and Contraindications to Lumbar Puncture

Indications

- Diagnosis of meningitis, encephalitis and subarachnoid haemorrhage (sometimes)
- Measurement of CSF pressure, for example, for idiopathic intracranial hypertension (IIH)
- Removal of CSF therapeutically (IIH)
- Diagnosis of conditions, for example, neoplastic involvement

Contraindications

- Raised intracranial pressure
- Local infections at site of puncture area
- Platelet count $<40 \times 10^9/L$ (check local guidance)
- Mass lesion in brain or spinal cord

CSF: Cerebrospinal fluid.

The CSF results sent through are:

- Protein: 1.5 g/L (normal range 0.2–0.4 g/L)
- Glucose: 1.5 mmol/L
- Leucocytes: 500/mm^3
- Pneumococcus is seen on Gram stain

HOW DOES THIS CHANGE YOUR MANAGEMENT PLAN?

Diagnosis: pneumococcal meningitis.

You should immediately start treatment with antibiotics as per local guidelines (e.g. IV cefotaxime 8 g daily in four divided doses) because there is a high incidence of penicillin-resistant pneumococcus (Table 7.1). Empirical intravenous dexamethasone should also be given to all adults with acute bacterial meningitis within 1 hour of presentation to hospital (ideally shortly after antibiotics).

WHAT ARE THE COMMON CAUSATIVE ORGANISMS?

These are listed in Box 7.5.

- **Pneumococcal meningitis** most commonly occurs in the debilitated or in those with a chest or sinus infection, valvular disease, splenectomy or a fistula from the paranasal air sinuses to the brain
- **Meningococcal meningitis** (see also p. 9) occurs in epidemics and is seen in young adults. It is sometimes associated with a petechial or purpuric rash and has a very rapid evolution. Nasopharyngeal swab culture is useful for typing meningococcus and *Haemophilus* (see later)
- ***Staphylococcus aureus* meningitis** generally occurs in the context of systemic infection, abscesses or neurosurgical procedures
- ***Pseudomonas*** and other Gram-negative enterobacilli are usually a consequence of surgical access to the CSF
- ***Listeria meningitis*** is quite common. It should be treated with amoxicillin and gentamicin. It is also associated with encephalitis
- ***Haemophilus influenzae*** type B used to be extremely common but has been substantially reduced in many countries by immunisation (Hib vaccine) in children

Progress. This male made an excellent recovery from his pneumococcal meningitis.

TABLE 7.1 ■ **Example Treatment Regimens: Antibiotics and Acute Bacterial Meningitis**

Organism	First choice	Alternative
Unknown	Cefotaxime	Benzylpenicillin + cefotaxime
Meningococcus	Benzylpenicillin	Cefotaxime
Pneumococcus	Cefotaxime	Penicillin if organism is sensitive
Haemophilus	Cefotaxime	Chloramphenicol
Listeria	Amoxicillin + gentamicin	–

This table demonstrates the value of cefotaxime in clinical practice.

BOX 7.5 ■ Causes of Meningitis

Bacterial

- *Meningococcus*
- *Pneumococcus*
- *Listeria* spp.
- *Staphylococcus aureus*
- *E. coli*
- *Pseudomonas* spp.

Viral

- Enteroviruses
- Mumps (meningoencephalitides)

Atypical

- Tuberculosis
- *Cryptococcus*
- Leptospirosis

Noninfective

- Subarachnoid haemorrhage
- Chemical meningitis

Recurrent

- Nasal sinus fistula
- Traumatic CSF leak
- Epstein–Barr virus
- Sarcoidosis, Behçet
- Mollaret meningitis (herpes simplex virus type 2)

E. coli, Escherichia coli; CSF, cerebrospinal fluid.

CASE HISTORY (2)

A 22-year-old male is admitted from the emergency department with an insidious 2-week history of malaise, headaches and marked confusion. He has recently had close contact with a family member who has been diagnosed with TB. **On examination**, he is pyrexial and drowsy and has neck stiffness and upgoing plantar responses. There is a concern that this patient has **tuberculous meningitis.**

WHAT ACTION WOULD YOU TAKE?

- Take bloods for U and Es, FBC, liver function test (LFT), CRP and clotting profile
- Chest X-ray: may show evidence of pulmonary TB
- Computed tomography scan: an immediate scan is done because, with this male's confusion and possible raised ICP, coning is a possibility following lumbar puncture. The CT scan is normal
- Lumbar puncture:

The CSF results (Table 7.2) sent back to your F1 junior doctor are:

- Glucose 1.8 mmol/L (blood level 6.5, i.e. low glucose)
- Protein 2.3 g/L (very high protein)
- White cell count (WCC) 250 (70% lymphocytes)

Note: the CSF protein can be so high as to cause the formation of a fine clot ('spider web').

TABLE 7.2 ■ **Typical Changes in the CSF in Meningitis**

	Normal	**Viral**	**Pyogenic**	**Tuberculosis**
Appearance	Crystal clear	Clear/turbid	Turbid/purulent	Turbid/viscous
Mononuclear cells	<5 mm^3	10–100 mm^3	<50 mm^3	100–300 mm^3
Polymorph cells	Nil	Nil[a]	200–300/mm^3	0–200/mm^3
Protein	0.2–0.4 g/L	0.4–0.8 g/L	0.5–2.0 g/L	0.5–3.0 g/L
Glucose	2/3–1/2 blood glucose	$>1/2$ blood glucose	$<1/2$ blood glucose	$<1/3$ blood glucose

CSF: Cerebrospinal fluid.
[a]Some polymorph cells may be seen in the early stages of viral meningitis and encephalitis.
(From Feather, A., Randall, D., Waterhouse, M., eds., 2021. Kumar and Clark's Clinical Medicine, tenth ed. London, Elsevier, 2021; Box 26.58.)

Note: tubercle bacilli are seen only occasionally in the CSF, and the CSF must be sent for culture, which takes 6 weeks

HOW WOULD YOU MANAGE THIS CASE?

Start antituberculous chemotherapy based on the clinical picture and high protein in the CSF, which strongly suggest tuberculous meningitis. Do not wait for the culture! Give therapy as per local guidelines (e.g. rifampicin, isoniazid, ethambutol and pyrazinamide) for 6 weeks until the culture and sensitivities come back. Three drugs should be given for 3 months, followed by rifampicin and isoniazid for 9 months, depending on sensitivities. Consider adjuvant corticosteroid – dexamethasone is the preferred agent. Specialist advice should be sought for treatment, notification and contact tracing.

Progress. This patient made a good recovery. Dexamethasone was given for the first 3 weeks.

Brain Abscess

A brain abscess is a suppurative collection of microbes (most commonly bacterial, fungal or parasitic) within a gliotic capsule in the brain parenchyma. They can be single or multifocal and they have a similar clinical and radiological presentation to central nervous system tumours.

CASE HISTORY

A 57-year-old male is brought to the emergency department by ambulance having been found unconscious at home by his family. They tell you he had been complaining of progressively worsening headaches over the last 2 to 3 weeks. He has been feeling generally unwell and feverish in the last week. After initial assessment, his GCS drops further, and he requires intubation to protect his airway. He is taken for a CT head, which demonstrates a right parietal ring enhancing lesion.

WHAT IS THE MOST LIKELY DIAGNOSIS?

Cerebral abscess. The associated symptoms from cerebral abscesses are related to infection (e.g. fevers) and/or mass effect. Neurological symptoms can be localising (e.g. hemiparesis) or related to increased ICP (e.g. reduced consciousness, vomiting).

WHAT ARE THE RISK FACTORS FOR THIS CONDITION?

Risk factors include:

- Immunocompromise: HIV, diabetes, immunomodulating therapy
- Ear, nose and throat infection: sinusitis, otitis media, recent dental procedure
- Recent neurosurgery or meningitis
- Intravenous drug abuse
- Endocarditis

WHAT IS THE POTENTIAL AETIOLOGY?

- Bacterial: commonly *Staphylococcus aureus*, *Streptococcus*, *Listeria* and *Bacteroides* with 40% associated with infection of adjacent structures (otitis media, sinusitis, mastoiditis
- Fungal: *Candida, Cryptococcus, Histoplasma, Aspergillus*. Incidence is increasing due to rising use of broad-spectrum antimicrobials and immunosuppressants
- Protozoa: *Entamoeba, Schistosoma, Toxoplasma*

INVESTIGATIONS

- Full blood count: typically shows a marked leucocytosis
- Urea and electrolytes: hyponatraemia can be caused by syndrome of inappropriate antidiuretic hormone secretion (SIADH)
- Erythrocyte sedimentation rate/CRP: raised
- Take 2 × blood cultures preferable before starting antibiotics
- Computed tomography brain: initial investigation of choice, typical 'ring enhancement' appears on contrast-enhanced studies as disease progresses
- Magnetic resonance imaging can provide greater contrast to detect early lesions
- Lumbar puncture is rarely helpful and contraindicated if there is raised ICP

HOW WOULD YOU MANAGE THIS PATIENT?

Treatment involves drainage of the intracranial collection, effective antibiotic therapy, and the removal of any primary source of infection:

- Commence empirical IV antibiotics based on local guidelines, for example, third-generation cephalosporin (such as ceftriaxone), metronidazole and vancomycin
- Add antifungal if fungal cause suspected (e.g. amphotericin)
- Refer for surgical decompression/ aspiration (send pus for culture)
- Commence anticonvulsant if seizure activity, for example, levetiracetam
- Consider corticosteroids if there is evidence of massive cerebral oedema

Traumatic Brain Injury

CASE HISTORY

A 25-year-old male is knocked unconscious by a blow from a sledgehammer. He regains consciousness after a few minutes and attends the emergency department. He is nauseated and in pain but reasonably alert, with a GCS (Table 7.3) of 14. His conscious level then rapidly deteriorates to a GCS of 5. A subsequent CT scan reveals a large extradural blood collection that requires emergency drainage by craniotomy.

TABLE 7.3 ■ Glasgow Coma Scale (GCS)

Parameter	Score
Eye opening (E)	
Spontaneous	4
To speech	3
To pain	2
No response	1
Motor response (M)	
Obeys	6
Localises	5
Withdraws	4
Flexion	3
Extension	2
No response	1
Verbal response (V)	
Orientated	5
Confused conversation	4
Inappropriate words	3
Incomprehensible sounds	2
No response	1

Glasgow Coma Scale = E + M + V (GCS minimum = 3; maximum = 15.)
(From Feather, A., Randall, D., Waterhouse, M., eds., 2021. Kumar and Clark's Clinical Medicine, tenth ed. London, Elsevier, 2021; Box 26.28.)

HOW DOES EXTRADURAL HAEMORRHAGE DIFFER FROM SUBDURAL?

Extradural haemorrhage is a serious secondary effect of head injury. These bleeds occur into a tight space, resulting in a rather long lucid interval as the blood slowly accumulates. Computed tomography reveals a convex, hyperdense collection in the acute phase. By contrast, subdural haemorrhages bleed more freely into a more easily opened space, so the shape is concave on CT, and there is little lucid interval.

Progress. Following his craniotomy and drainage, the patient gradually recovered over the next few days. However, 2 to 3 weeks later, he was still amnesic and needed constant attention. He is being followed up by the neurologists.

REMEMBER

- Always monitor head injuries carefully and record changes in GCS rather than simply considering one value in isolation
- The result of secondary swelling by haemorrhage or oedema (the latter is common in children) is raised ICP, leading to reduced perfusion pressure and coning

WHAT ARE THE COMPLICATIONS OF TRAUMATIC BRAIN INJURY?

Primary Effects

- Diffuse axonal injury
- Contusion
- Laceration
- Vascular lesions

Secondary Effects

- Extradural haemorrhage
- Subdural haemorrhage
- Cerebrospinal fluid leak, infection
- Hydrocephalus
- Compromised airway, respiration
- Hypotension

Late Sequelae

- Chronic daily headache
- Posttraumatic stress disorder
- Vertigo
- Cognitive impairment

> **REMEMBER**
>
> Posttraumatic amnesia of >24 hours indicates severe brain injury.

WHAT ACTION WOULD YOU TAKE IN A PATIENT WITH A HEAD INJURY?

- Attend first to any secondary or concomitant general problems, that is resuscitation, hypovolaemic shock, hypotension or compromised airway
- Assess severity, using circumstances of injury and period of amnesia as a guide
- Establish whether there is anterograde amnesia: the inability to form memories from the time of injury to the time of continuous normal memory is the most accurate guide
- Brainstem damage in head injury can affect central respiratory drive, bulbar function and pressor responses
- Regular GCS measurements; <5 at 24 h implies severe injury and 50% of such patients die
- Arrange a CT scan (Box 7.6)

HOW WOULD YOU MANAGE THE FOLLOWING PROBLEMS?

- If the patient is deteriorating or has evidence of raised ICP, consider insertion of a bolt, which is simply a tube into the ventricle through which ICP can be recorded
- If ICP is >20 mm Hg, there is a need to treat. Give mannitol or hypertonic saline. Hyperventilation with intermittent positive pressure ventilation (IPPV) will also lower the ICP
- If the patient has haemorrhages, a craniotomy may be indicated

---

BOX 7.6 ■ NICE Guidelines for Head Injuries: Criteria for Immediate Request for CT Scan of the Head (Adults)

GCS <13 on initial assessment in the emergency department
- GCS <15 at 2 h after injury on assessment in the A and E department
- Suspected open or depressed skull fracture
- Any sign of basal skull fracture (haemotympanum, 'panda' eyes, CSF leakage from the ear or nose, Battle sign)
- Posttraumatic seizure
- Focal neurological deficit
- More than one episode of vomiting
- Amnesia for events >30 min before impact

CSF: cerebrospinal fluid; GCS, Glasgow Coma Scale; NICE, National Institute for Health and Care Excellence.

FOLLOW-UP

Check for continued improvement in the weeks subsequent to the head injury. At 2 to 3 weeks post injury, the development of hydrocephalus is a major complication.

CASE HISTORY

A 30-year-old male falls from a second-storey building and is immediately unconscious. He is admitted comatose, GCS 5, although he is breathing spontaneously. There are no external injuries, and a CT scan of the head is normal. He does not regain consciousness.

WHAT IS THE LIKELY DIAGNOSIS?

Diffuse axonal injury is the primary effect of traumatic brain injury and a common cause of vegetative state. There is usually immediate loss of consciousness followed by prolonged coma.

Milder axonal injury is reversible, for example, in concussion. This damage occurs with brain accelerations or decelerations, such as hitting the floor or wall, rather than by a direct blow to the head. The mechanism of damage is due to stretching of axons, causing Ca^{2+} entry and neurofilament damage, and interrupting axonal transport over the next 12 hours. Certain areas are particularly vulnerable, such as the parasagittal white matter, internal capsule, cerebellar peduncles, posterior corpus callosum and dorsolateral midbrain.

Progress. This patient was in a coma for a week and never recovered. Consent was obtained for his organs to be used for transplantation.

Severe Brain Injury

CASE HISTORY

Your patient has had a severe hypoxic cerebral episode following a cardiac arrest. He is currently stable from a cardiac point of view but comatose (GCS 5) and requiring ventilatory support on the intensive care unit (ICU). He has been given 24 h of induced hypothermia 32°C to 34°C. The ITU staff and the patient's relatives want an indication of the likelihood of useful recovery.

WHAT ACTION WOULD YOU TAKE?

First, check for a remediable cause of coma or any confounding factors worsening the patient's responsiveness (see Investigations box). For example:

- Brain imaging may reveal a potentially treatable but unsuspected condition, possibly additional to the primary pathology, such as subdural or intracerebral haemorrhage or hydrocephalus
- An EEG may show abnormalities indicative of an unsuspected metabolic encephalopathy or subclinical seizure activity
- The patient may still be under the influence of long-acting anaesthetic agents or other sedative drugs

INVESTIGATIONS

- Review bloods – check for electrolyte imbalance or metabolic derangement
- Recent drug history
- Computed tomography or MRI brain
- Electroencephalography
- Echocardiography – assess cardiac output

WHICH ASPECTS OF EXAMINATION SHOULD BE ASSESSED ROUTINELY?

- Glasgow Coma Scale score (see Table 7.3)
- Eye movements:
    - Following, roving, conjugate
    - Optokinetic nystagmus (following a moving grid pattern)
    - Vertical and horizontal doll's head movement
- Pupils
- Corneal reflexes
- Bulbar function: is the patient tolerating the endotracheal (ET) tube?
- Respiratory function: level of ventilator support
- Tone and reflexes
- General examination, for example, chest, infected pressure sores, abdominal guarding

WHAT ARE YOUR PROGNOSTIC INDICATORS?

There are some prognostic values, depending on the time after the initial cerebral insult. The following criteria indicate **poor outcome**:

- Absent or extensor plantar response 72 h after cerebral insult
- Absent pupillary or corneal reflexes 72 h after cerebral insult

In general, every case must be assessed on its merits, especially with regard to the nature of the original insult and whether it was a discrete event or likely to result in ongoing brain injury.

Note: relatives should not be given conflicting or inaccurate information.

DETERMINATION OF BRAIN DEATH

Determination of brain death is made only by the appropriate consultant specialists who assess – on separate occasions – the various brainstem reflexes and responses listed under 'Aspects of examination', earlier. The nature of the insult must be clear and remediable causes must be excluded. Because the criteria for brain death are heavily weighted towards brainstem function and, in the UK, EEG corroboration is not required, locked-in syndrome should be excluded. In this state, a severe pontine lesion prevents access to or from the outside world. The only signs of relatively spared higher-level function may be preserved vertical optokinetic nystagmus or eye following and preserved vertical doll eye reflexes.

Fits and Faints

CASE HISTORY (1)

A 16-year-old young female is referred with a suspected seizure. She had begun feeling generally unwell and lightheaded then, on getting up from her chair, she suddenly lost consciousness without warning. She was incontinent of urine. She woke some minutes later but had nausea and malaise for the rest of the day. Witnesses said that, when unconscious, she was flaccid and pale, and her mouth, hands and feet were twitching.

IS THIS A 'FIT' OR A 'FAINT'?

The patient has probably suffered a 'faint' (vasovagal syncope). Some factors are good for distinguishing a fit from a faint (Table 7.4), whereas others are unreliable. In this case, it is noted that 'faints' (except for cardiac syncope) occur predominantly on standing, and the preceding symptoms are prolonged or ill defined. Twitching is not usually as violent as in a clonic seizure, and the underlying muscle tone is not increased.

Vasovagal faints are generally idiopathic, but there are often precipitating or predisposing factors.

INVESTIGATIONS

In suspected cardiac syncope include:
- Electrocardiogram
- Twenty-four hour ambulatory monitoring
- Echocardiogram

TABLE 7.4 ■ **Features of Fits and Faints**

	Fit (Seizure)	Faint (Syncope)
Prodrome	None or characteristic brief aura	Short or prolonged. Blood draining, visual darkening, rushing noise. Cardiac syncope may have no prodrome
Posture at onset	Any	Standing unless cardiac
Injury	Common	Rarer. Protective reflexes may act
Incontinence	Sometimes	Sometimes
Skin colour	Normal, flushed or pale	Pale
Recovery	Slow return of consciousness	Rapid, more physical weakness with clear sensorium
Frequency	Rare to many a day	Not repeated attacks each day
EEG	May be abnormal	Normal

EEG, Electroencephalography.

WHAT CAN INCREASE THE RISK OF VASOVAGAL SYNCOPE?

- Low baseline BP and/or postural hypotension
- Heavy periods
- Micturition with prostatic problems
- Hyperthermia
- Fasting, hypoglycaemia
- Dehydration
- Vagal stimuli such as distress or nausea

Vasovagal attacks must be distinguished from cardiac syncope (see p. 251). In the latter there is often no warning; there may be breathlessness and engorged jugular veins, and the heart rate may be faster than 140 or slower than 40.

Progress. This patient and her parents were reassured that she had had a simple vasovagal syncope.

CASE HISTORY (2)

A 16-year-old young male presents with repeated brief falls. He does not seem to lose consciousness but has been seen in the emergency department several times with severe head and facial injuries resulting from these episodes. Recovery, apart from associated injury, is immediate.

WHAT IS THE DIAGNOSIS?

This history is suggestive of **atonic seizures**. This seizure disorder usually presents in childhood, often as one aspect of a complex epileptic syndrome. Not all seizures resulting in falls are generalised tonic–clonic in nature.

The loss of tone is immediate and absolute so that no protective reflexes occur and injury can be severe. Some sufferers need to wear protective helmets.

Progress. The patient was referred to the neurologists for ongoing management of his epilepsy.

CASE HISTORY (3)

A 28-year-old male is brought to the emergency department because he was found to be unconscious, rigid, shaking, and foaming at the mouth in the high street. He stopped shaking but remained drowsy in the ambulance. You are then called to see him urgently because the shaking starts again on arrival.

WHAT IS THE DIAGNOSIS?

An epileptic seizure is a convulsion or transient abnormal event experienced by the subject as a result of a paroxysmal discharge of cerebral neurones. Epilepsy, by definition, is the continuing tendency to have such seizures. Recurrent seizures can be prevented in most cases by the use of anticonvulsant drugs.

REMEMBER

Status epilepticus exists when seizures follow each other without recovery of consciousness.

HOW WOULD YOU MANAGE THIS SITUATION?

General Measures

- Secure the airway
- Administer oxygen
- Secure venous access: many anticonvulsants cause phlebitis, so choose large veins and insert two
- Give glucose IV if hypoglycaemia is a possibility
- Give thiamine, 250–500 mg by slow IV injection, if patient is a chronic alcohol user or there is a suspicion of malnutrition

> **REMEMBER**
>
> Full ventilatory support must be available when treating status epilepticus.

Control of Seizures

- First administer an intravenous benzodiazepine (following local guidelines) for example lorazepam 0.1 mg/kg (max 4mg as single dose initially) by slow (2 mg/min) IV injection
- Give rectal diazepam (10–20 mg) or 10 mg buccal midazolam if IV access is difficult or in the community
- If seizures continue, give IV phenytoin or fosphenytoin or levetiracetam or sodium valproate. Choice depends on availability, local guidance, contraindications, type of epilepsy and usual antiepileptic medication (where applicable and known)
- If seizures continue (despite initial treatment), consider phenobarbital
- If seizures continue despite these measures, the patient is given a general anaesthetic, using thiopentone or propofol, and management is continued with full anaesthetic support

Progress. This patient had no further fits after being given phenytoin. He was known to have epilepsy and was referred back urgently to his normal consultant for the management of his drug therapy.

Headaches

CASE HISTORY (1)

A 72-year-old female is admitted to the emergency department with a very severe headache of explosive onset. She is slightly drowsy with a GCS of 13 and has photophobia and meningism.

A CT scan shows blood in the subarachnoid space (this has a 95% sensitivity in the first 24 hours).

HOW WOULD YOU ACUTELY MANAGE THIS PATIENT?

- Comprehensive ABCDE assessment and management – secure airway if required and carefully monitor GCS and pupillary reflexes
- Arrange CT angiography in patients with confirmed subarachnoid haemorrhage (SAH) to identify the causal pathology (consider MR angiography if CT is inconclusive and aneurysm is still suspected)
- Urgently discuss with a specialist neurosurgical centre
- **Nimodipine** (e.g. 60 mg orally 4-hourly for 2–3 weeks, or 1 mg/h IV) can reduce arterial spasm and reduce further cerebral infarction

- Avoid hypotension (it may worsen the ischaemic deficit), and treat hypertension if systolic pressure is persistently >180 mmHg (maintain the mean arterial pressure at least >90 mmHg). Aim for a very gradual decrease in BP with careful monitoring and frequent repeat neurological examination
- Supportive measures include bed rest, analgesia and laxatives (avoid sudden rises in ICP or BP)
- Watch for complications, including hyponatraemia/SIADH, hydrocephalus (obstruction of cerebral aqueduct by blood) and vasospasm-causing ischaemic deficits.

N.B. If the scan is negative and the history is highly suggestive of an SAH, a lumbar puncture is necessary

- A **lumbar puncture** can be performed to look for blood-stained CSF and xanthochromia (bilirubin discoloration of CSF due to cell lysis) if a CT head scan (performed >6 h after symptom onset) is negative or inconclusive. Xanthochromia may be detected from approximately 12 h to 3 weeks after SAH

> **REMEMBER**
>
> If two or more first-degree relatives have had a SAH, the rest of the family should be screened by MR angiography.

WHAT OTHER CONDITIONS CAN CAUSE AN ACUTE SEVERE HEADACHE?

Conditions that can mimic SAH include sudden onset of meningitis or viral meningism, migraine, spontaneous subdural haemorrhage and postcoital headache. The last of these is a headache of very sudden onset but is a benign self-limiting condition, perhaps a variant of migraine. With the availability of MR angiography, patients are now often scanned to exclude aneurysms. Finally, low-pressure headache may be of sudden onset. This is a poorly understood condition where headache may occur suddenly on standing and generally settles when lying down. There is meningeal enhancement on MRI and a low CSF pressure. The condition is again self-limiting. At least some cases relate to CSF leaks, sometimes from lumbar puncture (postlumbar puncture headache) and occasionally from Valsalva manoeuvres.

Progress. In this patient, a posterior communicating aneurysm was found. She was treated with an intravascular coil insertion and made a good recovery.

> **CASE HISTORY (2)**
>
> A 35-year-old male complains of continuous headache day and night. He used to have a different headache, which was episodic. This previous headache was unilateral, throbbing and would last a few hours. It was also associated with photophobia, visual scotomata and nausea. The new headache has no such features. He takes eight paracetamol tablets a day and codeine to try and control the pain.

WHAT IS THIS NEW HEADACHE MOST LIKELY CAUSED BY?

Chronic migraine headache. The headache associated with migraines sometimes becomes transformed into a more chronic headache, punctuated by migraine-like exacerbations. Often the patient is given regular analgesia, which has a well-known effect of perpetuating headache.

WHAT ACTION SHOULD YOU TAKE?

Other causes of new or persistent severe headache should be excluded (e.g. space-occupying lesion, haemorrhage, infection). It is important to take a proper history, perform a thorough examination and arrange appropriate imaging when required.

WHAT IS THE MANAGEMENT OF THIS CONDITION?

This is broadly similar to episodic migraine, sumatriptan prophylaxis is given if the sufferer has more than about two migraines a month or finds them very debilitating.

Progress. After appropriate investigations, this patient was reassured that he did not have a malignant or serious disease.

Chronic analgesia abuse should be stopped. This male was advised to reduce this gradually over a month. He was told to expect his headaches to be worse over this period but then improve.

INFORMATION

Calcitonin-gene-related peptide (CGRP) influences neuronal modulation of pain and this may play a role in migraine. Four monoclonal antibodies to the CGRP have been developed and are now being used in chronic migraine, that is erenumab, eptinezumab, fremanezumab and galcanezumab.

CASE HISTORY (3)

A 40-year-old male presents to the emergency department with a severe headache that then settles on arrival. This has happened before and he has always been discharged immediately. On taking a history, it transpires that an excruciating headache comes on gradually at about the same time every day. The headache is unilateral and pounding, involves the side of the face, and is associated with a watering eye and nose. He jumps up and down in agitation with the pain. The symptoms generally only last about an hour.

WHAT IS THE CAUSE OF THIS HEADACHE?

This description is typical of **cluster headache.** Each cluster may last a few weeks, with several months of relief in between.

Cluster headache is distinct from migraine and consists of recurrent bouts of excruciating unilateral pain that typically wake the patient. Attacks cluster around one eye. Cluster headache affects adults, mainly males aged 30 to 40 years. Alcohol and glyceryl trinitrate can provoke attacks. Severe pain can last for several hours and is associated with vomiting. One cheek and nostril become congested. Transient ipsilateral Horner syndrome is common. One bout of cluster attacks, with pain every few nights, usually lasts 1 to 2 months. Despite excruciating pain, there are no sequelae. Bouts recur at intervals over several years but tend to disappear after the age of 55.

Progress. In this patient, treatment with analgesics and prophylactic migraine drugs did not help. However, his attacks were attenuated with SC sumatriptan. Oxygen inhalation also helped on occasions. A short course of oral prednisolone reduced the frequency of attacks.

CASE HISTORY (4)

A 30-year-old female has a long history of short but severe headaches on one side of the face, lasting only a few minutes but occurring several times a day. There is considerable flushing and rhinorrhoea on the same side during each attack. There is no trigger to the attacks.

WHAT IS THE CAUSE OF THIS HEADACHE?

The patient has **paroxysmal hemicrania**; the attacks are longer in duration than in trigeminal neuralgia but shorter than in cluster headaches or migraine. There is generally some associated autonomic disturbance, as seen here. There is a specific and often extremely rewarding response to indometacin, as occurred in this female.

Some causes of acute, episodic and chronic headaches are given in Box 7.7.

Falls

CASE HISTORY (1)

A 70-year-old male presents with recurrent falls. **On examination**, he has a rigid increase in tone, worse in the trunk than the limbs, marked bradykinesia and extreme mental slowness. He is unable to move his eyes vertically or laterally. He walks with a rather upright gait. He is thought to have Parkinson disease but has had a poor response to levodopa (LD).

BOX 7.7 ■ Causes of Headache

Very Sudden
- Subarachnoid haemorrhage
- First migraine attack
- Subdural haemorrhage
- Meningitis, encephalitis
- Inflammatory meningoencephalitis, for example, systemic lupus erythematosus (SLE)
- Cerebral abscess
- Raised intracranial pressure
- Low-pressure headache

Episodic
- Tension headache
- Migraine
- Paroxysmal hemicrania
- Cluster headache
- Trigeminal/occipital neuralgia
- Giant cell arteritis (temporal or cranial arteritis)
- Postcoital headache

Chronic
- Tension headache
- Analgesia abuse
- Chronic hemicrania
- Chronic cluster headache
- Cervicogenic headache
- Space-occupying lesions
- Raised intracranial pressure
- Ongoing after many acute headaches
- Associated with depression/anxiety

WHAT IS THE DIAGNOSIS?

This patient has **progressive supranuclear palsy** (PSP; also known as Steele–Richardson syndrome). Parkinson disease usually results in falls late on in the disease. Early falls should lead to suspicion of PSP or multisystem atrophy (which does not cause early cognitive problems).

INFORMATION

Progressive Supranuclear Palsy

- Parkinsonism
- Axial rigidity
- Dementia
- Defective upward-and-lateral gaze

Some common causes of falls are listed in Box 7.8. Some simply relate to stance or gait difficulties.

Progress. This patient continued to deteriorate and died of pneumonia 6 months later.

CASE HISTORY (2)

A 65-year-old female is worried she has epilepsy. She suffers repeated falls when walking outside. There is no warning before falling and she recovers immediately in a state of embarrassment. If she loses consciousness at all, it could be for a split second only because she is certainly aware when she hits the ground.

There is no abnormality on examination.

BOX 7.8 ■ Causes of Falls

Preserved Consciousness

- Leg weakness
- Spasticity
- Extrapyramidal syndromes
- Ataxia, periodic ataxia
- Vertigo
- Drop attacks
- Cataplexy
- Epilepsy, myoclonus

Loss of Consciousness

- Epilepsy
- Faint
- Syncope (cardiac or vascular insufficiency)
- Vertebrobasilar TIA
- Intermittent hydrocephalus
- Metabolic, for example, hypoglycaemia
- Toxic encephalopathy
- Other encephalopathies

TIA, Transient ischaemic attacks.

WHAT IS THE DIAGNOSIS?

These episodes are most consistent with **drop attacks**. They are benign episodes that more commonly occur in women. There is no loss of consciousness and they are not considered epileptic. They are due to sudden changes in lower limb tone, presumably brainstem in origin.

Progress. This patient was reassured that she did not have epilepsy and was helped by using a walking stick.

Difficulty Walking

CASE HISTORY (1)

A 75-year-old male is referred with a 1-year history of progressive difficulty with his walking. He has hypertension, which is well controlled with ramipril 5 mg daily. His wife says that his memory has been progressively getting worse.

On examination, he has a Mini Mental State score of 22, indicating a cognitive impairment. His grasp and snout (pursing of lips on lightly tapping the closed lips) reflexes are present, indicating frontal lobe disease. His legs are stiff and his walking is disorganised. This is an apraxic gait.

An apraxic gait is typical of frontal lobe pathology and can be regarded as a problem with high-level programming and execution of gait. This male has vascular dementia (multiinfarct dementia). Patients with cerebrovascular disease should be imaged to exclude a frontal meningioma or other lesion.

HOW WOULD YOU MANAGE THIS PATIENT?

As with other dementias, the treatment is symptomatic and involves addressing the individual's main needs and supporting their carers.

It is also important to investigate and treat their individual cardiovascular risk factors in order to slow progression. This involves the use of antiplatelets for patients with previous stroke or TIA relating to atherosclerotic or small-vessel disease. It also involves management of risk factors such as diabetes, hypertension, diabetes and hyperlipidaemia.

CASE HISTORY (2)

A 70-year-old female has a 3-week history of progressive difficulty in walking and loss of bladder function. For the last 6 months, she has had problems with a stiff gait, numbness in the feet and pains down the left arm.

On examination, she has wasting and weakness of the hands and brisk triceps reflexes. In the legs, there are signs of an UMN lesion with brisk reflexes and an extensor plantar response. There is also patchy sensory loss in both arms and feet.

WHAT IS THE DIAGNOSIS?

Cervical myelopathy, which at this age is most commonly due to spondylitis. She requires an urgent MRI scan of her cervical spine with a view to early decompression because relatively, acute deficits are more potentially reversible. The MRI showed cord compression at the level of C5 to 6 (Fig. 7.10).

Walking difficulties with upper motor signs in the upper limbs should always be investigated by cervical imaging. Thoracic compression is relatively much less common in the elderly age group.

Other common causes of difficulty in walking are:

- Neurological:
  - Myopathy: proximal, Trendelenburg positive (pelvis drops on the side of the stance leg, suggesting weakness of abductor muscles of the hip), worse on stairs

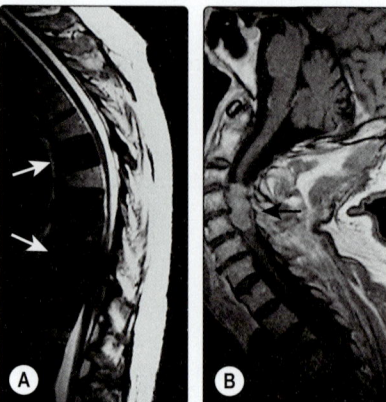

Fig. 7.10   Magnetic resonance imaging showing spinal cord compression. (A) Multiple vertebral metastases (*arrows*); (B) cervical compression caused by meningioma (*arrow*).

- Peripheral neuropathy: foot drop
- Extrapyramidal, for example, shuffling, stooped
- Spasticity: stiff, circumducting hip
- Apraxic: upright, high-stepping
- Ataxic: wide-based
- Rheumatological/orthopaedic:
  - Polymyalgia
  - Hip joint disease

Progress.   In view of this patients's serious disability and bladder problems, decompressive surgery was performed. This stabilised her condition but without improvement in her bladder function.

Movement Disorders

Typically categorised as follows (both may coexist):
- Hypokinesia – slowed movement with increased tone
- Hyperkinesia – added, uncontrollable movements

CASE HISTORY (1)

A 22-year-old female develops an acute gastrointestinal illness with abdominal pain, vomiting and diarrhoea. After 2 days, she becomes generally stiff and has prolonged episodes of painful spasm of the axial muscles with opisthotonic posturing. Her eyes periodically roll upwards involuntarily (oculogyric crises). She had been given metoclopramide for her vomiting.

WHAT IS THE LIKELY DIAGNOSIS?

Oculogyric crises from metoclopramide.

Acute dystonic reactions can occur in sensitive individuals after relatively modest doses of drugs with central antidopaminergic action, such as neuroleptics or certain antiemetics, for example, metoclopramide. Neuroleptic malignant syndrome can also occur.

Treatment of oculogyric crisis involves the identification and stoppage of the responsible agent. These acute dystonias respond generally to IV centrally acting antimuscarinics, for example, procyclidine 5 to 10 mg.

WHAT CONDITIONS TYPICALLY CAUSE HYPOKINESIA?

- Parkinson disease
- Multisystem atrophy
- Progressive supranuclear palsy
- Dementia with Lewy bodies
- Corticobasal degeneration
- Some frontal dementias, mass lesions
- Tardive dyskinesia (+ hyperkinetic)
- Psychomotor retardation

WHAT CAN CAUSE HYPERKINESIA?

- Choreo-athetosis
- Ballismus
- Dystonia
- Myoclonus
- Tics
- Tremor
- Psychogenic

Progress. This female was given IV procyclidine 5 mg IV. Her dystonia settled within 24 hours.

CASE HISTORY (2)

A 40-year-old male has a 1-year history of involuntary facial movements and a shuffling gait. He has a past history of schizophrenia, for which he was given haloperidol. **On examination**, he has intermittent involuntary protrusion of his tongue, grimacing and blepharospasm. He has some writhing movements of his left arm and repetitive rubbing of the soles of his feet on the floor when sitting. Voluntary arm movements are slow. He walks slowly with a shuffling gait and stooped posture.

WHAT IS THE DIAGNOSIS?

Tardive dyskinesia. This develops in patients previously, as well as currently, on antipsychotic medication. The movement disorder may be a complex mixture of hyperkinetic restlessness (akathisia), dystonia, choreo-athetosis and hypokinetic bradykinesia. They are late and difficult to reverse. The effects of antidopaminergics are thought to be due to long-term dysregulation of dopaminergic pathways. Sometimes, in the short term, increases in antipsychotic drug doses actually improve the hyperkinetic aspects temporarily (direct antidopaminergic action), but this is likely to lead to worsened long-term problems. The drugs that are good for avoiding acute extrapyramidal side effects are also good for minimising long-term side effects.

Progress. In this patient the haloperidol was gradually reduced and stopped. His symptoms improved. He has been told of the risk of recurrence on further antipsychotic therapy.

Parkinson's Disease

Parkinson's disease is a neurodegenerative disorder affecting nigrostriatal dopaminergic cells, as well as other brain cells. It causes a combination of tremor, rigidity and akinesia, developing slowly over many months or years.

CASE HISTORY

A 75-year-old male with Parkinson's disease presented with uncontrollable gyrating movements of his arms and legs. On obtaining a detailed history, it transpired that he was on levodopa (LD) therapy. This had recently been increased to cocareldopa 50/200 (a mixture of carbidopa and LD) three tablets × 4 daily.

WHAT IS THE PROBLEM?

This patient has dyskinesia – a common, late side-effect of LD therapy for Parkinsonism. About 10% of patients per year of therapy will develop such dyskinesias, involving uncontrollable choreoathetoid movements and dystonic posturing. At this stage in the illness, the severity of dyskinesia is dose-dependent and so a balance has to be struck between 'off' symptoms of bradykinesia and rigidity and 'on' dyskinetic symptoms. In this case the cocareldopa was prescribed at too high a dose.

When commencing LD therapy, patients are generally started on cocareldopa 25/100 or cobeneldopa (100 mg/25 mg tablets: a mixture of benserazide hydrochloride and LD in proportions of 1:4) × 3 daily. These drugs consist of a combination of LD and a peripheral DOPA decarboxylase inhibitor (DDI) to prevent inappropriate peripheral activation of dopamine. The dose of these drugs can be gradually increased in amount and frequency as the underlying disease worsens.

Alternatively, patients may receive a controlled-release preparation; cocareldopa 50/200 has nearly twice the bioavailable strength of straight careldopa, but the cobeneldopa (25/1000) preparation is a more equivalent dose. The controlled-release preparations may be given once at night to help with nocturnal or early morning 'off' symptoms or may be given 2 to 3 times a day alone or in combination with straight LD in an effort to smoothen fluctuating symptoms.

INFORMATION

Some physicians start off with controlled-release preparations. This is to minimise dose fluctuations that may result in dyskinesias later in the course of the disease, but there is no clear evidence for this protective effect.

Occasionally, dyskinesias occur in relation to dramatic fluctuations in LD levels rather than in relation to high peak levels; the solution in this situation is to place the patient on a higher dose of longer-acting medication.

WHAT ARE THE TREATMENT OPTIONS FOR PARKINSON DISEASE?

- Exercise and physiotherapy are useful
- Initiate pharmacological treatment when there is impairment/disability resulting from symptoms
- Early treatment with monoamine oxidase B (MAOB) inhibitors (**selegiline** or **rasagiline**) may delay the need for more definitive dopamine replacement therapy by several months

- **Dopamine agonists (DAs)** are used in patients <70 years. Although they are less effective and less well tolerated than LD, they are also associated with fewer long-term motor complications
- In older patients (i.e. those more severely affected at diagnosis), start LD + DDI (**cobeneldopa** or **cocareldopa**) because of fewer side-effects
- Nonergot DAs (**pramipexole** and **ropinirole** oral 3 times daily, or once daily with slow-release formulations, **rotigotine** via transdermal patch) are used in preference to ergot-derived drugs
- All patients with Parkinson disease will eventually require treatment with LD, often in combination with a DA.

Progress. This patient was put on a lower dose of cocareldopa and the dyskinesia settled.

Multiple Sclerosis (MS)

Multiple sclerosis is an autoimmune disease of unknown aetiology. It causes plaques of demyelination throughout the brain and spinal cord. Acute relapses are caused by focal inflammatory demyelination, which causes a conduction block. These plaques can be demonstrated using an MRI scan (Fig. 7.11).

CASE HISTORY (1)

A 28-year-old male presents with several days of pain and progressive loss of vision in one eye.
Examination showed diminished visual acuity 6/36 and disc swelling (papilloedema). He had previously had an episode of difficulty in walking and urinary incontinence, which had recovered fully after several weeks.

WHAT IS THE PROBLEM WITH HIS EYES?

The swelling of the disc, along with diminished visual acuity, suggests optic neuritis, as other causes of papilloedema do not usually give visual disturbance. Optic neuritis is a common early presentation of MS. The previous history, suggesting an episode of transverse myelitis (inflammation of the cord), indicates dissociation in space and time, providing strong clinical support for the diagnosis of MS.

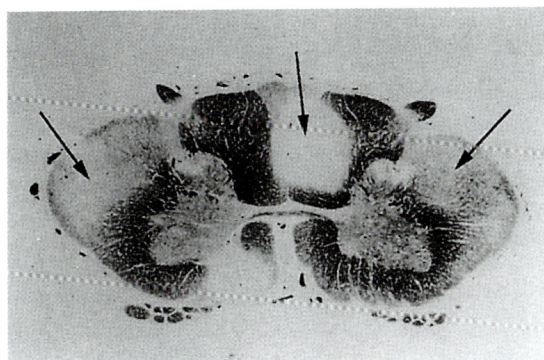

Fig. 7.11 Multiple sclerosis – showing plaques in the posterior column and lateral corticospinal tracts (*arrows*). (Courtesy the late Dr Ian MacDonald.)

WHAT ACTION WOULD YOU TAKE?

- An **MRI** should be performed to look for the demyelinating lesions of MS
- **Cerebrospinal fluid analysis** for oligoclonal bands is usually unnecessary to corroborate the diagnosis further
- **Visual evoked potentials** are likely to be delayed in the affected eye but may also reveal subclinical involvement of the other eye, providing evidence for dissociation in space
- **Medication**. Recovery after an episode of optic neuritis is aided by IV methylprednisolone, for example, 1 g/day for 3 days

Progress. This patient's vision improved following his steroid therapy. However, the MRI showed demyelinating lesions of MS and he is being followed up in the neurology clinic.

CASE HISTORY (2)

A previously well 25-year-old female develops double vision, vertigo and unsteadiness, as well as speech and swallowing problems, over 2 days. She is admitted to hospital, where she rapidly deteriorates, becoming confused and hypoxic. She requires ventilatory support. An MRI scan reveals a number of small bilateral periventricular white matter lesions, along with lesions in the brainstem and cerebellar peduncles. She is given IV methylprednisolone and recovers well over the next 2 weeks, apart from residual mild vertigo and intermittent diplopia.

REMEMBER

Multiple sclerosis may sometimes present dramatically as a brainstem syndrome with central respiratory problems and rapid severe bulbar failure. Early supportive management and steroids are essential in such cases. There may be excellent recovery following the relapse. Patients with known MS who suffer a relapse involving bulbar function or dysarthria should similarly be carefully observed.

CASE HISTORY (3)

A patient with known MS who has frequent severe relapses, bladder instability and incontinence, and painful leg spasms wonders if anything can be done for her incurable condition.

WHAT WOULD YOU SUGGEST?

Many forms of treatment are being used; as yet there is no evidence to support one over the other:

- **Acute relapses:** short courses of steroids, such as IV methylprednisolone 1 g/day for 3 days or high-dose oral steroids, are used widely in relapses that affect function and do sometimes reduce severity. They do not influence long-term outcome
- **Preventing relapse and disability.** Beta-interferon (both IFN β-1b and β-1a) by self-administered injection is used in relapsing and remitting disease. This is defined as at least two attacks of neurological dysfunction over the previous 2 or 3 years followed by a reasonable recovery. IFN β-1b is also used for secondary progressive MS. Interferon certainly reduces the relapse rate in some patients and prevents an increase in lesions seen on MRI. Unwanted effects are flu-like symptoms and irritation at injection sites. Beta-interferons are expensive

- **Glatiramer acetate**, an immunomodulator, has been shown to reduce relapse frequency in ambulatory patients with relapsing remitting MS – similar to beta-interferon
- **Natalizumab** is a monoclonal antibody that inhibits migration of leucocytes into the CNS by inhibitory α-4 integrins found on the surface of lymphocytes and monocytes. It is useful in severe, relapsing remitting MS that is unresponsive to other treatments. It is associated with a risk of progressive multifocal leucoencephalopathy (PML), and all patients need close surveillance for this and hypersensitivity reactions
- **Alemtuzumab**, an anti-CD52 monoclonal antibody that destroys T- and B-cells, reduces disease activity
- **Mitoxantrone** is sometimes used in primary progressive MS in specialist centres. It is potentially cardiotoxic and myelosuppressive
- **New oral disease-modifying drugs**, for example, **fingolimod**, a sphingosine-1-phosphate receptor modulator, and **cladribine** (both given orally), an immunomodulator of lymphocytes, have shown benefit in ongoing trials

Progress. This patient was admitted for reassessment. She was treated with baclofen for her spasms and spasticity and gabapentin for neuropathic pain. An antimuscarinic (oxybutynin) was tried for her urinary problems but eventually, she was taught to self-catheterise intermittently. The physiotherapists, occupational therapists and a social worker were also asked to review her. Disease-modifying therapy was thought to be inappropriate for her advanced condition.

Guillain–Barré Syndrome

This is an acute sensorimotor polyneuropathy that often follows a gastrointestinal infection, for example, *Campylobacter*, cytomegalovirus or a respiratory infection.

CASE HISTORY

A 34-year-old female is brought to the emergency department by her relatives; she has a 4-day history of difficulty walking. She had mild gastroenteritis due to *Campylobacter jejuni* about 5 weeks before but had recovered from this. Her relatives thought she was 'putting it on' but became a bit concerned when they found that she was unable to climb the stairs to her flat.

On examination, she looked well and was orientated but was extremely anxious because she thought she was becoming paralysed. She had a symmetrical weakness in her limbs, which was worse proximally. Reflexes were absent and she had normal plantar responses. There was a mild sensory deficit in a glove and stocking distribution.

WHAT IS THE DIAGNOSIS?

This could be the **Guillain–Barré syndrome.** *Do not* leave this patient unattended because the progression can be fast and her respiratory muscles can be affected within a few hours.

INVESTIGATIONS

- Blood tests: FBC, liver function tests (LFTs), glucose and renal function can help rule out other causes of acute flaccid paralysis. Hepatic aminotransferases may be very high in the first few days and are associated with more severe disease
- Electrocardiogram: check for conduction abnormalities
- Nerve conduction studies: the most useful test to support diagnosis
- Lumbar puncture: CSF protein is typically elevated with no elevation in CSF cell counts
- Spirometry: monitored forced vital capacity

WHAT SHOULD YOU DO?

Admit her. Once she is on the ward, perform a lumbar puncture. In this patient the CSF protein is raised. She gets progressively weaker and is having difficulty breathing.

HOW WOULD YOU NOW MANAGE THIS PATIENT?

- Admit her to high high-dependency unit (HDU) or ICU
- Regularly monitor her respiratory function with vital capacity
- Intubation and ventilation might be required – call for expert help
- Nursing care should take care to avoid pressure ulcers
- Give prophylaxis to prevent venous thrombosis (low-molecular-weight (LMW) heparin, for example, enoxaparin)
- Steroid therapy is ineffective
- Intravenous immunoglobulin (IVIG) given in the first 2 weeks reduces duration and severity of weakness. *Note:* Check IgA levels; severe allergic reactions occur (due to IgG antibodies) with IgA deficiency
- Plasma exchange and IVIG have been shown to be equally efficacious – choice is often institution dependent (combination therapy is not recommended)

Progress. This patient was given IVIG and gradually improved over the next few months.

INFORMATION

Eighty percent of patients make a full recovery and can walk independently 6 months after disease onset with specialist support. Recovery from severe disease may be more prolonged, but most patients regain the ability to walk again independently. Long-term neuropathic pain, fatigue and muscle weakness are often reported.

Spinal Cord Compression

This produces radicular pain at the level of the cord lesion with a spastic tetraparesis, or paraparesis, and sensory loss below the level of the lesion.

CASE HISTORY

A 56-year-old male is admitted with a 2-week history of weakness in his legs. He has no other complaints but admits that he is a heavy smoker.

On examination, there is weakness of both legs, which is more marked distally; the left leg is more severely affected. Knee and ankle jerks are slightly brisk and he has a bilateral extensor plantar response. He reports new incontinence of urine. There are no sensory signs. He has no neurological deficit in his arms.

INVESTIGATIONS

- Routine bloods show a haemoglobin (Hb) of 100 g/L
- Chest X-ray was normal, making carcinoma with secondaries unlikely, despite the patient being a heavy smoker
- Magnetic resonance imaging spine demonstrates an osteolytic lesion at T10
- Serum protein electrophoresis and immunofixation shows a monoclonal band
- Bence Jones protein is present in the urine
- Bone marrow shows infiltration with plasma cells

WHAT IS THE DIAGNOSIS?

Multiple myeloma. This is a haematological malignancy characterised by terminally differentiated plasma cells, infiltration of the bone marrow and the presence of a monoclonal immunoglobulin in the serum and/or urine. It is typically associated with osteolytic bone disease, anaemia, and renal failure. Spinal cord compression (SCC) is a devastating complication of multiple myeloma and has the potential to cause loss of neurological function. The most commonly reported presenting symptoms are back pain, motor weakness and sensory changes.

Progress. Urgent decompression was performed by a neurosurgeon and the patient subsequently received radiotherapy and chemotherapy. He still requires a catheter and is mobilising only slowly with a frame.

REMEMBER

Diagnosis is urgent with cord compression. Prompt diagnosis enables decompression to be performed before severe symptoms develop and potentially before urinary problems; if the latter are present, they are frequently permanent, even with decompression.

Further Reading

Diplopia

Gilhus, N.E., 2016. Myasthenia gravis. N. Engl. J. Med. 375 (26), 2570–2581.
Narayanaswami, P., et al., 2021. International consensus guidance for management of myasthenia gravis: 2020 update. Neurology 96 (3), 114–122.

Loss of Vision

Charles, A., 2017. Migraine. N. Engl. J. Med. 377 (6), 553–561.

Bell's Palsy

Baugh, R.F., et al., 2013. Clinical practice guideline: Bell's palsy, Otolaryngol. Head Neck Surg 149 (3 Suppl), S1–S27.
De Almeida, J.R., Al Khabori, M., Guyatt, G.H., et al., 2009. Combined corticosteroid and antiviral treatment for Bell palsy: a systematic review and meta-analysis. J. Am. Med. Assoc. 302, 985–993.

Stroke/TIA

Lioutas, V.A., Ivan, C.S., Himali, J.J., et al., 2021. Incidence of transient ischemic attack and association with long-term risk of stroke. JAMA 325 (4), 373–381.
NICE, CKS, 2022. Stroke and transient ischaemic attack in over 16s: diagnosis and initial management. NICE.
Royal College of Physicians; Scottish Intercollegiate Guidelines Network; Royal College of Physicians of Ireland, 2023. National clinical guideline for stroke for the United Kingdom and Ireland.

Parkinson's Disease

Bressman, S., Saunders-Pullman, R., 2019. When to start levodopa therapy for Parkinson's disease. N. Engl. J. Med. 380, 389–390.
Internation Parkinson and Movement Disorder Society, 2023. MDS position paper: diagnosis of Parkinson's disease.

Multiple Sclerosis

NICWE, CKS, 2022. Multiple sclerosis in adults: management.
Reich, D.S., Lucchinetti, C.F., Calabresi, P.A., 2018. Multiple sclerosis. N. Engl. J. Med. 378, 169–180.
Scolding, N., et al., 2015. Association of British Neurologists: revised (2015) guidelines for prescribing disease-modifying treatments in multiple sclerosis. Pract. Neurol. 15 (4), 273–279.

Falls

Brignole, M., Moya, A., de Lange, F.J.ESC Scientific Document Group, 2018. ESC guidelines for the diagnosis and management of syncope. Eur. Heart J. 39 (21), 1883–1948.
Dykes, P.C., Carroll, D.L., Hurley, A., et al., 2010. Fall prevention in acute care hospitals. J. Am. Med. Assoc. 304, 1912–1918.

Meningitis

McGill, F., Heyderman, R.S., Panagiotou, S., et al., 2016. Acute bacterial meningitis in adults. Lancet 388, 3036–3047.

McGill, F., et al., 2016. The UK joint specialist societies guideline on the diagnosis and management of acute meningitis and meningococcal sepsis in immunocompetent adults. J. Infect. 72 (4), 405–438.

Headaches

Lawton, M.T., Vates, G.E., 2017. Subarachnoid hemorrhage. N. Engl. J. Med. 377, 257–266.

NICE, CKS,, 2022. Subarachnoid haemorrhage caused by a ruptured aneurysm: diagnosis and management. NICE.

Spinal Cord Compression

Al-Qurainy, R., Collis, E., 2016. Metastatic spinal cord compression: diagnosis and management. BMJ 353, i2539.

NICE, CKS, 2023. Spinal metastases and metastatic spinal cord compression. NICE.

Ropper, A.E., Ropper, A.H., 2017. Acute spinal cord compression. N. Engl. J. Med. 376, 1358–1369.

CHAPTER 8

Psychiatry

Dementia

Dementia is the most common organic brain syndrome seen in elderly inpatients; 7% of people over the age of 65 and up to 33% over the age of 85. Treatable causes can be found in 10% of patients with definite dementia, but that figure is considerably higher if the 'pseudodementia' of depressive illness is included.

Dementia is a global, acquired, progressive deterioration of intellect, memory and personality. Altered ('clouded') consciousness is not usually involved, in contrast to delirium, although dementia often confers an underlying predisposition for delirium.

CASE HISTORY

A 74-year-old female is brought into the emergency department, having been found wandering in the street at night. She is poorly nourished and dishevelled and has several bruises on her arms and legs. You find out from her daughter that her husband died 6 months previously.

HOW DOES DEMENTIA PRESENT?

- Loss of memory, especially short-term
- Episodes of increasing 'confusion'
- Falls, with or without head injury
- Wandering and getting lost (getting into the wrong bed), especially at night
- Insomnia
- Weight loss
- Slow recovery and mobilisation after injury (e.g. hip fracture) or illness (e.g. myocardial infarct, pneumonia)
- Incontinence
- Difficulty dressing: parietal lesion of dressing dyspraxia
- Behavioural disinhibition: frontal lobe sign
- Severe extrapyramidal reaction to dopamine antagonists: Lewy body dementia

WHAT ARE THE CAUSES?

These are listed in Box 8.1.

DIFFERENTIAL DIAGNOSIS

- Delirium
- Amnestic syndrome: relatively specific memory loss, for example, Wernicke–Korsakoff syndrome
- Depressive 'pseudodementia'
- Learning disability ('amentia')

BOX 8.1 ■ Causes of Dementia

Common Causes

Over 65

- Alzheimer disease
- Multiinfarct dementia
- Lewy body disease
- Parkinson disease

Under 65

- Alzheimer disease
- AIDS
- Alcoholic dementia
- Head injuries

Less Common Causes

- Prion disease (Creutzfeldt–Jakob)
- Huntington's
- Fronto-temporal dementia (Pick's)
- Multiple sclerosis
- Wilson disease

INVESTIGATIONS

- A corroborative history: duration, presentation, mood, alcohol, past history
- A Mini-Mental State Examination (MMSE): a brief, structured bedside screening test of memory
- Intelligence quotient (IQ) (performed by a psychologist) to confirm cognitive decline
- Blood tests to consider (based on history):
  - Gamma-glutamyl transpeptidase and mean corpuscular volume (MCV): raised levels are evidence of excess alcohol consumption
  - Urea and electrolytes (U and Es), estimated glomerular filtration rate (eGFR)
  - Liver enzymes
  - Free T4 and thyroid stimulating hormone (TSH)
  - Venereal disease research (VDRL) test (syphilis screening)
  - Haemoglobin (Hb)
  - Erythrocyte sedimentation rate (ESR) or C-reactive protein (CRP)
  - Auto-immune screen to include antinuclear antibody (ANA)
  - Serum electrophoresis
  - Glucose levels
  - Vitamin B12 and red cell folate
  - Calcium
  - HIV testing after counselling in at-risk group
  - Mid-stream urine (MSU)
  - Chest X-ray (CXR)
- Computed tomography (CT)/MRI brain scan: tumour, subdural haematoma, normal pressure hydrocephalus and infarcts *might* confirm generalised cerebral atrophy
- Electrocardiogram (ECG): arrhythmias
- Electroencephalography (EEG): diffuse slow waves are rare before 75 in normal health
- Consider lumbar puncture, if diagnosis is unclear

EXAMINATION

- Cardiovascular, neurological and endocrine system: to exclude secondary causes
- Mental state examination
- Simple cognitive screening bedside tests: dementia may be suggested by the quality of the responses, for example, 'perseveration' (repeating a response beyond the relevant question), 'confabulation' (inventing recollections to compensate for memory loss)
- Look for depressed affect

INFORMATION

Simple Cognitive Screening

- Orientation in time, place and person: ask day, month, year, ward, hospital, town/city, country, identity of relatives or key ward staff
- Attention and concentration: ask patient to recite the days of the week or the months of the year backwards (should be 100% accurate)
- Verbal short-term memory: teach patient to recite immediately a name and address accurately (a test of registration: they should be able to do this in two attempts). Then ask the patient to recall the name and address 5 min later (test of memory recall; should recall 95% of the individual items)
- Long-term memory: tests of general information, for example, recent news, world events or on a subject of interest to them
- Premorbid intelligence (necessary to judge whether there has been a deterioration in intellect): establish the level of education achieved and occupation

HOW WOULD YOU MANAGE A CASE OF DEMENTIA?

- Treat any reversible cause
- Stop antimuscarinic drugs, if possible
- Involve a psychiatrist early regarding diagnosis and management
- Acetylcholinesterase inhibitors may be indicated in early Alzheimer disease (e.g. donepezil, galantamine or rivastigmine), as well as memantine (affects glutamate transmission), in conjunction with specialist advice from the old age psychiatry team
- While on the ward, ensure adequate fluids, nutrition, and treatment of constipation and any other reversible causes of incontinence
- If possible, discharge home as soon as possible to avoid disorientating experience of admission
- Involve the nearest relatives only
- Refer to old age psychiatry specialist dementia services

Progress. This patient improved considerably after a few days in hospital with care from a multidisciplinary team (MDT). Her daughter lived fairly nearby and so was able, with the occupational therapist, to arrange for aids at home to allow independent living. This patient was assessed by the psychogeriatrician, who thought her dementia symptoms might well be related to her depression (pseudodementia) following the death of her husband. She was started on citalopram (a selective serotonin reuptake inhibitor [SSRI]) 8 mg daily, with some improvement. She returned home but requires continual supervision.

Delirium Tremens

Delirium tremens (DTs) is the most severe form of alcohol withdrawal syndrome and is a medical emergency because of the major complications that can arise. It often occurs on the second or third day after admission due to stopping drinking suddenly, although it can occur after a significant reduction in drinking in those who are highly alcohol-dependent.

CASE HISTORY

A 49-year-old male was admitted via the emergency department to the orthopaedic ward, having had a fall and fracturing his pelvis. On the third day after admission, he became disorientated and restless with visual hallucinations. The orthopaedic junior doctor wants your advice.

A full history elicits that the patient had been a heavy drinker for 10 or more years and obviously has had no alcohol since the fall. You think he has DTs – particularly as he has had a similar episode in the past.

REMEMBER

Heavy drinkers underreport and conceal alcohol consumption. The problem is suggested by:
- Regular medical presentations
- Injuries/falls
- Anxiety/depression/self-harm
- Marital/family/financial/legal difficulties

WHAT ARE THE CLINICAL FEATURES OF DTs?

- Coarse tremor (which may affect the whole-body)
- Disorientation in place and time
- Anxiety (often severe)
- Motor restlessness
- Nausea and/or diarrhoea
- Insomnia
- Nightmares
- Excessive sympathetic drive:
  - Sweating
  - Tachycardia
  - Hypertension
  - Low-grade fever
- Reduced attention
- Illusions: visual
- Hallucinations: classically visual and frightening but may be tactile or auditory; small animals (insects, spiders, rats) advance menacingly towards and over the patient
- Persecutory delusions
- Convulsions in severe cases

REMEMBER

Complications of DTs
- Comorbid illness or trauma (infection, dehydration, head injury)
- Hypoglycaemia
- Electrolyte disturbances (sodium, potassium, magnesium)
- Convulsions
- Coma
- Death

- Serum U and Es (especially hypokalaemia)
- Calcium and magnesium
- Gamma-glutamyl transpeptidase (raised)
- Aspartate transferase
- Bilirubin
- Glucose
- Haemoglobin
- Mean corpuscular volume (raised)
- Mid-stream urine
- If necessary, appropriate X-rays to exclude infection (CXR) and trauma (CT brain scan if indicated: ?subdural)

HOW WOULD YOU TREAT DTs?

- Admit the patient to an acute medical bed
- General measures
- Treat electrolyte and fluid imbalances in particular
- Treat any comorbid disorder
- Parenteral thiamine (200–300 mg daily in divided doses) must be given early if long-term dementia is to be prevented

INFORMATION

Wernicke–Korsakoff Syndrome

Acute confusion, ocular palsies and nystagmus and ataxic gait, leading to chronic short-term memory loss and confabulation

SPECIFIC DRUG THERAPY

- Follow a protocol if your hospital has one
- Oral treatment is preferred, unless the patient is severely distressed and disturbed. Doses suggested here may not be adequate to control the initial condition, and more may be required:
    - Diazepam 10 mg × 4 daily orally or
    - Chlordiazepoxide 20 mg × 4 daily orally
    - Oxazepam is used in patients with severe liver disease
- Chlormethiazole capsules should be avoided because of problems with dependence and adverse effects
- Doses of chlordiazepoxide up to 200 mg spread over the first 24 h may be required initially in uncontrolled, severe, life-endangering withdrawal with fits. The patient must be monitored constantly, with resuscitation facilities available
- Prophylactic anticonvulsants (e.g. carbamazepine 200 mg × 2 daily) can be given when there is a previous history of withdrawal convulsions or if the current presentation has been complicated by fits

Progress. This patient improved after 3 days of diazepam treatment and the dose of the medication was tapered to nothing over the next 7 days. More gradual tapering is required in a patient with a history of convulsions, with a longer period (e.g. 3 months) on anticonvulsants. This patient was discharged from hospital and provision of long-term care was arranged.

LONG-TERM CARE

This primarily involves maintaining abstinence from alcohol. Referral to alcohol support agencies requires individual motivation. Acamprosate has been shown to be helpful in reducing craving in conjunction with support from addiction services or group therapy. Those with concurrent psychological problems (e.g. depression, psychosis) need psychiatric referral. This patient remains abstinent and still attends group therapy.

Depression

See also Chapter 15.

Depressive illness is common but often undetected or inadequately treated (see Information box). The central symptom is usually low mood. Associated symptoms reflecting effects on an individual's behaviour, thoughts, perceptions and cognition become more marked as the severity of the condition increases.

Whereas much depressive illness has an insidious onset and never reaches the attention of acute medical or specialist services, up to one-third of physically ill patients attending hospital have depressive symptoms.

INFORMATION

Depressive illness can be missed in medical patients for the following reasons:
- Depression is considered 'understandable' in those physically unwell
- Symptoms of depression are attributed entirely to an underlying medical condition
- Negative attitude to diagnosis of depression and reluctance to report symptoms
- Limited opportunity to discuss emotional issues in a medical setting

---

ASSOCIATIONS OF DEPRESSION IN PATIENTS PRESENTING ACUTELY

- Suicide attempt or deliberate self-harm (DSH)
- Concurrent physical illness (particularly chronic, painful, life-threatening or disfiguring)
- Unpleasant and demanding treatment for physical illness
- Destabilisation of a chronic condition, exacerbation of physical symptoms or excessive functional impairment
- Medical treatment refusal or poor compliance
- Weight loss, poor nutrition, self-neglect or unusual behaviour (e.g. heavy drinking)
- Increased somatic concern and unexplained physical symptoms

---

CASE HISTORY

A 66-year-old female is admitted to a medical assessment unit (MAU) for investigation of anaemia, which had made her breathless and tired so that she was unable to cope on her own. Her husband died 6 months previously. The ward nurses have noted that she has been despondent and reluctant to care for herself, and her nutritional intake has been poor. You suspect she may be depressed.

BOX 8.2 ■ Assessment of Mental State: Key Areas

Appearance/Behaviour
- General state of health, self-care, facial expression, eye contact, rapport, cooperation, posture and movement

Speech
- Rate, tone, quantity, volume, spontaneity and form

Mood
- Sustained disturbance: depressed, elated, anxious, irritable
- Reactivity: reduced 'blunted', increased 'labile'
- Congruity: appropriateness to circumstances or theme of discussion

Thoughts
- Preoccupations, predominant concerns
- Mood-congruent ideas (e.g. suicidal)
- Delusions: abnormal unshakeable beliefs inconsistent with sociocultural context

Perceptions
- Auditory or visual hallucinations (a perception in the absence of a stimulus), presence of which may be suggested by abnormalities of general behaviour

Insight
- Recognition and attribution of illness/awareness of merits of treatment

---

INFORMATION

Depression can be broadly categorised as follows:
- Mild: low mood often associated with anxiety symptoms
- Moderate: increasingly low mood, depressive thinking (e.g. suicidal) with biological symptoms (sleep disturbance with early morning waking, mood worse in the morning, reduced appetite, weight and libido)
- Severe: more intense low mood, suicidal thoughts with development of psychotic symptoms, including delusions and hallucinations (most often associated with suicide)

HOW WOULD YOU ASSESS THIS CASE?

A summary of the key areas of observation and enquiry is provided in Box 8.2.

INVESTIGATIONS

- Full blood screen, including full blood count (FBC), U and Es, creatinine (eGFR), thyroid function tests (TFTs), liver biochemistry, serum calcium
- Accurate diagnosis requires a detailed history, with a reliable corroborative account if possible, and a mental state examination
- Factors that increase vulnerability to developing depression:
  - Previous history of depression
  - Family history of depression or suicide
  - Stress/life events, particularly with separation or loss
  - Social isolation or adversity
  - Physical illness and its treatment
  - Medication that can cause depression
  - Alcohol/substance misuse

DIFFERENTIAL DIAGNOSIS

- Dementia
- Delirium
- Alcohol or substance misuse
- Chronic dysthymia
- Grief (normal or pathological)

HOW DO YOU IDENTIFY A SEVERE CASE?

In moderate to severe depression, mental state examination may reveal:
- Depressed facial appearance, tearfulness, reduced expression, poor eye contact, retardation of movement or agitation
- Speech: may be slow and impoverished
- Persistent, pervasive low mood worse in the morning, anhedonia (loss of interest in pleasure), abulia (inability to make decisions), reduced motivation or energy. *Note:* these complaints are not usually attributable to physical illness alone – psychologically healthy people often cope resiliently with physical illness
- Suicidal thoughts may be present and should always be enquired about and explored carefully:
    - Have you had any desperate thoughts?
    - Do you feel that life is not worth living?

Biological symptoms are often present. You should ask about feelings of hopelessness (often associated with suicidal contemplation). Other mood-congruent thoughts that might be present include pessimism, feelings of guilt, worthlessness, self-reproach, persecution and impoverishment. In severe depression, thoughts can reach delusional intensity and may be associated with perceptual abnormalities, for example, condemnatory auditory hallucinations. Tests of cognitive function may be poorly performed due to impaired memory and concentration. In the elderly with fragile but intact cognitive function, severe depression may suggest a dementia ('depressive pseudodementia').

Diagnosis. This patient has moderate depression.

HOW WOULD YOU MANAGE THIS CASE?

- Exclude an organic cause: this patient has anaemia. Investigations show an Hb of 76 g/L, MCV of 101, ESR of 31 mm/h and white cell count (WCC) of 4200
- **Diagnosis:** A macrocytic anaemia that is probably due to her poor nutritional state and likely to be caused by folate deficiency. You do not want to treat her with folate until you have excluded B_{12} deficiency
- The laboratory says that the serum levels will be available tomorrow; when they arrive, they show a serum B_{12} of 150 pmol/L, a serum folate of 6 nmol/L and a red cell folate of 70 μg/L, indicating **folate deficiency.** You start her on folic acid 5 mg daily with regular blood monitoring
- Consider other possible organic causes of depressive symptoms (Box 8.3)
- Specific management depends on the severity:
    - Mild depression may respond to counselling and attempts to resolve problems leading to depression
    - Mild to moderate depression can respond well to cognitive behavioural therapy, which requires time and available resources

---

BOX 8.3 ■ Organic Causes of Depressive Symptoms

Endocrine
- Hypothyroidism
- Cushing syndrome
- Hyperparathyroidism
- Addison disease
- Hypercalcaemia

Infections
- Viral illness
- Hepatitis
- HIV

Metabolic
- Anaemia (particularly vitamin B_{12} and iron deficiency)
- Renal disease
- Cancer

Neurological
- Multiple sclerosis
- Brain tumour
- Parkinson disease
- Poststroke
- Dementias

Drugs
Many drugs have the potential to cause depressive symptoms: check data sheet. Examples include:
- Steroids
- Antihypertensives, beta-blockers, digoxin
- Levodopa, methyldopa
- Cimetidine, metoclopramide
- Aminophylline, theophylline
- Regular use of stimulants

- Moderate to severe depression is more likely to present and be detected acutely and often responds well to medication
- Establish whether the patient is at risk
- Refer to the Psychiatric team, but explain this to the patient first
- Assess capacity if the patient is refusing treatment
- Psychiatric treatment can usually be managed by the liaison team on the medical ward: this is preferable if medical problems require treatment. A Psychiatric Nurse is required to observe the patient
- The patient will require regular review
- Psychiatric treatment or admission using the Mental Health Act is considered on the basis of severity and risk
- Identify aftercare support from family or professionals, having discussed this with the patient
- Inform her primary care physician

WHAT MEDICATION WOULD YOU CONSIDER AND HOW WOULD YOU BEGIN TREATMENT?

When prescribing antidepressants:

- A psychiatric opinion is usually obtained
- Medication is most effective in moderate and severe depression
- Compliance is essential and enhanced by good communication. Good prescribing practice includes explanation of:
  - The diagnosis
  - The likelihood of response to treatment (around two-thirds respond well)
  - Common side effects, which often precede benefits
  - A delay of 2–3 weeks before therapeutic effect
  - The fact that antidepressants are not addictive (a common misconception)
- Older tricyclic antidepressants (TCAs) have proven efficacy but significant side effects (e.g. antimuscarinic, postural hypotension, cardiotoxic in overdose) and have largely been super-seded by newer drugs. TCAs are still useful if newer agents are not tolerated, sedation is desirable, or the patient has had a previous effective response. Avoid prescribing large quan-tities for outpatients and on discharge
- The most commonly prescribed newer antidepressants are SSRIs, which can cause nausea but, in general, are better tolerated, cause fewer problematic interactions with other drugs and are less toxic in overdose
- It is difficult to predict which antidepressant will be best tolerated in view of the range of side effects and significant individual variation
- Elderly patients often require a lower starting dose and a more gradual dose increase
- As a general rule, treatment should continue for at least 6 months after recovery from the acute episode

Progress. This patient's depression responded to a mixture of bereavement counselling and drug therapy with an SSRI (escitalopram 10 mg daily). Her anaemia was due to dietary folate defi-ciency and responded well to treatment with oral folic acid, which was continued at home. She is being seen regularly by her general practitioner (GP) and her Hb levels are being checked. She is still on escitalopram.

REMEMBER

- Severe depression can be life-endangering (e.g. acutely suicidal, not eating or drinking)
- Refer to the mental health team who may consider the use of electroconvulsive treatment (ECT)

Suicide and Deliberate Self-Harm (DSH)

Presentation to hospital after an attempt to self-harm is a frequent cause of acute medical admis-sions. The most common method is drug overdose, which is associated with recent alcohol con-sumption in up to 50% of cases.

The majority of DSH does not represent a serious suicide attempt. Motivations include:

- Escape from overwhelming stress
- Desire to effect a change in personal circumstances ('cry for help')
- Wish to die: serious suicidal intent is evident in up to one-fifth of DSH presentations

Many of the components of the assessment of DSH can be applied to patients who describe having 'suicidal thoughts'.

CASE HISTORY

You are called to see a 24-year-old female who is accompanied by a friend that called an ambulance to bring the patient to the emergency department. The patient is tearful, smells of alcohol, and says that she took a handful of paracetamol 4 hours previously after a violent argument with her partner. She tells you that her mother died 3 months ago and that she wants to join her. She has seen her doctor recently, complaining of poor sleep.

REMEMBER

- Dependants might be at risk (e.g. young children at home): inform a social worker if necessary
- Some hospitals have dedicated staff who assess all patients. In these situations, your task is to identify those who are in need of immediate attention or treatment

HOW WOULD YOU MANAGE THIS CASE OF DSH?

- Examine the patient and check conscious level (Glasgow coma scale [GCS] 15), respiratory rate (15/min) and BP (104/72 mm Hg)
- Attend to immediate medical requirements. Most patients will be admitted to hospital after overdose for specific treatment or observation. They may underestimate or understate the number of tablets taken
- When the medical condition is stable, interview the patient, if possible with a collateral history from reliable informants, and aim to cover the following aspects

Identify Mental Illness

- Most completed suicides are associated with a psychiatric diagnosis, most often a depressive illness. Many suicide victims have seen their doctor in the preceding weeks
- Conversely, clear psychiatric illness is evident in less than one-third of DSH presentations. Most occur after a 'life event', with up to half following a relationship problem
- The most common diagnoses include depression, alcohol dependence and personality disorders (borderline, antisocial)

Detect Patients at Risk of Completed Suicide

- Serious suicide attempts form a minority of DSH presentations, but individuals who harm themselves have a greatly increased risk of suicide compared to the general population
- A high proportion of suicide victims have a previous history of DSH
- An indication of risk should be documented in the notes with an appropriate plan of action

---

INFORMATION

Features Associated With Increased Suicide Risk

- Demographic: socially isolated (divorced, widowed, never married); male (rates in young males are increasing steeply), older age, minority groups (e.g. young Asian women), unemployed, low socioeconomic class, certain professions (doctors, dentists, vets, farmers), individuals with access to means (drug users, gun owners)
- Attempt:
  - Planning: taking care of affairs (cancelled appointments, final acts, e.g. suicide note – the content of which can be helpful)
  - Circumstances: performed in isolation, steps to avoid detection

- Method: violent, severe overdose or believed likely to be lethal
- History: present or previous psychiatric diagnosis (particularly depression, schizophrenia), recent hospital discharge, previous DSH, recent life event (e.g. bereavement, retirement, divorce), physical illness (chronic painful illness, CNS disorders [multiple sclerosis, epilepsy], cancer, HIV), family history of psychiatric illness/suicide, alcohol/drug misuse, impulsive personality
- Mental state: agitation, depressed mood, suicidal thoughts, hopelessness, delusions, hallucinations, insight in early schizophrenia

Explore Suicidal Thoughts

- Never avoid detailed but tactful questions concerning suicidal ideas and intentions
- Responses need to be assessed in the context of the overall presentation, especially if the patient is unforthcoming
- Establish the patient's thoughts about the episode of self-harm
- Find out if the patient wishes to die. Ask questions to assess underlying mental state, for example,
- How does the patient see the future?
- Does the patient see life as completely hopeless?
- Does the patient feel he/she would be better off dead?
- Assess plans for further attempts: method, circumstances
- Identify protective factors: reasons for not wishing to die, for example, change in circumstances, family, dependants

Identify Means of Preventing Recurrence

The most significant factor predictive of repetition is the number of previous episodes. Assess:

- Current and previous coping resources
- Level of support: identify important relationships
- Possible precipitants (current problems, recent events) and means of addressing them
- Alternative methods of dealing with distress

FURTHER MANAGEMENT: PSYCHIATRIC LIAISON REFERRAL

- Many hospitals have dedicated staff to assess all DSH presentations in liaison with the psychiatric team. Learn to recognise individuals in need of immediate attention or treatment
- Most patients do not require further psychiatric intervention
- If a significant psychiatric disorder is identified, management can be initiated as an inpatient or outpatient in communication with the patient's doctor
- High-risk cases or those with severe symptoms will require psychiatric admission – if necessary, using compulsory detention. Level of risk and nursing observation required should be communicated and documented

DIFFICULT MANAGEMENT PROBLEMS

Repeated Presenters (e.g. Self-laceration, Overdose, Actual or Threatened)

- Behaviour often associated with personality-related vulnerabilities (e.g. borderline personality), dysfunctional coping and intermittent stress in the absence of other clear psychiatric diagnosis

- A planned, consistent multidisciplinary response coordinated through the Psychiatric team can sometimes help provide containment
- Reduction in the maladaptive expression of distress may occur with support from a key worker, counselling, psychotherapy or enhanced social support
- Occasional, psychiatric crisis admissions may be required but these should be kept to a minimum in favour of longer-term strategies
- Low-dose antipsychotic medication may help to reduce arousal and subjective distress, avoiding prescriptions for large quantities and identifying a care professional or other reliable, willing carer to help supervise the medication initially if required

Refusal of Medical Treatment

- Involve senior colleague and/or psychiatrist (to determine if mental disorder impairs capacity)
- Explain clearly the risks of not having treatment
- Assess capacity to make informed decision and record it (see Information box)
- If treatment is considered necessary, attempt persuasion/negotiation, if possible, including a friend or relative the patient trusts
- Continue trying to gain the patient's trust, explaining merits of treatment and risks of refusal. A patient who is frightened, angry or presenting in crisis may choose to cooperate as his/her distress settles
- If the patient has capacity and refuses treatment, a second opinion from a senior is advisable
- It is essential for discussions with the patient, management decisions and their reasons to be clearly documented in detail and discussed with a senior colleague
- The Mental Health Act can be used to detain a patient who is refusing medical treatment in hospital if the patient is exhibiting symptoms of mental disorder that places their health, safety or that of others at risk and provides for the administration of treatment for a mental disorder that might be impairing a patient's capacity to decide on their medical treatment

INFORMATION

Assessing Capacity to Withhold Consent to Examination, Investigation or Treatment

- Adults are presumed competent to refuse medical advice and treatment
- Decisions with more serious implications require greater capacity
- A patient lacks capacity if some impairment or disturbance of mental functioning causes an inability to decide whether to consent to or refuse treatment, which is determined by:
  - Inability to comprehend and retain information on indications and benefits of proposed treatment and in particular the possible risks of refusing it
  - Being incapable of weighing up the information in order to arrive at a decision
  - Temporary incapacity (e.g. due to head injury, altered mood, alcohol) may permit essential life-saving treatment without consent

Patients Unwilling to Remain in Hospital for Further Assessment

- The patient's capacity to make this decision should be documented
- If the patient is considered at risk, appropriate staff should attempt to detain him/her in hospital under common law to permit an urgent mental health assessment by a psychiatrist and approved social worker. Reasons relating to the patient's behaviour, mental state and possible risks should be carefully documented

Intoxicated or Violent Patients

- The assistance of hospital security or the police might be necessary

- Assessment will be more productive if the patient is given time to sober up (in which case, the behaviour may completely settle), as long as the patient or others are not put at risk
- Consider a psychiatric opinion if an underlying psychiatric disorder is thought likely

---

REMEMBER

Enforced physical treatment is given under common law and is not sanctioned by use of the Mental Health Act. The decision to go ahead depends on consideration of:

- The patient's capacity to refuse treatment
- Reasonable professional practice and a doctor's duty of care to the patient
- Necessity of the treatment to save life or to prevent a serious incident or a deterioration in health
- The decision to treat being in the patient's best interests

---

Progress. This patient had taken approximately 20 tablets of paracetamol (10 g) and was given N-acetylcysteine IV, her liver function remained normal. This was her first episode of DSH, and she realised the seriousness of what she had done and the necessity for future counselling.

Acute Anxiety

CASE HISTORY (1)

You are called to the emergency department to see a breathless young female patient. She is acutely distressed and breathing rapidly. She feels light-headed and has paraesthesiae in her hands and feet.

Differential diagnoses, such as a respiratory emergency (e.g. asthma, pulmonary embolus and pneumothorax), must first be excluded. Panic attacks are suggested by:

- Extreme fear
- Subjective complaint of difficulty breathing in rather than out
- Respiratory alkalosis (causing tetany and relative hypocalcaemia)
- Arterial blood gases (ABGs) showing hypocapnia but normal oxygen levels
- Sweating
- Emotional trigger (shock)
- Environmental trigger (crowd phobia)

MANAGEMENT

Provide reassurance that the symptoms are not dangerous and try and find a quiet space for the patient. Patients frequently hyperventilate as part of the attack, which is felt subjectively as shortness of breath. This should be explained to the patient and they should be supported with calm breathing exercises. In the emergency setting benzodiazepines can be used to terminate an acute attack but they should only be for short term use. This patient was able to return home and underwent a course of cognitive behavioural therapy.

CASE HISTORY (2)

The nursing staff inform you that a 55-year-old male is refusing to have any more haemodialysis, having just started this treatment. A phobic reaction to dialysis is suggested by avoidance, abnormal fear and sympathetic overdrive, during dialysis or talking about it.

Depressive illness is a common association of anxiety and should always be excluded. These phobias are also common in oncology (vomit phobia with chemotherapy).

HOW WOULD YOU MANAGE THIS PATIENT?

- Support and sympathy with explanation of the phobia
- Consider short-term use of benzodiazepines (e.g. diazepam) in emergent circumstances
- Ask a psychologist to consider graded exposure therapy
- A sertraline, citalopram, paroxetine, or fluoxetine (SSRI) is often required in the presence of comorbid depressive illness

WHEN SHOULD PHARMACOTHERAPY BE CONSIDERED IN THE TREATMENT OF ANXIETY?

Pharmacotherapy should be considered if there is a marked functional impairment or if symptoms have not improved following low-intensity psychological interventions.

INFORMATION

Patients should be educated about panic attacks. Guidance should be provided on how to manage them, prevent them, and how to access support services.

WHAT ARE THE PHYSICAL SYMPTOMS AND SIGNS OF ANXIETY?

- Dilated pupils
- Photosensitivity: patient might be wearing dark glasses
- Phonosensitivity: patient cannot bear any noise
- Dry mouth
- Flushed face and neck
- Sweating
- Hyperventilation
- Associated hypocapnia and respiratory alkalosis: cause relative hypocalcaemia (tingling or numbness) in extremities and face, light-headedness and tetany
- Tachycardia (pulse may be as high as 140 beats per minute [bpm])
- Nausea
- Diarrhoea
- Frequency of micturition
- Increased muscle tension

WHAT ARE THE PSYCHOLOGICAL SYMPTOMS OF ANXIETY?

- Excessive fear
- Derealisation (patient feels that the environment is less real and solid, with a feeling of detachment)
- Fear of collapse
- Catastrophic thinking ('I am about to die from a heart attack')

ALWAYS LOOK FOR THE FOLLOWING ASSOCIATIONS

- Phobias: abnormal fear and avoidance of particular situations or things
- Depressive illness
- Obsessive–compulsive disorder: repetitive ruminations that are inconsistent with the personality, along with repeated behaviours; checking excessively or hand-washing because of fear of germs

Progress. This patient settled quickly with counselling and 5 mg of diazepam. He subsequently continued dialysis without any problems.

Opiate Dependence

Drugs in this group include diamorphine (heroin), morphine, pethidine, methadone, dihydrocodeine, buprenorphine, oxycodone and fentanyl.

EFFECTS OF OPIATE USE

- Euphoria
- Analgesia
- Relaxation
- Drowsiness

Heroin addicts are 16 times more likely to die than individuals of equivalent age, chiefly as a result of overdose. They frequently present in the acute hospital setting.

CASE HISTORY (1)

You are called to see a 23-year-old male admitted 24 h previously following a road traffic accident. He is verbally abusing nursing staff and wants to leave against medical advice. He is demanding methadone, stating that he is a **heroin addict**.

HOW WOULD YOU ASSESS THIS PATIENT?

- Attempt to defuse the situation and prevent an escalation of disturbed behaviour
- Take a history of drug use, including each drug taken, amount and route
- Obtain information from other sources:
  - Previously or currently attended drug support agencies if patient admits to having received help. They may be able to tell you if the patient has a regular prescription for methadone
  - Corroborative history from other reliable informant with patient's consent
- Examine for evidence of opiate use: withdrawal symptoms begin within 12 h of last use and increase in severity over the first 48 h. With longer-acting opioids, such as methadone, onset of withdrawal symptoms can be delayed and their duration increased. Opiate withdrawal that is uncomplicated by other drugs is subjectively unpleasant but not life-threatening, and can present with:
  - Agitation
  - Anxiety
  - Low mood
  - Restlessness
  - Tachycardia
  - Sweating

- 'Goose flesh'
- Dilated pupils
- Yawning
- Sneezing
- Vomiting
- Lacrimation
- Rhinorrhoea
- Look for evidence of recent drug use, for example, needle marks, phlebitis, skin abscesses. Subjective complaints include craving, poor sleep (which can last months), abdominal cramps, nausea, diarrhoea and musculoskeletal pain

HOW WOULD YOU INVESTIGATE THIS PATIENT?

- Send urine for drug screen
- Infection screen (risk of hepatitis B, C, HIV)

HOW WOULD YOU MANAGE AND TREAT THIS PATIENT?

Prescribing Methadone

- Oral methadone mixture should be given if you are satisfied a significant habit exists, and this is confirmed by reliable sources or objective evidence of use or withdrawal symptoms
- If possible, seek advice from a local specialist drug unit
- There are published guidelines on clinical management of drug use and dependence – a copy should be available in the hospital pharmacy
- Any registered medical practitioner can prescribe methadone
- Methadone tablets should not generally be prescribed because of their potential for misuse
- Dose required to control withdrawal can be carefully titrated in hospital. Start at low dose of methadone, for example, 10 mL (1 mg per 1 mL mixture). A further 10 mL at 4-hourly intervals is used until objective signs of withdrawal are controlled. Establish daily requirement
- Doses >40 mL (40 mg) daily should be taken only if there is reliable information that the patient has been receiving higher regular prescription, but even in this case, dose should be gradually titrated upwards

REMEMBER

Avoid high doses. Methadone overdose causes respiratory arrest – patients can overstate their requirements and physical tolerance of opiates can change quickly.

Symptomatic Treatment of Withdrawal Symptoms

This may be indicated and includes the following:

- Give loperamide for diarrhoea
- Patients may demand more methadone than required to control withdrawal symptoms in order to promote sleep. This should be avoided. Short-term use of hypnotic medication is an alternative. Diazepam also helps with muscle spasm and anxiety
- Observe for evidence of withdrawal from other drugs, for example,
  - Alcohol: DTs
  - Benzodiazepines: risk of convulsions

- Comorbid psychiatric disorder can be present:
  - Depressive illness
  - Psychotic symptoms (if polydrug use includes stimulants or hallucinogenic drugs)

When Condition is Stable

Gradually reduce methadone by 10% per day if aiming for abstinence. This patient wishes to remain on methadone in the longer term and was already receiving regular prescription prior to admission. He requests referral to the local drug support service. The reduction regimen may require some flexibility to promote cooperation.

> **REMEMBER**
>
> Patients should be warned of the risks even of relatively low doses of methadone and be cautioned about its safe-keeping, particularly if there are children at home (5–10 mL could be lethal for a child).

Progress. On discharge, as drug service support is required, arrange planned transfer of care and be specific about who will prescribe and when. The patient's doctor should be informed and may be willing to prescribe. Avoid giving large prescriptions. Methadone should generally be prescribed for collection on a daily basis but drug services can advise on this. This patient continues on methadone supplied by the local drug support service.

> **CASE HISTORY (2)**
>
> A young male is rushed to the emergency department in a comatose state. His friend tells you he used heroin after an abstinence of 4 weeks.

HOW DO YOU PROCEED?

- Careful history: dose, timing and type of heroin used:
  - Two doses of heroin were obtained from an illicit source, dose unknown. The patient's friend says that a number of tablets were obtained and she was fairly certain that they were not only heroin because they were cheap. The patient had been at a drug help clinic while abstinent and was aware of fentanyl being contaminated with illicit supplies of heroin
- Urgent cardiorespiratory support should be available
- Assess evidence of opiate toxicity (an acute medical emergency):
  - Conscious level – GCS 13
  - Respiratory depression – 12 bpm
  - Bradycardia – 52/min
  - Miosis – present
  - Hypothermia – 36.4°C
- Examine for other causes of impaired consciousness (e.g. head injury)
- Administer the opiate antagonist naloxone (0.4–2 mg):
  - Intravenous naloxone has a high affinity for opiate receptors and reverses the signs of toxicity by displacing ingested opiates
  - Life-threatening symptoms may recur in view of the relatively short half-life (minutes) of naloxone, which may need to be readministered, depending on the half-life of the opiate taken (e.g. half-life of methadone is >24 h)

INFORMATION

Naloxone is an opioid antagonist that often requires repeated doses if respiratory depression continues. Naloxone must be readily available for use in the community.

Heroin overdose, causing life-threatening respiratory depression, can occur after a period of abstinence as physical tolerance is reduced. Prior overdose is a strong predictor of further overdoses and of overdose death.

Clinicians are well aware of the potency of fentanyl; it binds the Mu-receptor 50 to 100 times more strongly than morphine.

REMEMBER

All patients need to be monitored in hospital for at least 24 hours, even if they make a brisk recovery.

Progress. This patient made a rapid recovery with the use of repeated naloxone and agreed to be referred back to the Drug Dependency Unit.

The Disturbed Patient

A behaviourally disturbed patient is often distressed and frightened by their subjective experiences or the circumstances in which they find themselves. The behaviour may place the individual or others at risk.

TYPICAL PRESENTATIONS

- Agitation and restlessness
- Overactivity
- Communication of distress, for example, self-injury or mutilation, threats to harm self
- Fluctuating and unpredictable behaviour
- Intimidating, defensive or over-sensitive behaviour
- Verbally loud, aggressive or violent conduct

UNDERLYING CAUSES OF BEHAVIOURAL DISTURBANCES

Organic Mental Disorders

- Dementia: patients can be restless and aggressive and may wander because of disorientation. Their dementia may be exaggerated by coexistent physical conditions, for example, acute infection, constipation
- Delirium: arising from a number of causes and commonly associated with disturbed behaviour due to misinterpretation of surroundings. Conscious level is impaired, often with fearfulness, perceptual abnormalities (visual or auditory hallucination) and abnormal thinking (e.g. persecutory delusions)
- Epilepsy: ictal (e.g. temporal lobe) or postictal

Other Psychiatric Disorders

- Major psychoses:
  - Schizophrenia: delusional thinking or abnormal sensory experience (e.g. auditory hallucination) may be driving behaviour

- Manic psychosis: elevation in mood can be associated with hyperactive and disorganised behaviour
- Anxiety and depression: can be associated with agitation, restlessness and high arousal. Major depression is associated with suicidality and self-harm

Substance Use

This includes alcohol intoxication or withdrawal and use of other drugs, for example, stimulants, hallucinogens, solvents.

Physical Illness

Individuals may have a physical cause to explain their disturbed behaviour, for example, chronic pain, side effects of medication.

Personality Factors in the Absence of Physical or Psychiatric Disorder

Personality vulnerabilities or 'disorders' can give rise to several distinct patterns of problematic behaviour, which may be associated with circumstances, crises, stress or intoxication. This can include exaggerated propensities to express anger, violent, explosive or antisocial conduct, or self-mutilating and cutting.

CASE HISTORY

A young male walks into the emergency department. He is unkempt, preoccupied and suspicious. His behaviour is bizarre, disorganised and unpredictable. He has been argumentative and is threatening physical violence, causing distress to staff and other patients.

MANAGEMENT

- Aim to identify the cause and take control of the situation
- Of paramount concern is the safety of the patient, other patients, yourself and colleagues
- Disturbed patients should be assessed in a safe area with adequate staff support (medical, nursing, security) and access to a panic alarm
- Consider the possibility that the patient might be concealing a weapon
- Specific management depends on the severity of the disturbed behaviour and the cause
- Clues to the diagnosis can often be found by carefully observing an uncooperative patient, even from a distance while awaiting staff support, for example, impairment of the conscious level may suggest delirium or drug intoxication; a smell of alcohol may be apparent. A major psychotic mental illness may be suggested from the appearance, behaviour and speech, for example, preoccupation, suspiciousness, overactivity, thought disorder, delusional ideas
- Additional background information from reliable informants is invaluable but not always possible

After an initial assessment of the situation and with appropriate staff support, a further attempt to calm this patient should be made.

Use Interpersonal Skills/De-Escalation

- Approach the patient in a nonconfrontational manner, avoiding invasion of their personal space. Disturbed patients may misinterpret their surroundings and the motives of others, and whereas their behaviour can create fear in those around them, they are often defensive and frightened themselves. The likelihood of cooperation is enhanced if the patient feels safe

- Clear communication with sensitive statements and questions is often helpful
- Ask the patient what he/she wants; listen and offer advice and reassurance
- Attempt to interview the patient in a safe, relaxed setting
- If initial attempts to engage the patient fail, and providing the situation has not escalated, give the patient some space and time before trying again. Make sure the patient is appropriately observed. The time can be used to consider alternative management

If the Patient Remains Uncooperative

An uncooperative patient whose behaviour is of concern and suggests a mental health problem will require an urgent mental health assessment. An approved 'clinician' – under the Mental Health Act (often the duty Psychiatrist) – is required to sign a medical recommendation that the patient be detained on mental health grounds. If this is appropriate, the patient will be transferred to the psychiatric team. Should the patient's behaviour be considered to present a risk to him/herself or others before this can be completed, the use of restraint and possibly medication under common law should be considered. The reasons for this course of action should be clearly documented and suitable staff should be available.

Following Implementation of the Mental Health Act

As the patient's behaviour remains disturbed and he is a risk to himself and others, safe restraint can be used (as a last resort) by suitably trained staff.

Medication

- Reduction in arousal can be achieved by a carefully planned regimen of antipsychotic medication, preferably given orally and in liquid form in the first instance
- Before IM medication is decided on, all noninvasive measures to calm the patient and secure cooperation should be attempted. Even patients who present as highly disturbed initially may agree to take oral medication when it becomes clear that the situation is under control
- Giving IM medication to a potentially resistive and aroused patient is not without risk, which must be outweighed by risks of inaction and clearly documented
- Resuscitation equipment must be available
- The dose of antipsychotic medication can be reduced by combination with a sedating benzodiazepine in the short term
- Follow local guidance and start at low doses, oral if possible, and increase gradually, depending on response. An suitable example regimen is:
  - Haloperidol oral 2.5–5 mg
  - Lorazepam oral 1–2 mg, IM 0.5–1 mg
- Vital signs (pulse, temperature, BP, conscious level) should be monitored every 15 min
- While the behaviour continues to present a risk, the dose may be repeated at intervals of 30 min to 1 h until the patient is settled, subject to regular monitoring of vital signs

---

REMEMBER

Particular caution should be used in patients who have never received antipsychotic medication previously ('neuroleptic-naïve') because of the possibility of adverse effects, such as a hypersensitivity reaction or acute dystonia.

When the Patient is More Settled

Further assessment can be carried out to establish an accurate diagnosis prior to starting regular treatment.

Progress. This patient's doctor is eventually contacted and you are told that a diagnosis of schizophrenia was made 5 years ago. The patient had been well, but the doctor said he had not attended the clinic (despite reminders) in the last 3 months and suspects he has run out of medication. He has been on olanzapine 10 mg daily. This information is passed on to the psychiatric team, who continue his management.

Further Reading

Suicide and Deliberate Self-Harm

Fazel, S., Runeson, B., 2020. Suicide. N. Engl. J. Med. 382, 266–274.

Acute Anxiety

Craske, M.G., Stein, M.B., 2016. Anxiety. Lancet 388, 3048–3059.
NICE, CKS, 2023. Generalized anxiety disorder. NICE.

Opiate Dependence

Babu, K.M., Brent, J., Juurlink, D.N., 2019. Prevention of opioid overdose. N. Engl. J. Med. 380, 2246–2255.
Bisaga, A., 2019. What should clinicians do as fentanyl replaces heroin?. Addiction 114 (5), 782–783.
Wood, E., 2018. Strategies for reducing opiate overdose deaths. N. Engl. J. Med. 378, 1565–1567.

CHAPTER 9

Rheumatology and Bone Disease

Osteoarthritis (OA)

CASE HISTORY

A 75-year-old female attends the emergency department with pain in the left groin. The pain has been present for several months, but she has not sought medical advice until now. The pain is now so severe that she is unable to walk more than a few yards, and it is keeping her awake at night. She lives alone and is unable either to manage her pain or to cope alone at home.

On examination, movements at the left hip were decreased compared to the right and movement was painful, compatible with OA of the hip.

The assessing doctor has arranged for a pelvic X-ray, which shows OA of the left hip. You are asked to see her for possible admission.

DESCRIBE THE MAIN RADIOLOGICAL FEATURES OF OA OF THE HIP

The X-ray shows joint space narrowing, periarticular sclerosis, cyst formation and osteophytes. These are the four classic features of OA (Fig. 9.1).

HOW WOULD YOU ASSESS THIS PATIENT?

The long-standing history suggests a gradual onset of the pain. A more acute history of systemic symptoms might have indicated joint sepsis or a pathological fracture.

The main site of the pain – especially in the left groin radiating into the left thigh/knee – indicates that the hip is the source of the pain. Beware referred pain either from the lumbar spine (common) or the knee (less common).

A full musculoskeletal examination is needed. The gait, arms, leg and spine (GALS) is a useful screen (see Further reading) (Fig. 9.2).

Diagnostic Clues

Look for Heberden's nodes (distal interphalangeal [DIP] joints), Bouchard's nodes (proximal interphalangeal [PIP] joints), 'square' hands, painful thumb and carpometacarpal joints. These can indicate primary nodal OA. Fig. 9.3 shows the distributions of generalised OA and pyrophosphate arthropathy.

Examine

- Other joints for evidence of inflammatory arthritis, for example, psoriatic arthritis, rheumatoid arthritis (RA)
- Lumbar spine for referred pain
- Hips:
  - Ask patient to walk to assess gait
  - Measure leg lengths
- Assess range of all movements fully and compare with right hip. Examine from behind to look for pelvic tilt and perform Trendelenburg test

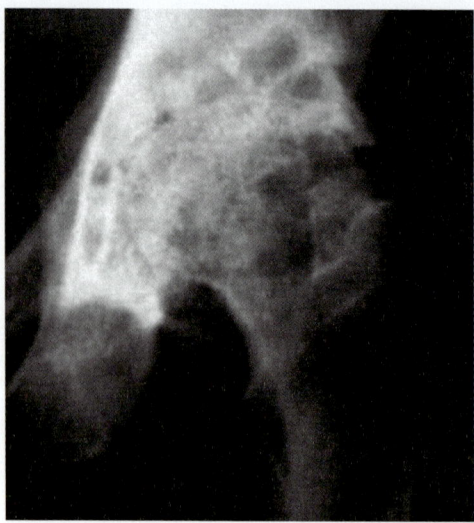

Fig. 9.1   Severe osteoarthritis (OA) of the hip.

WHAT POINTS WOULD YOU CONSIDER WHEN DECIDING IF ADMISSION IS APPROPRIATE?

Full general medical examination is essential because comorbid conditions in this age group are common. For example, in a patient with significant disability, consider the possibilities of pneumonia, cardiac disease or urinary tract infection. The patient's nutrition might be poor, raising the possibility of osteomalacia – a well-described problem in the elderly.

A full assessment of the patient's ability to cope at home is essential and you should ask her about her ability to wash, dress and feed herself. This disability assessment will weigh strongly when discussing admission to hospital.

HOW WOULD YOU INITIALLY MANAGE THIS PATIENT?

- Admit because:
  - The patient lives alone
  - She needs pain control
  - She is unable to manage her activities of daily living
- Give analgesia:
  - Paracetamol can be used for occasional short-term pain relief (or when other options are contraindicated); however, trials have shown little or no effect on pain in OA
  - Topical NSAIDs and/or topical capsaicin may be useful for hand and knee OA and can be considered for OA of other joints
  - A short course of an NSAID can be started if topical treatment is effective (e.g. ibuprofen, naproxen). There is a high risk of gastrointestinal (GI) toxicity with long-term NSAID use in this patient's age group. A gastroprotective agent (proton pump inhibitors, e.g. lansoprazole) should be coprescribed. NSAIDs should be avoided in patients with renal impairment (estimated glomerular filtration rate [eGFR] <60 mL/min/1.73 m^2). Diclofenac and high-dose ibuprofen are contra-indicated in people with cardiovascular disease
  - Opiates should be avoided unless other analgesia has not worked because of sedation/confusion and constipation

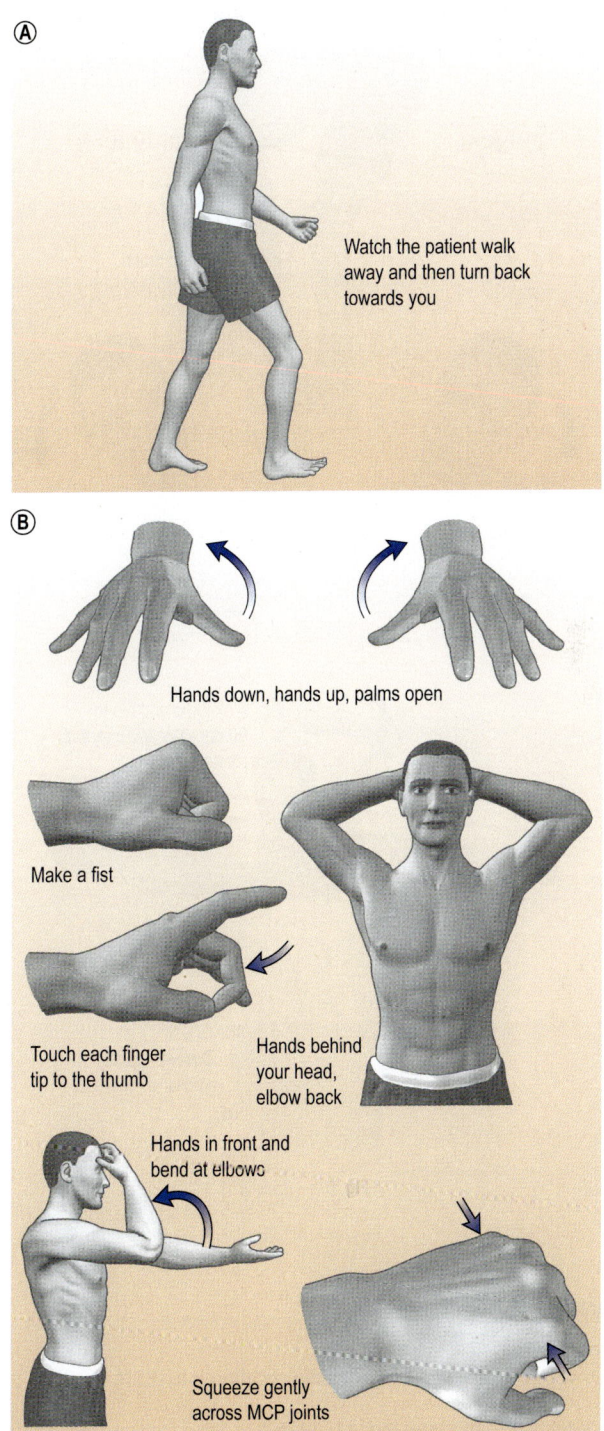

Watch the patient walk away and then turn back towards you

Hands down, hands up, palms open

Make a fist

Touch each finger tip to the thumb

Hands behind your head, elbow back

Hands in front and bend at elbows

Squeeze gently across MCP joints

Fig. 9.2 (A–D) Musculoskeletal examination: gait, arms, leg, spine. MCP, metacarpophalangeal; MT, metatarsal.

Ⓒ

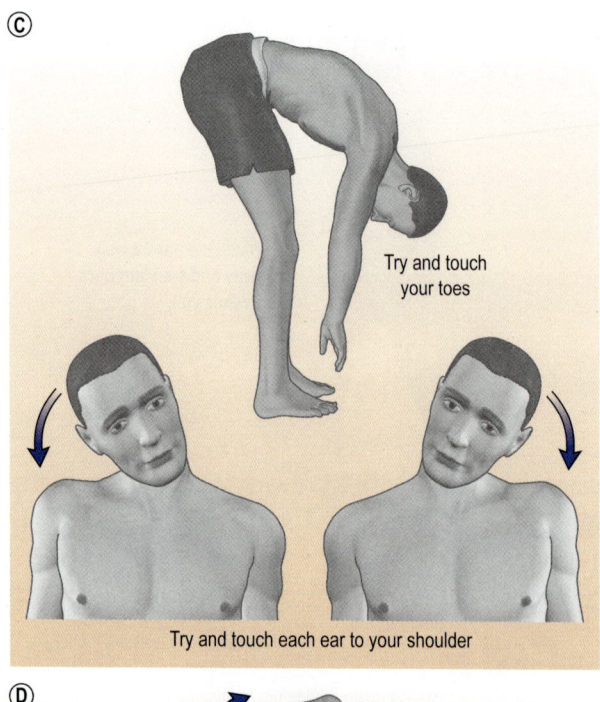

Try and touch
your toes

Try and touch each ear to your shoulder

Ⓓ

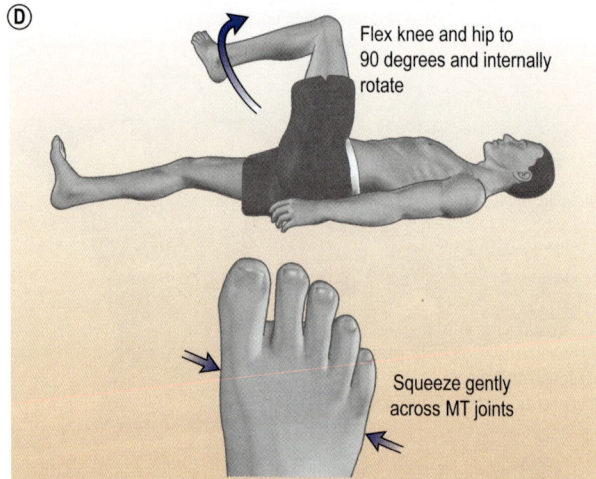

Flex knee and hip to
90 degrees and internally
rotate

Squeeze gently
across MT joints

Fig. 9.2 *cont'd*

INVESTIGATIONS

- Full blood count (FBC)
- C-reactive protein (CRP) or erythrocyte sedimentation rate (ESR)

Note: If she had been febrile, blood cultures would have had to be taken.

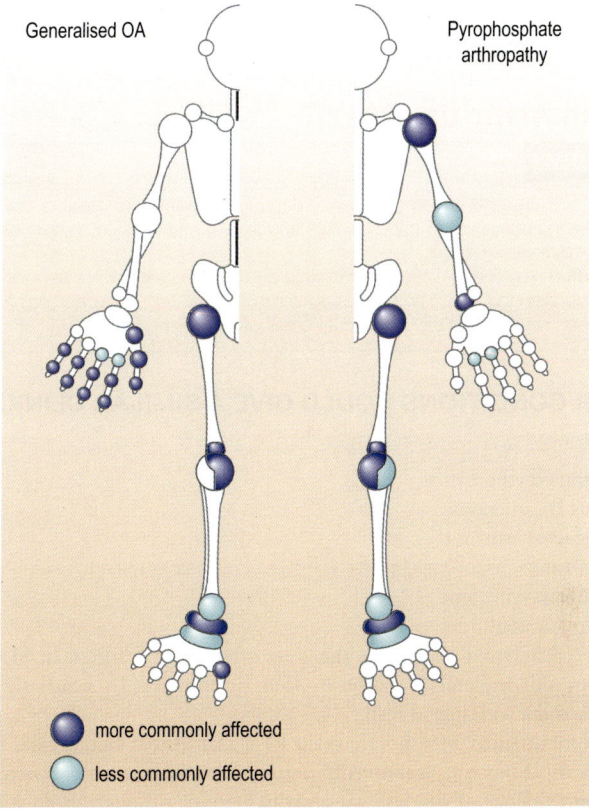

Fig. 9.3   Generalised nodal osteoarthritis (OA) and pyrophosphate arthropathy.

LATER MANAGEMENT

Refer to a rheumatologist or medicine for the elderly consultant. In the meantime, organise:
- Physiotherapy:
  - Mobilise hip, joint protection exercises
  - Assess walking aids, for example, stick, Zimmer frame
  - Hydrotherapy
- Occupational therapy and social work assessments

There should be detailed planning before discharge, including liaison with her doctor and a home visit.

WHAT ARE THE INDICATIONS FOR SURGERY?

Referral to orthopaedics for surgery:
- Severe pain, especially at night
- Substantial impact on quality of life
- Poor mobility

Note: Intra-articular corticosteroid injections can be trialled if other treatments are ineffective or unsuitable; patients must be informed that this only offers short-term relief.

Progress. The general health of the patient was good, and hip surgery is a very effective treatment. She was therefore booked for a total hip replacement (THR). Her postoperative recovery was excellent and she was able to walk without pain.

Rheumatoid Arthritis (RA)

CASE HISTORY

A 26-year-old female presents to the emergency department with rapid onset of severe, widespread joint pain and swelling affecting her hands, wrists and feet symmetrically. She has lost half a stone in weight and feels systemically unwell.

On examination, you find that she has hot joints with a symmetrical synovitis, joint restriction of the wrists, metacarpophalangeal (MCP) and proximal interphalangeal (PIP) joints, and painful metatarsophalangeal (MTP) joints. You suspect this is an acute onset of RA.

WHAT OTHER CONDITIONS COULD GIVE A SIMILAR CLINICAL PICTURE?

- Systemic lupus erythematosus (SLE)
- Erythrovirus B_{19} infection
- Poststreptococcal arthritis
- Psoriatic arthritis
- Primary Sjögren syndrome
- Some systemic vasculitides

In the first two differential diagnoses, there are often other features. In SLE, photosensitive rashes, hair loss, serositis and oral ulceration are seen. Erythrovirus B_{19} nearly always presents with flu-like symptoms and a widespread rash.

Poststreptococcal arthritis may be preceded by a sore throat but is rare. Psoriatic arthritis is usually asymmetrical but can occasionally present with a symmetrical pattern. Psoriatic nail changes and other evidence of psoriasis are usually present, although these might develop after the onset of arthritis.

Sjögren syndrome can be associated with intermittent parotid swelling and sicca symptoms: dry eyes (keratoconjunctivitis sicca) and dry mouth (xerostomia).

HOW WOULD YOU MANAGE THIS PATIENT?

REMEMBER

Rheumatoid arthritis is a multisystem disease, so look carefully for pulmonary, cardiac or neurological involvement, although these are less common at presentation.

A full history and general medical examination are essential. Specific points are as follows:
- Look for nodules or vasculitis: uncommon at first presentation
- Perform a full musculoskeletal examination, noting the symmetry of the joint involvement
- Look for persistent inflammatory symmetrical arthritis (PISA). The most common cause of this is RA

The most commonly involved joints at onset in RA are the wrists, MCP, PIP and MTP joints.

Admission is necessary to manage a patient who is very unwell systemically and to exclude other pathology.

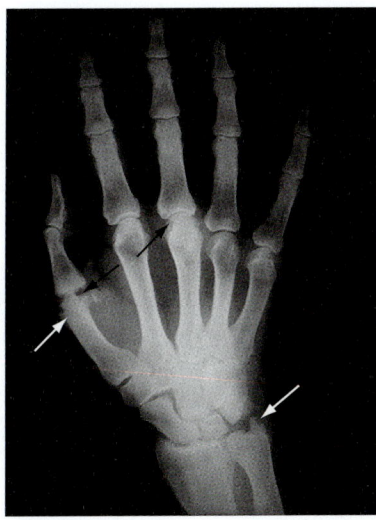

Fig. 9.4 X-ray of early rheumatoid arthritis (RA) showing typical erosions at the thumb and middle metacarpophalangeal (MCP) joints and at the ulnar styloid (*arrows*).

INVESTIGATIONS

- Full blood count/ESR, biochemistry, including globulin level, CRP
- Antinuclear antibodies (ANA)/rheumatoid factor (RhF)
- Anticitrullinated peptide antibodies (ACPA) are positive early in the disease
- X-ray hands and feet for erosions, periarticular osteopenia (Fig. 9.4) (MRI if necessary)
- ASO titre if sore throat
- Blood cultures if febrile
- Erythrovirus B_{19} titres if the ANA/RhF are negative

HOW WOULD YOU INITIALLY MANAGE THIS PATIENT?

- NSAIDs for symptoms control (e.g. ibuprofen or naproxen) – consider the risk of GI toxicity (although this patient is young) and cardiovascular risk factors
- Disease-modifying antirheumatic drugs (DMARDs): these should be given at the earliest opportunity because RA is a systemic disease that leads rapidly to joint damage and disability. It is not acceptable to treat RA with NSAIDs alone. There is accumulating evidence to show that early DMARD use delays joint damage and functional disability. Initial DMARDs commonly used include hydroxychloroquine, sulfasalazine, methotrexate or azathioprine. Hydroxychloroquine is often recommended for patients with low disease activity as it is better tolerated and has a more favourable risk profile. Methotrexate is more effective for moderate to severe disease; however, it is associated with more adverse effects. Folic acid supplementation has been shown to reduce the risk of some of these effects
- Biologics, such as anti-TNF-α agents (e.g. infliximab and etanercept) and IL-6 inhibitors (e.g. tocilizumab), are effective when initial DMARD therapy has failed. Infectious complications, such as tuberculosis (TB), are a concern with these agents
- Targeted synthetic DMARDs (ts DMARD) are also available, for example, baricitinib (a Janus kinase inhibitor)
- Combination therapy has been shown to be effective for severe or resistant disease activity

LATE MANIFESTATIONS OF RA

Changes in the hand are shown in Fig. 9.5. Other joints, such as knees and hips, become involved later in the disease course.

All drugs need careful explanation to the patient and close monitoring for toxicity

Consider short courses of corticosteroids (e.g. oral prednisolone up to 20 mg daily then taper) alongside DMARDs for patients with early disease or as a management for acute flares.

Progress. This patient had a high ESR of 60 mm/h and a CRP of 90 mg/L, indicating active disease. Her ACPA and RhF were positive in the serum, typical of RA. The X-rays of her hands showed soft tissue swelling only. An MRI was therefore performed and showed early erosions, confirming the diagnosis.

This patient was admitted and treated symptomatically with analgesics. She was started on prednisolone and methotrexate. The pain and swelling improved and she was discharged, still with some residual problems. She was given a follow-up appointment for clinic in 2 weeks' time.

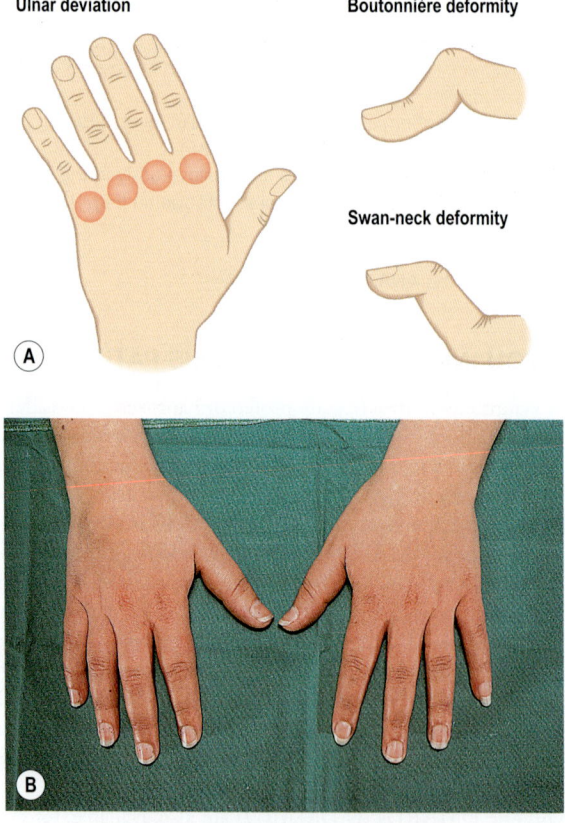

Fig. 9.5 (A–B) RA: late manifestations.

Systemic Lupus Erythematosus (SLE) and Vasculitis

CASE HISTORY

A 28-year-old female is referred to you by her doctor. Six weeks ago, she delivered her first baby and the pregnancy and delivery were uneventful. Two weeks after delivery, she developed a widespread polyarthritis affecting her hands, feet and knees, and a photosensitive rash on her face. In the last week or two, she has become extremely unwell with weight loss and painful lesions on her hands and feet.

On examination, she is clearly unwell, with a facial rash and severe oral ulceration. Examination of her hands and feet shows extensive digital infarcts with necrotic ulceration on the palms, finger pulps and soles of the feet. There are splinter haemorrhages and nail-fold infarcts.

WHAT ARE YOUR DIFFERENTIAL DIAGNOSES?

The differential diagnosis includes an inflammatory autoimmune rheumatic disease, such as SLE, which has developed after delivery of her baby. The lesions on her hands (Fig. 9.6) and feet are strongly suggestive of vasculitis, which is a serious prognostic factor that requires immediate therapy.

REMEMBER

The major risk of vasculitis is organ involvement, including renal, cerebral and pulmonary disease, which can be life-threatening.

HOW WOULD YOU INVESTIGATE AND MANAGE THIS PATIENT?

Investigations (Table 9.1) are performed to look for the possibility of major organ involvement, which might be vasculitic. Her urine must be tested immediately for blood and protein and sent for urine cytology to look for fragmented red cells and/or casts. The presence of an 'active' urine sediment with fragmented or dysmorphic red cells and granular casts has a >90% specificity for glomerulonephritis.

Progress. The patient was found to be anaemic with an Hb of 50 g/L, a raised ESR of 80 mm/h, normal CRP, a raised ANA and antidsDNA autoantibodies. A diagnosis of SLE was reached.

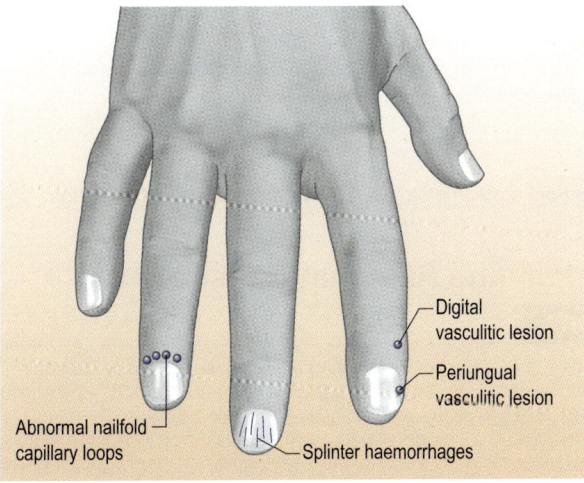

Fig. 9.6   Vasculitic lesions seen in the fingers.

TABLE 9.1 ■ Investigations for SLE and Vasculitis

Investigation	Typical Finding
FBC	Immune cytopenias, especially neutropenia and thrombocytopenia, are common in SLE
	There may be anaemia of chronic disease or haemolytic anaemia – check Coombs' test
ESR and CRP	The pattern of a high ESR but normal CRP is characteristic of SLE
Renal function	U and Es, 24-h urine protein/eGFR
Liver biochemistry	Hypoalbuminaemia is common
Lupus serology	
ANA	Present in 95% of SLE patients
dsDNA	Specific marker for SLE; a negative dsDNA, however, does not exclude SLE
ENA	Ro/La photosensitivity/Sjögren's
	RNP/Sm often seen in severe SLE
Complement	Low values indicate activation of complement or, rarely, congenital deficiency
ANCA	A marker of vasculitis: a systemic vasculitis is an alternative to SLE

ANA, Antinuclear antibodies; ANCA, antineutrophil cytoplasmic antibody; CRP, C-reactive protein; eGFR, estimated glomerular filtration rate; ENA, extractable nuclear antigen; ESR, erythrocyte sedimentation rate; FBC, full blood count; SLE, systemic lupus erythematosus.

Once the diagnosis of lupus is established on clinical and serological grounds, therapy consists of simple analgesia (including NSAIDs) and additional treatment depending on the individual systems involved. This can consist of hydroxychloroquine and, if required, corticosteroids (e.g. oral prednisolone 5-60 mg daily or IV pulse methylprednisolone 500 mg on alternate days for three doses). Corticosteroids should be used at the lowest possible dose to control symptoms for the shortest period of time. Methotrexate, azathioprine or mycophenolate mofetil can also be considered depending on disease severity.

Immunosuppressive therapy is commonly used to treat vasculitis. One approach is IV cyclophosphamide therapy given 2-weekly or monthly. The patient should be carefully counselled about the risks and benefits of cyclophosphamide; these include adverse effects, such as cytopenias, haemorrhagic cystitis and infections, including herpes zoster and infertility. If the patient is breastfeeding, she should stop because cyclophosphamide and other immunosuppressives, such as azathioprine, are excreted in breast milk.

On treatment with steroids (see earlier), her symptoms settled and a decision was taken to delay immunosuppressive therapy until after she had stopped breastfeeding.

REMEMBER

Specialist advice from a rheumatologist or immunologist should be sought.

Acute Autoimmune Rheumatic Disease

CASE HISTORY

A 33-year-old female of African origin is admitted through the emergency department, complaining of breathlessness and swollen legs. Two years ago, she was admitted with a psychotic illness that had features of schizophrenia and improved with antipsychotic medication.

In the last 6 months, she has developed a symmetrical small joint inflammatory arthritis, mouth ulcers and photosensitive facial rashes. Over the last 2 weeks, she has become breathless and her legs have become severely swollen.

On examination, she is anaemic and has a pulse rate of 120/min with pulsus paradoxus. Her BP is 90/60. She has bilateral pleural effusions, a raised jugular venous pressure (JVP) with a sharp rise and y descent (Friedreichs sign) and pitting oedema to her waist. There is synovitis of the small joints of her fingers, and she has florid splinter haemorrhages. Her urine showed heavy proteinuria.

WHAT IS THE LIKELY DIAGNOSIS?

Diagnosis is likely to be **SLE complicated by nephrotic syndrome**. In addition, she may have cardiac tamponade from a pericardial effusion.

Systemic lupus erythematosus is nine times more common in females than in males and is found more often in people of African-Caribbean descent; it is also often more severe in these groups.

This patient has many characteristic features of SLE: inflammatory polyarthritis, mouth ulcers, photosensitive rashes, psychotic illness, serositis with pleural and probably pericardial effusions, and renal disease with nephrotic syndrome (Fig. 9.7). The high JVP might indicate early tamponade.

HOW WOULD YOU MANAGE THIS PATIENT?

The most urgent priority is to establish whether this patient has cardiac tamponade. The low BP and the presence of pulsus paradoxus, tachycardia and raised JVP, with increased distension during inspiration and cardiomegaly on CXR, are strong pointers to this. An echocardiogram is performed

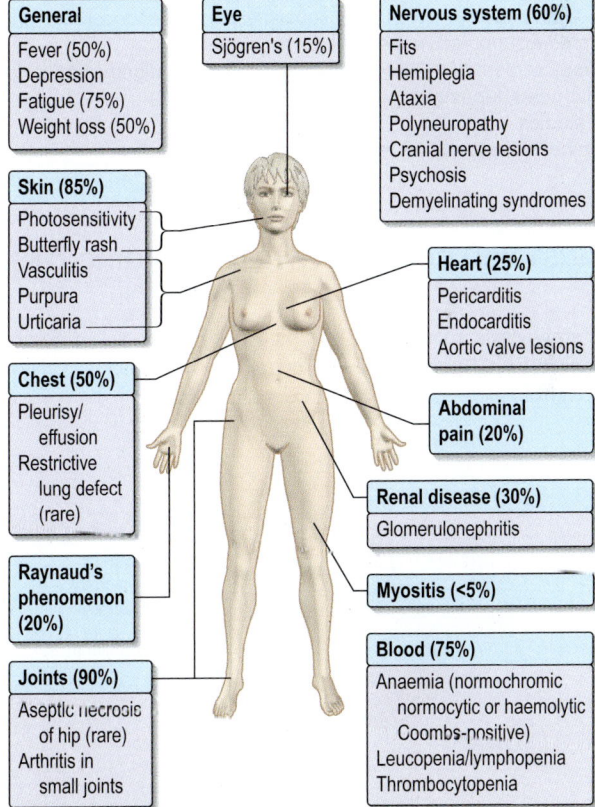

Fig. 9.7 Clinical features of systemic lupus erythematosus (SLE).

urgently, which shows an echo-free region between the myocardium and the intense echo of the parietal pericardium. This confirms the effusion and the clinical signs confirm tamponade.

The overwhelming majority of patients with lupus who have cardiac tamponade associated with a pericardial effusion respond to high-dose oral corticosteroids and do not need pericardiocentesis. This should be performed, however, if the patient deteriorates despite corticosteroid therapy or if sepsis is present.

The next priority is to determine the extent and severity of the renal disease. Serum creatinine, eGFR, albumin and 24-h urine protein are essential. If there is an 'active' urine sediment, e.g. fragmented red cells and granular casts, indicating glomerulonephritis, renal biopsy is required.

INVESTIGATIONS

- Full blood count with reticulocyte count, Coombs' (direct antiglobulin test) if positive: the anaemia is haemolytic
- Urea and electrolytes (U and Es) (eGFR): renal impairment may be present
- Biochemistry: serum albumin will be low
- Twenty-four-h urine protein should be started
- Urine cytology for fragmented red cells and granular casts: a useful marker of glomerulonephritis
- Chest X-ray: to document pleural effusions and cardiomegaly (Fig. 9.8)
- Echocardiogram: to document pericardial effusion and possible valve lesions
- Electrocardiogram
- Blood gases
- Blood cultures/urine cultures: to exclude sepsis, especially endocarditis, prior to corticosteroid and immunosuppressive therapy
- Full autoantibody screen: ANA, DNA, extractable nuclear antigens (ENA), RhF, ACPA, anticardiolipin antibodies, lupus anticoagulant, ANCA (Table 9.2)
- Complement studies
- A diagnostic renal biopsy may be required later

WHAT ELSE MUST YOU CONSIDER WHEN MANAGING THIS PATIENT?

- Thrombosis prophylaxis: this patient is at high risk of deep vein thrombosis (DVT)/pulmonary embolus (PE). Thromboembolic deterrent (TED) stockings and prophylactic low-molecular-weight heparin should be given

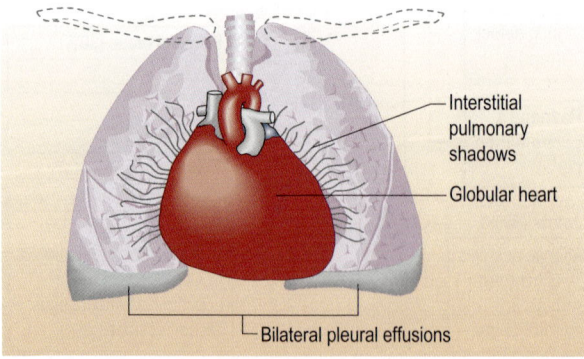

Interstitial pulmonary shadows

Globular heart

Bilateral pleural effusions

Fig. 9.8 Diagram of a chest X-ray (CXR) showing pleural effusions and cardiomegaly.

TABLE 9.2 ■ **Antinuclear Autoantibodies and Disease Associations**

Antibody	Disease	Prevalence
ds-DNA	SLE	70%
Antihistone	Drug-induced lupus	–
Anticentromeric	Limited scleroderma	70%
Anti-Ro (SS-A)	SLE	40%–60%
	Primary Sjögren's	60%–90%
Anti-La (SS-B)	SLE	15%
	Primary Sjögren's	35%–85%
Anti-Sm	SLE	10%–50% (higher prevalence in West Africa and Asia)
Anti-UI-RNP	SLE	30%
	Overlap syndrome	–
Anti-Jo-1 (antisynthetase)	Polymyositis	30%
	Dermatomyositis	–
Anti-topoisomerase-1 (Scl-70)	Diffuse cutaneous SSc	30%

RNP, Ribonucleoprotein; Ro, La, first two letters of name of patients; Sm, Smith, patient's name; SS-A, SS-B, Sjögren syndrome A and B; SSc, systemic scleroderma; SLE, systemic lupus erythematosus.
From Feather, A., Randall, D., Waterhouse, M., eds., 2021. Kumar and Clark's Clinical Medicine, tenth ed. Elsevier, London; Box 18.38.

- Is the anaemia haemolytic? If so, it should respond to corticosteroids
- Angiotensin-converting enzyme (ACE) inhibition: when the BP has normalised as a result of treatment of the tamponade, start an ACE inhibitor. This is especially useful in protein-uric patients
- If renal biopsy confirms proliferative glomerulonephritis, the treatment of choice is cortico-steroid therapy and intermittent IV cyclophosphamide, followed by azathioprine
- This patient's lipid profile might well be deranged, especially in the nephrotic syndrome: this will need to be assessed and managed actively. Measurement of serum lipids is per-formed and the patient started on a statin immediately if hypercholesterolaemia is present
- Prophylaxis against corticosteroid-induced osteoporosis: a baseline dual-energy X-ray absorp-tiometry (DXA) scan should be performed and calcium supplementation should be started

WHAT IS THE LONG-TERM PROGNOSIS?

The majority of patients with SLE have a good prognosis, although clearly, this patient has a serious disease with life-threatening complications. Mortality in SLE occurs at two peak periods: those patients who die from overwhelming disease, thrombosis or sepsis, and those who die pre-maturely from accelerated atherosclerosis. Prognosis has been considerably improved by earlier recognition and effective therapy.

Progress. This patient had several problems. Her cardiac effusion gradually responded to high-dose oral steroids and her BP improved. She had a haemolytic anaemia of 95 g/L. She was dis-charged on steroids and an ACE inhibitor after an inpatient stay of 2 weeks. She later had a renal biopsy, which confirmed a proliferative glomerulonephritis and was seen by the nephrologists for treatment. A DXA scan did not show osteoporosis.

Reactive Arthritis

Reactive arthritis is an inflammatory arthritis occurring after exposure to certain GI and genito-urinary infections. It is associated with a triad of urethritis, arthritis and conjunctivitis (Fig. 9.9).

CASE HISTORY

A 21-year-old male presents with pain and swelling of his left knee and pain in his left heel. The pain started acutely, but there was no history of trauma. He was seen in the genitourinary medicine clinic around 6 weeks ago as he developed dysuria after having unprotected sexual intercourse with a new partner. He has no relevant past medical history.

On examination, there is a warm effusion over the left knee and tenderness over the left Achilles' insertion. You suspect a diagnosis of **reactive arthritis**

WHAT OTHER DIAGNOSES MUST YOU CONSIDER?

Always exclude septic arthritis if there is any diagnostic uncertainty. Other differentials include ankylosing spondylitis, psoriatic arthritis, RA, and gout.

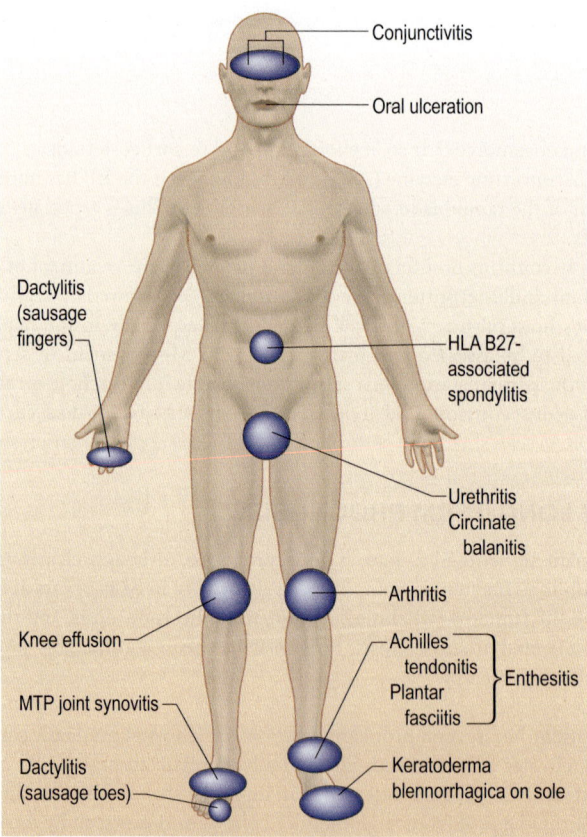

Fig. 9.9   Clinical features of reactive arthritis.

WHAT ORGANISMS ARE COMMONLY RESPONSIBLE FOR THIS CONDITION?

Reactive arthritis can be divided into two main subgroups:

- Postenteric infection: most commonly *Campylobacter*, *Salmonella* and *Shigella* species
- Postvenereal: following *Chlamydia trachomatis infection* or with human immunodeficiency virus (HIV)

INVESTIGATIONS

- Full blood count (white cell count (WCC) typically elevated), U and E, liver function tests
- C-reactive protein/ESR – typically elevated (nonspecific)
- Blood cultures – if possibility of septic arthritis
- Urogenital and stool cultures – usually negative after the onset of arthritis
- HLA-B27 is positive in the majority of those affected
- Rheumatoid factor and antinuclear antibodies are absent
- X-rays – often normal in early stages, in advanced or long-term disease may show periosteal reaction and proliferation
- Joint aspiration and synovial fluid aspiration – may be required to rule out septic or crystalline arthritis

HOW WOULD YOU MANAGE THIS PATIENT?

Treatment is focused on symptomatic relief and halting joint damage:

- NSAIDs (e.g. naproxen) are first line – consider gastroprotection as well as renal and cardiovascular risks. No NSAID has been found to be superior to any other
- Corticosteroids (e.g. prednisolone 0.5 mg–1 mg/kg/day orally) can be used if there is no response to NSAIDs or in acute flares
- Disease-modifying antirheumatic drugs can be considered when other treatments fail or if aggressive treatment is required to prevent joint destruction

Progress. This patient's symptoms improved with NSAIDs and resolved within 3 months.

Crystal Arthritis

Two main types of crystal account for the majority of crystal-induced arthritis. They are (1) sodium urate (gout) and (2) calcium pyrophosphate (pseudogout) and are distinguished by their different shapes and refringence properties under polarised light with a red filter. Rarely, crystals of calcium apatite or cholesterol cause acute synovitis.

CASE HISTORY

A 73-year-old female was admitted a week ago to the stroke unit with a right hemiparesis. She has developed a hot, swollen right knee. You have been asked to see the patient for your advice on whether this might be a septic arthritis.

On further questioning, you discover that the patient has attended the hypertension clinic for many years and has been taking bendroflumethiazide. She has also complained of knee pain intermittently over the last 5 years, but the joint has never previously swelled up. She is making a reasonable recovery from her stroke, and there is no other relevant history.

Clinically, there is no evidence of tophi. The knee is hot and movement is restricted due to a large tense effusion. She is afebrile.

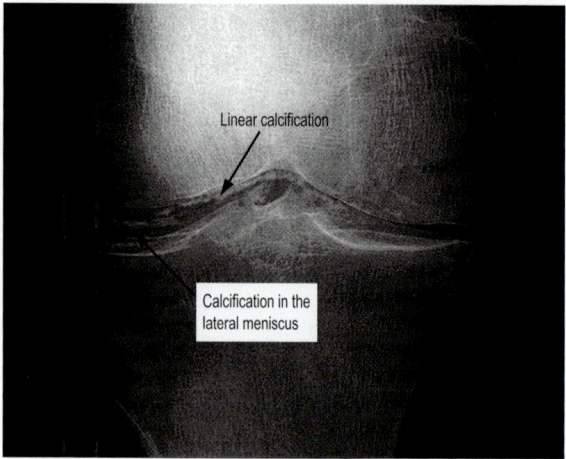

Fig. 9.10 Chondrocalcinosis of the knee. Note the linear calcification in the hyaline cartilage and calcification of the lateral meniscus (plus mild secondary OA). OA, Osteoarthritis.

HOW WOULD YOU MANAGE THIS PATIENT?

The X-ray showed chondrocalcinosis (Fig. 9.10) and patello-femoral and tibio-femoral OA. The serum uric acid was elevated (520 μmol/L); she is taking a thiazide diuretic. The differential diagnosis thus includes gout or pseudogout, of which pseudogout is probably more likely in this clinical context. The uric acid level, although high, is usually >600 μmol/L with gout.

INVESTIGATIONS

- Full blood count, U and Es, ESR/CRP
- Bone and liver biochemistry
- Serum urate
- X-ray of affected joint(s) – exclude other causes, cartilage calcification is suggestive but not diagnostic and detects only about 40% of articular crystal deposits
- Blood cultures
- Aspiration of the joint using a sterile technique; fluid should be sent for cells, crystals and culture

HOW DOES PSEUDOGOUT TYPICALLY PRESENT?

This patient has the typical presentation of pseudogout: an acute onset of a swollen joint in an elderly patient who has been admitted for other reasons, usually a stroke, myocardial infarction (MI), or chest infection.

Calcium pyrophosphate is the most common crystal associated with pseudogout (Fig. 9.11). The crystals are diagnosed on synovial fluid analysis using polarised light microscopy. They are rhomboidal and positively birefringent and can be idiopathic or associated with OA. A number of metabolic conditions are also associated with calcium pyrophosphate deposition; these include hypothyroidism, hyperparathyroidism, acromegaly, Wilson disease, haemochromatosis, hypophosphatasia and hypomagnesaemia.

The differential diagnosis of gout is also confirmed on crystal examination. These urate crystals are negatively birefringent needle-shaped crystals.

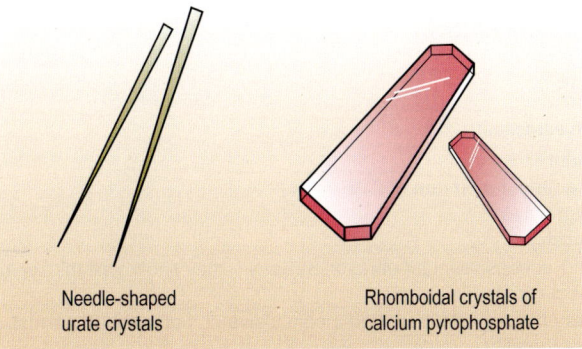

Needle-shaped
urate crystals

Rhomboidal crystals of
calcium pyrophosphate

Fig. 9.11 Urate and calcium pyrophosphate crystals.

HOW WOULD YOU MANAGE THIS PATIENT?

Septic arthritis, although unlikely, should be excluded, and providing joint aspiration and synovial fluid culture and blood cultures are all negative, the knee should be aspirated to dryness and injected with a steroid, for example, dexamethasone.

Risk factors should be minimised and the thiazide diuretic (which can precipitate gout) should be switched to an alternative antihypertensive medication. Intensive physiotherapy is necessary, with particular attention to quadriceps exercises and maintenance of mobility and hydration in the patient.

Progress. This patient's pain improved and she was able to be gradually mobilised with the help of physiotherapy. Her speech improved over the first 2 weeks, but she was left severely disabled by her right-sided weakness. She was eventually transferred to long-term care.

Polymyalgia Rheumatica/Giant Cell Arteritis

Polymyalgia rheumatica (PMR) and giant cell (cranial) arteritis (GCA) are systemic vasculitides affecting people over 50 years of age. Both are associated with the finding of a giant cell arteritis on temporal artery biopsy.

CASE HISTORY

A 73-year-old female presents to the emergency department feeling nonspecifically unwell. On further questioning, she has a headache and joint aches, particularly of her shoulders and hips, in addition to widespread aches and pains. She has marked joint stiffness, particularly of the shoulders and hips, lasting for several hours each morning and occasionally all day. The headache is predominantly right-sided and the patient says that it is painful when she brushes her hair. In addition, she has pains in the left jaw on talking or eating.

On examination, the scalp is tender and it is difficult to palpate the temporal arteries. The rest of the examination is normal. Her shoulders and hips ache at the extremes of the range of movement but are otherwise normal.

WHAT IS THE LIKELY DIAGNOSIS?

The most likely diagnosis in a patient over 50 years is temporal arteritis (giant cell arteritis) with PMR, and there is therefore a significant risk of blindness from arteritis of the ophthalmic artery. A differential diagnosis includes malignancy of any cause and myeloma, which can, rarely, mimic

PMR. The ESR is nearly always significantly elevated, but approximately 1% to 5% of patients with PMR have a normal ESR.

INVESTIGATIONS

The following are essential:

- Full blood count
- Erythrocyte sedimentation rate or CRP
- Urea and electrolytes
- Liver biochemistry
- Consider rapid-access vascular ultrasonography – may show wall thickening (halo sign), stenosis or occlusion
- Temporal artery biopsy – if ultrasound inconclusive or if ultrasound normal, but there is a high pretest probability

---

HOW WOULD YOU MANAGE THIS PATIENT?

This patient should be commenced on 60 mg of prednisolone immediately and a temporal artery biopsy should be arranged within the next 24 h. The clinical diagnosis is **giant cell arteritis.**

The histological features of GCA are shown in Box 9.1.

The response to steroids is usually dramatic in these patients and a response is often seen within 24–48 h. The steroid therapy can then be reduced reasonably quickly, over a few months, to 15–20 mg daily; if this is not possible, a steroid-sparing agents such as tocilizumab or methotrexate should be added to achieve this (specialist use only).

Aspirin is considered for patients with vascular ischaemic complications.

This patient is also at high risk of osteoporosis and subsequent vertebral fractures, and calcium and vitamin D supplementation should be coprescribed routinely. A baseline DXA should be requested. If there is already osteoporosis, bisphosphonates should be given.

Progress. This patient's headache quickly disappeared on steroid therapy, and in 6 months she was well on prednisolone 10 mg daily with a normal ESR. Her steroids will be continued for at least 1 year, with regular checks of her ESR.

PATIENTS WHO FAIL TO RESPOND TO STEROIDS

Such patients should be investigated in detail for an underlying malignancy, especially multiple myeloma. Occasionally, other conditions such as severe hypothyroidism might also present with similar joint aches but the clinical picture of temporal arteritis with a good response to steroids is usually characteristic enough to establish the diagnosis.

BOX 9.1 ■ Histological Features of Cranial Arteritis

- Intimal hypertrophy
- Inflammation of the intima and subintima
- Breaking up of the internal elastic lamina
- Giant cells, lymphocytes and plasma cells in the internal elastic lamina

Polymyositis and Dermatomyositis

CASE HISTORY

A 64-year-old female presents to her GP with weakness and fatigue that has gradually worsened over the last 5 weeks. It predominantly affects her thighs, and she struggles to get out of a chair without help. Over the last 3 to 4 months, she has also noticed a rash develop over her face, elbow and hands, as well as some facial swelling.

On examination, she has violaceous plaques over the extensor surfaces of the elbows and a periorbital heliotrope rash. Dilated capillary loops are noted at the base of her fingernails. Fine bibasal crepitations are noted on auscultation of her chest.

WHAT IS THE LIKELY DIAGNOSIS?

Diagnosis: dermatomyositis.

Dermatomyositis and polymyositis are idiopathic inflammatory myopathies that present with proximal skeletal muscle weakness and muscle inflammation. Dermatomyositis is also associated with a variety of characteristic skin manifestations.

INFORMATION

Features of dermatomyositis on examination:

- Gottron papules (Fig. 9.12) – typically present over dorsal surface of MCP joints (pathognomonic of dermatomyositis)
- Heliotrope rash (with/without periorbital oedema) – symmetrical periorbital dusky/red rash
- Periungal erythema and nail-fold capillary dilation – common but also seen in some other connective tissue disorders
- Proximal muscle weakness with preserved sensation and normal tendon reflexes

WHAT ARE THE RISK FACTORS FOR THIS CONDITION?

Key risk factors include:

- Family history of autoimmune disease
- Children or age >40 years
- Female sex
- Ultraviolet radiation exposure

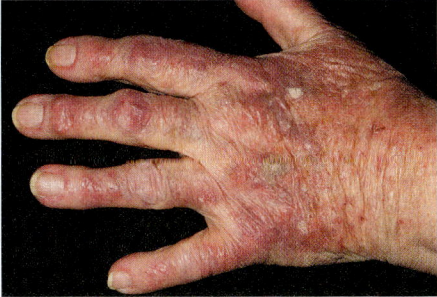

Fig. 9.12 Gottron papules over the bony prominences of the fingers (they can also be found on the elbows, knees and feet). A violaceous rash, with or without scale, may appear on the back of the hands and palm as well. (From Habif, T.P., Dinulos, J.G., Shane Chapman, M., et al., 2018. Skin Disease: Diagnosis and Treatment, fourth ed. Connective Tissue Diseases, Fig. 14.22, Elsevier Ltd., London.)

WHAT FURTHER INVESTIGATIONS WOULD YOU REQUEST?

- The diagnosis is established by electromyography (EMG) and confirmed by muscle biopsy
- Creatine kinase – rarely normal in active disease, and the level can be a good indicator of disease activity
- About 20% have antiJo-1 antibodies – indicates a poor prognosis with interstitial lung disease
- Autoantibody testing for myositis-specific antibody (MSA) and myositis-associated auto-antibodies (MAA) can be useful to differentiate the patients with underlying malignancy
- Echocardiography – perform in all patients as myocardial involvement can cause congestive cardiac failure (indicates a poor prognosis but only occurs in <5% of patients)
- High-resolution CT chest – should be performed in all patients with respiratory symptoms or examination

HOW WILL YOU MANAGE THIS PATIENT?

The goal of treatment is to achieve disease remission. Dermatomyositis is often the most responsive to therapy out of the inflammatory myopathies.

Nonpharmacological

- Sun-blocking agents
- Engage with physiotherapy as able to maintain muscle strength
- Speech and language therapy input can help with difficulties in swallowing

Pharmacological

- Steroids are the primary treatment for acute flares – if mild topical steroids may be enough, but for more severe disease, high doses of systemic steroids are required to gain control (e.g. methylprednisolone 1 g once daily for 3–5 days)
- This is then converted to oral steroids (e.g. prednisolone 1 mg/kg/day) for 2–4 weeks and tapered
- Intravenous immunoglobulin (IVIG) can be used with steroids initially for patients who have significant muscle weakness
- If steroids are insufficient, immunosuppressants such as azathioprine, cyclophosphamide or methotrexate can be used
- If there is lung involvement, then an aggressive regimen combining ciclosporin A or tacrolimus with cyclophosphamide is recommended alongside steroids

WHAT ARE THE POTENTIAL COMPLICATIONS OF THIS CONDITION?

- Dysphagia secondary to muscle weakness
- Gastrointestinal ulceration can cause melaena or haematemesis
- Increased risk of malignancy
- Cardiac disease occurs in 50% of cases but is rarely symptomatic except in advanced disease: atrioventricular defects, tachyarrhythmias, infarction, dilated cardiomyopathies, pericarditis
- Interstitial lung disease can occur in up to 40% of patients (drug-induced pneumonitis can also be caused by treatment with methotrexate)
- Complications of steroid therapy, for example, osteoporosis

Acute Back Pain

CASE HISTORY

A 36-year-old pub owner presents to the emergency department having experienced severe back and buttock pain after lifting a barrel of beer. The pain radiated down the left leg to the sole of the foot with associated paraesthesia. On further questioning, he finds that it is extremely painful to move his back and that the pain is worse on coughing or sneezing. The pain is also worse in the leg than in the back. He says that he has not passed any urine for 6 h.

On examination, he is found to be in severe pain and is lying flat on the examination couch. He finds it too painful to stand up, but his hips, knees and other joints are all normal on examination. Straight-leg raising on the right is 40 degrees, but on the left is only 10 degrees, with a strongly positive sciatic stretch test. The femoral nerve stretch test is also strongly positive on the left and neurological examination reveals an absent left ankle jerk and sacral anaesthesia.

WHAT IS THE LIKELY DIAGNOSIS? WHAT INVESTIGATION WOULD YOU REQUEST?

The history and clinical examination are almost diagnostic for a large L5/S1 disc protrusion with compromise of the cauda equina, which can lead to urinary retention. This is therefore a neurosurgical emergency.

The most urgent investigation is imaging (MRI) of the lumbar spine and pelvis (Fig. 9.13). The patient should be catheterised and analgesia should be given. This includes IM non-steroidals, such as IM diclofenac, or opiate analgesics, including morphine, if needed. The patient should be referred immediately to a neurosurgeon or orthopaedic surgeon with an interest in acute spinal

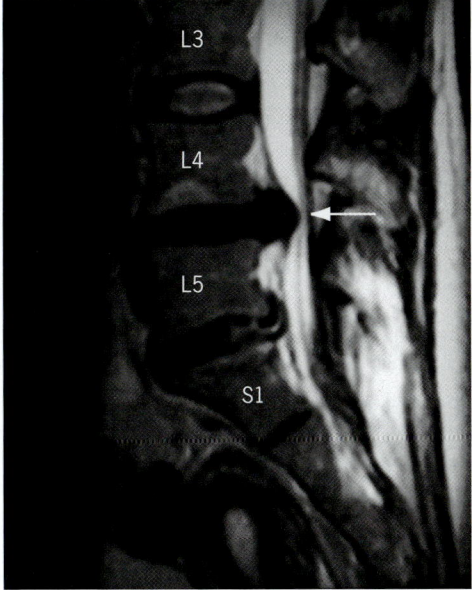

Fig. 9.13 Magnetic resonance imaging of the lumbar spine showing a central disc prolapse at the L4/L5 level (*arrow*). The signal from the L4/L5 and L5/S1 discs indicates dehydration, whereas the appearance of the L3/L4 signal is normal.

problems for urgent decompressive surgery with a laminectomy and discectomy. Any delay in diagnosis or decompression might lead to a permanent neurological deficit.

Progress. This patient required urgent surgery, as the MRI showed a large L5/S1 disc protrusion. He made a good recovery and had no permanent neurological deficit.

Severe Back Pain/Osteoporosis

Osteoporosis is characterised by reduced bone density and microarchitectural deterioration of bone tissue, leading to increased bone fragility and the susceptibility to fracture.

CASE HISTORY

A 71-year-old female presents with severe thoracic spinal pain, which came on suddenly 6 h previously. The pain is severe and radiates around the thoracic spine and front of the chest; it is worse on coughing or sneezing. In the past medical history, she has had RA for the last 25 years and is currently taking 7.5 mg of prednisolone daily. Her RA has been in remission for 5 years on this therapy, and she is on no other medication. Disease-modifying drugs used in the past either have induced toxicity or have been ineffective.

On examination, there is evidence of quiescent RA with classic rheumatoid deformities, nodules and synovial thickening, but no active synovitis. On examination of the thoracic spine, there is a marked kyphosis and she is exquisitely tender over T8. The thoracic spine is markedly restricted on rotation, reproducing her pain radiating around the chest to the anterior aspect of the chest.

WHAT IS THE LIKELY DIAGNOSIS?

The most likely diagnosis is steroid-associated osteoporosis with an acute vertebral fracture. The differential diagnosis should include myeloma and other malignancies because these can also present with vertebral fractures.

WHAT INVESTIGATIONS WOULD YOU DO?

INVESTIGATIONS

- Full blood count
- Erythrocyte sedimentation rate
- Renal function
- Bone and liver biochemistry
- C-reactive protein
- X-ray chest and thoracic spine
- Consider CT or MRI if further evaluation is needed, for example, preprocedural planning

Imaging should include a CXR and specific views of the dorsal spine, which are likely to show one or more vertebral crush fractures. Crush fractures have a characteristic appearance, and on the AP view of the thoracic spine, all the pedicles should be visible. Should any pedicles be missing, this should immediately raise the suspicion of metastatic malignancy as a cause of the vertebral fracture.

Later, a myeloma screen, including protein immunofixation, serum light chain assay and urine for Bence Jones protein, should be done.

A DXA scan is performed to establish the degree of osteoporosis (Fig. 9.14). This gives an accurate index of bone mineral density in relation to the normal range for an age-, sex- and race-matched population. The World Health Organization definition of osteopenia is a T score

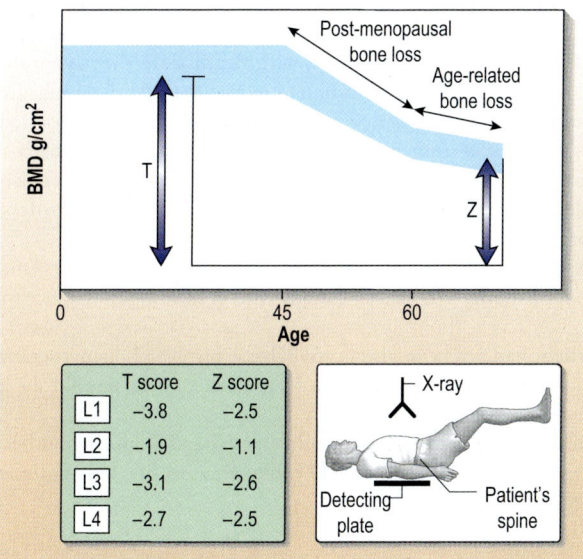

Fig. 9.14 Dual energy X-ray absorptiometry (DXA) scan. Graph showing bone mineral density (BMD; vertical axis) against age. T score is the number of standard deviations by which the patient's BMD differs from the population average for a healthy young adult. Z score is as the T score but BMD deviations from the population average for the patient's age.

of –1.5 to 2.5. The definition of osteoporosis is a T score of greater than –2.5 standard deviations below the mean and established or severe osteoporosis is a T score of greater than –2.5 with an established fracture.

HOW WOULD YOU INITIALLY MANAGE THIS PATIENT?

In the acute setting of a recent vertebral fracture, give strong analgesia. This usually consists of paracetamol, NSAIDs such as naproxen or diclofenac (caution in older people due to an increased susceptibility to GI bleeding and cardiovascular events), and opioids if required (e.g. oxycodone).

After an initial short period of bed rest, mobilisation should be encouraged.

Progress. This patient's pain proved difficult to control and kyphoplasty was performed. This involves injecting methyl methacrylate through a needle placed directly into the damaged vertebra. This allowed mobilisation with physiotherapy help.

WHAT LONG-TERM TREATMENT DOES THIS PATIENT REQUIRE?

This patient should commence specific therapy for osteoporosis:
- Ensure adequate calcium intake and vitamin D levels – prescribe supplements if required. Other lifestyle modifications include smoking cessation, keeping alcohol intake to a moderate level and encouraging active weight-bearing exercise
- Oral bisphosphonates (e.g. alendronate or risedronate) are the first line treatment and reduce the risk of further fractures. These therapies are well tolerated in this age group, but

alendronate and risedronate are associated with a small but significant risk of oesophagitis. All the bisphosphonate drugs are poorly absorbed and should be taken at least 2 h before a meal with a full glass of water; particularly with alendronate, the patient should not lie down for at least 2 h after taking the medication to reduce the risk of oesophagitis. These medications increase bone mineral density over a 3- to 5-year period and also reduce fracture risk

■ Raloxifene, a selective oestrogen-receptor modulator (SERM), has been shown to increase bone mineral density. The main adverse effects of raloxifene include a risk of thrombosis and possible endometrial/uterine malignancy. There is evidence that raloxifene protects against the risk of breast cancer

■ Denosumab (a human monoclonal antibody that inhibits osteoclasts) may also be a treatment option for patients who cannot comply with or have an intolerance to bisphosphonates

Progress. This patient had not been given prophylactic bisphosphonate therapy, which is usually necessary in addition to calcium for patients on long-term steroids, nor did she have regular DXA scans to assess the development of osteoporosis.

Her prednisolone 7.5 mg daily was gradually tapered and stopped, and her RA remained in remission, with some analgesia and an NSAID being required. She has continued on alendronate calcium and has regular DXA scans.

Osteomyelitis

CASE HISTORY

A 56-year-old female presents with a 2-month history of upper back pain and weight loss. She has just arrived home after visiting relatives in Bangladesh for the last year.

There is no relevant past history, and she is taking no medication.

On examination, she is in pain and looks thin. Her pulse is 110/min and regular; her temperature is 38°C. Cardiovascular, respiratory and abdominal examinations are all normal and neurological examinations, including power, tone and reflexes, are within normal limits. There are no sensory signs.

All her joints are normal, but she is tender over the thoracic spine, which is exquisitely painful on rotation of the thoracic spine.

INVESTIGATIONS

- Haemoglobin 106 g/L, mean corpuscular volume (MCV) 83
- Erythrocyte sedimentation rate 102 mm/h, CRP 94
- Urea and electrolytes normal
- Biochemistry: serum Ca 2.3 mmol/L; phosphate 1.2 mmol/L; serum alkaline phosphatase 103 IU/L
- Thoracic spine X-ray was normal
- Chest X-ray showed no evidence of TB

WHAT ARE THE POTENTIAL DIAGNOSES?

The differential diagnosis is **spinal tuberculous osteomyelitis** (Pott's disease), despite the normal CXR. A differential diagnosis would include *Staphylococcus aureus* discitis, although this tends to affect the lumbar spine, whereas tuberculous spinal disease characteristically affects the thoracic spine or the thoraco-lumbar junction.

WHAT FURTHER INVESTIGATION WOULD YOU REQUEST?

The most useful investigation is an MRI scan of the thoracic spine. This showed destruction of the T4 vertebral body with evidence of discitis at T4/T5. A paravertebral abscess accompanied the bone destruction. These findings are typical of thoracic spine TB. There was no evidence of cord compression.

Progress. Aspiration of the vertebral abscess was carried out to culture the tubercle bacillus and to obtain the sensitivities. She was commenced on isoniazid, pyrazinamide, rifampicin and ethambutol, to be given for 9 months (reducing drugs when sensitivities are known). Other risk factors should always be considered, such as immunosuppression and HIV disease.

As vertebral collapse was not present, the prognosis is usually excellent in these patients if the organism is fully sensitive to therapy and compliance with therapy is maintained.

This patient made an excellent recovery and was left with no sequelae from her spinal abscess.

Septic Arthritis

Septic arthritis is due to haematogenous spread from skin or a respiratory tract infection. It is also seen after surgery or sometimes following trauma to the joint.

> **CASE HISTORY**
>
> A 38-year-old male presents with a 3-day history of pain and swelling in his right knee. His right arm is swollen from the thigh downwards and there is a large effusion on the right knee with overlying erythematous skin. On further inspection, you notice injection sites in the right antecubital fossa, and the patient admits to intravenous drug use. You suspect **septic arthritis**.

WHAT ARE THE RISK FACTORS FOR THIS CONDITION?

- Advanced age
- Prior joint inflammation – for example, RA, gout, systemic connective tissue disorders
- Previous surgery/prosthesis
- Overlying skin infection
- Diabetes
- Immunodeficiency – for example, HIV
- Intravenous drug use

HOW WOULD YOU FURTHER INVESTIGATE THIS PATIENT?

- Take blood for FBC (WCC may be elevated), U and Es, CRP/ESR and blood cultures (positive in approx. 30% of patients if taken before antibiotics)
- Consider X-ray to exclude other diagnoses
- Ultrasound can show the presence of effusion and guide aspiration
- Consider CT and/or MRI scanning if there is diagnostic uncertainty – these are the most sensitive methods for diagnosing periarticular abscesses, joint effusions and osteomyelitis
- The joint should be aspirated using a sterile technique, and the fluid sent for microscopy, culture and crystals

TABLE 9.3 ■ **Examination of Synovial Fluid**

Characteristics of Synovial Fluid	Diagnosis	WCC/mm³
Clear, yellow and viscous	Osteoarthritis	<3000
Translucent and thin	Rheumatoid arthritis	3000–40,000
Very cloudy	Seronegative arthritis	
	Reactive arthritis	
	Crystal arthritis	
	Sepsis	750,000

Polarised light microscopy with a red filter needs to be undertaken by an expert:

- Gout: negatively birefringent, needle-shaped crystals of sodium urate
- Pyrophosphate arthropathy (pseudogout): rhomboidal, weakly positively birefringent crystals of calcium pyrophosphate

Gram staining is essential if septic arthritis is suspected and may identify the organism immediately. Joint fluid should be cultured and antibiotic sensitivities requested

The fluid can be examined directly in a clear syringe or sterile pot. The characteristics of synovial fluid show a trend from clear to purulent, which roughly indicates the type of arthritis

---

INFORMATION

Knee Aspiration

- Explain procedure and obtain consent
- Strict aseptic technique
- Two percent lidocaine as local anaesthetic
- Medial or lateral approach 0.5–1 cm below the patella
- Use a white needle to ensure that even viscous or purulent fluid can be aspirated easily
- Caution in anticoagulated patients

The most common organism is *S. aureus*, which is seen in 40–70% of patients. Gram-negative organisms are the next most common. *Neisseria gonorrhea* is the most common cause of a nontraumatic acute monoarthritis in young sexually active patients.

This patient is at risk for HIV and an HIV test is performed. Should HIV be proven, microbiology assessment of the synovial fluid is crucial, particularly for atypical organisms, such as *Mycobacterium avium intracellulare* and other forms of TB.

Progress. A septic arthritis due to *S. aureus* infection was confirmed on blood and synovial fluid culture (Table 9.3). The patient was commenced on IV flucloxacillin. Arthroscopic drainage and washout of the joint were performed at 48 h, which minimised joint damage. He made a good recovery.

Metabolic Bone Diseases

CASE HISTORY (1)

An 84-year-old female presents to the emergency department following a fall. Initial X-rays show a right-sided femoral fracture. She is also complaining of diffuse tenderness along all long bones and proximal muscle weakness. She has a history of advanced chronic kidney disease and she is predominantly housebound.

On examination, she has generalised tenderness of the long bones and proximal muscle weakness.

A more detailed inspection of the X-rays reveals multiple cortical infractions (transverse lucencies with sclerotic borders, also known as Looser zones – Fig. 9.15). Based on this, you suspect an underlying diagnosis of **osteomalacia**.

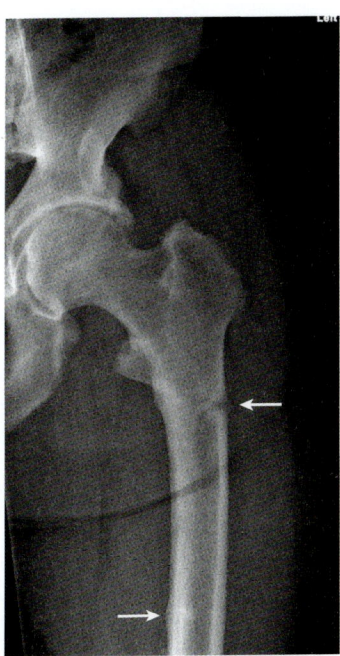

Fig. 9.15 Frontal radiograph of the left proximal femur in a patient with osteomalacia demonstrating axial migration, Looser zones in the medial and lateral cortex (*arrows*), and enthesopathy. (From Resnick, D.L., Jacobson, J.A., Christine Chung, B., et al., 2025. Resnick's Bone and Joint Imaging, fourth ed. Rickets and Osteomalacia, Fig. 30.10, Elsevier INC, Philadelphia, PA. Courtesy Dr. Rick Whitehouse, Manchester, UK.)

WHAT IS THE AETIOLOGY OF THIS CONDITION?

Osteomalacia is a metabolic bone disease defined by incomplete mineralisation of the mature bone matrix (osteoid) following growth plate closure in adults.

This is most commonly caused by vitamin D deficiency either due to insufficient sunlight exposure or malabsorption. It can also be caused by liver disease due to malabsorption of vitamin D and reduced 25-hydroxycholecalciferol synthesis.

Certain drugs (e.g. phenytoin, carbamazepine, rifampicin) can also cause low vitamin D levels.

Rarer causes include hypophosphataemia, renal tubular acidosis and Fanconi syndrome.

Chronic kidney disease (CKD) mineral bone disorder is a term applied to pathological fractures associated with renal disease causing defective 1,25-dihydroxyvitamin D synthesis.

HOW DOES OSTEOMALACIA DIFFER FROM RICKETS?

Rickets and osteomalacia are caused by the same underlying disease process. Rickets is characterised by defective mineralisation of the epiphyseal growth plate cartilage in children. This results in skeletal deformities and growth restriction.

> **REMEMBER**
>
> Osteoporosis differs from osteomalacia as it involves normal bone mineralization but overall bone loss.

INVESTIGATIONS

- Bone profile: typically low vitamin D, low/normal calcium, low phosphate, high alkaline phosphatase
- Parathyroid hormone: typically high (secondary hyperparathyroidism) but not in all patients
- Check renal function
- X-ray: loss of cortical bone, Looser/milkman pseudofractures (partial undisplaced fractures) – Fig. 9.15

HOW WOULD YOU MANAGE THIS PATIENT?

- Lifestyle changes: improve diet, safe sun exposure
- Calcium-vitamin D3 supplementation (if diet is insufficient)
- If secondary to severe liver disease or end-stage CKD, then specialist treatment with activated vitamin D metabolites may be needed:
  - Alfacalcidiol or calcitriol for renal disease (monitor for hypercalcaemia)
  - Calcifediol for hepatic disease or malabsorption

CASE HISTORY (2)

A 68-year-old male presents to his doctor with chronic anterior thigh pain and difficulty walking. He has a background of carpal tunnel syndrome and hearing loss. He takes no regular medication. As part of his initial investigations, he was sent for a routine X-ray, which demonstrated tibial bowing and defects in the cortical and cancellous bone (Fig. 9.16).

Based on this, you suspect a diagnosis of Paget disease.

WHAT IS THE UNDERLYING PATHOPHYSIOLOGY OF THIS DISEASE?

Paget disease is a chronic localised bone remodelling disorder associated with abnormal osteoclast activity and increased osteoblast activity. This results in rapid formation of disorganised and mechanically weaker bone, causing deformity and increasing the risk of pathological fractures. It can occur in any bone but has a predilection for the axial skeleton.

Most patients are asymptomatic, symptomatic patients typically experience pain localised to the bone or neurological symptoms caused by nerve impingement by bone overgrowth (e.g. hearing loss, facial pain, spinal stenosis).

The aetiology is not fully understood, but there are genetic associations and certain viral infections (paramyxoviruses, RSV) have been implicated.

INVESTIGATIONS

- Serum alkaline phosphatase is elevated in up to 85% of patients
- Calcium, phosphate and parathyroid hormone (PTH) are typically normal
- X-rays may show (Fig. 9.16):
  - Osteolysis (radiolucency) and excessive formation can both occur
  - 'Blade of grass' lesions: V-shaped pattern between affected and healthy bone
  - 'Cotton-wool' pattern: multifocal sclerotic areas in the skull
- Radionuclide bone scans can help define the extent of metabolically active disease

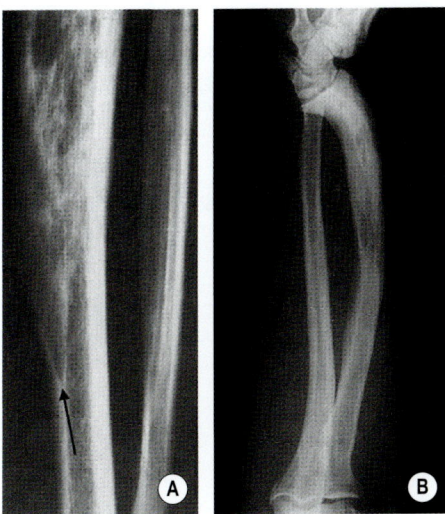

Fig. 9.16   Radiographs demonstrating features associated with Paget disease: (A) shows sharply demarcated lysis along the distal anterior cortex (*arrow*) of the tibia ('blade of grass' appearance). The proximal tibia shows bony expansion and has a mixed sclerotic and lytic appearance, indicating a more advanced disease. (B) shows cortical expansion, sclerosis, and bowing of the radius. (From Grant, L.A., Griffin, N., 2019. Grainger & Allison's Diagnostic Radiology Essentials, second ed. Benign Bone Tumours, Elsevier Ltd., London.)

WHAT IS THE MANAGEMENT?

- Physiotherapy and orthotics can be helpful
- Analgesia – paracetamol and NSAIDs (avoid opioids if possible)
- **Bisphosphonates** (e.g. zoledronic acid, alendronic acid) are recommended for symptomatic patients or for patients with asymptomatic disease in areas at high risk for complications

> **REMEMBER**
>
> Calcium and vitamin D deficiency must be corrected before starting a bisphosphonate to avoid hypocalcaemia.

Further Reading

Osteoarthritis

Bruyère, O., et al., 2019. An updated algorithm recommendation for the management of knee osteoarthritis from the European Society for Clinical and Economic Aspects of Osteoporosis, Osteoarthritis and Musculoskeletal Diseases (ESCEO). Semin. Arthritis Rheum. 49 (3), 337–350.

Doherty, M., Dacre, J., Dieppe, P., et al., 1992. The GALS locomotor screen. Ann. Rheum. Dis. 51, 1165.

NICE, CKS, 2022. Osteoarthritis in over 16s: diagnosis and management. NICE.

Rheumatoid Arthritis

NICE, CKS, 2020. Rheumatoid arthritis in adults: management. NICE.

Smolen, J.S., et al., 2023. EULAR recommendations for the management of rheumatoid arthritis with synthetic and biological disease-modifying antirheumatic drugs: 2022 update. Ann. Rheum. Dis. 82 (1), 3–18.

SLE and Vasculitis

British Society for Rheumatology, 2018. The British Society for Rheumatology guideline for the management of systemic lupus erythematosus in adults.

Salmon, J.E., Niewold, T.B., 2020. A successful trial for lupus. N. Engl. J. Med. 382, 287–288.

Tsokos, G.C., 2011. Systemic lupus erythematosus. N. Engl. J. Med. 378, 1949–1961.

Crystal Arthritis

Mulay, S.R., Anders, H.J., 2016. Crystallopathies. N. Engl. J. Med. 374, 2465–2476.

CHAPTER 10

Endocrinology and Diabetes

Diabetes Mellitus

Diabetes mellitus is a syndrome of chronic hyperglycaemia due to relative insulin deficiency or resistance or both.

CASE HISTORY (1)

You are phoned by a general practitioner (GP) who has seen a 50-year-old male in his surgery, complaining of thirst and polyuria. His blood glucose is 24 mmol/L. He is tired but otherwise well. He has no other medical problems.

WHAT ARE THE KEY CLINICAL DECISIONS?

- Does this patient need admission?
- Does he need insulin?
- What is the immediate management?

WHAT IS THE LIKELY DIAGNOSIS?

The likelihood is that this patient has **type 2 diabetes** (Table 10.1). The risk of ketoacidosis is small and he will not need admission unless he is either ketotic (ketonuria +++) or is very dehydrated.

This patient should be advised to avoid sweet drinks (especially sweetened canned drinks) and an appointment arranged for him to attend a diabetic outpatient clinic. Contact the diabetic liaison nurse in your hospital and arrange for the patient to be seen urgently.

WHAT ARE THE INDICATIONS FOR ADMITTING A DIABETIC PATIENT?

- Severe dehydration (may have hyperosmolality)
- Intercurrent illness such as pneumonia or urinary tract infection (UTI)
- +++ ketonuria
- Tachycardia or tachypnoea

INFORMATION

WHO Diagnostic Criteria for Diabetes Mellitus

- Fasting venous plasma glucose >7.0 mmol/L (126 mg/dL) after 8 h fast*
- Random venous plasma glucose >11.1 mmol/L (200 mg/dL)*
- Glycated haemoglobin (HbA1c) of >6.5% (48 mmol/mol) (Table 10.2)

*Two readings are required for asymptomatic individuals. Note also:

- Impaired fasting glucose: 5.6–6.9 mmol/L
- Impaired glucose tolerance: >7.8 and <11.1 mmol/L, 2 h after 75 g oral glucose tolerance test (GTT)

An oral GTT is required only for borderline cases.

TABLE 10.1 ■ **The Spectrum of Diabetes: A Comparison of Type 1 and Type 2 Diabetes Mellitus**

—	Type 1	Type 2
Epidemiology	Younger (usually <30 years of age)	Older (usually >30 years of age)
	Usually lean	Often overweight
	Increased in those of Northern European ancestry	All racial groups. Increased in peoples of Asian, African, Polynesian and American Indian ancestry
	Seasonal incidence	—
Heredity	HLA-DR3 or DR4 in >90%	No HLA links
	30%–50% concordance in identical twins	~50% concordance in identical twins
Pathogenesis	Autoimmune disease	No immune disturbance
	Islet cell autoantibodies	Insulin resistance
	Insulitis	—
	Association with other auto-immune diseases	—
	Immunosuppression after diagnosis delays beta-cell destruction	—
Clinical	Insulin deficiency	Partial insulin deficiency initially
	May develop ketoacidosis	May develop hyperosmolar state
	Always need insulin	Many come to need insulin when beta-cells fail over time
Biochemical	Eventual disappearance of C-peptide	C-peptide persists

HLA, Human leukocyte antigen.
Note: there is a significant rise in the incidence of young patients with type 2 diabetes mellitus, especially in the obese and in Asian populations.

TABLE 10.2 ■ **HBA1c – Conversion of Percentage Values to mmol/mol**

Diabetes Control and Complication Trial (HbA1c %)	International Federation of Clinical Chemistry (HbA1c mmol/mol)
4.0	20
5.0	31
6.0	42
6.5	48
7.0	53
7.5	59
8.0	64
9.0	75
10.0	96

HBA1c, Glycated haemoglobin.

Progress. At the diabetic clinic, the diabetic specialist nurse explained lifestyle changes that are an essential part of treatment, that is, stopping smoking and losing weight via diet and exercise. The nurse arranges for an appointment for this patient to be checked by the doctor and for eye testing. He was also started on metformin 500 mg daily, increasing to 1.5 g daily.

CASE HISTORY (2)

You are telephoned by a GP who has seen a 17-year-old male in his surgery, complaining of thirst and polyuria. He has recently lost 8 kg in weight. His blood glucose is 31 mmol/L.
    The key decisions are again:
    • Does this patient need admission?
    • Does he need insulin?
    • What is the immediate management?

WHAT WOULD YOU RECOMMEND FOR THIS PATIENT?

This patient is much more likely to be presenting with early **type 1 diabetes** and might not be ketotic yet because he could still have a degree of residual beta cell function (the 'honeymoon' phase). Again, assessment of ketosis, acidosis and dehydration must be made to determine whether he needs admission. He should be seen within 24 hours either by the diabetic liaison nurse or in hospital to commence insulin. If there is any doubt, the patient should be seen in the emergency department immediately.

Progress. At the diabetic clinic the patient was found to be dehydrated with mild ketosis. He was admitted to the medical assessment unit (MAU) to commence insulin therapy.

Diabetic Ketoacidosis (DKA)

CASE HISTORY

A 21-year-old female presents to the emergency department, having been generally unwell for 2 weeks and having been treated for a UTI by her doctor.
    On examination, severe dehydration, a tachycardia of 120 beats per minute (bpm), and a BP of 90/50 mm Hg are noted. The nurses have checked the patient's finger-prick blood glucose and found it to be 30 mmol/L.

What is the Most Likely Diagnosis?

Diabetic ketoacidosis.

HOW DO PATIENTS PRESENT WITH KETOACIDOSIS?

- Unwell ± intercurrent illness (e.g. bacterial or viral infection)
- Polyuria and polydipsia
- Hyperventilation or dyspnoea
- Vomiting ± abdominal pain
- Impaired conscious level

Patients known to have type 1 diabetes mellitus most commonly develop ketoacidosis when insulin is omitted because of missed meals during an intercurrent illness (e.g. gastroenteritis). Patients become rapidly dehydrated (Fig. 10.1) and acidotic (over hours). Tachypnoea or Kussmaul respiration (a deep, sighing respiration) is prominent, with the smell of ketones on the breath. It is the fall in pH that causes coma.

The blood glucose might not be particularly high and severe acidosis may be present, with glucose values as low as 10 mmol/L. This might be due to recent self-administration of insulin, which is insufficient alone to correct the acidosis in the presence of dehydration.

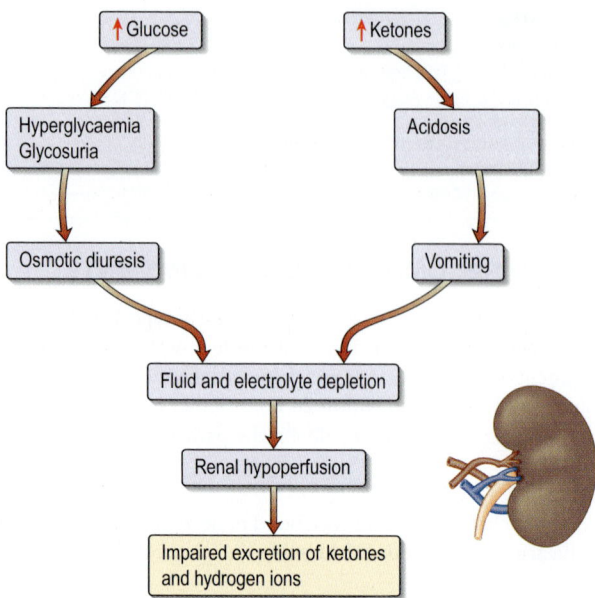

Fig. 10.1   Dehydration occurs during ketoacidosis as a consequence of two parallel processes. Hyperglycaemia results in osmotic diuresis, and hyperketonaemia results in acidosis and vomiting. Renal hypoperfusion then occurs and a vicious circle is established as the kidney becomes less able to compensate for the acidosis.

WHAT FEATURES INDICATE SEVERE DKA?

Poor prognostic features include:

- Impaired conscious level (indication for urgent intubation)
- pH < 7.0 (anion gap >16)
- Oliguria
- Low serum potassium at presentation

INVESTIGATIONS

- Blood glucose
- Venous blood gas (arterial if results do not match clinical condition or concerns about oxygenation) and pH – assess severity of acidosis
- Urea and electrolytes (U and Es)– hyperkalaemia common, hypernatraemia may be present due to dehydration, acute kidney injury (AKI) common, calculate plasma osmolality
- Urinalysis (ketones strongly positive +++)
- Plasma ketones
- Full blood count (FBC) – raised white cell count (WCC) common
- Blood ± urine cultures
- Electrocardiogram (ECG)

HOW WOULD YOU MANAGE THIS PATIENT?

General Measures

- Admission to high dependency unit (HDU)/intensive care unit (ICU)

- Consider a central line in patients with a history of cardiac disease/renal impairment/autonomic neuropathy, or in the elderly
- Consider placing an arterial line to monitor arterial blood gases (ABGs) and plasma potassium
- Nasogastric tube: if there is an impaired conscious level, to prevent vomiting and aspiration
- Urinary catheter: if there is no urine for 2 h or serum creatinine is high
- Thromboprophylaxis with thromboembolic deterrent (TED) stockings and low molecular weight heparin (LMWH) unless contraindicated

REMEMBER

Management of DKA requires fluid, insulin, potassium and *care.*

Fluid Replacement

Start intravenous fluids as soon as DKA is confirmed. Table 10.3 shows examples of blood values in severe ketoacidosis and compares these with the values seen in the hyperosmolar, hyperglycaemic state (see p. 396).

The guidelines for fluid replacement are shown in Table 10.4. These are applicable to young patients.

- When blood glucose falls to <14 mmol/L, give 10% glucose in addition to normal saline. This will enable the insulin infusion to be continued. Continued insulin is required to inhibit ketone production
- Continue with IV fluids 1 L every 4–6 h until the patient is rehydrated and ketosis resolves (~24 h). Monitor fluid status closely.

TABLE 10.3 ■ **Examples of Blood Values**

	Severe Ketoacidosis	Hyperosmolar, Hyperglycaemic state
Na^+ (mmol/L)	140	155
K^+ (mmol/L)	5	5
Cl^- (mmol/L)	100	110
HCO_3^- (mmol/L)	5	25
Urea (mmol/L)	8	15
Glucose (mmol/L)	30	50
Arterial pH	7.0 (H^+ > 100 nmol/L)	7.35

The normal range of osmolality is 285–300 mOsmol/kg. It can be measured directly, or can be calculated approximately from the formula:

Osmolality = $2(Na^+ + K^+)$ + glucose + urea

For example, in the patient with severe ketoacidosis described above:

Osmolality = $2(140 + 5)$ + 30 + 8 = 328 mOsmol/kg

In the example of nonketotic hyperosmolar coma:

Osmolality = $2(155 + 5)$ + 50 + 15 = 385 mOsmol/kg

The normal anion gap is <17. It is calculated as $(Na^+ + K^+) - (Cl^- + HCO_3^-)$.

In the example of ketoacidosis, the anion gap is 40.

In the example of nonketotic hyperosmolar coma, the anion gap is 20.

Mild hyperchloraemic acidosis may develop in the course of therapy. This will be shown by a rising plasma chloride and persistence of a low bicarbonate, even though the anion gap has returned to normal.

TABLE 10.4 ■ Guidelines for Average Fluid Replacement in Young Patients

Volume	Duration/Timing
1 L 0.9% saline + 20 mmol/KCl	Over the first 30 min
1 L 0.9% saline + 20 mmol/KCl	Over next 1 h
1 L 0.9% saline + 20 mmol/KCl	Over next 2 h
1 L 0.9% saline + 20 mmol/KCl	Over next 4–6 h

KCl, Potassium chloride.

TABLE 10.5 ■ Potassium Replacement in Patients With Diabetic Ketoacidosis

Serum Potassium (mmol/L)	Amount of KCl (mmol/h)
<3	40
3–4	30
4–5	20
5–6	10
>6	Stop KCl

KCl, Potassium chloride.

Insulin Regimen

- Always follow local protocols
- Add 50 units of soluble insulin to 50 mL 0.9% saline and administer by IV infusion; this equates to 1 U/mL
- Commence at 6 U/h and continue at 3 U/h after venous glucose falls to <11.5 mmol/L (this varies between guidelines and can be adjusted based on body weight)
- Glucose must then be administered to prevent hypoglycaemia
- Continue IV insulin infusion until ketosis resolves and the patient is eating, and for 2–4 h after the first SC dose of soluble insulin

Potassium Replacement (Table 10.5)

Total body potassium can be depleted by approximately 1000 mmol, and the plasma potassium falls rapidly as potassium shifts into the cells under the action of insulin. Use less potassium in patients with renal impairment or oliguria.

- Monitor serum (K$^+$) every 2 h initially, then every 4 h until stable
- Use premixed potassium-containing infusions wherever possible

Acidosis

- If the pH is <7.0, consider isotonic (1.26%) sodium bicarbonate given at a rate of 500 mL over 4 h (seek senior advice)
- If the pH is >7.0, bicarbonate need not be given

ASSESSMENT DURING TREATMENT

- Remember that the role of insulin is primarily to suppress ketogenesis rather than to lower blood glucose
- Blood glucose (bedside testing every hour, laboratory blood glucose 4-hourly)

- Plasma potassium every 4 h; the main risk is hypokalaemia
- Repeat ABGs after 2 h. A calculated anion gap (needs chloride estimation) may be adequate for monitoring

---

REMEMBER

Causes of Death in DKA

- Hyperkalaemia
- Aspiration due to gastric stasis
- Cerebral oedema due to acidosis ± overhydration
- Hypokalaemic respiratory arrest

Progress. This patient started eating and receiving treatment with subcutaneous (SC) insulin after 48 h. She was helped with her insulin injections and discharged on the sixth day with support from the community diabetic nurse.

Hyperosmolar Hyperglycaemic State

CASE HISTORY

A 60-year-old female was brought to the emergency department following a collapse. She has been generally unwell for the last year. Her husband confirms that she has had polyuria and polydipsia with nocturia of 3 to 4 times every night. Over the last month, she has started using sugar drinks to build herself up because she has been losing weight.

Examination reveals an extremely dehydrated female with increased tissue turgor. Pulse 100 regular, BP 100/60, jugular venous pressure (JVP) not visible, Glasgow coma scale (GCS) 12.

Investigations revealed:

Na^+ 165, K^+ 5.9, U 24.7, Cr 170, bicarbonate 20, glucose 64 mmol/L, pH 7.31, pCO_2 4.7 kPa, pO_2 11.2 kPa, plasma osmolality $2 \times (165 + 5.9) + 64 + 24.7 = 429.7$ mOsmol/kg.

WHAT IS THE DIAGNOSIS?

These findings are typical of a **hyperosmolar hyperglycaemic state (HHS)** – see Table 10.3. This most commonly occurs in older patients with type 2 diabetes. It is characterised by a very high glucose, a relatively normal acid–base balance and high plasma osmolality. These patients are also at increased risk of venous and arterial thromboses. The mortality is higher than for DKA. This patient's biochemistry has been slowly getting worse over many weeks, so normalisation must be equally slow.

INFORMATION

Calculation of Osmolality

$2 \times ((Na^+ \text{ mmol/L}) + (K^+ \text{ mmol/L})) + (\text{urea mmol/L}) + (\text{glucose mmol/L})$ – normal range 285 to 300 mOsmol/kg

---

REMEMBER

Ketones can be found in the urine of any starved person.

HOW DO PATIENTS WITH HHS TYPICALLY PRESENT?

- Middle-aged or elderly patient
- Insidious onset of polyuria and polydipsia
- Severe dehydration
- Altered conscious level
- Most middle-aged or elderly patients have not previously been diagnosed with diabetes
- Respiration is usually normal
- Presentation is usually precipitated by infection, stroke or myocardial infarction

WHAT FURTHER INVESTIGATIONS WOULD YOU REQUEST?

- Plasma glucose: usually >40 mmol/L
- Urea and electrolytes: significant hypernatraemia occurs, but this is masked by the high glucose. The Na^+ usually increases as the venous glucose, and therefore the extracellular colloid osmotic pressure fall, and water moves into the intracellular space
- Arterial blood gases: pH usually >7.3 with a normal anion gap
- Plasma osmolality: typically >320 mOsmol/kg
- Estimated corrected sodium: to evaluate water loss as a result of hyperglycaemia (see Information box)
- Full blood count: may show polycythaemia, dehydration or a leucocytosis from infection
- Creatine kinase: if rhabdomyolysis suspected
- Troponins: if cardiac ischaemia suspected
- Electrocardiogram: for myocardial infarction or ischaemia
- Chest X-ray: for signs of infection
- Urine: for urinalysis, microscopy and culture

INFORMATION

Calculation of Corrected Sodium Concentration

Add 2.0 mmol/L to the measured serum sodium for every 5 mmol/L increase in glucose concentration.

REMEMBER

The principal cause of death and morbidity in HHS is arterial and venous thrombosis due to the hyperosmolar state.

Assessment of Severity

- The degree of consciousness correlates most closely with plasma osmolality. Coma is usually associated with an osmolality of >400 mOsmol/kg
- A coexistent lactic acidosis considerably worsens the prognosis

HOW WOULD YOU MANAGE THIS PATIENT?

General Treatment Measures

- Aim to correct the high osmolality with fluid and insulin over 48–72 h
- Manage as for DKA, except:
  - 0.9% saline is the standard fluid for replacement given slowly – aim to achieve a positive balance of 3–6 L by 12 h and the remaining replacement of estimated fluid losses within next 12 h

- Ensure slow correction of serum sodium. The sodium should not fall faster than 10 mmol/L in 24 hours
- Start insulin at a slower rate (e.g. 3 U/h) as patients are often sensitive to insulin (follow local protocols). The fall in blood glucose should be no more than 5 mmol/L/h.
- Anticoagulate with LMWH unless contraindicated
- Insert a urinary catheter if oliguria is present or serum creatinine is high
- Once stable, stop insulin therapy and commence oral hypoglycaemic agents or manage by diet alone

Progress. This patient was discharged on metformin 1 g daily and instructed on lifestyle changes, for example, controlling weight; an urgent appointment was made with the community diabetic nurse.

Hypoglycaemic Coma

CASE HISTORY

A 25-year-old male is brought to the emergency department by the police, having been found behaving abnormally. He is aggressive and irrational and attempts to punch the staff. He is restrained and a MedicAlert bracelet is found under his shirt, indicating that he has diabetes.

WHAT DIAGNOSIS MUST YOU CONSIDER?

Hypoglycaemia

Always consider hypoglycaemia in confused patients and check a blood glucose. The most common cause of coma in a patient with diabetes is hypoglycaemia due to drugs. The long-acting sulphonylureas, such as glibenclamide, or long-acting insulins, such as isophane, are prone to do this. Patients who are *not* known to have diabetes but who are hypoglycaemic should have a laboratory-determined blood glucose test, and blood saved (serum) for determination of insulin and C-peptide, the fragment of pro-insulin that is found in endogenous insulin (to diagnose insulinoma or factitious drug administration).

HOW DO HYPOGLYCAEMIC PATIENTS PRESENT? (BOX 10.1)

Patients with tightly controlled diabetes can have frequent episodes of hypoglycaemia and can become desensitised to sympathetic activation. These patients can develop neuroglycopenia before sympathetic activation and complain of 'loss of warning'. Use of beta-blockers can also minimise the warning signs of hypoglycaemia by blocking the features of an activated sympathetic nervous system.

Conversely, patients with poorly controlled diabetes can develop sympathetic signs early and avoid these by running a high blood glucose.

INVESTIGATIONS

Patients With Diabetes Who Have Frequent Hypoglycaemic Attacks

- Urea and electrolytes: hypoglycaemia is more common in diabetic nephropathy because the kidney is one of the sites of insulin metabolism
- Thyroid function tests (TFTs): hypothyroidism is associated with type 1 diabetes mellitus and impairs counter-regulation
- 09:00 cortisol ± short adrenocorticotrophic hormone (ACTH; tetracosactide) stimulation test: hypoadrenalism reduces hepatic glycogen stores
- Take an alcohol history
- Consider deliberate self-harm

BOX 10.1 ■ Presentation of Patients With Hypoglycaemic Coma

Sympathetic Overactivity (Glucose <3.5 mmol/L)

- Tachycardia
- Palpitations
- Sweating
- Anxiety
- Pallor
- Tremor
- Cold extremities

Neuroglycopenia (Glucose <2.6 mmol/L)

- Confusion
- Slurred speech
- Localised neurological impairment
- Coma

HOW WOULD YOU MANAGE HYPOGLYCAEMIA?

Conscious Patient

- Treat with 15–20 g carbohydrate, that is, four glucose tablets, or a glucose drink

Unconscious Patient

- Take blood sample
- Give:
    - 75 mL 20% glucose IV or
    - 1 mg glucagon IM if IV access not rapidly established
- Do not use 50% glucose in peripheral veins
- Once recovered, give carbohydrate as above
- Admit the patient if the cause is a long-acting sulphonylurea or a long-acting insulin, and give a continuous infusion of 10% glucose (e.g. 1 L 8-hourly) and check glucose hourly or 2-hourly
- Patients should regain consciousness or become coherent within 10 min, although complete cognitive recovery might lag by 30–45 min. Do not give further boluses of IV glucose without repeating the blood glucose. If the patient does not wake up after 10 min or more, repeat the blood glucose and consider another cause of coma – stroke or a head injury during their confused state

HYPOGLYCAEMIA IN THE NONDIABETIC PATIENT

Hypoglycaemia in patients without diabetes is rare and always needs investigation – usually as an inpatient. Always:

- Confirm the hypoglycaemia with a laboratory sample before treatment
- Take a simultaneous serum sample for insulin and C-peptide, and send it urgently to the laboratory for centrifugation and separation

WHAT CAN CAUSE NONDIABETIC HYPOGLYCAEMIA?

- Drugs:
    - Surreptitious insulin or sulphonylurea ingestion
    - Ethanol

- ■ Quinine
- ■ Pentamidine
- ■ Disopyramide
- ■ Prescription errors, for example, chlorpropamide for chlorpromazine (ask for all drugs to be brought in)
- ■ Tumours:
  - ■ Insulinoma
  - ■ Retroperitoneal sarcomas and other malignancies
- ■ Liver failure
- ■ Hypopituitarism, causing ACTH, growth hormone (GH) and thyroid stimulating hormone (TSH) deficiency

Progress. This patient responded to IV glucose and quickly returned to normal. He explained that he was out with friends last night and forgot to eat but continued to drink alcohol. He thinks he may have given himself the wrong amount of insulin, as he overslept and was late for work.

The Sick Diabetic Patient

CASE HISTORY

A 40-year-old male with a 15-year history of type 1 diabetes mellitus and previously documented proteinuria is referred from the emergency department with vomiting and a feeling of being generally unwell. Glucose was 20 mmol/L, electrolytes were normal and blood gases did not support DKA (pH 7.4; bicarbonate 20 mmol/L). An ECG shows evidence of evolving anterior myocardial infarction (MI). This is the typical presentation of a 'silent MI'. Chest pain is frequently atypical or absent in diabetes due to small-fibre neuropathy. The other major cause of this type of nonspecific presentation is occult infection and often further investigations are required.

INVESTIGATIONS

- • Full blood count
- • Urea and electrolytes
- • Arterial blood gases
- • Chest X-ray
- • Mid-stream urine (MSU)
- • Electrocardiogram
- • Blood cultures

Other investigations to consider later if occult infection is suspected:

- • Abdominal ultrasound or abdominal CT scan
- • Tc bone scanning
- • Labelled white cell scan

HOW WOULD YOU MANAGE THIS PATIENT?

This patient has a diagnosis of ST-elevation myocardial infarction (STEMI) and requires immediate therapy with aspirin 300 mg chewed and a P2Y12 inhibitor, for example, prasugrel or clopidogrel. He was immediately transferred to the coronary care unit for further assessment and possible percutaneous coronary intervention (see chapter 2). His diabetes was initially controlled on insulin infusion because he was kept nil by mouth for the cardiac procedures (Table 10.6). The infusion was continued until the patient was eating and drinking. Insulin treatment has been proven to improve outcome in patients with diabetes in the immediate period after MI.

TABLE 10.6 ■ Example of a Variable Rate Insulin Infusion for Type 1 Diabetic Patients in Hospital

Level of Blood Glucose (Measured Hourly)	Insulin Infusion (units/h)
<4.0 mmol/L	0.5
4.0–7.0 mmol/L	1
7.1–9.0 mmol/L	2
9.1–11.0 mmol/L	3
11.1–14.0 mmol/L	4
14.1–17.0 mmol/L	5
17.1–28 mmol/L	6
>28 mmol/L	8

Note: this is only a guide and insulin doses should be adjusted upwards if the patient is known to have a high insulin requirement, and always reviewed regularly to see if the doses are appropriate. The aim is to keep blood glucose in the 7 to 9 region.

Once eating and drinking, the patient can be converted back to his/her usual insulin regimen or, if tight glycaemic control is essential, on to × 4 daily insulin, which gives greater ease of adjustment.

HOW WOULD YOU CONVERT A DIABETIC PATIENT FROM IV TO SC INSULIN?

- Follow local guidelines
- An example of a suitable regime would be:
  - Calculate total dose over last 24 h
  - Give 25% of total as soluble insulin 30 min before each meal (i.e. × 3 daily)
  - Give 25% of total dose as intermediate-acting isophane insulin at 22:00
- Monitor blood glucose fasting and 2 h after meals (postprandial) – each finger-prick glucose measures the adequacy of the previous dose
- Aim for glucose <10 mmol/L postprandial and <8 mmol/L fasting
- Do not discontinue IV insulin until 1–2 h *after* the first SC insulin dose is administered because IV insulin has a half-life of only 3 min

Management of Diabetic Patients Presenting for Surgery

CASE HISTORY

You are asked to see a 50-year-old male with no previous history of diabetes who is admitted for coronary artery bypass graft (CABG) surgery and found to have a blood glucose of 13 mmol/L. This patient has suffered from angina for 5 years and still has symptoms on maximal medical therapy. He has had coronary angiography, which shows triple-vessel disease, and his cardiologist has recommended surgery rather than percutaneous coronary intervention.

HOW WOULD YOU MANAGE THIS PATIENT?

- Ask about symptoms of diabetes, for example, thirst, polyuria, lack of energy
- Check that a laboratory glucose has been sent to confirm the diagnosis of diabetes (random glucose 13.4 mmol/L)

- Discuss the patient's angina symptoms and the urgency of CABG surgery with the cardiologist
- It is agreed by all, including the patient, that his diabetes should be treated and blood sugar controlled before surgery is performed
- He is referred to the diabetic liaison nurse for assessment and discussion of treatment as an outpatient

---

REMEMBER

Always bring diabetes under control before patients undergo surgery unless it is an emergency.

INFORMATION

Assessment of New Patients With Diabetes

- Carry out a biochemical assessment of long-term glycaemic control (e.g. HbA1c)
- Measure body weight
- Measure blood pressure
- Measure plasma lipids
- Measure visual acuity
- Examine the retina through dilated fundi (ophthalmoscope initially, followed by retinal photo)
- Test urine for protein
- Test blood for renal function (creatinine and estimated glomerular filtration rate [eGFR])
- Check general condition of the feet, peripheral pulses and sensation
- Review cardiovascular risk factors
- Introduce self-monitoring and injection techniques if insulin is required
- Review dietary knowledge

Progress. This patient was managed with lifestyle changes and metformin, initially 500 mg daily. He will undertake surgery when his HbA1c is <7% (53 mmol/mol).

MANAGEMENT OF DIABETIC PATIENTS UNDERGOING SURGERY

- Non-insulin treated patients should stop any SGLT-2 inhibitors the day before surgery and the day of surgery. Sulphonyureas (e.g. gliclazide), acarbose and meglitinides should also be stopped on the day of surgery
- Metformin can be given on the day of surgery (check local protocols); however, if on TDS dosing, the lunchtime dose should be omitted
- Patients with mild hyperglycaemia (fasting blood glucose <8 mmol/L) can be treated as nondiabetic
- Those with higher levels are treated with soluble insulin prior to the procedure/surgery, and with glucose, insulin and potassium infusion during and after the procedure. Be careful of hypoglycaemia due to the additive effect of medications taken previously
- Postoperatively, patients should return to their normal management regimen when they begin eating and drinking

WHO NEEDS VARIABLE RATE INSULIN PERIOPERATIVELY?

VRII is the preferred method for:

- Patients with Type 1 or 2 diabetes undergoing surgery with a fasting period > one missed meal

- Patients with Type 1 diabetes undergoing surgery who have not received background insulin
- Patients with suboptimal diabetes management (HbA1c > 69 mmol/mol [>8.5%])
- Most diabetic patients requiring emergency surgery
- Patients with persistent hyperglycaemia (capillary blood glucose [CBG] >12 mmol/L) in the perioperative period

Note: If the patient is already on a long-acting insulin analogue (e.g. LEVEMIR, LANTUS or TRESIBA), these should be continued at 80% of the usual dose (follow local guidelines)

URGENT SURGERY IN PATIENTS WITH DIABETES

Surgery requires patients to fast for several hours. In addition, a general anaesthetic and surgery themselves place significant stresses on an individual. The hormonal response to stress involves a significant rise in counter-regulatory hormones to insulin, in particular cortisol and adrenaline (epinephrine). For this reason, patients with diabetes undergoing surgery often require an increased dose of insulin, despite their fasting state. If possible, long-acting hypoglycaemic agents are reduced to 80% of the normal dose the night before surgery because hypoglycaemia might otherwise occur.

The procedure for insulin-treated patients is:

In patients whose diabetic control is poor and who are not undergoing emergency surgery, diabetic control should be reassessed and therapy adjusted to achieve an HbA1c < 8.5% (70 mmol/mol) preoperatively

Preoperative glucose levels should be in the range of 6–11 mmol/L

The patient's usual insulin is given the night before the operation and, whenever possible, diabetic patients should be first on the morning procedure/operating list

An variable rate insulin infusion with glucose and potassium can be given during the procedure/surgery. The insulin can be mixed into the glucose solution or administered separately by syringe pump

Postoperatively, the infusion is maintained until the patient is able to eat. Other fluids needed in the perioperative period must be given through a separate IV line and must not interrupt the glucose/insulin/potassium infusion. Glucose levels are checked every 2 to 4 hours and potassium levels are monitored. The amount of insulin and potassium in each infusion is adjusted either upwards or downwards, according to the results of regular monitoring of the blood glucose and serum potassium concentrations

The same approach is used in the emergency situation, with the exception that a separate variable-rate insulin infusion may be needed to bring blood glucose under control before surgery

The Diabetic Foot

CASE HISTORY

The chiropodist in the diabetic clinic asks you to review an 84-year-old female who is complaining of severe pain in her big toe. She had attempted to cut a toe nail a week ago and the toe had become painful and infected. She is known to have type 2 diabetes, for which she takes metformin and gliclazide. She does not have regular supervision of her diabetes.

On examination, she has a 2 cm ulcer on the medial side of her big toe with swelling and erythema.

WHAT FURTHER POINTS WOULD BE HELPFUL IN THE HISTORY?

- Is there a previous history of foot problems?
- Does she regularly inspect and wash her feet? Is she careful about buying shoes of the correct size?
- How good is her sight?
- Does she live alone? Does she have any help?
- Is there any suggestion of peripheral vascular disease, for example, intermittent claudication?
- Is there any suggestion of peripheral sensory problems? Does she complain of numbness or burning in her feet?

WHAT PARTICULAR POINTS DO YOU LOOK FOR ON EXAMINATION?

- Inspect the lesion. Take a swab for culture
- Look for signs of neuropathy:
  - Dry skin
  - Evidence of sensory loss to pin-prick/light touch/vibration
  - Check ankle jerks – absent knee and ankle jerks and sensory loss indicate a neuropathy
- Look for signs of vascular insufficiency:
  - Check peripheral pulses
  - Are the toes cold?

PATHOGENESIS OF FOOT ULCERS

- Most ulcers occur as a result of trauma
- Neuropathy causes:
  - Reduced sensitivity
  - Altered proprioception with 'high pressure' on parts of the foot
  - Autonomic dysfunction, leading to dry skin with cracks and fissures
- Peripheral vascular disease:
  - Very common
  - Leads to ischaemic ulcers (pure ischaemic ulcers in 10%). Ninety percent of ulcers are due to neuropathy alone, or a combination of neuropathy and ischaemia

HOW WOULD YOU MANAGE THIS PATIENT?

- Admit the patient
- Take swabs for microbiology
- Arrange an urgent X-ray to look for foreign bodies, gas and osteomyelitis
- Early effective antibiotic treatment is essential:

- Use broad-spectrum antibiotic cover until cultures are available, for example, flucloxacillin, amoxicillin and metronidazole
- Discuss with a microbiologist
- Control the diabetes with insulin until the foot is healed when oral treatment can be restarted
- Establish the presence of other diabetic complications (see earlier)
- Ask the diabetic team to carry out a full assessment and arrange for future follow-up care

---

INFORMATION

According to the International Working Group on the Diabetic Foot, a diabetic foot infection is defined by the presence of at least two of the following:

- Local swelling or induration
- Erythema (>0.5 cm around the wound)
- Local tenderness or pain
- Local warmth
- Purulent discharge

Progress. This patient was admitted and seen by the tissue viability nurse for daily dressing of her foot ulcer. The inflammation settled and she was discharged after 6 days with full nursing care at her own home. Note that 40% of patients have a recurrence within 1 year after ulcer healing.

Diabetes in Pregnancy

CASE HISTORY (1)

You are asked to see a 28-year-old female who is 18 weeks pregnant and has been found to have a blood glucose of 10 mmol/L. She is asymptomatic and gives no history of diabetes.

You suspect a diagnosis of **gestational diabetes.**

HOW SHOULD THIS PATIENT BE MANAGED?

Meticulous glycaemic control is of paramount importance in pregnancy. The patient should initially be taught to monitor her blood glucose levels and be advised on lifestyle changes, including diet. Blood glucose levels should be measured 1 hour after each meal. If blood glucose is <7 mmol/L, then insulin is not required.

Always check your local protocol as guidelines vary regarding the use of oral antihyperglycaemic agents (e.g. metformin). There is a lack of data regarding long-term offspring outcomes, but in practice, they are widely used.

High levels of glucose are associated with a risk of neonatal macrosomia, fetal death and postnatal hypoglycaemia. Thus the patient should be commenced on soluble insulin with each meal and a long-acting insulin at night if glucose is not controlled to <7 mmol/L with diet ± metformin.

INFORMATION

- It is normal to have a lower blood glucose during pregnancy
- Thresholds vary between diabetic units, but a fasting glucose >6 mmol/L or a random/postprandial glucose >7.8 mmol/L is an indication for home blood glucose monitoring
- Diet should be healthy but not restricted
- Pregnant females have a low threshold to start insulin

Progress. This patient required insulin therapy, which was continued until she delivered at normal term.

CASE HISTORY (2)

You are called to the labour ward to see a patient who is on insulin. She has been on soluble insulin 12 U three times daily and isophane insulin 18 U last thing at night, with very good control of her blood sugar. She is now in labour and her blood glucose levels are not well controlled.

WHAT IS YOUR IMMEDIATE MANAGEMENT OF THIS PATIENT?

A variable rate insulin infusion as per local protocols.

The dose of insulin is adjusted with hourly glucose assessment to a target blood glucose of 4 to 8 mmol/L. The infusion is maintained until the patient is able to eat and drink.

It is essential to determine whether the patient had type 1 diabetes before pregnancy (in which case, insulin should never be stopped) or whether she has gestational diabetes when insulin therapy can be stopped after delivery. The placental hormones cause insulin resistance and, after the third stage of labour, gestational diabetes can disappear.

Progress. This mother has type 1 diabetes, so she was commenced on her pre-pregnancy dose of insulin when she started eating. Intravenous insulin must be continued until 4 hours after the first dose of SC insulin. She is followed up at her doctor's diabetic clinic.

Cushing Syndrome

Cortisol is the principal endogenous glucocorticoid secreted from the adrenal glands, the amount is controlled by the level of plasma ACTH.

Cushing syndrome is caused by excess glucocorticoids for the reasons shown in the Information box, of which exogenous corticosteroid administration is the most common.

Patients have undiagnosed Cushing syndrome for some time, and present because of metabolic decompensation due to either hypokalaemia (which can be severe), or hyperglycaemia and resultant dehydration.

Other complications follow, including secondary infection, bruising and bleeding, uncontrollable hypertension and osteoporotic fractures (Fig. 10.2).

INFORMATION

Causes of Cushing Syndrome

(Percentages in brackets refer to incidence of the primary cause)

- Excess corticosteroid administration
- Pituitary-dependent Cushing disease (85%)
- Adrenal adenoma (10%)
- Ectopic ACTH protection (5%)

CASE HISTORY

A 55-year-old female presents with a 2-year history of atypical depression and 3 weeks of confusion, altered behaviour and an inability to climb stairs due to muscular weakness. Her weight has increased marginally, but she has lost muscle bulk from the arms and legs.

On examination, she was obese and plethoric, with a moon face and buffalo hump. Her skin was thin with multiple striae over her breasts, abdomen and thighs.

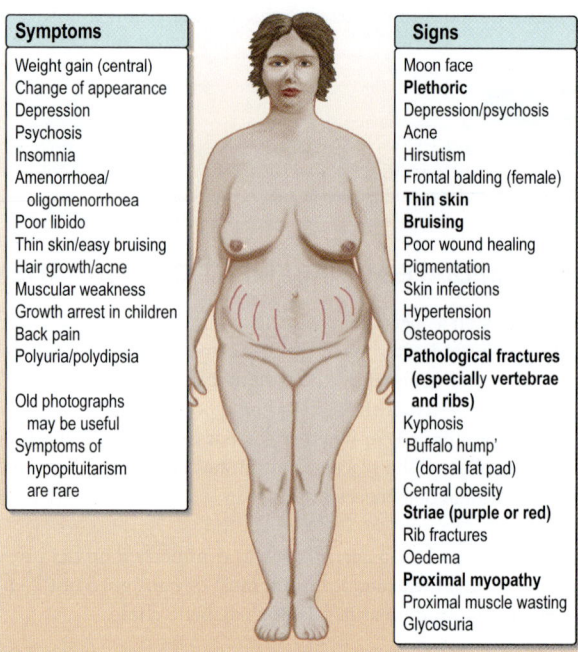

Symptoms	Signs
Weight gain (central)	Moon face
Change of appearance	**Plethoric**
Depression	Depression/psychosis
Psychosis	Acne
Insomnia	Hirsutism
Amenorrhoea/	Frontal balding (female)
oligomenorrhoea	**Thin skin**
Poor libido	**Bruising**
Thin skin/easy bruising	Poor wound healing
Hair growth/acne	Pigmentation
Muscular weakness	Skin infections
Growth arrest in children	Hypertension
Back pain	Osteoporosis
Polyuria/polydipsia	**Pathological fractures**
	(especially vertebrae
	and ribs)
Old photographs	Kyphosis
may be useful	'Buffalo hump'
Symptoms of	(dorsal fat pad)
hypopituitarism	Central obesity
are rare	**Striae (purple or red)**
	Rib fractures
	Oedema
	Proximal myopathy
	Proximal muscle wasting
	Glycosuria

Fig. 10.2 Symptoms and signs of Cushing syndrome. Bold type indicates the signs of most value in discriminating Cushing syndrome from simple obesity and hirsutism.

WHAT IS THE LIKELY DIAGNOSIS?

Cushing Syndrome

The patient was dehydrated and was found to have glycosuria, with a blood glucose of 30 mmol/L. Arterial blood gases reveal:

- pH 7.60
- pO_2 12.0 kPa
- pCO_2 5.4 kPa

This patient has a metabolic alkalosis due to the chronic hypokalaemia found in Cushing. Electrolytes came back from the laboratory, confirming your suspicions:

- Na^+ 145 mmol/L
- K^+ 2.5 mmol/L
- Urea 15.0 mmol/L
- Creatinine 120 µmol/L
- Bicarbonate 37 mmol/L
- Glucose 27 mmol/L

HOW WOULD YOU MANAGE THIS PATIENT?

The hypokalaemia and hyperglycaemia need prompt treatment. Total body potassium is likely to be extremely low, and as potassium is replaced, the initial effect will be to reduce the bicarbonate rather than to increase the extracellular (serum) potassium.

- Start potassium replacement both orally and IV (not more than 20 mmol in any 3 h)
- Rehydrate the patient with 0.9% saline + potassium chloride (40 mmol/L) added to each bag with 2-hourly K^+ monitoring

- Start an IV infusion of insulin titrated to blood glucose level. This might exacerbate the fall in serum potassium
- After 48 h, the patient was rehydrated and had a serum K⁺ of 4.5 mmol/L
- *Confirm the diagnosis of Cushing syndrome*
  - Collect 24 h urine for urinary free cortisol (normal <700 nmol in 24 h)
  - Measure midnight cortisol (normal <50 nmol/L)
  - Give 8 h low-dose dexamethasone suppression (0.5 mg 6-hourly for 48 h at 09:00, 15:00, 21:00, 03:00 followed by 09:00 cortisol)

Progress. Cushing is confirmed and the patient is referred for specialist investigation. These investigations will include determination of ACTH dependence, pituitary and adrenal CT scanning and localisation procedures.

Hyperthyroidism

CASE HISTORY (1)

A 65-year-old female is brought to the emergency department with acute breathlessness and cough, producing frothy, blood-tinged sputum.

On examination, she had profuse sweating with rapid severe breathlessness. She has atrial fibrillation (AF), and auscultation reveals wheezes and crackles throughout the chest. Your diagnosis of **pulmonary oedema** is confirmed by the CXR, which shows bilateral perihilar shadowing and Kerley B lines of interstitial oedema.

The ECG shows fast AF (160/min), but there is no evidence of cardiac ischaemia or other abnormality (Fig. 10.3).

HOW WOULD YOU ACUTELY MANAGE THIS PATIENT?

Admit the patient to the HDU and start treatment of acute heart failure, oxygen, IV furosemide 50 mg and vasodilatation therapy, for example, a glyceryl trinitrate infusion.

Progress. She responds well but still has fast AF. Thyroid function tests reveal a free T4 of 45 pmol/L (normal range 9.0–23) with a suppressed TSH.

WHAT IS THE DIAGNOSIS AND WHAT TREATMENT IS INDICATED?

Diagnosis – hyperthyroidism.
  Treatment:
- Control the heart rate using beta-blockers (e.g. propranolol 60-80 mg every 4–6 h), and digoxin if required
- Avoid amiodarone, as this will potentially interfere with further management

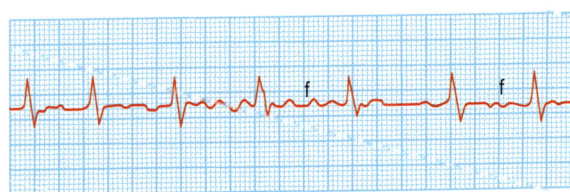

Fig. 10.3 Electrocardiogram showing atrial fibrillation. Note the absolute rhythm irregularity and baseline undulations (f waves). (From Kumar, P., Clark, M. (Eds.), 2017. Kumar and Clark's Clinical Medicine, ninth ed. Elsevier, Edinburgh; Fig 23.46A.)

■ Anticoagulate the patient (heparin and warfarin, or thrombin inhibitors, e.g. rivaroxaban)
■ Start antithyroid medication, for example, carbimazole 40 mg daily (or methimazole)
■ Determine the cause of the hyperthyroidism

Beta-adrenoreceptors are sensitised to normal circulating catecholamines by high levels of thyroxine and beta-blockade is useful in achieving symptom control in hyperthyroidism; it is also helpful in treating high-output heart failure and achieving rate control. Propranolol is used in high doses because, being lipid-soluble, it crosses the blood–brain barrier.

REMEMBER

- Thyroid stimulating hormone is invariably suppressed in hyperthyroidism (except for the exceptionally rare TSH-secreting pituitary adenoma)
- Hyperthyroidism often presents in the elderly with AF and few other features

INVESTIGATIONS

- Thyroid antimicrosomal auto-antibodies and antithyroglobulin antibodies (in the serum): positive in up to 90% of patients with Graves disease
- Thyroid technetium scan to distinguish a 'hot nodule' (focal uptake) from Graves disease (uniform uptake) and from viral thyroiditis (zero uptake)

Progress. This patient was confirmed as having Graves disease. She was followed up for her hyperthyroidism with a reduction of her carbimazole dosage. A cardiologist advised her to stay on digoxin and warfarin, and she remained in AF at 6 months.

CASE HISTORY (2)

A 75-year-old female is referred with weight loss, general malaise and apathy.
Clinical examination is unremarkable, except for a mild tachycardia of 100 bpm.
Routine investigations (remembering to include TFTs) (Table 10.7) have now been phoned through by the laboratory with the following results:
- Free T_4: 56 pmol/L (normal range 9–23 pmol/L)
- Thyroid stimulating hormone <0.1 mU/L (normal range 0.3–5.5 mU/L)

Elderly patients can have atypical presenting features of hyperthyroidism, which may be dominated by weight loss, apathy and fatigue.

REMEMBER

Weight loss without obvious cause always requires a TSH measurement.

INFORMATION

Hyperthyroidism in the Elderly

- Weight loss
- Atrial fibrillation
- Lethargy
- Proximal myopathy

TABLE 10.7 ■ Characteristics of TFTs in Common Thyroid Disorders[a]

—	TSH (0.3–3.5 mU/L)	Free T4 (10–25 pmol/L)	Free T3 (3.5–7.5 pmol/L)
Thyrotoxicosis	**Suppressed (<0.05 mU/L)**	**Increased**	**Increased**
Primary hypothyroidism	**Increased (>10 mU/L)**	Low/low–normal	Normal or low
TSH deficiency	Low–normal or subnormal	**Low/low–normal**	Normal or low
T3 toxicosis	Suppressed (<0.05 mU/L)	Normal	**Increased**
Compensated euthyroidism	**Slightly increased (5–10 mU/L)**	**Normal**	Normal

[a]The clinically most informative tests in each situation are shown in bold.
TFTs, Thyroid function tests; TSH, thyroid stimulating hormone; T3, triiodothyronine.

WHAT ARE THE POTENTIAL CAUSES OF HYPERTHYROIDISM?

Common Causes

- Graves disease
- Multinodular goitre
- Toxic solitary nodule
- Viral thyroiditis
- Amiodarone

Rare Causes

- Thyroid stimulating hormone-secreting pituitary adenoma
- Choriocarcinoma
- Factitious (self-medication)

WHAT TESTS WOULD YOU ORDER FOR A PATIENT WITH A GOITRE?

- **Thyroid function tests:** TSH plus free T_4 or T_3
- **Thyroid antibodies:** to exclude auto-immune aetiology
- **Ultrasound:** ultrasound with high resolution is a sensitive method for delineating nodules and can demonstrate whether they are cystic or solid. In addition, a multinodular goitre may be demonstrated when only a single nodule is palpable. Unfortunately, even cystic lesions can be malignant and thyroid tumours may arise within a multinodular goitre; therefore fine-needle aspiration (FNA) (see next point) is often required and is performed under ultrasound control at the same time as the scan
- **Fine-needle aspiration (FNA):** In patients with a solitary nodule or a dominant nodule in a multinodular goitre, there is a 5% chance of malignancy; in view of this, FNA should be performed. This can be done in the outpatient clinic. Cytology in expert hands can usually differentiate the suspicious or definitely malignant nodule. Fine-needle aspiration reduces the necessity for surgery, but there is a 5% false-negative rate, which must be borne in mind (and the patient appropriately counselled). Continued observation is required when an isolated thyroid nodule is assumed to be benign without excision

■ **Thyroid scan** (99ᵐ technetium): This can be useful to distinguish between functioning (hot) or nonfunctioning (cold) nodules. A hot nodule is only rarely malignant; however, a cold nodule is malignant in only 10% of cases and FNA has largely replaced 99ᵐ technetium scans in the diagnosis of thyroid nodules

WHAT ARE THE PHARMACOLOGICAL TREATMENT OPTIONS IN HYPERTHYROIDISM?

■ Rapid symptomatic treatment (if necessary): propranolol 40–80 mg 8-hourly
■ Control thyroid overactivity, for example:
  ■ Carbimazole 40 mg once daily *or*
  ■ Propylthiouracil (PTU) 200 mg × 3 daily

The last two drugs inhibit the formation of thyroid hormones (Fig. 10.4). Carbimazole and PTU will induce hypothyroidism after 4 to 8 weeks at these doses, and either treatment should be titrated down to a maintenance level (e.g. carbimazole 10 mg daily) or thyroxine should be added back at a dose of 100 to 150 µg in a 'block and replace' regimen. Patients are typically treated for 6 to 18 months with antithyroid drugs. All patients commencing antithyroid drugs should be warned about possible rashes, which are common and usually self-limiting without discontinuation, and severe sore throats or mouth ulcers, which may indicate a dangerous fall in neutrophils.

Treatment with radio-iodine is frequently employed if patients relapse after medical treatment but may also be used as primary treatment, particularly in multinodular goitres or toxic adenomas. Surgery is reserved for large goitres or for patient preference after relapse.

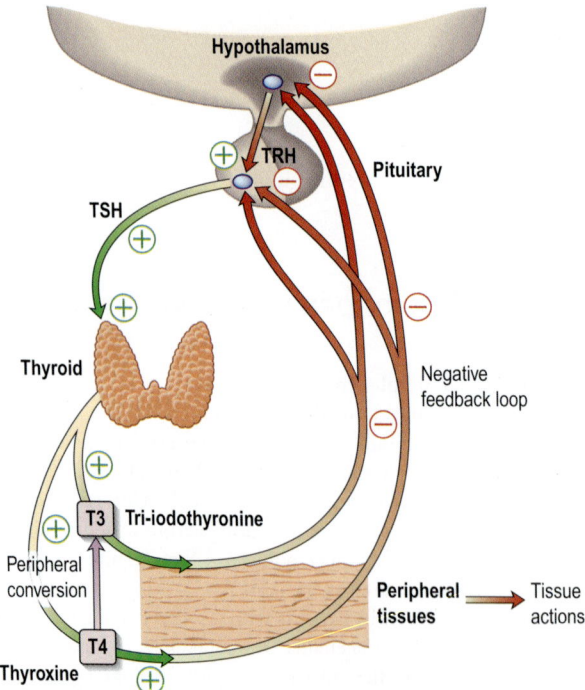

Fig. 10.4 The hypothalamic–pituitary–thyroid axis. Pituitary thyroid stimulating hormone (TSH) is secreted in response to hypothalamic thyrotropin releasing hormone (TRH) and stimulates secretion of T4 and T3 from the thyroid. T4 and T3 have actions in peripheral tissues and exert negative feedback on the pituitary and hypothalamus.

INFORMATION

Investigation of a Solitary Nodule

- All solitary nodules >1 cm should be evaluated, as should 'dominant' nodules in nodular goitres
- Fine-needle aspiration cytology is the first-line investigation to identify a papillary carcinoma or follicular neoplasm
- Ultrasound is used to diagnose multinodular goitre
- Isotope scanning might identify a toxic 'hot' solitary nodule; these are almost always benign

Progress. This patient was treated with carbimazole and at 3 months was euthyroid.

CASE HISTORY (3)

You have been phoned by a doctor who has received the results of some TFTs on one of his patients. The blood test report showed a high free T4: 45 pmol/L (normal range 10–25) with a suppressed TSH (<0.1 mU/L). On further questioning, it transpires that the test was performed in a patient who was unwell with a painful neck. You recommend a thyroid technetium uptake scan, which shows minimal uptake, and arrange for the patient to come to outpatients in 2 weeks.

When you see the patient, he is better but still clinically hyperthyroid. Repeat TFTs are as follows: free T4 7.0 pmol/L; TSH 25 mU/L.

WHAT IS THE LIKELY DIAGNOSIS?

This patient is now biochemically hypothyroid, although the initial biochemistry demonstrated hyperthyroidism.

This presentation is strongly suggestive of **viral thyroiditis (de Quervain)**. Thyroid hormones are released in the early stage (when the patient is thyrotoxic) and patients typically become biochemically, and later clinically, hypothyroid. The tissue effects of high levels of thyroxine last longer than their serum levels and symptoms often lag behind the biochemical changes.

Progress. Viral thyroiditis does not usually require treatment; hypothyroidism is often transient, although a short course of thyroxine (3–6 months) should be used if high TSH persists. Autoantibodies might be positive because of the viral damage and do not necessarily predict long-term thyroid dysfunction. Thyroid function tests at 6 to 12 months were normal in this patient.

INFORMATION

Features of Viral (de Quervain) Thyroiditis

- Neck discomfort or pain on swallowing, a short course of prednisolone is used if pain is severe
- History of viral illness
- Hyperthyroidism (usually 1–3 weeks), followed by hypothyroidism, and then resolution
- Disparity between clinical features and biochemistry
- High erythrocyte sedimentation rate (ESR)
- Reduced uptake on technetium uptake scan
- Weakly positive antithyroid antibodies

CASE HISTORY (4)

A 42-year-old female was brought to the emergency department with a 24-hour history of vomiting, diarrhoea and two seizures. She had become confused and was now very drowsy.

She was accompanied by her partner, who explains that she has been unwell for 6 months with a thyroid problem, for which she takes tablets. Following a severe cold 7 days ago, he thinks that she has stopped her therapy.

On examination, she has a GCS of 8 with the following findings:
- Tachycardia >145–bpm, AF
- Hyperpyrexia >41°C
- Heart failure
- Jaundice

Patients who have two or more of the above have a high mortality. Symptoms can also include psychosis, vomiting, diarrhoea, seizures and coma.

WHAT IS THE LIKELY DIAGNOSIS?

Thyroid Storm

This is defined as being present in a patient with biochemical hyperthyroidism and any two of the above features. It is a rare medical emergency because thyrotoxicosis is now easy to diagnose biochemically and can be treated earlier.

It can be precipitated by thyroid surgery, the administration of radioiodine, the withdrawal of or noncompliance with antithyroid medication and by acute illness.

HOW WOULD YOU TREAT THIS PATIENT?

- Cooling of the patient with tepid sponging and a fan. Do not use aspirin as an antipyretic – this is contraindicated in thyroid storm (it displaces thyroxine from its binding globulin and increases the free T4)
- Beta-blockers (e.g. IV propranolol titrated up to maximum total dose of 10 mg then 60–80 mg 4–6 hourly orally) unless contraindicated by asthma. (*Note*: heart failure is not a contraindication to beta-blockers)
- Fluid replacement – this needs careful assessment. Heart failure will rapidly come under control once the patient's heart rate is lowered
- Hydrocortisone (e.g. 300 mg IV loading dose then 100 mg IV 8-hourly) - this blocks T4 to T3 conversion
- Propylthiouracil (e.g. 500–1000 mg orally as a loading dose then 250 mg 4-hourly)
- Potassium iodide as iodine blocks thyroxine synthesis and release. This should be given at least 1 h after the PTU, which blocks iodine incorporation but not uptake

Progress. This patient responded to her emergency treatment and was referred back to the endocrine team, who have now recommended radioactive thyroid treatment.

Amiodarone and Thyroid Function

CASE HISTORY

A 45-year-old female presents to the emergency department with increased breathlessness over the last few days. On direct questioning, she says that she has been losing weight (8 kg) for 4 months. She gives a past history of heart problems for which she is under the care of a cardiologist. She is unsure of the exact problem but says that she does take tablets for an irregular pulse and has brought them with her. She is on amiodarone and also takes warfarin and a diuretic.

On examination, she has an irregular pulse of 120/min and a raised JVP with crackles at both bases. You diagnose mild heart failure with AF, which is confirmed by ECG.

HOW WOULD YOU INITIALLY TREAT THIS PATIENT?

You increase her diuretic to furosemide 80 mg daily and start her on enalapril at a small initial dose of 2.5 mg daily.

Progress. On the post-take ward round, your consultant is pleased with your summary of the patient's condition and your initial management. He asks you about the weight loss, which you have noted but so far have no explanation for. Fortunately, you have done many blood tests, including TFTs, the results of which are now available. These show a free T4 30.7 pmol/L and a TSH < 0.1 mU/L.

HOW SHOULD YOU PROCEED?

- Confirm how long the patient has been on amiodarone and check the clinical record to establish whether there are any previous TFT results, particularly those before amiodarone therapy was commenced
- Amiodarone can cause hypo- or hyperthyroidism. In patients who have nodular thyroid disease, the synthesis of thyroxine may be autonomous and is limited only by iodine availability: thyrotoxicosis may be precipitated. In others, the Wolff–Chaikoff effect may result in hypothyroidism. Amiodarone also blocks T4 to T3 conversion, causing a high T4 and normal T3
- Examine the patient for clinical evidence of hyperthyroidism
- The patient is clinically as well as biochemically thyrotoxic, so start carbimazole 40 mg daily and ask the patient's cardiologist to discontinue amiodarone and use other therapy for her AF. Amiodarone-induced thyrotoxicosis can require high doses of carbimazole and sometimes prednisolone is helpful in controlling the condition. Because amiodarone contains large amounts of iodine, radioiodine cannot be used.

INFORMATION

Amiodarone contains a substantial amount of iodine and has a half-life of about a month. Thus amiodarone behaves like slow-release iodine. Thyroid function tests on amiodarone:

- Normal
- High free T4, normal TSH due to reduced conversion: monitor
- Subclinical thyrotoxicosis, that is suppressed TSH: change therapy
- Clinical thyrotoxicosis: change treatment and control overactivity
- Hypothyroidism: titrate thyroxine very gradually, starting at 25 µg daily

Progress. The cardiologists agreed that this patient should stop amiodarone and start verapamil. They said that two attempts at direct current (DC) conversion had failed in the past and DC was unlikely to be successful now. The patient became euthyroid after 3 months' carbimazole therapy.

INFORMATION

Wolff and Chaikoff first noted that excessive iodine suppresses thyroid function and causes short-term atrophy of the thyroid gland. Surgeons use this effect by administration of potassium iodide for 10 days before surgery. This is also why potassium iodide is used in thyroid storm.

Hypothyroidism

CASE HISTORY

A 42-year-old female is seen in clinic because she is having irregular periods that are sometimes very heavy. She thinks she has become menopausal and wonders about hormone replacement therapy (HRT). A more detailed history reveals that she has general malaise, weight gain (5 kg in 6 months), constipation and a hoarse voice.

On examination, she is overweight with a body mass index (BMI) of 35. There is no palpable goitre, but she does have swollen, nonpitting oedema of her legs and slow relaxation of her ankle jerks.

You suspect a diagnosis of **hypothyroidism**.

Investigations show a raised TSH (30 µg/L) and free T4 of 4.2 pmol/L, confirming hypothyroidism. Interpretation of TFTs is shown in Fig. 10.5.

Hypothyroidism is now diagnosed by a multitude of practitioners:

- Lipid clinic: cause of hypercholesterolaemia
- Psychiatrists: organic psychosis or depression
- Neurologists: ataxia
- Ear, nose and throat (ENT) surgeons: dysphonia or deafness
- Cardiologists: during follow-up of amiodarone treatment
- Dermatologists: dry skin or hair
- Gynaecologists: menorrhagia, oligo- or amenorrhoea, infertility
- Geriatricians: screening test
- Diabetologists: screening test in diabetes

In primary hypothyroidism the TSH will *always* be elevated and often very high.

Adult-onset primary hypothyroidism is usually due to auto-immune disease unless there has been:

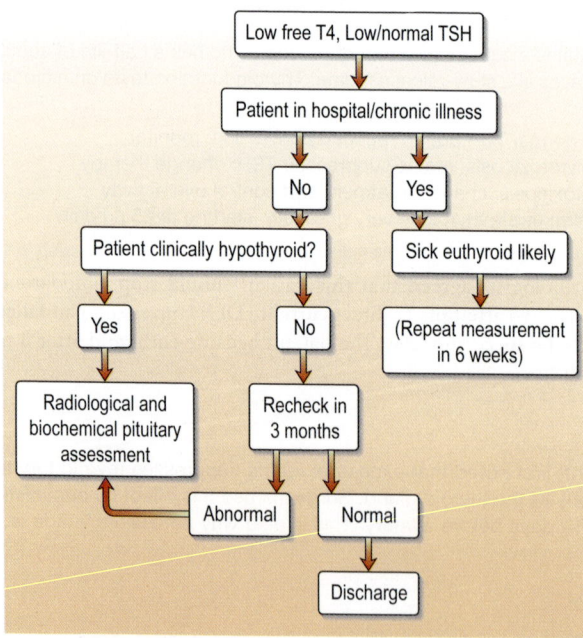

Fig. 10.5   Interpretation of thyroid function tests. TSH, thyroid stimulating hormone.

- Amiodarone treatment
- Previous thyroid surgery
- Previous radioiodine treatment
- Viral or postpartum thyroiditis

HOW WOULD YOU TREAT THIS PATIENT?

The patient, who is otherwise fit and not at risk of ischaemic heart disease, is started on 100 µg levothyroxine daily.

It takes about 6 weeks for a steady state to be reached. Aim to increase the levothyroxine dose in 25 µg increments every 6 weeks until the TSH is within or just below the normal range (3–3.5 mU/L). Occasionally, patients require only 50 to 75 µg daily, although usually 100 to 150 µg daily is required. Think about associated auto-immune diseases:

- Vitamin B_{12} deficiency
- Myasthenia gravis
- Addison disease
- Coeliac disease
- Other organ-specific auto-immune diseases

If the patient has angina, be very careful indeed. Many clinicians start at 25 µg per day (or even alternate days) and increase every 4 to 6 weeks. With hypothyroidism or when attempting thyroxine replacement with unstable angina, treat the heart disease first.

WHAT IS COMPENSATED HYPOTHYROIDISM?

Early in the course of hypothyroidism, the TSH is elevated (4–20 mU/L), but T4 and T3 are normal. Opinion differs as to the need for treatment. Most endocrinologists replace with levothyroxine:

- If autoantibodies are present in high-titre
- If the patient has typical symptoms of hypothyroidism
- In the presence of a high cholesterol
- If TSH is >10 mU/L

Progress. The patient made a complete recovery on levothyroxine therapy and did not require HRT.

Addison Disease

> **CASE HISTORY**
>
> A 35-year-old teacher has been under the care of a gynaecologist for amenorrhoea and menopausal symptoms. She has been increasingly tired and has lost weight over a 6-month period. She presents acutely to the emergency department with a 2-day history of vomiting and postural hypotension.
>
> **On examination**, she has a dull, slightly grey/brown pigmentation, easily seen on her palmar creases. Her blood pressure is 80/60 with a postural drop.
>
> Electrolytes:
> - Sodium: 127 mmol/L
> - Potassium: 5.2 mmol/L
> - Urea: 16 mmol/L
> - Creatinine: 140 µmol/L

WHAT IS THE DIAGNOSIS?

The clinical presentation and electrolytes indicate **adrenal insufficiency.** Treatment with gluco-corticoids (e.g. hydrocortisone) and IV 0.9% saline is life-saving in this situation and should be started immediately after a blood sample is taken for plasma cortisol/ACTH measurements.

Adrenal insufficiency presents gradually—over months—but also, as in this case, with acute haemodynamic collapse, often precipitated by infection, trauma or surgery. Crises can also occur in patients with known Addison disease during relatively trivial episodes such as a viral infection; for this reason, patients are advised to increase (typically double) the dose of hydrocortisone during illness.

Patients who are on long-term steroids for inflammatory conditions, such as asthma, also have pituitary-adrenal suppression but do not develop the same pattern of electrolyte disturbance and rarely become so unwell because they have preserved mineralocorticoid (i.e. aldosterone) secretion.

WHAT ARE THE TYPICAL CLINICAL FINDINGS IN ADDISON DISEASE?

Acute

- Hypotension (may be severe or postural)
- Nausea and vomiting
- Diarrhoea
- Hyponatraemia and hyperkalaemia
- Metabolic acidosis
- Hypercalcaemia
- Mild elevation of TSH

Chronic

- Weight loss and anorexia
- Fatigue
- Generalised weakness
- Hyperpigmentation
- Arthralgia and myalgia
- Depression, apathy and confusion

INFORMATION

Common Causes of Adrenal Failure

Primary

- Auto-immune: often associated with other auto-immune disease (e.g. type 1 diabetes mellitus, hypothyroidism, premature ovarian failure)
- Tuberculous adrenalitis: consider in immigrant populations/developing countries
- Drugs (e.g. ketoconazole, metyrapone)

Secondary (i.e. Due to ACTH Deficiency)

- Long-term glucocorticoid therapy (oral, inhaled, topical or intranasal steroids)
- Hypopituitarism

HOW WOULD YOU ACUTELY MANAGE THIS PATIENT? (FIG. 10.6)

General

- Give IV 0.9% saline
- Correct hypoglycaemia with 5% glucose
- Identify and treat a precipitating cause

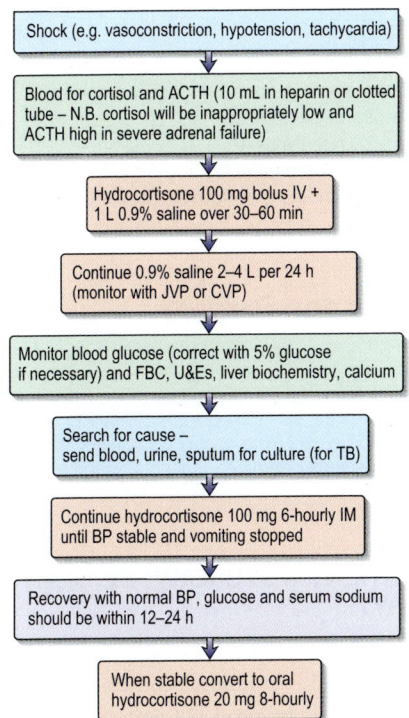

Fig. 10.6   Management of acute adrenal failure. (From Kumar, P., Clark, M. (Eds.), 2011. Kumar and Clark's Medical Management & Therapeutics. Elsevier, Edinburgh; Fig. 20.19.)

Specific

- Take samples for cortisol and ACTH
- Hydrocortisone (100 mg IV or IM); the intramuscular route gives sustained plasma levels
- Continue hydrocortisone 50–100 mg IV/IM × 4 daily

INVESTIGATIONS

Further Investigations

- Full blood count (anaemia, normochromic normocytic)
- Glucose (hypoglycaemia)
- Serum calcium (might be high)
- Arterial blood gases (acidosis)
- Chest X-ray (tuberculosis [TB], carcinoma)
- Short tetracosactide test (see Information box) if necessary to confirm diagnosis
- Pituitary MRI if hypopituitarism suspected

The initial cortisol in this female was <100 nmol/L, and so Addison disease is confirmed. In a less clear-cut case, use a tetracosactide test.

Progress. Once the patient had recovered and was eating and drinking, hydrocortisone replacement was rapidly tapered to 20 mg daily, given as 10 mg (06:00) + 5 mg (12:00) + 5 mg (18:00) to try to mimic the physiological circadian rhythm. Fludrocortisone was commenced at 100 µg daily.

Patients on Steroids for Surgery

CASE HISTORY

A 50-year-old female who is known to have chronic asthma and who has been on oral prednisolone between 10 and 40 mg for at least the last 10 years is admitted for a right hemicolectomy for a caecal carcinoma. Her asthma has been difficult to control on inhalers alone and she finds that it worsens whenever her dose of oral prednisolone is reduced to 10 mg, which she is on at present.

HOW SHOULD THE PATIENT'S STEROIDS BE CONTINUED FOLLOWING SURGERY?

Patients who have been on prednisolone for more than 3 months are likely to have a suppressed pituitary–adrenal axis (Fig. 10.7). Adrenal mineralocorticoid production will be normal so that the risks of a typical Addisonian crisis are small, but nevertheless, this patient will not be able to

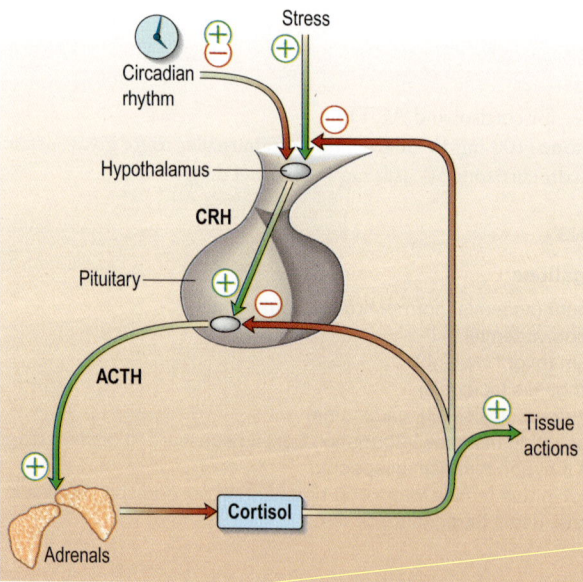

Fig. 10.7 Control of the hypothalamic-pituitary-adrenal axis. Pituitary adrenocorticotrophic hormone (ACTH) is secreted in response to hypothalamic corticotrophin-releasing hormone (CRH) triggered by circadian rhythm, stress and other factors, and stimulates secretion of cortisol from the adrenal. Cortisol has multiple actions in peripheral tissues and exerts negative feedback on pituitary and hypothalamus.

mount the normal cortisol response to surgery. Glucocorticoid replacement should be given as follows:

- At induction: hydrocortisone 100 mg IV; *then*
- Continue infusion of hydrocortisone 200 mg/24 h

An IV infusion of hydrocortisone (25–100 mg over 24 h, i.e. 1–4 mg/h) should be given to all patients who will have a prolonged period nil by mouth or who are on the intensive care unit (ICU). The pharmacokinetics of hydrocortisone are such that a continuous infusion of 4 mg/h will achieve a steady-state plasma cortisol level of >500 nmol/L, similar to patients on the ICU with normal adrenals. A serum cortisol sample after 12 hours of infusion can be used to titrate the hydrocortisone infusion down to achieve a cortisol level of 500 to 750 nmol/L.

Resume oral steroids when possible – double hydrocortisone doses for 48 hours or for up to a week following major surgery.

> **INFORMATION**
>
> Once-daily steroids are used in pharmacological doses to treat inflammatory conditions. Such treatment is not appropriate for hydrocortisone replacement in patients with Addison disease or congenital adrenal hyperplasia (who might not be able to synthesise any adrenal steroids), or following adrenalectomy, when there is a risk of true Addisonian crises. These patients need twice-daily treatment.

Progress. This patient's postoperative period was prolonged due to her asthma and she spent 48 hours in the ICU. She eventually made a good recovery but continues to need oral steroids.

Hypercalcaemia

> **CASE HISTORY**
>
> A 56-year-old female patient who has been found to have fibroids has been admitted for a hysterectomy. She has been treated for hypertension but no other known illness, and no symptoms other than menorrhagia. A routine biochemical screen has revealed a corrected calcium of 2.75 mmol/L (normal range 2.20–2.60 mmol/L).

> **INFORMATION**
>
> An incidental finding of a raised serum calcium is a common presentation of hypercalcaemia and should be evaluated.

WHAT IS THE APPROPRIATE MANAGEMENT OF THIS CASE WITH MILD HYPERCALCAEMIA?

In mild to moderate hypercalcaemia with a corrected calcium <3.00 mmol/L:

- Ensure breast examination and CXR are reviewed
- Ensure adequate hydration preoperatively
- Continue IV 0.9% saline (1 L 8-hourly) postoperatively until patient is drinking freely
- Urea, electrolytes and calcium postoperatively
- Follow-up with full investigation

INVESTIGATIONS

- Urea and electrolytes and eGFR
- Serum parathyroid hormone (PTH)
- Erythrocyte sedimentation rate
- Serum electrophoresis and immunofixation for paraprotein
- Serum-free light chain assay
- Twenty-four-hour urine collection for calcium estimation
- Chest X-ray
- Thyroid function tests
- Serum angiotensin-converting enzyme (ACE) levels (for sarcoidosis)

WHAT ARE THE CLINICAL FEATURES OF MODERATE/SEVERE HYPERCALCAEMIA?

- Malaise, tiredness, fatigue
- Anorexia and weight loss
- Thirst and polyuria
- Nonspecific musculoskeletal symptoms
- Renal calculus (stones)
- Osteoporosis ('bones')
- Abdominal pain ('groans')
- Confusion ('psychic moans')

WHAT ARE THE POTENTIAL CAUSES OF HYPERCALCAEMIA?

INFORMATION

- Primary hyperparathyroidism is the most common cause of mild to moderate hypercalcaemia
- Malignancy accounts for 50% of severe hypercalcaemia and is usually apparent with physical examination + CXR and breast examination

PTH-dependent

- Primary hyperparathyroidism (the most common cause of mild hypercalcaemia)
- Tertiary hyperparathyroidism (in the context of chronic kidney disease)
- Familial hypocalciuric hypercalcaemia (FHH) (slightly raised PTH)

Parathyroid Hormone-independent

- Myeloma
- Solid tumours: breast, bronchus, kidney, lymphoma
- Vitamin D excess (especially the 1 alpha analogues of vitamin D)
- Sarcoidosis
- Thyrotoxicosis
- Glucocorticoid insufficiency

WHAT ARE THE BIOCHEMICAL FEATURES OF PRIMARY HYPERPARATHYROIDISM?

- Elevated PTH in the presence of hypercalcaemia. High normal PTH with hypercalcaemia also suggests hyperparathyroidism because any other cause of hypercalcaemia should suppress the PTH

- Elevated or high/normal 24 h urinary calcium excretion (normal range 2–8 mmol/24 h)
- Low bicarbonate 15–20 mmol/L (PTH excess causes a mild renal tubular acidosis)
- Moderately elevated ESR
- Normochromic anaemia

Familial hypocalciuric hypercalcaemia (FHH) is a benign, familial, autosomal dominant condition caused by a mutation of the calcium-sensing receptor in the kidney and parathyroid gland. It is not associated with renal calculi and is asymptomatic. It can be difficult to distinguish from asymptomatic primary hyperparathyroidism. A low urinary calcium suggests the diagnosis, which is confirmed by examining family members.

TREATMENT OF PRIMARY HYPERPARATHYROIDISM

Patients who are symptomatic or who have complications should all be referred for parathyroid surgery, whatever the serum calcium level.

Most authorities suggest that the majority of asymptomatic patients should also be treated surgically because they are at risk of developing complications, and should certainly be referred for specialist opinion.

Progress. This patient had an uneventful postoperative recovery following her hysterectomy but did not want to consider any further surgery unless it became absolutely necessary. She is being followed with regular serum calcium levels.

Severe Hypercalcaemia

CASE HISTORY

A 72-year-old female is referred with a working diagnosis of 'recurrent hyperparathyroidism'. She had a history of primary hyperparathyroidism, treated surgically 10 years previously.

Three months prior to admission, she had become generally unwell, weak and lethargic. She reported a weight loss of 5 kg. The GP had performed blood tests: corrected calcium 3.5 mmol/L, urea 16 mmol/L, creatinine 150 µmol/L. Renal function was previously normal. The patient arrived dehydrated and vomiting. She was found to have a fungating breast carcinoma, which she had kept secret.

- Recurrence of hyperparathyroidism after surgical cure is unusual and suggests a familial cause of hyperparathyroidism (e.g. multiple endocrine neoplasia) or an alternative cause, for example, breast cancer
- Hypercalcaemia causes dehydration by creating a secondary type of nephrogenic diabetes insipidus (DI). As calcium clearance is itself dependent on GFR, hypercalcaemia can rapidly decompensate in the presence of fluid depletion

INFORMATION

Severe hypercalcaemia is defined as corrected calcium >3.5 mmol/L or >3.0 with evidence of dehydration.

HOW WOULD YOU MANAGE THIS PATIENT'S SEVERE HYPERCALCAEMIA?

- Aggressive rehydration with 0.9% saline – initial bolus of 1–2 L followed by 200–500 mL/h depending on volume status, cardiac function, and renal function. This reverses the dehydration caused by hypercalcaemia-induced nephrogenic DI and promotes calciuresis
- Bisphosphonate: treatment of choice for hypercalcaemia of malignancies or of undiagnosed cause; 60–90 mg infusion of disodium pamidronate via a cannula in a large vein causes normalisation of serum calcium in 80% of patients after 48–72 h

Other treatments:

- Zoledronic acid: 4 mg infusion over 15 mins
- Denosumab: consult a specialist before use
- Glucocorticoids (e.g. prednisolone 60 mg daily is used in sarcoidosis or vitamin D toxicity)
- In life-threatening hypercalcaemia, haemodialysis may be necessary

Progress. This patient's calcium level remained within the normal range for 2 weeks. She was referred to the oncology department for treatment of the breast cancer and was started on an oral bisphosphonate, as skeletal secondaries were demonstrated.

Hypocalcaemia

CASE HISTORY

A 32-year-old patient develops tingling and numbness around the mouth and in the extremities 3 days after a total thyroidectomy. She has become emotionally labile.

On examination, tapping the facial nerve (Chvostek sign) causes her upper lip to twitch. A serum calcium is 1.82 mmol/L corrected.

The patient's parathyroid glands might have been inadvertently removed. Before the plasma calcium result was available, an urgent assessment of the patient was made to determine the severity.

WHAT ARE THE CLINICAL FEATURES OF HYPOCALCAEMIA?

- Abnormal neurological sensations and neuromuscular excitability
- Numbness around the mouth and paraesthesia of the distal limbs
- Hyperreflexia
- Carpal and pedal spasms
- Tetany contractions (may include laryngospasm)
- Generalised seizures
- Chvostek sign is elicited by tapping the facial nerve just anterior to the ear, causing ipsilateral contraction of the facial muscles (positive in 10% of normal people)
- Trousseau sign is elicited by inflating a BP cuff for 3 min at the level of systolic BP. This causes mild ischaemia, unmasks latent neuromuscular hyperexcitability and enables carpal spasm to be observed
- Electrocardiogram: prolonged QT interval

INFORMATION

Causes of Tetany

In the Presence of Alkalosis

- Hyperventilation
- Excess antacid therapy
- Persistent vomiting
- Hypochloraemic alkalosis, for example, primary hyperaldosteronism

In the Presence of Hypocalcaemia

- See following section

HOW DO YOU ASSESS SEVERITY?

The symptoms and signs described are a much better guide to prognosis than the absolute value of the plasma calcium. In the presence of a low calcium (corrected calcium <2.0 mmol/L), any of the above features should be taken as evidence that urgent treatment is required.

HOW WOULD YOU TREAT THIS PATIENT? (TABLE 10.8)

- Administer 10 mL calcium gluconate (10 mL of 10% calcium gluconate (2.20 mmol)) before the plasma calcium result is back
- Repeat as necessary or proceed with an infusion of calcium gluconate 10% 40 ml over 24 hours
- Monitor serum calcium concentrations regularly
- If hypomagnesaemic, you may need to correct the magnesium level before the hypocalcaemia will resolve
- Hypocalcaemia is usually transient

INVESTIGATIONS

- Plasma calcium (and albumin) and phosphate
- Plasma magnesium
- Urea and electrolytes
- Plasma PTH level (low in hypoparathyroidism, high in vitamin D deficiency
- Vitamin D level
- Skull X-ray (intracranial calcification of chronic hypocalcaemia)

TABLE 10.8 ■ **Management of Symptomatic Hypocalcaemia**

Severity of Hypocalcaemia	Recommended Action
Emergency	
Spontaneous tetany, laryngospasm, seizures	Give 10 mL calcium gluconate 10% over 5 min IV, then proceed as below
Acute Severe Hypocalcaemia	
Frequent spasms/distressing symptoms and corrected calcium <2.00 mmol/L *or*	Calcium infusion: calcium gluconate at 15 mg/kg IV over 4 h in 1 L 0.9% saline. This is equivalent to ((weight in kg) × 1.7) mL of 10% calcium gluconate
Mild symptoms and corrected calcium of <1.90 mmol/L	ECG monitoring is essential for patients with arrhythmias
	Check magnesium level and correct if low
Acute Mild Hypocalcaemia	
Mild symptoms with calcium 1.90–2.20 mmol/L	Oral calcium supplements
	Calcium carbonate (600 mg Ca^{2+} daily) 1–2 tablets 2–3 × daily. Preferably between meals to increase availability of calcium for intestinal absorption
	If hypocalcaemia is associated with insufficient vitamin D, give calcium carbonate with colecalciferol 1 tablet 2–3 × daily (Ca^{2+} 600 mg)
Chronic Hypocalcaemia	
Symptoms frequently mild unless accompanied by osteomalacia	Oral calcium supplements (as above)
	If due to dietary vitamin D deficiency, use oral calcium as previous
	With hypoparathyroidism, either primary, secondary or persisting following thyroid/parathyroid surgery: add alfacalcidol 1 µg daily. This medication requires careful monitoring and usually endocrine follow-up

WHAT ARE THE POTENTIAL CAUSES OF HYPOCALCAEMIA?

- Hypoparathyroidism (primary, secondary or, most commonly, postsurgical)
- Renal failure (associated hyperphosphataemia)
- Vitamin D deficiency (giving rickets and osteomalacia)
- Pseudo-hypoparathyroidism (resistance to PTH)
- Severe magnesium deficiency (causes both reduced PTH secretion and resistance to PTH action)
- Acute pancreatitis
- Rhabdomyolysis

HOW DO YOU MANAGE SYMPTOMATIC HYPOCALCAEMIA?

The aim of acute management is not to return the calcium to normal but to ameliorate the acute manifestations of hypocalcaemia (see Table 10.8).

Progress. This patient's serum calcium was normal on the fourth postoperative day and she made an uneventful recovery.

INFORMATION

Administration of alfacalcidol (0.5–1.0 µg), together with oral calcium gluconate, is used for chronic hypoparathyroidism with regular calcium monitoring.

Phaeochromocytoma and Paraganglioma

Phaeochromocytomas are rare catecholamine-producing tumours derived from neuroendocrine cells, usually involving the adrenal glands (90%) or elsewhere in the sympathetic chain (paragangliomas).

CASE HISTORY

Three hours after a surgical procedure for colonic malignancy, a 62-year-old female becomes hypertensive, tachycardic and hyperglycaemic and develops an inappropriate lactic acidosis. When you review the notes, you discover that she has a 3 cm adrenal mass seen on a CT scan preoperatively, which was felt to be an incidental finding by the surgical team. On further questioning, you determine that she has had a history of paroxysmal palpitations, flushing, sweating attacks and headaches for years.

This history and CT findings would be compatible with a phaeochromocytoma.

Phaeochromocytoma is known as the 10% tumour (see Information box). It can be diagnosed during routine screening of hypertensive patients (found in only 0.1% of hypertensive subjects), the investigation of unusual episodes or cardiac events of uncertain aetiology. Phaeochromocytomas are usually associated with hypertension, 'attacks' and/or headache. They secrete adrenaline (epinephrine) or noradrenaline (norepinephrine) (Fig. 10.8).

INFORMATION

Phaeochromocytoma – the 10% Tumour

- Ten percent are bilateral
- Ten percent are extra-adrenal, usually around the sympathetic chain, when they are known as paragangliomas
- Ten percent are malignant

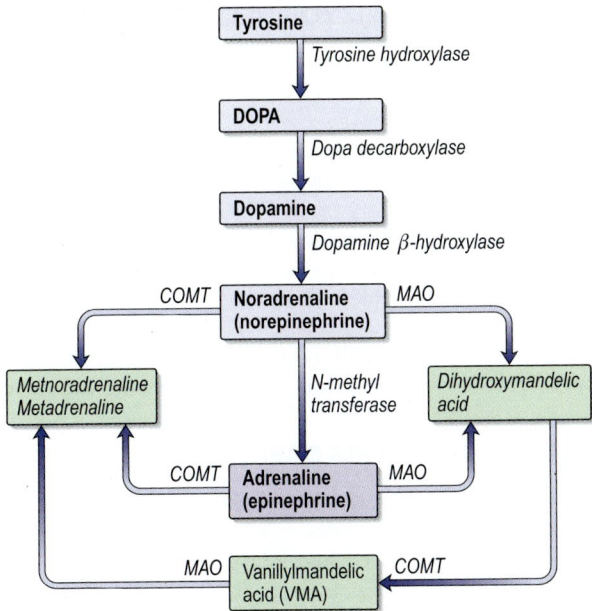

Fig. 10.8 The synthesis and metabolism of catecholamines. COMT, Catechol-O-methyl transferase; DOPA, dihydroxyphenylalanine; MAO, monoamine oxidase.

HOW DO THESE TUMOURS PRESENT?

Symptoms and signs of catecholamine excess include:
- Hypertension (sustained or paroxysmal)
- Anxiety attacks
- Palpitations and tachycardia
- Cold extremities
- Cold sweats, tremor, pallor
- Cardiac arrhythmias, including atrial and ventricular fibrillation
- Hypertensive crises, which may be precipitated by intercurrent illness, surgery or drugs (e.g. beta-blockers, tricyclic antidepressants, metoclopramide and naloxone)
- Pulmonary oedema with normal left ventricular (LV) function
- Unexplained lactic acidosis
- Apparent type 2 diabetes

ASSOCIATIONS

A family history is vital, particularly in young patients, and might reveal the following autosomal dominant conditions:
- Neurofibromatosis type I (neurofibromata, café-au-lait spots, Lisch nodules (iris hamartomas) and axillary freckling)
- von Hippel–Lindau disease (cerebellar haemangioblastomas, retinal haemangiomas and renal cell carcinoma)
- Multiple endocrine neoplasia type 2 (medullary thyroid carcinoma and hyperparathyroidism)
- Hereditary paraganglioma syndromes (phaeochromocytoma, carotid body tumour)

WHAT INVESTIGATIONS WOULD YOU REQUEST?

These include:

- Urea and electrolytes: potassium is often low; urea may be high if dehydrated
- Glucose: hyperglycaemia
- Urinary catecholamines (adrenaline, noradrenaline and dopamine) are measured by most laboratories. Two sets of normal 24-hour urinary catecholamines make a phaeochromocytoma very unlikely
- Plasma (heparinised) catecholamines (adrenaline, noradrenaline and dopamine) are specific but not sensitive tests. The blood must be taken directly to the laboratory for centrifugation
- MRI/CT scan of the adrenals should be delayed until biochemical diagnosis but is useful in localising the lesion
- ^{131}I-Meta-iodobenzylguanidine (MIBG) scan: MIBG is taken up selectively by adrenal tissue and is useful for localisation of tumour, particularly in extra-adrenal sites

HOW WOULD YOU MANAGE THIS CASE?

- Give adequate fluid replacement with 1 L 0.9% saline initially over 1 h, then 1 L 8-hourly
- Initiate oral alpha-blockade: e.g. phenoxybenzamine 10 mg orally twice daily initially, increase by 10 mg/day increments every other day according to response, maximum 120 mg/day. However, a disadvantage of phenoxybenzamine is that it also blocks presynaptic alpha-2 receptors enhancing the release of noradrenaline which can cause a reflex tachycardia. Selective Alpha-1 blockers such as doxazosin or prazosin are increasingly used instead.)
- When the BP is controlled after alpha blockade add a beta-blocker, for example, atenolol: 25–100 mg orally once daily, propranolol 30–60 mg/day orally (immediate-release) given in 2–3 divided doses (avoid labetalol)
- Surgery: hypotension commonly occurs intraoperatively when the tumour is removed, and this should be managed with blood, plasma expanders and inotropes as required. Inotropes should be used only when the patient is appropriately fluid-replete. Expansion of intravascular volume 12 h before surgery significantly reduces the frequency and severity of postoperative hypotension
- In an emergency (hypertensive crisis), IV phentolamine 5–20 mg (as a single dose) should be used, but great care should be taken to rehydrate the patient adequately in order to prevent severe hypotension

Progress. This patient improved with alpha- and beta-blockade and her BP stabilised. She was referred to the endocrine department, which, after further investigations, recommended surgical removal of the tumour.

Hypopituitarism

PATHOPHYSIOLOGY

Deficiency of hypothalamic-releasing hormones or of pituitary trophic hormones can be selective or multiple. Thus isolated deficiencies of GH, luteinising hormone/follicle-stimulating hormone (LH/FSH), ACTH, TSH and vasopressin are all seen; some cases are genetic and congenital, while others are sporadic and auto-immune or idiopathic in nature.

Multiple deficiencies usually result from tumour growth or other destructive lesions. There is generally a progressive loss of anterior pituitary function. Growth hormones and gonadotrophins are usually first affected. Hyperprolactinaemia, rather than prolactin deficiency, occurs relatively early because of loss of tonic inhibitory control by dopamine. Thyroid stimulating hormone and ACTH are usually last to be affected.

CASE HISTORY

A 60-year-old male is admitted with a sudden onset of explosive headache and a left III nerve palsy. A CT scan showed no evidence of an intracranial haemorrhage. A lumbar puncture showed a mild lymphocytosis.

Viral meningitis is suspected but his recovery is slow. He is noted to have small testes and a hypogonadal appearance. Six weeks later, he is readmitted with weight loss and a chest infection. Endocrine screening shows a low 09:00 serum cortisol and undetectable serum testosterone.

WHAT IS THE LIKELY INITIAL DIAGNOSIS?

Hypopituitary coma and apoplexy.

Pituitary apoplexy occurs with infarction or haemorrhage into an undiagnosed pituitary tumour. It produces severe headache with sudden visual field defects or ocular palsy. Axial CT scanning can miss pituitary apoplexy but MRI usually shows the tumour.

WHAT ARE THE CLINICAL FEATURES OF PITUITARY APOPLEXY?

Pituitary infarction can be silent. Apoplexy implies the presence of symptoms:

- Headache occurs in 75% of cases (may be of sudden onset, and very severe or mild)
- Visual disturbance (compression of the optic tract, usually causing bitemporal hemianopia)
- Ocular palsy present in 40% of cases: unilateral or bilateral
- Nausea/vomiting
- Meningism
- Hemiparesis

Clinically, pituitary apoplexy can be very difficult to distinguish from subarachnoid haemorrhage, bacterial meningitis, mid-brain infarction (basilar artery occlusion) and cavernous sinus thrombosis.

WHAT INITIAL INVESTIGATIONS WOULD YOU REQUEST?

An MRI of the pituitary reveals a tumour mass. *Note*: MRI will often reveal a pituitary tumour, although it cannot distinguish between recent and old haemorrhage (CT might help).

A single clotted blood sample should be taken to measure cortisol, thyroid function, prolactin, GH, testosterone (in men) and the gonadotrophin hormones.

ASSESSMENT OF SEVERITY: PITUITARY APOPLEXY

The course of pituitary apoplexy is variable. Headache and mild visual disturbance can develop slowly and persist for several weeks. In the acute form, apoplexy might cause optic nerve compression, haemodynamic instability and coma and is potentially fatal. Neurosurgical advice should always be sought. Residual endocrine disturbance invariably occurs. Panhypopituitarism is the usual result. Table 10.9 shows an example replacement therapy.

INFORMATION

- Neurosurgical decompression via a trans-sphenoidal route is the definitive treatment for pituitary apoplexy
- Obtundation and visual deterioration are absolute indications for neurosurgery
- Patients without confusion or visual disturbance generally do well without surgery

TABLE 10.9 ■ **Replacement Therapy for Hypopituitarism**

Axis	Usual Replacement Therapies
Adrenal	Hydrocortisone 15–40 mg daily (starting dose 10 mg on rising/5 mg lunchtime/5 mg evening)
	(Normally no need for mineralocorticoid replacement)
Thyroid	Levothyroxine 100–150 μg daily
Gonadal	—
Male	Testosterone IM, orally, transdermally or implant
Female	Cyclical oestrogen/progestogen orally or as patch
Fertility	HCG plus FSH (purified or recombinant) or pulsatile GnRH to produce testicular development, spermatogenesis or ovulation
Growth	Recombinant human growth hormone used routinely to achieve normal growth in children
	Also advocated for replacement therapy in adults where growth hormone has effects on muscle mass and well-being
Thirst	Desmopressin 10–20 μg 1–3 times daily by nasal spray or orally 100–200 μg 3 times daily
	Carbamazepine, thiazides and chlorpropamide are very occasionally used in mild diabetes insipidus
Breast (prolactin inhibition)	Dopamine agonist (e.g. cabergoline 500 μg weekly)

FSH, Follicle-stimulating hormone; GnRH, gonadotrophin-releasing hormone; HCG, human chorionic gonadotrophin.

HOW WOULD YOU MANAGE THIS PATIENT'S ACUTE HYPOPITUITARISM?

- Diagnostic samples for cortisol, TFTs and prolactin (single plain venous sample)
- Hydrocortisone 100 mg should be administered when the diagnosis is suspected
- Give glucose if the patient is hypoglycaemic
- Investigate and treat his chest infection

HOW DO PATIENTS WITH HYPOPITUITARISM TYPICALLY PRESENT?

- Patients present at times of stress (e.g. following a general anaesthetic) with hypoglycaemia due to the combination of a lack of GH, cortisol and thyroxine, all of which have a counter-regulatory effect on insulin
- Postpartum infarction of the gland occurs following postpartum haemorrhage and vascular collapse during a difficult delivery (Sheehan syndrome). This diagnosis should be suspected with failure to lactate, amenorrhoea and general ill-health postpartum
- Other features of hypopituitarism are nonspecific and include tiredness, weakness, loss of body hair, loss of libido (sexual interest) and features of hypothyroidism
- Note that patients with ACTH deficiency have no postural BP drop and normal electrolytes, as adrenal mineralocorticoids (aldosterone) are unaffected

ASSESSMENT OF SEVERITY: ACUTE HYPOPITUITARISM

The degree of hypopituitarism bears little relationship to the clinical state of the patient. In the absence of stress, patients with severe hypopituitarism might have few complaints. Examination in males might reveal small testes and women can demonstrate either amenorrhoea or inappropriately low postmenopausal gonadotrophins. Patients with mild hypopituitarism might become profoundly unwell at times of stress, such as during an intercurrent infection.

WHAT ARE THE POTENTIAL CAUSES OF ACUTE HYPOPITUITARISM?

- Destruction of the pituitary gland by primary or metastatic tumour
- Ischaemic necrosis after postpartum haemorrhage
- Pituitary apoplexy
- Postpituitary surgery or radiotherapy
- Primary empty sella syndrome

HOW CAN YOU INVESTIGATE ANTERIOR PITUITARY FUNCTION?

- Baseline blood samples must be taken for cortisol, free thyroid hormone levels, testosterone luteinising hormone (LH), follicle-stimulating hormone (FSH), prolactin and GH levels
- Dynamic investigation of pituitary function can be deferred and the patient should be treated expectantly with hydrocortisone (e.g. 10 mg × 2 daily once stable)
- Imaging using CT with fine cuts through the pituitary or MRI is indicated to find any space-occupying lesion

Progress. This patient's hypopituitarism improved without surgery, and at 3 months his serum hormone levels were normal. He was evaluated further for possible treatment of his pituitary adenoma.

Diabetes Insipidus

Transient diabetes insipidus (DI) often occurs after pituitary surgery because of vasopressin deficiency and can also occur acutely following head injury. Consider DI if asked to see a patient with polyuria and polydipsia who has normal blood glucose. Diabetes insipidus is also a cause of hypernatraemia.

CASE HISTORY

You are called to see a patient who had a trans-sphenoidal hypophysectomy the day before for a non-functioning pituitary adenoma. He has made a good recovery from surgery but now complains of severe thirst and is passing large volumes of dilute urine.

Results of his **investigations:**

- Na$^+$: 146
- K$^+$: 4.0
- Urea: 4.7
- Creatinine: 90
- Urine specific gravity (dipstick): 1.001

WHAT IS THE LIKELY DIAGNOSIS?

This patient probably has transient DI.

HOW WOULD YOU MANAGE THIS PATIENT?

- Ensure adequate access to water or commence IV glucose 5% and 0.45% saline to match urine output if the patient cannot drink enough
- Make sure an accurate fluid balance chart is being maintained
- If urine output is >200 mL/h for 2 consecutive hours, check plasma and urine osmolality
- Diabetes insipidus is confirmed by the presence of a high plasma osmolality (>290) in the presence of an inappropriately low urine osmolality (<500 mOsmol/kg)
- Start desmopressin: 2–4 micrograms/day IV/SC given in 2 divided doses (can also be given nasally 10–40 micrograms/day in 1–3 divided doses)
- If the plasma osmolality is low, the patient might be overdrinking due to a dry mouth, and a low urine osmolality is appropriate. In this circumstance, administration of desmopressin will cause a further fall in plasma osmolality and can be dangerous

WHAT ELSE CAN CAUSE DIABETES INSIPIDUS?

Diabetes insipidus is either cranial (Cranial Diabetes Insipidus [CDI]) or nephrogenic (Nephrogenic Diabetes Insipidus [NDI]) due to the inability of anti-diuretic hormone (ADH) to act on the kidney (Box 10.2).

Progress. This patient's DI was transient and he improved with IV fluids.

Syndrome of Inappropriate Antidiuretic Hormone (SIADH)

Inappropriate secretion of ADH results in retention of water and subsequent hyponatraemia. Mild symptoms of confusion, irritability and nausea occur as sodium levels fall below 125 mmol/L (125 mEq/L); fitting and coma occur as the sodium falls below 115 mmol/L. A diagnosis of SIADH can be made only in a patient who is clinically normovolaemic with normal thyroid and adrenal function.

BOX 10.2 ■ Cranial and Nephrogenic Causes of Diabetes Insipidus (DI)

Cranial DI
- Hypothalamic tumour
- Basal skull fracture
- Neurosarcoidosis
- Other hypothalamic diseases
- Idiopathic
- Infection
- Inflammatory

Nephrogenic DI
- Drugs:
- Diuretics
- Lithium
- Hypercalcaemia
- Hypokalaemia
- Kidney disease, for example, renal tubular acidosis
- Idiopathic

CASE HISTORY

A 65-year-old smoker complained of a chronic cough and haemoptysis. A CXR revealed a hilar mass. He was referred to the chest clinic for further investigation.

Electrolytes: Na$^+$ 118, K$^+$ 4.4, urea 3.3, creatinine 100, glucose 4.9, measured plasma osmolality 255.

In view of the low plasma osmolality, a spot urine was also sent to the biochemistry department: urinary sodium 30 mmol/L, urinary osmolality 350 mOsmol/kg.

This patient's urinary osmolality is high for his current plasma osmolality. Normally, the kidney can make urine as dilute as 100 mOsmol/kg (urine specific gravity (SG) = 1.0001) or as concentrated as 1300 mOsmol/kg in a patient who is dehydrated (urine SG = 1.4000). The current urinary osmolality has to be interpreted with knowledge of the current plasma osmolality.

This patient does indeed have **inappropriate ADH**. He was put on 1 L fluid restriction daily and commenced on demeclocycline.

Mild hypovolaemia is a potent stimulus for vasopressin (ADH) release, and volume-depleted patients given hypotonic fluid will frequently become hyponatraemic. Evaluation of volume status and recent fluid charts is essential in assessing hyponatraemia.

INFORMATION

Syndrome of Inappropriate Antidiuretic Hormone (SIADH)
- Dilutional hyponatraemia due to excessive water retention
- Low plasma osmolality with higher 'inappropriate' urine osmolality
- Continued urinary sodium excretion >30 mmol/L
- Absence of hypokalaemia (or hypotension)
- Normal renal, adrenal and thyroid function

HOW DOES SIADH TYPICALLY PRESENT?

Most commonly, patients with true SIADH present with incidentally discovered hyponatraemia. Alternatively, they might present with a fit or episodes of confusion.

WHAT ARE THE POTENTIAL CAUSES?

- Small-cell lung carcinoma (commonest)
- Drugs (e.g. carbamazepine, selective serotonin reuptake inhibitors (SSRIs))
- Pneumonia
- Tuberculosis
- Intracranial pathology
- Other neuroendocrine tumours

WHAT OTHER CAUSES OF HYPONATRAEMIA SHOULD YOU THINK OF?

It is essential for other causes of hyponatraemia (in particular, diuretics) to be excluded. The diagnosis of SIADH cannot be made in a patient who is on diuretics. The differential diagnosis of hyponatraemia includes hypothyroidism, adrenal and renal insufficiency, and chronic states such as cirrhosis and congestive cardiac failure.

HOW WOULD YOU FURTHER INVESTIGATE HYPONATRAEMIA?

- Take a drug history, for example, diuretics, SSRIs or carbamazepine
- Urea and electrolytes and plasma osmolality: hyponatraemia will be seen

- Urinary electrolytes and osmolality
- The patient will have a low plasma osmolality (<280) and an inappropriately concentrated urine (>300)
- Free T4 and TSH to exclude hypothyroidism
- Cortisol and short ACTH test to exclude Addison disease
- Chest X-ray and chest CT (tuberculosis, carcinoma)
- Computed tomography/MRI brain to exclude intracranial pathology

HOW COULD YOU TREAT THIS PATIENT?

- Fluid restriction – 1–1.5 L/day
- Tolvaptan: selective V2 receptor antagonist.
- Demeclocycline: reduces responsiveness of the collecting tubule to ADH. Side effects such as skin photosensitivity and nephrotoxicity limit use. Requires close monitoring

Progress. On fluid restriction and tolvaptan, this patient's serum Na$^+$ returned to normal levels. He was referred to the oncologists for management of his bronchial carcinoma.

Further Reading

Diabetic Ketoacidosis, Hyperosmolar Hyperglycaemic State and Hypoglycaemic Coma

Joint British Diabetes Societies for Inpatient Care. 2023. The Management of Diabetic Ketoacidosis in Adults.
NICE, CKS. 2022. Type 1 Diabetes in Adults: Diagnosis and Management.
Umpierrez, G., Korytkowski, M., 2016. Diabetic emergencies – ketoacidosis, hyperglycaemic hyperosmolar state and hypoglycaemia. Nat. Rev. Endocrinol. 12 (4), 222–232.

Management of Diabetic Patients Presenting for Surgery

Centre for Perioperative Care. 2023. Guideline for Perioperative Care for People with Diabetes Mellitus Undergoing Elective and Emergency Surgery.

The Diabetic Foot

Armstrong, D.G., et al., 2017. Diabetic foot ulcers and their recurrence. N. Engl. J. Med. 376 (24), 2367–2375.
NICE, CKS. 2019. Diabetic Foot Problems: Prevention and Management.

Cushing's Syndrome

Fleseriu, M., et al., 2021. Consensus on diagnosis and management of Cushing's disease: a guideline update. Lancet Diabetes Endocrinol. 9 (12), 847–875.
Loriaux, D.L., 2017. Diagnosis and differential diagnosis of Cushing's syndrome. N. Engl. J. Med. 376 (15), 1451–1459.

Hyperthyroidism

Franklyn, J.A., Boelaert, K., 2012. Thyrotoxicosis. Lancet 379 (9821), 1155–1166.
Kahaly, G.J., et al., 2018. European Thyroid Association Guideline for the management of Graves' hyperthyroidism. Eur. Thyroid. J. 7 (4), 167–186.
NICE, CKS. 2019. Thyroid Disease: Assessment and Management. National Institute for Health and Care Excellence (NICE), London.

Addison's Disease

Betterle, C., Presotto, F., Furmaniak, J., 2019. Epidemiology, pathogenesis, and diagnosis of Addison's disease in adults. J. Endocrinol. Invest. 42 (12), 1407–1433.
Husebye, E.S., et al., 2021. Adrenal insufficiency. Lancet 397 (10274), 613–629.

Hypercalcaemia

Bilezikian, L., et al., 2018. Hyperparathyroidism. Lancet 391 (2018), 168–178.

Phaeochromocytoma and Paraganglioma

Neumann, U.P.H., et al., 2019. Pheochromocytoma and paraganglioma. N. Engl. J. Med. 381 (2019), 552–565.

CHAPTER 11

Haematology and Oncology

Microcytic and Macrocytic Anaemia

DEFINITION OF ANAEMIA

Anaemia is present when the level of haemoglobin (Hb) in the blood is below the normal range (NR). The NR varies at different ages and between males (130–170 g/L) and females (115–150 g/L).

> **REMEMBER**
>
> An accurate result depends on a correctly taken blood sample:
> - Avoid prolonged venous occlusion
> - Do not take the sample from an arm with an IV infusion
>
> If the Hb concentration does not fit the clinical picture, consider taking another sample

ASSESSMENT

The impact of anaemia on an individual is variable and will depend on:
- The degree of anaemia
- The speed of onset
- Age
- Cardiovascular reserve

Symptoms are nonspecific and clinical signs are easily overlooked:
- Tiredness, lack of energy
- Shortness of breath on exercise
- Palpitations
- Ischaemic pain

> **INVESTIGATIONS**
>
> The **classification of anaemia** (Fig. 11.1) is based on the mean corpuscular/red cell volume (MCV; NR 80–96 fL).
>
> Further investigation is determined by whether the anaemia is microcytic (<80 fL), macrocytic (>96 fL) or normocytic.

> **CASE HISTORY (1)**
>
> A 45-year-old female of African origin presents to the emergency department with chest pain that is suggestive of cardiac ischaemia.
>
> **On examination**, she looked well. Cardiovascular examination showed a pulse of 82/min, a blood pressure of 140/80 and no abnormal signs. General examination was normal.

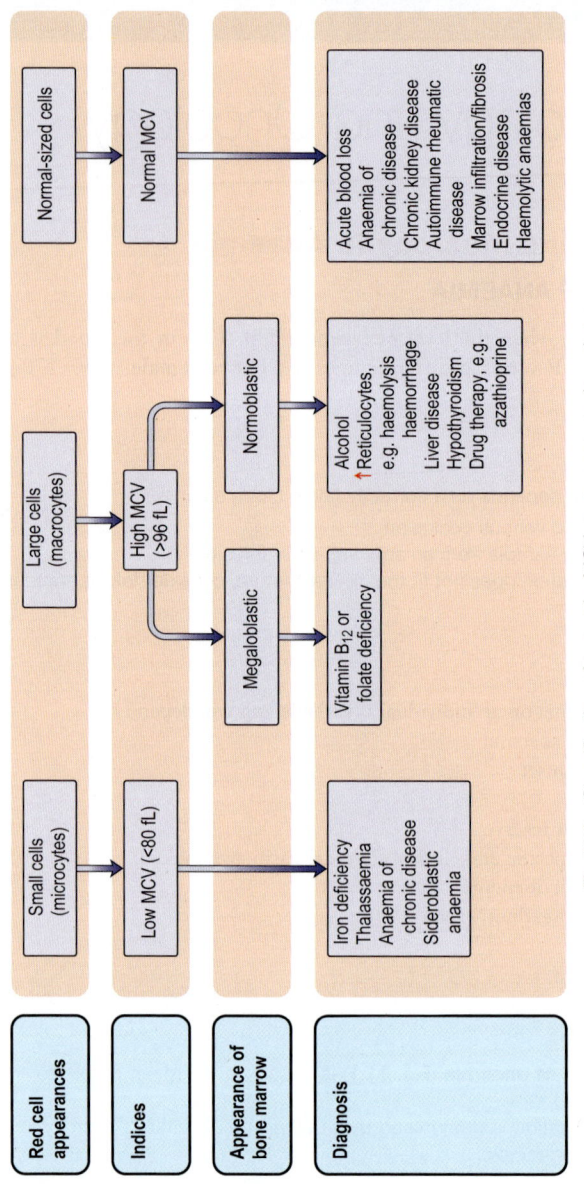

Fig. 11.1 Classification of anaemia. MCV, mean corpuscular volume.

INVESTIGATIONS

- Haemoglobin 99 g/L
- MCV 59 fL
- Red cell distribution width (RDW) 14%
- White cell count (WCC) 6.4 × 10⁹/L
- Platelets 273 × 10⁹/L
- Erythrocyte sedimentation rate (ESR) 10 mm/h
- Anisocytosis, poikilocytosis +
- Target cells ++

These are the features of a microcytic anaemia.

WHAT IS THE REASON FOR HER ANAEMIA AND IS IT RELEVANT TO HER PRESENTATION?

The first thing to exclude is iron deficiency, commonly due to uterine or gastrointestinal (GI) bleeding. Iron deficiency is unlikely in this patient:

- Very low MCV with only moderate anaemia
- Minimal variation in red cell size (anisocytosis) and shape (poikilocytosis)
- The serum ferritin (30 μg/L) was normal, indicating normal tissue stores of iron. (*Note:* ferritin can be high because it is an acute-phase protein that rises whenever the ESR or C-reactive protein (CRP) is elevated)

The anaemia of chronic disease, a form of functional iron deficiency, is also unlikely without an obvious underlying illness and a normal ESR.

REMEMBER

- Ferritin is an acute-phase protein. Iron deficiency can therefore be difficult to diagnose in the presence of inflammatory disease, and tissue iron stores might need to be examined directly by bone marrow aspiration
- Serum transferrin receptor assay does help to differentiate between these conditions

A common cause of a microcytic anaemia in patients of certain ethnic groups is β-thalassaemia trait. This is common in people from Africa, the Mediterranean, the Middle East, India and SE Asia.

Characteristically, β-thalassaemia trait results in a marked microcytosis with only a moderate anaemia, as shown in this patient. In addition, the RDW is normal. (*N.B.* It is high in iron deficiency.)

Beta-thalassaemia trait is confirmed by measuring glycated haemoglobin (HbA₂), which is normally <3.4% of total Hb.

Progress. The HbA₂ in this patient was 5.2%, confirming a diagnosis of β-**thalassaemia trait**.

Patients are asymptomatic and require no treatment. *Note*: Do not give iron. The anaemia is therefore not likely to be the cause of this patient's cardiac ischaemia. The patient was referred to the cardiac department for further investigation and management of her chest pain.

REMEMBER

The anaemia of β-thalassaemia trait is:

- Life-long
- Stable

CASE HISTORY (2)

An 81-year-old female presents to the emergency department with recent-onset congestive cardiac failure. **On examination**, she is mildly jaundiced and anaemic. Her pulse was 88/min, BP 120/90. She had signs of heart failure with a raised venous pressure, a third heart sound, basal crackles and marked lower leg oedema.

INVESTIGATIONS

- Haemoglobin 32 g/L
- Mean cell volume 121 fL
- White cell count 1.5×10^9/L
- Platelets 64×10^9/L
- Anisopoikilocytosis +++
- Hypersegmented neutrophils present

The findings indicate a severe macrocytic anaemia with a moderate neutropenia and thrombocytopenia. The diagnosis could be **pernicious anaemia**.

Vitamin B_{12} or folate deficiency impairs DNA synthesis and affects all rapidly dividing cells, particularly in the bone marrow, resulting in pancytopenia when severe. The anaemia is slow to develop and elderly patients, in particular, often do not present until very late.

Avoid blood transfusion, if at all possible, because there is a risk of volume overload and acute left ventricular failure.

Make a precise diagnosis by measuring serum vitamin B_{12}, serum and red cell folate:

- In vitamin B_{12} deficiency the serum vitamin B_{12} concentration is always reduced; in folate deficiency the red cell folate concentration is always reduced
- Severe vitamin B_{12} deficiency can be associated with a low red cell folate and a normal or high serum folate. Vitamin B_{12} is the cofactor in the reaction that cycles 5-methyl-tetrahydofolate. This allows folic acid to be retained within the cells

REMEMBER

Drugs and rare metabolic defects can result in megaloblastic anaemia with normal vitamin levels:

- Methotrexate induces functional folate deficiency
- Transcobalamin II deficiency results in intracellular vitamin B_{12} deficiency (but is very rare)

Bone marrow aspiration (not generally necessary since modern analysers can provide rapid vitamin B_{12} levels):

- Confirms megaloblastic erythropoiesis
- Documents pretreatment iron stores
- Excludes other conditions – myelodysplasia, acute leukaemia and aplastic anaemia – all of which can present with a macrocytosis and pancytopenia

CAUSES

- **Folate deficiency?** Nutritional deficiency is almost always a factor in any cause of folate deficiency, whether this is due to increased requirements (e.g. myelofibrosis, haemolysis) or excess alcohol use. In malabsorption, for example, coeliac disease, there is also poor dietary intake of folate

■ **B$_{12}$ deficiency?** Most cases of vitamin B$_{12}$ deficiency are due to malabsorption, either gastric (because of intrinsic factor deficiency) or intestinal (due to small bowel disease). Pernicious anaemia (antibodies against intrinsic factor) is the most common cause

ADDITIONAL INVESTIGATIONS

■ Intrinsic factor antibody assay (positive in 50% of patients with pernicious anaemia)
■ Antitissue transglutaminase antibodies and/or jejunal biopsy (to exclude coeliac disease)
■ Barium meal and follow-through (to exclude small bowel disease, e.g. Crohn disease); in a female of this age, only after the other causes have been excluded

Many patients with moderate vitamin B$_{12}$ or folate deficiency have a normal Hb with a raised MCV. Vitamin assays should be performed if the clinical picture is suggestive of a deficiency.

■ Gastrointestinal disease or surgery, including glossitis, malabsorption or diarrhoea
■ Neurological disease, including visual loss, a peripheral neuropathy or evidence of demyelination
■ Psychiatric disorders, including dementia, confusion or depression
■ Malabsorption or restricted diets, including vegans and those with anorexia nervosa
■ Alcohol excess
■ Infertility
■ Autoimmune endocrine disease
■ Family history of pernicious anaemia
■ Drug therapy, particularly anticonvulsants

Diagnosis. This patient had megaloblastic anaemia secondary to severe vitamin B$_{12}$ deficiency.

Pernicious Anaemia

■ Serum B$_{12}$: 25 ng/L (NR 160–960 ng/L)
■ Serum folate: 14.6 µg/L (NR 4.0–18.0 µg/L)
■ Red cell folate: 86 µg/L (NR 160–640 µg/L)

MANAGEMENT

When possible, treat with a single haematinic. In this case, administer hydroxocobalamin 1000 µg IM daily for 3 days, then 1000 µg every 3 months for life.

> **REMEMBER**
>
> Never give folate alone because, although it might partially correct the blood abnormalities associated with vitamin B$_{12}$ deficiency, it will also cause the B$_{12}$ level to drop even further and might precipitate severe neuropathy.

Do full blood counts (FBCs) with reticulocytes and U and Es initially daily (in a severely anaemic patient – as in this case) to look for:

■ Hypokalaemia, which can occasionally develop 1–2 days post therapy
■ Reticulocyte count, which starts to increase 2–3 days after treatment and reaches a peak on days 5–7
■ Haemoglobin concentration, which often falls further before starting to rise

Stay calm! Avoid blood transfusion. Failure of the reticulocyte count and Hb to rise in the predicted manner might be due to:

■ Incorrect diagnosis and/or treatment: review laboratory data
■ Coexistent iron deficiency: check iron stores, for example, ferritin levels

- Intercurrent infection: review patient – chest infection, urinary tract infection?
- Coexistent hypothyroidism

> **REMEMBER**
>
> Pernicious anaemia is an autoimmune disease; 1% to 2% of patients will also develop thyroid disease. Gastric cancer is also slightly more common (1%–3% of cases).
> The majority of patients with vitamin B_{12} deficiency have vitamin B_{12} malabsorption and require life-long treatment with vitamin B_{12}.

Treatment

For vitamin B_{12} deficiency, hydroxocobalamin 1000 µg IM every 3 months is standard. High doses of vitamin B_{12} (2 mg daily) orally are also effective. Nutritional deficiency of vitamin B_{12} is uncommon, however a vegan diet increases the risk significantly.

ANAEMIA DUE TO FOLIC ACID DEFICIENCY

These patients need 6 months' treatment with folic acid 5 mg daily after the cause (e.g. coeliac disease) has been defined and treated. Folic acid is ineffective, however, in the treatment of methotrexate toxicity therefore IV folinic acid is given.

Haemolytic Anaemia

Haemolytic anaemias are caused by increased destruction of red cells in two sites: intravascular or extravascular.

> **CASE HISTORY**
>
> A 60-year-old female presents with a history of feeling tired and exhausted for the last week. She is normally well but is under the care of the haematologists with chronic lymphocytic leukaemia (CLL). She knows all about the condition, having been diagnosed 4 years ago. She is not on any treatment but is under regular follow-up.
> **On examination**, she is clinically jaundiced, with cervical lymphadenopathy and a just palpable spleen.

> **INVESTIGATIONS**
>
> - Haemoglobin 68 g/L
> - Mean cell volume 90 fL
> - White cell count 30×10^9/L
> - Platelets 172×10^9/L
> - Reticulocytes 18.8%
> - Anisopoikilocytosis ++
> - Polychromasia ++
> - Spherocytes present
> - Lymphocytosis with smear cells
>
> She has a normocytic anaemia with a raised WCC and a reticulocytosis.

A normocytic anaemia can be due to:
- Acute blood loss
- Lack of erythropoietin (Epo) – chronic kidney disease (CKD)

- Bone marrow infiltration, for example, carcinoma
- Haemolysis

The patient described is anaemic and jaundiced with splenomegaly, suggesting a haemolytic anaemia. To confirm this, you need to demonstrate:

- Increased red cell production
- A reduced red cell lifespan

INCREASED RED CELL PRODUCTION

- Reticulocytosis: reticulocytes are immature red cells newly released from the bone marrow. They are larger than mature red cells, contain mRNA and appear polychromatic on standard blood films
- Bone marrow aspiration: erythroid hyperplasia

REMEMBER

Cortisol, androgens and thyroxine are all required for optimal erythropoiesis.

REDUCED RED CELL LIFESPAN

- Acholuric jaundice: unconjugated hyperbilirubinaemia, urobilinogen but no bilirubin in the urine (as unconjugated bilirubin is not hydrophilic)
- Abnormal red cell morphology: this might also indicate the specific cause of the haemolytic anaemia
- Demonstrated directly by radioactive isotope studies: reduced survival of ^{51}Cr-labelled autologous red cells (performed only if the diagnosis of haemolysis is in doubt)

There are many specific causes of haemolysis. The diagnosis can often be made by review of the blood film. Speak to the Haematology medical staff.

FEATURES OF HAEMOLYSIS ON BLOOD FILM

- Spherocytes: autoimmune haemolytic anaemia (AIHA), hereditary spherocytosis, *Clostridium welchii* septicaemia, extensive burns
- Red cell fragments: leaking mechanical heart valve, disseminated malignancy
- Sickled cells: sickle-cell anaemia, sickle-cell–HbC disease
- Bitten-out red cells: glucose-6-phosphate dehydrogenase (G6PD) deficiency, unstable Hb, oxidative drug therapy, for example, dapsone
- Malaria parasites

INVESTIGATIONS

- Antibody screen and direct antiglobulin test (DAT): in AIHA, autoantibodies to red cell membrane antigens are present in serum and on the red cell surface
- Urinary haemosiderin: positive in chronic intravascular haemolysis, such as paroxysmal nocturnal haemoglobinuria (PNH, very rare) and leaking mechanical heart valves
- Flow cytometry with antibodies against CD55 and CD59 antigens for PNH
- Glucose-6-phosphate dehydrogenase assay: common enzyme deficiency in particular ethnic groups (African, Mediterranean, SE Asian)

This patient had a strongly positive DAT with anti-IgG (see Fig. 11.2). The antibody eluted from her red cells was also present free in her serum and did not have any easily definable antigen

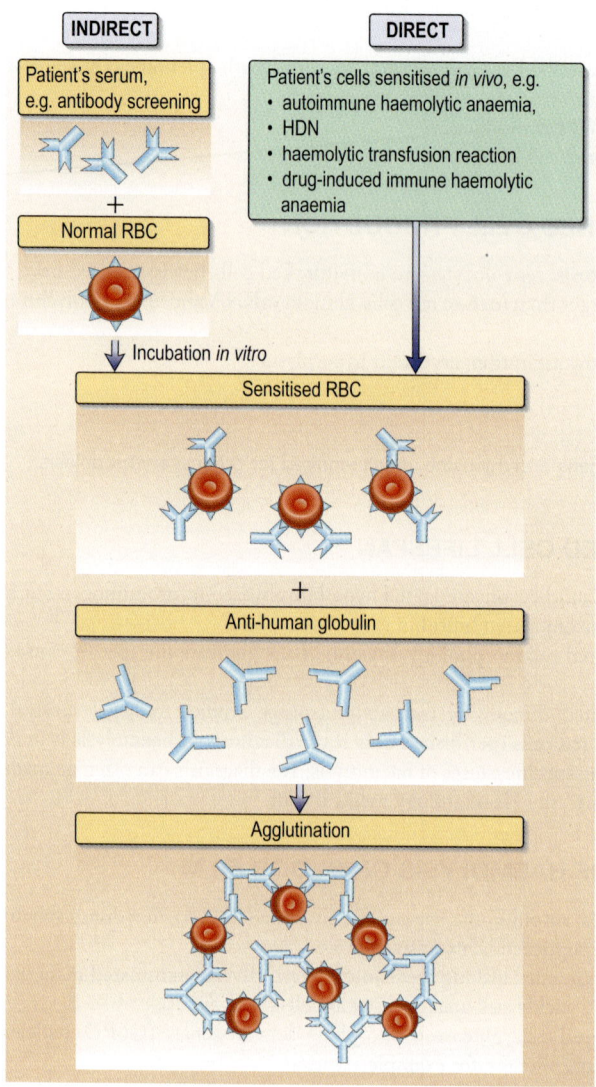

Fig. 11.2 Antiglobulin (Coombs') tests. The antihuman globulin forms bridges between the sensitised cells, causing visible agglutination. The direct test detects patients' cells sensitised in vivo. The indirect test detects normal cells sensitised in vitro. HDN, Haemolytic disease of the newborn; RBC, red blood cell.

specificity. She therefore has AIHA due to an IgG red cell autoantibody active at 37°C. AIHA can be primary or secondary. This patient is known to have CLL and has lymphadenopathy and a lymphocytosis with small, mature lymphocytes. Her AIHA is secondary to the underlying CLL; 10% to 15% of patients with CLL develop AIHA.

Diagnosis

Autoimmune haemolytic anaemia (secondary to underlying CLL).

MANAGEMENT

- Start oral prednisolone (e.g. 60 mg/day). This usually produces a remission. Corticosteroids reduce the production of antibodies and also destroy antibody-coated red cells
- Blood transfusion is necessary if the Hb continues to fall. Compatibility testing is complex because the autoantibody interferes with the cross-match; the laboratory could carry out autoabsorption studies to exclude additional alloantibodies. Transfuse slowly
- Refer the patient to her consultant in haematology to discuss further management

REMEMBER

Autoimmune haemolytic anaemia can develop acutely with a rapid fall in Hb. This patient has a short history. Check the Hb concentration at least once a day.

Progress. This patient went into remission on the steroids. Steroids are effective in about 80% of cases. The haematologists gradually reduced her steroids over 3 months and she was started on azathioprine. A year later, her CLL became active and she is now on rituximab and fludarabine.

Elevated Haemoglobin (Polycythaemia)

CASE HISTORY (1)

A 70-year-old male was admitted with breathlessness, wheeze, fever and cough productive of sputum. As a long-standing smoker, he suffers bouts of bronchitis but is otherwise in reasonable health.

On examination, he was not breathless at rest. Pulse was 82/min with no evidence of cardiac failure. Auscultation of the chest showed scattered wheeze and a few crackles at both bases. Peak flow was 350 L/min.

Initial investigations showed a haemaglobin (Hb) of 230 g/L, packed cell volume (PCV) 0.62, WCC $12 \times 10^9/L$, a mild neutrophilia and platelets $200 \times 10^9/L$.

CASE HISTORY (2)

In the next bed a 54-year-old male has been admitted with chest pain and a suspected myocardial infarct. His general health is reasonable, but he has developed severe night sweats and has lost 7 kg over the last 3 months. He denies smoking cigarettes and does not have any previous history of chest problems.

On examination, he looked well. Pulse and BP were normal. There were no abnormal signs in the cardiac or respiratory system.

Investigations show his Hb was 220 g/L with PCV 0.58, WCC $20 \times 10^9/L$ and platelets $600 \times 10^9/L$. Lactate dehydrogenase (LDH) was 740 U/L.

THESE TWO CASES BOTH HAVE ELEVATED HB BUT IS THEIR CAUSE THE SAME?

Haemoglobin (in red blood cells [RBCs]) is required for oxygen transport and, like most things, too much Hb has serious consequences and needs appropriate management (Fig. 11.3).

How to visualise the Hb level:

- Hb is expressed as a concentration, that is, g/L blood, but blood = plasma + solids (RBCs mainly). Thus Hb level must be related to the level of the plasma

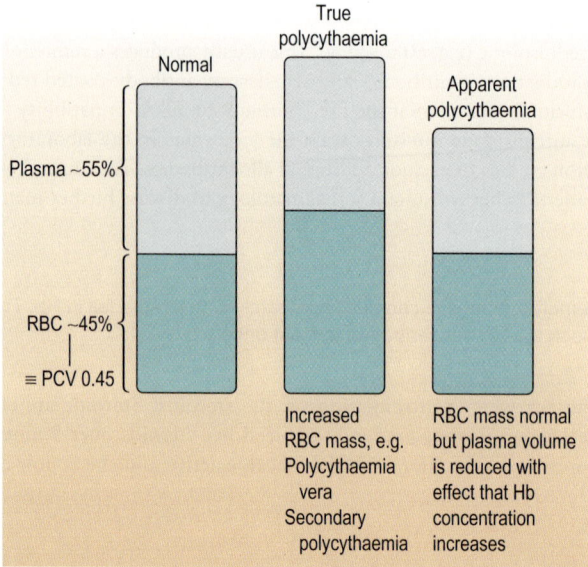

Fig. 11.3 Alteration of haemoglobin in relation to plasma. PCV, Packed cell volume; RBC, red blood cells.

PRELIMINARY MANAGEMENT

- Ensure that there are no hyperviscosity symptoms or signs:
  - Confusion
  - Visual disturbance
  - Peripheral circulatory disturbance
- Ensure that the patient is adequately hydrated
- Treat infection (if present)
- Identify correctable causes, for example, chronic hypoxia

Having made sure that the patients are stable, the next step is to determine the cause of the high Hb concentration. Before carrying out extensive investigation, it is sensible to contact the haematology team, who will either advise on further tests or take over each patient's care.

INFORMATION

Conditions in Which Hb Might Be High

- Primary proliferative polycythaemia (polycythaemia vera [PV])
- Secondary to an underlying hypoxic state: raised Hb serves a purpose:
  - Chronic lung disease
  - Cyanotic heart disease
- Inappropriately high level of Epo production: raised Hb serves no purpose:
  - Renal cell carcinoma
  - Uterine tumours
  - Cerebellar haemangioblastoma
- Relative/apparent polycythaemia:
  - Where the plasma component is reduced with the effect that Hb concentration rises, for example, dehydration, associated with obesity, hypertension, diuretics, smoking

---

The haematology registrar advises you to arrange some investigative tests.

INVESTIGATIONS

- Repeat FBC (to check that the result is correct or that the Hb has normalised with some oral/IV fluid).
- Biochemistry screen: renal function – is it normal? Uric acid – might be high in some types of polycythaemia
- Blood film: these patients had elevated platelets and WCC – make sure these are normal peripheral blood cells, with no evidence of leukaemia
- Presence of *JAK2* mutation (see Remember box)
- Bone marrow (see Remember box)
- Erythropoietin levels (normal or low in PV)

REMEMBER

Criteria for Polycythaemia Vera

Modified from revised WHO criteria.

Major Criteria

- Haemoglobin >185 g/L in men, >165 g/L in females or other evidence of increased red cell volume
- Presence of *JAK2* tyrosine kinase V617F or other functionally similar mutation, for example, *JAK2* exon 12

Minor Criteria

- Bone marrow biopsy, showing hypercellularity for age with tri-lineage growth (panmyelosis) with prominent erythroid, granulocytic and megakaryocytic proliferation
- Serum Epo level below the reference range for normals
- Endogenous erythroid colony (EEC) formation in vitro*

Diagnosis requires the presence of both major criteria and one minor criterion, or the presence of the first major criterion together with two minor criteria.

---

*EEC is not routinely available, but colony formation in the absence of exogenous erythropoietin in vitro is 100% specific and sensitive in patients without previous treatment.

For Diagnosis of Secondary Cases

- Blood gases or pulse oximetry (the latter is painless and quite adequate to exclude hypoxia only)
- Chest X-ray: emphysema, other lung pathologies
- Abdominal ultrasound: is the spleen enlarged? Remember renal and uterine causes of polycythaemia
- Bone marrow: not diagnostic in isolation but gives additional information
- Erythropoietin levels raised

Note: It is not necessary to carry out blood viscosity and red cell volume studies.

CLASSIC FEATURES OF POLYCYTHAEMIA VERA

- Weight loss, sweats, pruritus (itching is typically much more pronounced after a warm bath) (Fig. 11.4 shows erythromelalgia)
- High Hb and perhaps raised WCC + platelets
- Splenomegaly ± hepatomegaly
- Other causes (e.g. hypoxia) excluded
- Increased red cell mas
- Plasma volume normal

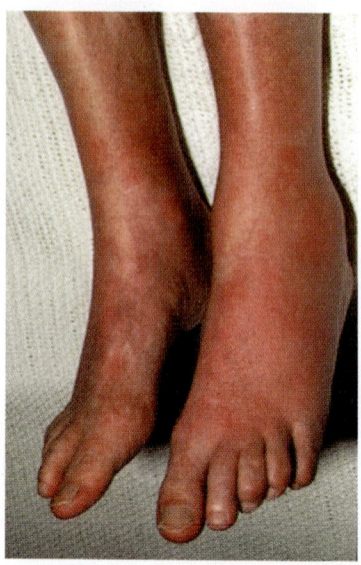

Fig. 11.4 Erythromelalgia of the toes. This is a painful complication in which the skin becomes suffused and red, as in this patient.

SECONDARY POLYCYTHAEMIA

- As for PV, but generally with no hepatosplenomegaly and no thrombocytosis
- Usually, a secondary cause is found, for example, cyanotic heart disease, lung disease, renal disease

APPARENT (OR RELATIVE) POLYCYTHAEMIA

- Red cell mass normal
- Reduced plasma volume
- No hepatosplenomegaly

MANAGEMENT AND PROGRESS

This is where knowledge of the underlying cause becomes crucial.

Your FIRST Patient Has Secondary Polycythaemia Due to Lung Disease

This is a physiological rise in Hb. Reducing the Hb to normal could have serious consequences because the rise in Hb is a compensatory mechanism.

The initial aim is to reduce the Hb to a safe level. Generally, this is achieved by venesection (removal of ~400–500 mL blood) every 2 days. In males the PCV is reduced to <0.5 and in females to <0.45.

All cases of secondary polycythaemia should be treated with venesection and treatment of the underlying cause, if possible. This patient's raised Hb was due to chronic lung disease, with the high Hb due to hypoxia.

Your SECOND Patient Has Polycythaemia Vera

(See Remember box above.)

- Venesect 400–500 mL weekly

- Then control marrow activity with hydroxycarbamide
- Use targeted therapy with *JAK1* and *JAK2* agonists in patients who do not respond to first-line therapy

LONG-TERM COMPLICATIONS

Up to 30% of patients with PV will develop intense marrow fibrosis and 5% develop acute myeloid leukaemia (AML). The other polycythaemias do not transform.

Elevated White Blood Cell Count

CASE HISTORY

A 17-year-old male who has ulcerative colitis was admitted to the medical assessment unit (MAU) because he felt unwell with a headache, sore throat and a temperature. He had also developed diarrhoea, but there was no blood in the stools. He was not on steroids but was on azathioprine 100 mg daily.

On examination, his tonsils were enlarged and inflamed; he had palatal petechiae and cervical lymphadenopathy.

Investigations showed an Hb of 124 g/L, MCV 98 fL and WCC 16×10^9/L with abnormal lymphocytes in the peripheral blood. A Monospot test is positive.

Diagnosis: Infectious mononucleosis.

There are many causes of a raised WCC (Box 11.1), and there is overlap with haematological malignancies, many of which present with WCC elevation. As a nonspecialist confronted with a patient who has an elevated WCC, the key question for you is: does this elevation represent a haematological malignancy or is it reflecting some other process?

A thorough history and examination will usually allow you to determine the cause of the elevated WCC. 'Alert' features suggesting a possible malignant cause include:

- Ill patients
- Those with bleeding/bruising
- Fever
- Enlargement of liver or spleen, or lymphadenopathy
- Weight loss
- Lymphocytes or bizarre/abnormal cells on blood film

BOX 11.1 ■ Causes of High White Blood Cell Counts

Patients With Haematological Malignancies Likely to Have High WCC

- Acute myeloid leukaemia
- Acute lymphoblastic leukaemia
- Chronic lymphocytic leukaemia
- Chronic myeloid leukaemia
- Lymphoma
- Other infiltrations: myeloma, myelofibrosis

Situations in Which a Reactive High WCC Occurs

- Infection
- Corticosteroid therapy
- Brisk GI tract bleeding
- 'Stress', for example, postoperative
- Post splenectomy

GI, Gastrointestinal; WCC, white cell count.

IS IT GLANDULAR FEVER OR ACUTE LEUKAEMIA?

The atypical lymphocytes seen in this patient with infectious mononucleosis can be confused with leukaemic blasts because the lymphocytes are large, often have nucleoli and resemble lymphoblasts. Specific tests, such as the Monospot, help confirm the diagnosis of infectious mononucleosis. In general, the haematology department will advise on further investigation, for example, cell marker analysis to exclude leukaemia.

Progress. This patient quickly improved, with no significant flare-up of his colitis. He was sent home after 72 hours, continuing on azathioprine.

REMEMBER

If in doubt, contact haematology. Early intervention in a patient with acute leukaemia is advised, and if you are not confident that the WCC rise is 'benign', seek expert help. There is less urgency if there is:

- A patient who is obviously well
- Isolated WCC only (Hb/platelets normal)
- Obvious infection
- Simple neutrophilia

Elevated Platelet Count

CASE HISTORY

A 75-year-old female was admitted with acute ischaemia of the toes in both feet.

On examination, she was found to have dusky skin on both feet, with evidence of early gangrene in the toes. Full blood count showed normal Hb, WCC 18×10^9/L (neutrophilia) and platelet count 1500×10^9/L.

Other significant features in this patient:
- Evidence of weight loss
- Splenomegaly 4 cm below the costal margin

You need to decide whether the marked elevation of the platelet count is likely to be *reactive* to some underlying process/disorder, or whether she has a *primary* marrow disorder because the management is dictated by the underlying cause.

WHY DOES THE PLATELET COUNT RISE IN A REACTIVE MANNER?

In simplistic terms, any acute stress (bleeding, operative surgery, severe infection) causes intense marrow activity with elevation of white cells and platelets in a nonspecific way.

Reactive thrombocytosis does not usually exceed 1000×10^9/L, whereas primary thrombocytosis is often >1000×10^9/L, but does not rely on platelet count alone. A reactive thrombocythaemia will resolve when the underlying problem, for example, infection, is treated.

IMMEDIATE ACTION

- Contact the haematologist
- Check end organs – are they threatened?
- Look at the fundi: vascular occlusion?
- Extremities: too late at this point because there is vascular damage to the feet in this patient
- Renal function.

- Is there a secondary (reactive) cause?
- Infection
- Bleeding
- Malignancy (breast, lung, bowel)
- Autoimmune rheumatic diseases

If none is obvious, check again for splenomegaly, as was found in this case.

If platelets are raised and there is splenomegaly, then the cause is likely to be a myeloproliferative disorder.

Diagnosis. This patient has a myeloproliferative disorder.

IS THERE A TEST THAT WILL CONFIRM A PRIMARY BONE MARROW PATHOLOGY?

Unfortunately not. The *JAK2* tyrosine kinase mutation is present in only 50% of cases (see PV). Bone marrow trephine biopsy can help because increases in the numbers of megakaryocytes (the cells that make platelets; Fig. 11.5) with clustering favour a diagnosis of essential thrombocythaemia (ET), but often it is a diagnosis of exclusion. Blood film examination may show marked variation in size and shape of the platelets (platelet anisocytosis; Fig. 11.6) in primary thrombocythaemia – but this is not diagnostic.

INFORMATION

Myeloproliferative Disorders Associated With Thrombocytosis

- Primary (essential) thrombocythaemia
- Polycythaemia vera
- Chronic myeloid leukaemia (CML)
- Myelofibrosis

MANAGEMENT

- Low-dose aspirin 75–200 mg/day (or dipyridamole if aspirin contraindicated)
- Plateletpheresis (using cell separator) if organ function is threatened and a rapid reduction in platelet count is needed
- Oral hydroxycarbamide to suppress bone marrow production of platelets (but beware of neutropenia if the dose is too high). Anagrelide and busulfan can also be used

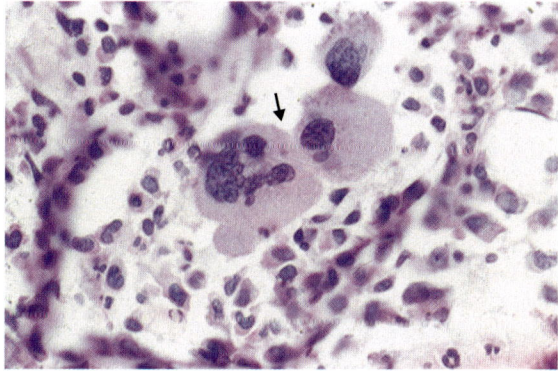

Fig. 11.5   Bone marrow in essential thrombocythaemia: clusters of megakaryocytes (from which platelets bud off) are seen in the centre of the field (*arrow*).

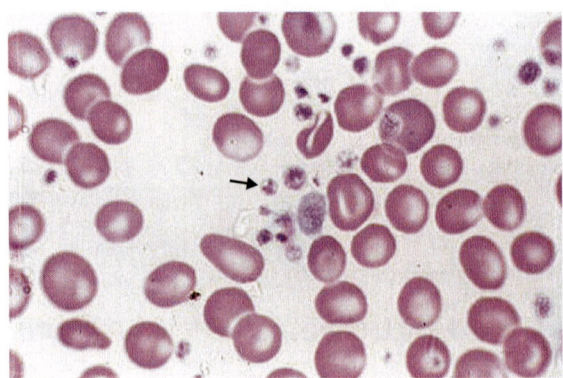

Fig. 11.6 Large numbers of platelets (small purple cells, arrow) in the blood film of a patient with essential thrombocythaemia.

COMPLICATIONS

■ Primary thrombocythaemia: generally indolent course but might transform to polycythaemia myelofibrosis in approximately 5% (occasionally transforms to AML)

Progress. This patient was referred to the vascular surgery department, which carried out Doppler and duplex imaging of her peripheral arteries but found no lesion amenable to surgery.

Platelet Disorders

CASE HISTORY (1)

You are asked to see a 24-year-old female who is in the emergency department. She has presented with petechiae scattered over her body. The doctor has found that she has a platelet count of 10×10^9/L. This female seems very well and tells you that she has had the petechiae for at least a week. She has no other symptoms. She is on the contraceptive pill but is taking no other tablets. She does not smoke and drinks wine (6 units) at the weekend only.

On examination, she has petechiae over her trunk, arms and legs. She has no other abnormal signs.

INVESTIGATIONS

You note the platelet count and also that all the other parameters in her blood count are normal. She also has a normal routine biochemistry.

REMEMBER

Meningococcal septicaemia has a purpuric rash and/or petechiae.

There are multiple causes of thrombocytopenia (Box 11.2). Thrombocytopenia may be the presentation of another disorder rather than a primary platelet disorder. All patients with severe thrombocytopenia (defined as $<20 \times 10^9$/L, which produces spontaneous haemorrhage) require admission for investigation/treatment.

BOX 11.2 ■ Causes of Thrombocytopenia

Failure of Platelet Production

Marrow Aplasia

METABOLIC DEFECTS
- Vitamin B_{12}/folate deficiency
- Uraemia
- Alcohol excess
- Liver disease

Drugs
- Chemotherapy ± radiation

Marrow Infiltration
- Leukaemia
- Lymphoma
- Myeloma
- Myelofibrosis
- Carcinoma

Decreased Platelet Survival

Immune
- Immune thrombocytopenic purpura (ITP)
- Systemic lupus erythematosus (SLE)
- Chronic lymphocytic leukaemia (CLL)
- Hodgkin lymphoma
- Drug-related

Infection
- Malaria
- Virus infection

Consumption
- DIC
- Extracorporeal circulation
- Haemolytic uraemic syndrome (HUS)
- Thrombotic thrombocytopenic purpura (TTP)

Loss From Circulation
- Splenomegaly
- Massive transfusion

DIC, Disseminated intravascular coagulation.

REMEMBER

The list of causes (Box 11.2) is not comprehensive and excludes inherited thrombocytopenia or causes that would present in childhood.

QUESTIONS THAT NEED TO BE ANSWERED IMMEDIATELY

- Does this patient have immune thrombocytopenic purpura (ITP)? Normal Hb, normal WCC, no hepatosplenomegaly or lymphadenopathy
- Does she have acute leukaemia? High WCC, abnormal white cells on film, lymphadenopathy, hepatosplenomegaly (occasionally)
- Does she have aplastic anaemia? Low Hb, low WCC, no lymphadenopathy, no hepatosplenomegaly

The **diagnosis** appears to be **ITP**. You are called back to see the patient 20 minutes later, as she has had a massive haematemesis. You think the diagnosis is ITP because there are no other features to make you think it is aplastic anaemia or acute leukaemia.

Major bleeding in ITP is not common but can be a serious complication. Treatment approaches should be decided by a haematologist.

MANAGEMENT FOR THIS PATIENT

- Adequate and secure IV access
- ABO and Rh(D) group and cross-match six units of blood
- Fluid and blood replacement as appropriate
- Start high-dose IV immunoglobulin infusion
- Platelet transfusion: 2 units immediately
- Oral prednisolone: 0.5–2 mg/kg daily

Progress. She had no further haematemesis and her platelet count rose to $50 \times 10^9/L$ on day five but remained at that level. After discussion, she was referred for splenectomy, which produced a good response in her platelet count.

LEARNING POINTS

- High-dose immunoglobulin elevates the platelet count by macrophage Fc receptor blockade of the reticuloendothelial system
- Endogenous platelets usually rise after 24–48 hours; the survival of exogenous platelets is improved
- Platelet transfusion is usually not necessary in ITP, except in the situation of life-threatening haemorrhage, such as in this case
- Seventy-five percent of patients respond to oral steroids, but the full therapeutic effect may take 2–4 weeks to develop

REMEMBER

Thrombocytopenic purpura might become chronic and might require long-term treatment ± splenectomy. Romiplostim and eltrombopag, thrombopoietin receptor agonists, are used if splenectomy has no effect.

CASE HISTORY (2)

You are asked to see a 50-year-old male on a surgical ward, who has come into hospital for an elective hernia repair. He is found on a routine preoperative FBC to have a platelet count of $90 \times 10^9/L$. His Hb and WCC count are normal.

This chronic presentation of mild thrombocytopenia is reasonably common. To establish the cause, you should systematically go through the causes of thrombocytopenia from an initial clinical history and examination.

CAN HE GO AHEAD AND HAVE HIS HERNIA REPAIR?

It might take a while to get to the bottom of his thrombocytopenia. Elective surgery can be performed, as the platelet count is $>80 \times 10^9/L$.

Avoid any NSAIDs as postoperative analgesia; make sure aspirin has not been taken within the last 10 days.

This male was discharged following a successful surgical repair, and 1 week later, his platelet count was 96×10^9/L. By 1 month the platelet count was normal. No clear reason for the thrombocytopenia was found but a **viral cause** seemed the most likely.

CASE HISTORY (3)

A 28-year-old female has had a dilation and curettage (D and C) for long-standing menorrhagia. It is now 5 days after the procedure, and she is still bleeding. She has been back in theatre and no local defect has been found. She says she had problems in the past with bleeding after dental extractions. Her prothrombin time (PT), activated partial thromboplastin time (APTT) and platelet count are normal.

DIAGNOSIS

This is the typical picture of an **inherited platelet disorder**. Severe platelet function disorders present in childhood, but milder versions do not usually present until surgery in adulthood. Clues here are bleeding after dental extraction and long-standing menorrhagia.

MANAGEMENT

Assess the extent of bleeding. Treatment options include:
- Tranexamic acid 1 g × 3 daily if mild bleeding
- Platelet transfusion if severe bleeding

In a classic platelet function disorder, the bleeding time is prolonged, but this test is difficult to perform. If you suspect a platelet function disorder, organise platelet function studies with your haematological laboratory.

Progress. This patient stopped bleeding following a platelet transfusion. She was referred to the haematology department for follow-up.

Bleeding Disorders

These can be due to inherited or acquired causes. They are due to haemolysis (either intra- or extravascular) or disorders of coagulation. Always take a good history and use your common sense, as illustrated in the case here.

CASE HISTORY (1)

You are phoned by a surgical specialist registrar, who is asking for your advice. He has just finished a bilateral hernia repair on a 50-year-old male and the right side is bleeding briskly. The patient has required a transfusion with 2 units of blood in the last 30 min. The surgeon tells you that the surgery has gone well and wants you to sort out his clotting.

WHAT DO YOU THINK ABOUT THIS CASE?

This patient is most likely to be **bleeding from a surgical cause**: 2 units in 30 minutes is far in excess of what you would expect to give in a patient with a clotting disorder, and he is bleeding from only one of the repair sites, not both. Best to advise the registrar to find the bleeding vessel!

Although this might seem like a somewhat silly example, it shows that not all bleeding is due to abnormal clotting. Look at the whole picture before jumping in with fresh frozen plasma (FFP).

INHERITED BLEEDING DISORDERS

You are far more likely to see acquired bleeding disorders than inherited ones. Inherited disorders are uncommon, but must be identified.

> **REMEMBER**
>
> Management of inherited disorders is complex: always seek specialist support.

HOW CAN I IDENTIFY THE INHERITED DISORDERS?

Most inherited disorders of any severity present in childhood, and hence most, if not all, patients will be able to tell you about their problem. They should carry a medical card with them, identifying the problem and their haematology consultant. It should be easy to sort out these patients and get in touch with the appropriate specialist. Always take any suggestion of an inherited bleeding disorder seriously (Figs. 11.7 and 11.8).

HOW CAN I IDENTIFY MILDER FORMS?

Milder inherited disorders might not present until later in life and usually do so after surgery or other interventions.

ACQUIRED BLEEDING DISORDERS

As mentioned, these are far more common than inherited problems and are usually seen in particular clinical settings. These common scenarios will be outlined later. Most acquired disorders involve multiple and complex defects of coagulation.

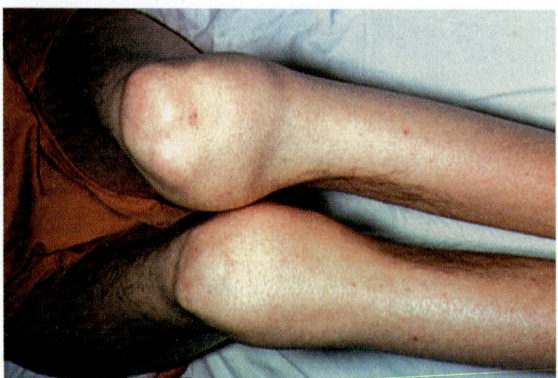

Fig. 11.7   Gross arthritis in a patient with haemophilia (inherited factor VIII or IX deficiency).

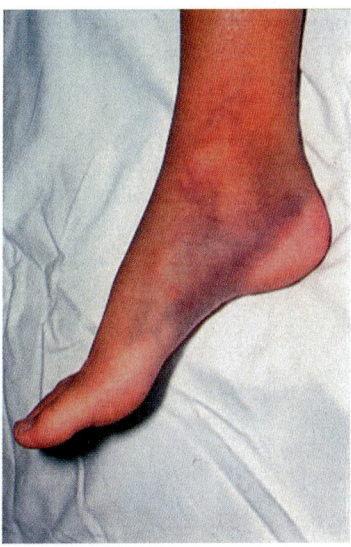

Fig. 11.8 This patient with haemophilia A has bled into his foot (note the *discoloration* of the foot below the medial malleolus).

INVESTIGATION OF A SUSPECTED BLEEDING DISORDER

Should I Check the Clotting in Everyone Who Bleeds?

Probably, although this is not absolutely necessary; however, it is best to have a low threshold. A normal set of results might help you be more secure that you are not overlooking something. Remember, though, always to take a full history and family history to try to identify any underlying inherited coagulation defect. For example, if a patient:

- Had excessive bleeding after a previous haemostatic challenge such as:
  - Operation
  - Dental extraction
  - Trauma
- Needed a previous blood transfusion for bleeding
- Gave a family history of bleeding
- Frequent epistaxis and/or easy bruising

WHAT SHOULD I REQUEST?

You request a basic coagulation screen:

- Full blood time to check platelet count
- Prothrombin time (PT)
- Activated partial thromboplastin time (APTT)

REMEMBER

Even a 2-second prolongation might indicate an inherited clotting problem of significance and should be investigated more fully.

These are the minimum number of tests to start with. If you really want to check that a clotting disorder exists, then the following should also be performed:

- Fibrinogen level
- Thrombin time (TT)

These tests form your baseline investigations or screening tests.

Acquired disorders are relatively easy because clotting times are usually notably prolonged.

There is a whole range of specialist investigations for the complete study of a coagulation disorder: it is best to seek specialist advice.

CASE HISTORY (2)

You are called to see a patient in the emergency department who is bleeding excessively from a dental extraction. The doctor thinks that the patient has liver disease and asks you for some help. There is nothing in the history to indicate what the liver problem might be, and the patient denies excess alcohol consumption.

On examination, you notice spider naevi, liver palms and splenomegaly. You agree that the excess bleeding is probably due to liver disease.

BLEEDING IN LIVER DISEASE

This causes widespread coagulation and bleeding problems. Always be aware that significant liver dysfunction can result in a potentially severe bleeding disorder. The components of liver-related bleeding are:

- Reduced synthesis of coagulation factors: the liver is the source of all coagulation factors (apart from factor VIII)
- Associated vitamin K deficiency: coagulation proteins might be synthesised but will not be active because of vitamin K deficiency
- Thrombocytopenia: frequently secondary to splenomegaly from portal hypertension
- Chronic low-grade disseminated intravascular coagulation (DIC)
- Abnormal fibrinogen synthesis: in liver disease, excess sialic acid residues are added to fibrinogen and hence an acquired dysfibrinogenaemia occurs

The classic laboratory defects would be:

- Prothrombin time prolonged due to decrease in factor II, V, VII or X
- Activated partial thromboplastin time prolonged due to decrease in all factors
- Thrombin time prolonged due to abnormal fibrinogen
- Fibrinogen degradation products (FDPs) increased (due to failure to remove from circulation ± chronic DIC)

INFORMATION

Causes of Vitamin K Deficiency

- Biliary obstruction
- Oral warfarin anticoagulant
- Liver disease
- Malabsorption states
- Inflammatory bowel diseases (with ileal resection)

MANAGEMENT

- Give 10 mg vitamin K daily IV for 3 days
- For acute bleeding, give 10–20 mL/kg FFP to replace all coagulation proteins
- If the fibrinogen level is low or TT prolonged, give cryoprecipitate to supply fibrinogen

Progress. This patient's bleeding stopped with help from the dental surgeons. The patient has been referred to the liver clinic for investigation and management of his chronic liver disease.

CASE HISTORY (3)

A 49-year-old male has been on treatment for hypertension for years. His renal function has gradually deteriorated, despite reasonable control of his blood pressure (now 130/80), stopping smoking and taking statin therapy (his present cholesterol level is 3.2 mmol/L).

His glomerular filtration rate (GFR) is 32 mL/min/1.73m². He has recently suffered from bruising around his upper arms and shins.

DIAGNOSIS: CHRONIC KIDNEY DISEASE

Anyone with significantly impaired renal function can have an acquired bleeding disorder. The major cause is toxic metabolites impairing platelet function, as is the case in this patient.

IS THE APTT OR PT ABNORMAL IN RENAL DISEASE?

No. As mentioned, the major defect is an acquired platelet disorder. The clotting times are usually normal.

SHOULD THE BLEEDING TIME BE MEASURED REGULARLY IN PATIENTS WITH RENAL DISEASE?

No, but remember that renal disease is a cause of an acquired bleeding disorder, and if you are planning surgery on the patient, there might be a bleeding problem.

WHAT CAN WE DO IN RENAL DISEASE?

There are several approaches to treatment, but sorting out the renal problem first is the best option. Dialysis will improve platelet function; this is why few stable dialysed/controlled patients actually bleed. The real risk group is those with a very high serum creatinine/urea.

Other treatments for bleeding include:
- Synthetic vasopressin analogue (desmopressin)
- Cryoprecipitate
- Platelet transfusion

These are all used in bleeding episodes.

Disseminated Intravascular Coagulation (DIC)

This is the most complex of the acquired bleeding disorders.

Disseminated intravascular coagulation is inappropriate and continued activation of coagulation leads ultimately to both bleeding and thrombosis.

The initial phase of DIC is thrombosis. This is why DIC is associated with end-organ damage leading to multiorgan failure.

REMEMBER

Disseminated intravascular coagulation is always secondary to some other major clinical problem.

Bleeding arises as a secondary phenomenon due to consumption of coagulation factors and platelets (caused by continued activation of clotting), and the activation of fibrinolysis (breaking down any fibrin that is laid down).

CASE HISTORY (1)

A 29-year-old male is brought to the trauma unit with severe injuries to his abdomen and legs as a result of a road traffic accident. Initial examination and CT scanning confirm that he has fractured both femurs and his pelvis. He has fluid in his abdomen on CT, suggesting internal organ damage.

He is resuscitated and taken to the intensive care unit (ICU), where he needs ventilation, volume replacement and cardiovascular support with inotropes. His leg fractures are stabilized, and he undergoes emergency laparotomy with resection of damaged small bowel. He initially improved, but then his renal and liver function deteriorated and he was diagnosed as having multiorgan failure. He was then noted to be bleeding from his laparotomy wound.

WHAT ACTION SHOULD YOU TAKE?

- Always think about DIC in a bleeding patient
- Try to make the diagnosis

WHAT ARE THE CAUSES OF DIC?

- Infection
- Obstetric complications (for females)
- Surgery
- Trauma
- Malignancy
- Liver disease
- Transfusion reactions

If someone is bleeding and you always think about DIC, you will not go wrong. In many ways, the long list of causes is academic when you first see the patient – but if they have DIC, you must identify the cause.

HOW DO YOU MAKE THE DIAGNOSIS?

Send off all the screening tests and FDPs. The pattern is:
- Platelets low: consumption
- Prothrombin time prolonged: consumption
- Activated partial thromboplastin time prolonged: consumption
- Thrombin time prolonged: consumption of fibrinogen and FDPs
- Fibrinogen low: consumption
- Fibrinogen degradation products high: breakdown of fibrin

Why Are FDPs Measured?

Fibrinogen degradation products tell you that fibrin is being broken down. The most specific test is the D-dimer, which tells you that cross-linked fibrinogen has formed and has then been broken down.

HOW DO YOU MANAGE DIC?

- Treat the underlying disorder
- Treat the underlying disorder!

- Treat the underlying disorder!!
- Support with FFP, cryoprecipitate and platelets

You must aim to treat the underlying disorder! DIC is always secondary. As mentioned, it is due to inappropriate and continued activation of clotting. Until you stop this by treating the underlying problem, it will not get better.

Blood component therapy is purely supportive. Give:

- 10–20 mL/kg FFP + cryoprecipitate
- Platelets
- Blood as required

Aim to restore the fibrinogen concentration to normal and the PT/APTT to within 4 s of normal.

Progress. Despite all efforts, the patient died.

CASE HISTORY (2)

A 50-year-old patient has carcinoma of the lung with a prolonged PT, APTT, TT, low fibrinogen and platelet count, and high FDPs, but he is not bleeding.

DOES THIS PATIENT HAVE DIC?

This is the picture of subclinical DIC – laboratory abnormalities but no bleeding. It is seen in chronic DIC, for example, in liver disease or malignancy. DIC ranges from florid bleeding to abnormalities that are picked up only by laboratory testing.

ANTICOAGULANT OVERDOSAGE

An obvious cause of bleeding. Do not forget to look for warfarin/heparin usage.

ACTION

Confirm anticoagulant overdosage by finding a prolonged PT (warfarin) or APTT (heparin). The treatment of bleeding depends on the problem, but in essence:

If Due to Warfarin: STOP WARFARIN

- Minor bleeding: if international normalised ratio (INR) >6.0. Restart warfarin when INR < 5.0; check INR daily. If INR > 8.0, give vitamin K 2.5 mg oral or 0.5 mg IV
- Major bleeding: give prothrombin complex concentrate 50 units/kg or FFP 15 mL/kg, give vitamin K 5 mg IV

If Due to Heparin: STOP HEPARIN

If bleeding is excessive or uncontrolled:

- Protamine reversal (1 mg IV neutralises 100 units of heparin – maximum dose 50 mg). Protamine only partially reverses low-molecular-weight heparin (LMWH)
- Seek advice
- Heparin excess will correct in a few hours

Surgical Cause

Suspect if there is rapid blood loss at operation. Do not underestimate the number of times this is forgotten and people chase a medical cause for bleeding when a vessel has a hole in it.

If you have a hole in a vessel, bleeding will not stop until the hole is fixed, however, good the coagulation system is.

> **REMEMBER**
>
> Surgical and medical bleeding might coexist. If you correct the coagulation and the patient is still bleeding, think surgical, whatever the surgeon says!

Thrombosis

CASE HISTORY (1)

You are asked to see a 24-year-old female who has had a life-threatening pulmonary embolus (PE). She received fibrolytic therapy on the intensive care unit (ICU). Her condition stabilised and she is now on warfarin following initial treatment with LMW heparin. She wants to know why she has had a PE. She has a family history of deep vein thrombosis (DVT).

ARE INVESTIGATIONS INDICATED?

Thrombosis is common but relatively uncommon under the age of 45 years unless there is a precipitating event. In such patients with a family history, about 50% have a definable underlying prothrombotic state. It is well worth investigating her formally for a prothrombotic state.

Attempt to identify any precipitating event, such as:

- Taking the combined oral contraceptive pill
- Immobility and/or recent surgery/fracture/injury
- Long-haul flight
- Obesity
- Malignancy

SHOULD SHE BE INVESTIGATED NOW OR LATER?

She is on warfarin, which can interfere with thrombotic investigations. Identifying an underlying thrombotic state acutely will not change the immediate management.

> **REMEMBER**
>
> - An abnormal result after an acute thrombosis does not mean an abnormality genuinely exists
> - It must be rechecked
> - However, a normal result is normal

She is on warfarin, so formal studies must be delayed. Refer her to a specialist for follow-up and investigation.

WHAT INVESTIGATIONS WILL BE REQUESTED AFTER STOPPING WARFARIN?

INVESTIGATIONS

- Lupus anticoagulant
- Antiphospholipid antibody
- Protein C deficiency
- Protein S deficiency
- Antithrombin deficiency
- Factor V Leiden
- 3′ prothrombin UTR variant
- *JAK2* mutation

These aim to look for an inherited deficiency of natural anticoagulants, mutations leading to increased thrombin generation or acquired causes of a prothrombotic state.

Progress. This patient has factor Leiden deficiency. She is referred to a specialist for long-term follow-up, counselling and family studies.

CASE HISTORY (2)

You are asked to see a 70-year-old male who had a DVT after a knee replacement, despite DVT prophylaxis. He has no family history of venous thrombosis. At present, he is on rivaroxaban 10 mg daily for 3 months.

SHOULD HE BE INVESTIGATED FOR THROMBOPHILIA?

No! At this age and in this setting, it is likely that a DVT has been precipitated by the surgery. The pick-up rate for a significant thrombotic disorder is very low in this setting. When asked to assess the thrombotic status, balance the likelihood of finding a defect against the value of identifying the exact defect.

CASE HISTORY (3)

You are called to see a 45-year-old male who is being anticoagulated for acute iliofemoral vein thrombosis with heparin. His APTT remains normal on 28,000 units of heparin per 24 h. The dose of heparin has been progressively increased over the last 3 days, but his leg swelling is worse.

WHAT DO YOU ADVISE?

The target APTT for heparin for an acute thrombosis is 1.5 to 2.5 times the mid-point of the NR. The most common reasons for failure are:
- Undermonitoring
- Underdosing
- Not actually receiving dose of heparin prescribed

ACTION

- Ensure prescribed dose is being given
- Increase dose by 10% per 24 hours (always check local guidelines)
- Recheck APTT in 4 hours
- If still low, repeat 10% increase in heparin dose and recheck at 4-hourly intervals

Heparin monitoring is notoriously bad in most hospitals. If IV heparin is being used, it should be monitored as per local guidelines, for example:

- Check APTT every 4 hours until target reached
- Increase dose in 10% increments
- Once target APTT reached, repeat at 4 h
- If APTT is stable, repeat 12-hourly

REMEMBER

- Outcome is dependent on the effectiveness of anticoagulation within the first 48 h
- Heparin resistance is rare, poor heparin control is very common

FOR HOW LONG SHOULD A PATIENT WITH VENOUS THROMBOEMBOLIC DISEASE BE ANTICOAGULATED WITH WARFARIN?

The duration and target INRs for various thrombotic conditions are listed in Table 11.1.

Recurrent venous thromboembolism (VTE) is essentially two or more events. The more events there are, the greater the likelihood of recurrence.

Long-term anticoagulation carries the risk of major haemorrhage (4% per annum) and death (~0.5% per annum). These must be balanced against recurrence prevention. Complications are far more common in older patients.

Recurrence is much higher in patients anticoagulated for 6 weeks rather than 6 months.

REMEMBER

- Drug interactions with warfarin
- Need to amend dosage in patients undergoing invasive procedures
- Regular anticoagulant clinic follow-up

TABLE 11.1 ■ Duration and Target INRs for Thrombotic Conditions

Condition	Duration	INR Target
Uncomplicated DVT	6 months	2.5
Complex DVT	6 months	2.5
Pulmonary embolus	6 months	2.5
Recurrent VTE	Indefinite	2.5; if the recurrent event occurs while taking warfarin, the intensity of anticoagulation is increased to a target of 3.5
Atrial fibrillation	Indefinite	2.5
Mechanical heart valves	Indefinite	3.5

DVT, Deep vein thrombosis; INR, international normalised ratio; VTE, venous thromboembolism.

Thrombosis and the Antiphospholipid Syndrome

CASE HISTORY

A 25-year-old female presents with a 2-day history of left leg swelling, and on the day of admission, she notices breathlessness and chest pains that are worse on deep inspiration.

In her past medical history, you find that she has had three miscarriages and one successful pregnancy. This pregnancy was complicated by hypertension and intra-uterine growth retardation, with a premature delivery at 31 weeks. On further questioning, you note that she has had oral ulceration, with rashes that are worse in the sunlight and has also been having headaches.

Drug history: she is on the oral contraceptive pill.

On examination, she has extensive splinter haemorrhages on most fingers. Her pulse is 100 and BP 110/70, but she is not cyanosed. Her heart sounds are normal, but there is a soft murmur of mitral regurgitation. She also has a soft left pleural rub.

Abdominal examination and neurological examination are normal. The left calf is swollen and the calf circumference is 3 cm greater than on the right. You note extensive livedo reticularis on her arms, thighs and knees.

WHAT IS THE DIFFERENTIAL DIAGNOSIS AND WHAT INVESTIGATIONS ARE REQUIRED?

This young patient (who is on the oral contraceptive pill) is deemed to have a DVT and a PE until it is proved otherwise.

An FBC revealed thrombocytopenia, which is commonly seen in the anti-phospholipid syndrome.

INVESTIGATIONS

- Electrocardiogram (ECG): look for the classic (but seldom seen) S1, Q3, T3 pattern of PE
- Chest X-ray: likely to be normal. However, it is useful to exclude other causes of pleuritic chest pain, including infective causes
- Ultrasound scan of the leg veins: to document the extent of the left calf thrombosis
- A V̇/Q̇ scan: to show the extent of the pulmonary emboli: still useful
- Plasma D-dimers: if these are undetectable, the diagnosis of PE and DVT is excluded
- Multidetector CT with contrast: good specificity 96% and sensitivity 85% for medium-sized pulmonary emboli

Choose the imaging techniques according to local availability.

DIFFERENTIAL DIAGNOSIS

In this case, this includes the antiphospholipid syndrome with a DVT and pulmonary emboli, along with an increased risk of thrombosis from the oral contraceptive pill. The history is rather suggestive of systemic lupus erythematosus (SLE), and this should be investigated further with autoantibodies to antinuclear antibodies (ANA), DNA and extractable nuclear antigens (ENA) and complement studies. The features favouring a diagnosis of the antiphospholipid syndrome, in this case, would include the three previous miscarriages and one pregnancy complicated by intra-uterine growth retardation and premature delivery. There is accumulating evidence in the literature to suggest that intrauterine growth retardation is due to recurrent placental thrombosis and this is often manifested by reduced umbilical artery flow patterns on Doppler studies, with an increased resistance index, notching or even reversed flow in the umbilical vessels.

THE ANTIPHOSPHOLIPID SYNDROME

Anticardiolipin antibodies and the lupus anticoagulant should be measured. Both of these are antiphospholipid antibodies and both tests should be requested because a small percentage of patients have either one or the other antibody but not both. A thrombophilia screen can exclude other factors, including the factor V Leiden mutation. Patients with the antiphospholipid syndrome also have reduced protein C and S levels, which are associated with the lupus anticoagulant.

LIBMAN–SACKS ENDOCARDITIS

Splinter haemorrhages and a mitral murmur could indicate Libman-Sacks endocarditis, a feature of antiphospholipid syndrome and SLE. These patients have mucinous degeneration of the mitral valve leaflets, and occasionally thrombus (which might embolise) is seen on the damaged valves. Similarly, the damaged valves might become secondarily infected, leading to infective endocarditis. The splinter haemorrhages could represent microemboli and are a feature of both the antiphospholipid syndrome and infective endocarditis.

HOW WOULD YOU MANAGE THIS PATIENT?

This patient should be admitted and commenced on heparin. This can be given intravenously as a continuous infusion, but many hospitals use once-daily LMW heparin. Warfarin should be commenced, and the eventual target INR should be 2.5.

Progress. The diagnosis of the antiphospholipid syndrome was confirmed and therapy with life-long warfarin at the target INR was started. These patients are often resistant to warfarin and occasionally require high doses.

In terms of the mitral valve disease, the patient needed counselling about appropriate antibiotic therapy for any infection. Prophylactic antibiotics are not required. Infective endocarditis was excluded, and she was monitored regularly because a small percentage of these patients require mitral valve replacement.

Sickle-Cell Disease

CASE HISTORY

An 18-year-old female of African origin came to the emergency department with severe pains in her right leg, left hip, chest and back. She was well known to many of the staff, as she had attended on many occasions with **painful sickle crises.**

The examination should initially be brief until adequate pain control has been achieved.

INVESTIGATIONS

Performed in the MAU, and aimed at assessing the severity of the crisis and determining any treatable cause:

- Full blood count plus reticulocytes
- Urea and electrolytes
- Liver biochemistry
- Group and save
- Monitor pulse oximetry

Compare values with normal steady-state values, which should be in the patient's notes. Remember that many nucleated red cells can result in an erroneously high WCC count. Infection is a frequent precipitant of a painful crisis, if suspected send:

- Mid-stream urine (MSU)
- Blood cultures

QUESTIONS TO ASK PATIENTS PRESENTING WITH SICKLE-CELL CRISES

Distribution of Pain? Any Bone Tenderness?

- Lumbar back pain can be particularly severe
- Rib, sternal or thoracic vertebral pain can impair respiratory effort and predispose to the acute chest syndrome

Any Precipitating Factors?

- Exposure to cold/skin chilling (might apply to this patient)
- Dehydration (could also apply to this patient)
- Hypoxia
- Infection

INFORMATION

A low O_2 saturation might reflect acute lung pathology, for example, pneumonia or the acute chest syndrome, or chronic sickle cell-related lung damage.

Chest X-ray and arterial gases are indicated only if there is:

- Rib, sternal and thoracic vertebral pain
- Signs of consolidation
- Tachypnoea (>25/min)
- O_2 saturation <80% on air or <95% on maximal supplementary O_2

Any Fever?

- Fever ± leucocytosis can indicate an underlying infection but is also compatible with ischaemic tissue necrosis secondary to intravascular sickling alone

Any Hepatosplenomegaly?

- Splenomegaly is unusual in adults with sickle-cell anaemia (HbSS) or HbS/β^0 thalassaemia; splenic atrophy is more common
- A larger spleen than normal for the patient (ask the patient or parents/consult medical notes) might indicate acute splenic sequestration

Compliance With Hyposplenic Prophylaxis?

- Patients with HbSS and HbS/β^0 thalassaemia have severe hyposplenism and are susceptible to overwhelming sepsis, particularly with *Streptococcus pneumoniae*
- Prophylaxis includes penicillin V 500 mg × 2 daily and vaccination with polyvalent pneumococcal, Hib and meningococcal vaccines

TREATMENT OF ACUTE PAINFUL SICKLE-CELL CRISES

Analgesic Regime Examples

Morphine

- 0.1 mg/kg IV/SC every 20 min until pain is controlled, *then*
- 0.05–0.1 mg/kg IV/SC (or oral morphine) every 2–4 h
- Patient-controlled analgesia (PCA) when pain controlled

Note: Ask the patient about previous morphine dosages. Check medical records and discharge summaries. Higher doses may be required in cases who have previously received opioids.

Patient-Controlled Analgesia (PCA) (Example for Adults >50 kg)

Morphine

- Patient-controlled analgesia bolus dose: 1 mg
- Lockout time: 5 minutes

When setting up a PCA always follow local protocols. Other options include oxycodone and fentanyl. When parenteral opiates are used, the following parameters must be monitored regularly on an hourly basis:

- Pain score
- Respiratory rate
- O_2 saturation on air
- Analgesia consumption.

Adjuvant Oral Analgesia

- Paracetamol 1 g 6-hourly
- ± Ibuprofen* 400 mg 8-hourly
- *or* Diclofenac* 50 mg 8-hourly.

Other Adjuvants

- Antipruritics e.g:
  - Hydroxyzine 25 mg × 2 as required
- Antiemetics e.g:
  - Prochlorperazine 5–10 mg × 3 per day as required
  - Ondansetron 4–8 mg x 3 per day as required
- Cyclizine 50 mg × 3 per day as required
  - Laxatives, e.g. macrogol 1–2 sachets per day

> **REMEMBER**
>
> Failure to maintain oxygenation can:
> - Exacerbate the painful crisis
> - Indicate the development of the acute chest syndrome

Hydroxycarbamide is useful in increasing HbF. It should be prescribed by haematologists and often takes months to have an effect. It reduces the episodes of pain, the acute chest syndrome and the need for blood transfusions. The overall mortality has also been shown to be reduced.

Supportive Measures

- Keep warm: use heat pads
- Hydration: aim for 3 L/24 h – orally if possible

---

*Caution advised against using NSAIDs in renal impairment.

- Venous access is often very difficult in these patients; the repeated insertion of IV lines should be avoided to conserve peripheral veins
- Intravenous hydration is indicated if:
  - Nausea/vomiting is uncontrolled
  - The patient is sedated
  - The serum urea and creatinine are rising
- Oxygenation: aim for O_2 saturation 95%
- Monitor the Hb concentration daily and transfuse if it falls to 150 g/L. All transfused blood should be matched for minor blood group antigens Kell and Rh (c and e, as well as d antigens)

> **REMEMBER**
>
> Do not use transfusions in this steady-state anaemia, in an uncomplicated painful episode and for minor surgery.

THE ACUTE CHEST SYNDROME

Most painful sickle-cell crises resolve without complications within 7 to 10 days. Development of the acute chest syndrome is the most common cause of death in adults with sickle-cell disease.

The syndrome is characterised by:

- Rib, sternal and/or thoracic vertebral pain
- Bilateral basal chest signs with new infiltrates on CXR
- Tachypnoea
- Deteriorating oxygenation
- Falling Hb concentration
- Fever and leucocytosis

Pathophysiology of Acute Chest Syndrome

- Infection
- Fat embolism from necrotic bone marrow
- Pulmonary infarction due to sequestration of sickled red cells

Treatment of Acute Chest Syndrome

- Exchange blood transfusion to reduce the amount of HbS to <20%
- Maintenance of oxygenation: this might include, for example, continuous positive airway pressure (CPAP) via a tight-fitting mask, or intermittent positive pressure ventilation (IPPV).
- Aggressive pain relief
- Intravenous antibiotic therapy

The majority of patients with a sickle-cell crisis present with severe, acute bone pain secondary to ischaemic bone marrow necrosis. Beware the patient with sickle-cell disease who presents unwell but without pain. Such patients might have other, less common, complications of sickle-cell disease, which can progress very rapidly (Figs. 11.9 and 11.10).

> **REMEMBER**
>
> **Other Complications of Sickle-Cell Disease Include**
>
> - Pneumococcal septicaemia
> - Splenic sequestration
> - Erythrovirus infection associated with marrow aplasia
> - Acute folate deficiency

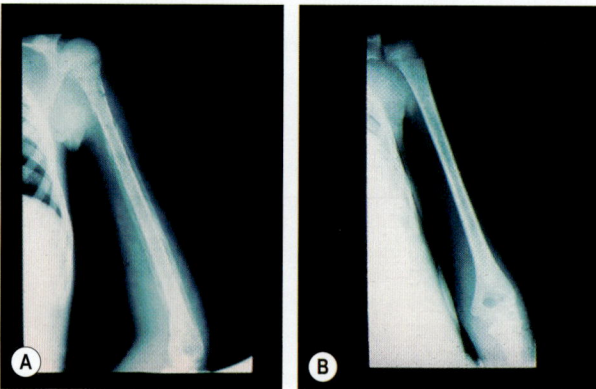

Fig 11.9   (A) Osteomyelitis of the humerus in a sickle patient (pretreatment). Note the elevation of the periosteum at the distal part of the humerus. (B) The same patient showing normal periosteum following treatment.

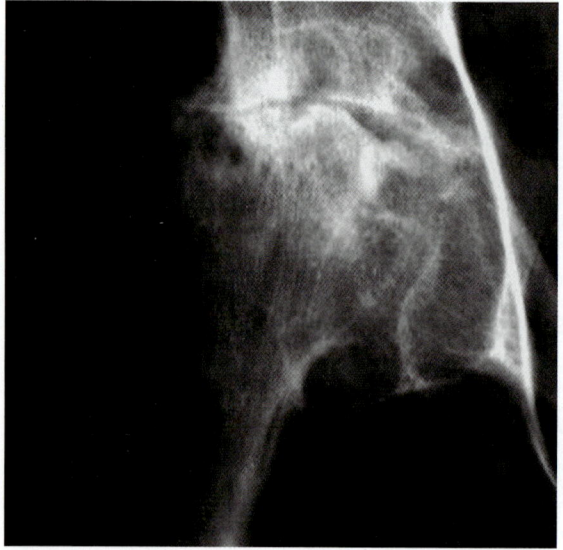

Fig. 11.10   Avascular necrosis of the femoral head in a patient with homozygous sickle-cell disease. There is a loss of joint space and distortion of the head of the femur and acetabulum.

Progress. This patient's current crisis was more severe than her previous ones and she went on to develop an acute chest syndrome requiring supplemental oxygenation.

Types of Sickle-Cell Disease

- Sickle-cell anaemia (HbSS)
- Sickle-cell–haemoglobin C disease (HbSC)
- Sickle-cell β-thalassaemia
- Rare compound heterozygotes, for example, HbSD

DIAGNOSIS IN THE EMERGENCY DEPARTMENT

- Information from patient
- Haemoglobinopathy card
- Blood count, reticulocyte count and blood film review
- Serum bilirubin
- Sickle solubility test (commercial kits are available)

Later:

- Hb electrophoresis (Fig. 11.11) on cellulose acetate membrane (CAM) at an alkaline pH, *or*
- High-performance liquid chromatography (HPLC)

Typically, the patient will be anaemic with evidence of haemolysis (elevated bilirubin and reticulocyte count). The blood film will show sickled red cells in variable numbers (Fig. 11.12). The

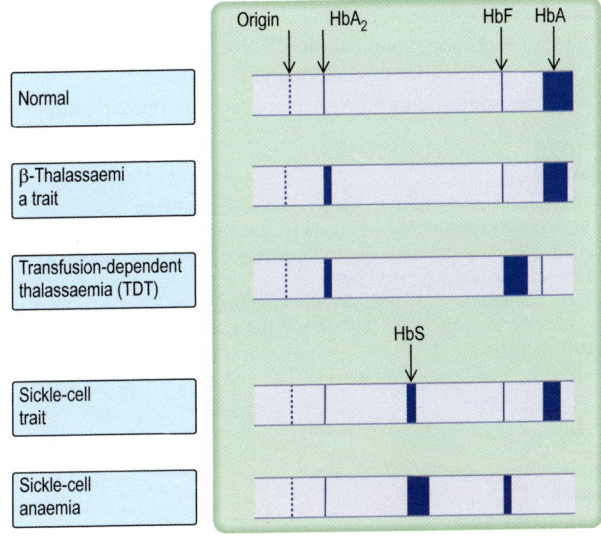

Fig. 11.11   Patterns of haemoglobin electrophoresis.

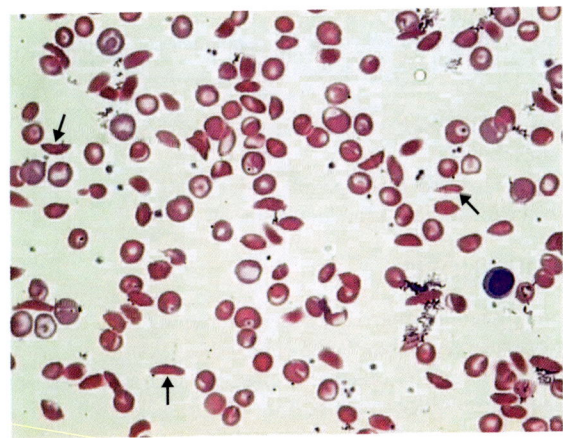

Fig. 11.12   Blood film in sickle-cell disease showing numerous sickle-shaped red cells (*arrows*).

sickle solubility test will be positive and CAM electrophoresis or HPLC will confirm the presence of HbS ± HbC or HbD with no HbA (except in HbS/β⁺ thalassaemia).

BEWARE

- In HbSC and HbS/β⁺ thalassaemia, the Hb concentration, reticulocyte count and serum bilirubin can be virtually normal
- The sickle solubility test is a qualitative test only and will be positive in any individual where the amount of HbS is >10%. This will include both sickle-cell trait and sickle-cell disease

Glucose-6-Phosphate Dehydrogenase Deficiency

DEFINITION

Glucose-6-phosphate dehydrogenase (G6PD) is an enzyme in the hexose-monophosphate pathway. It is responsible for generating nicotinamide adenine dinucleotide phosphate (NADPH). In the red cell, NADPH is a major source of reduction in the potential required to maintain the iron atoms of Hb in the ferrous state and to prevent membrane lipid peroxidation.

CASE HISTORY

A 30-year-old Nigerian male was brought to the emergency department having collapsed in the street. He had returned from a 3-month holiday in Nigeria 6 days previously. Two days before admission, he had developed central colicky abdominal pain and diarrhoea; 1 day before admission he began to feel weak and noticed his urine was discoloured red.

On examination, he was pyrexial (37.8°C), anaemic and jaundiced. There was no hepatosplenomegaly. Dipstix testing of urine was negative for bilirubin but positive for urobilinogen and blood. Urine microscopy revealed no red cells.

INVESTIGATIONS

- Haemoglobin 54 g/L
- Mean cell volume 91 fL
- White cell count 15.8 × 10⁹/L
- Platelets 249 × 10⁹/L
- Reticulocytes 11.61%

Blood film showed polychromasia, irregularly contracted and bitten-out red cells. There were no malaria parasites or Heinz bodies.

The patient has a normocytic anaemia with a reticulocytosis, suggesting **acute haemolysis or haemorrhage.**

Polychromasia refers to the appearance of reticulocytes, or immature red cells, when stained by using standard stains.

The appearance of the red cells is compatible with oxidative red cell damage. It is unusual to see Heinz bodies when patients have a functional spleen.

DIFFERENTIAL DIAGNOSIS

Malaria is a common cause of haemolysis in patients returning from the tropics. Other evidence to suggest acute intravascular haemolysis is shown in Table 11.2.

Haemoglobin electrophoresis on cellulose acetate membrane (CAM) and agar gel demonstrates sickle-cell trait but no other structural Hb variant. Sickle-cell trait does not result in a haemolytic anaemia.

TABLE 11.2 ■ **Evidence to Show Intravascular Haemolysis**

Test	Result
Serum bilirubin	65 µmol/L
Serum haptoglobins	Undetectable
Serum LDH	587 U/L
Schumm's test	Positive

LDH, Lactate dehydrogenase.

The negative isopropanol stability test excludes an inherited, unstable Hb variant.

The negative DAT (or Coombs' test) excludes immune-mediated red cell destruction.

Glucose-6-phosphate dehydrogenase was assayed by two methods that confirmed G6PD deficiency. The most common G6PD variant in individuals of African descent is G6PD A⁻.

> **REMEMBER**
>
> - Glucose-6-phosphate dehydrogenase deficiency will be present in all (homozygous) males who carry an affected X chromosome
> - Heterozygous females will have a dual population of red cells
> - Because X chromosome inactivation is random (lyonisation), some heterozygous females will demonstrate clinical G6PD deficiency

Deficiency of G6PD arises from a large number of different mutations in the *G6PD* gene, the majority of which are point mutations resulting in single amino-acid substitutions. Glucose-6-phosphate dehydrogenase deficiency is widespread in many tropical and subtropical populations where malaria was, or is, endemic. Frequencies of 20% of the population in Southern Europe and Africa, and 40% in SE Asia and the Middle East have been reported.

Glucose-6-phosphate dehydrogenase deficiency can present as:

- Neonatal jaundice
- Chronic haemolytic anaemia
- Acute haemolytic anaemia

An acute haemolytic crisis is the most common presentation, and most affected individuals are asymptomatic until this happens. Acute haemolysis occurs when an exogenous factor imposes an extra oxidative stress, which overwhelms the limited supply of NADPH in the red cells. Acute haemolysis can be precipitated by:

- Infection
- Drugs
- Fava beans (as either lightly cooked food or a pollen)

Many drugs (Table 11.3) have been implicated in attacks of acute haemolysis in susceptible individuals.

> **REMEMBER**
>
> - Some drugs (e.g. primaquine, aspirin and vitamin K) can be given safely in reduced doses
> - Some agents (e.g. dapsone and naphthalene) in sufficient amounts will cause haemolysis in individuals with normal levels of G6PD

Favism is a form of severe, acute, intravascular haemolysis, often with massive haemoglobinuria, precipitated by exposure to fava beans (*Vicia faba*) in individuals with G6PD deficiency. It is most common in children, following the ingestion of fresh, raw beans. Haemolysis is probably

TABLE 11.3 ■ Drugs That Commonly Cause Acute Haemolysis in Patients with G6PD

Type	Example
Antimalarials	Primaquine
–	Pyrimethamine
–	Chloroquine
–	Quinine
Sulfonamides	Sulfasalazine
	Dapsone
	Cotrimoxazole
Other antibacterials	Nitrofurantoin
–	Nalidixic acid
–	Quinolones, e.g. ciprofloxacin
Analgesics	Aspirin (>1 g per day)
Miscellaneous	Vitamin K analogues
–	Naphthalene
–	Probenecid
–	Dimercaprol
–	Methylene blue

G6PD, Glucose-6-phosphate dehydrogenase.

precipitated by divicine, a glucoside constituent in fava beans, which generates free oxygen radicals when oxidised.

DIAGNOSIS OF G6PD DEFICIENCY

Clinical Features

- Sudden onset
- Severe malaise and pallor often with fever and abdominal pain
- Dark urine
- Jaundice

REMEMBER

- The jaundice of haemolysis is prehepatic, and the bilirubin is unconjugated and therefore does not appear in the urine
- The dark urine is due partly to haemoglobinuria and partly to increased urobilinogen, which oxidises and darkens on standing

Laboratory Features

Blood count:
- Normocytic anaemia
- Reticulocytosis
- Bitten-out and irregularly contracted red cells

The spleen 'bites out' Heinz bodies, which are aggregates of oxidised methaemoglobin, from affected red cells.

Features of Intravascular Haemolysis

- Decreased haptoglobins

TABLE 11.4 ■ **Test Results Confirming the Cause of Intravascular Haemolysis**

Test	Result
Haemoglobin electrophoresis	HbA + HbS
Direct antiglobulin test (DAT)	Negative
Isopropanol stability test	Negative
G6PD assay	1.9 IU/g Hb

HbA, Haemoglobin A; HbS, haemoglobin S; G6PD, glucose-6-phosphate dehydrogenase.

- Increased LDH
- Haemoglobinaemia
- Haemoglobinuria
- Positive Schumm test due to methaemalbumin

One of the isoenzymes of LDH is found in high concentrations in red cells and is released in red cell damage.

Rapid depletion of haptoglobin with the formation of methaemalbumin is typical of intra-vascular haemolysis. In the absence of other scavenging serum proteins, excess haem binds to albumin and the ferrous iron is subsequently oxidised to ferric iron to give methaemalbumin and a positive Schumm test. The cause of the intravascular haemolysis in this patient was established by further tests (Table 11.4).

Haemoglobinuria might result in acute kidney injury, particularly in adults – monitor urine output, urea and creatinine.

REMEMBER

- Old red cells have less G6PD than young red cells and are destroyed first during a haemo-lytic attack
- Newly formed reticulocytes have relatively high concentrations of G6PD
- As a result of these two factors, the concentration of G6PD in an affected individual may rise during an acute haemolytic episode to within the NR
- If in doubt, retest 1 month later

Assessment of G6PD Activity

- Qualitative screening tests, for example, cresyl blue decolorisation test
- Quantitative enzyme assay by spectrophotometry

TREATMENT

- Stop any drug that could have precipitated the acute haemolysis
- Search for and treat any infection
- Monitor Hb concentration twice daily until stable
- Bed rest; urgent blood transfusion may be required in severe cases
- Patient education:
- Issue G6PD deficiency card and information leaflet
- Discuss avoidance of specific drugs and fava beans
- Offer family screening

WHAT HAD PRECIPITATED A HAEMOLYTIC CRISIS IN THIS MALE WITH G6PD DEFICIENCY?

This was initially obscure. He denied any drug ingestion but he had been repeatedly exposed to an oily liquid used for anointing at his church. When he produced the bottle, it smelt strongly of mothballs, and ultraviolet spectrophotometry confirmed the presence of naphthalene. Naphthalene is well known to cause acute haemolysis. It was first described in the 19th century after the introduction of β-naphthol to treat hookworm infestations. Many cases of affected infants have been described where the naphthalene was used as a moth repellent in clothes. The presence of G6PD deficiency greatly increases sensitivity to the oxidative red cell damage mediated by naphthalene.

Progress. The patient's Hb concentration did not fall any further but rose slowly, reaching 92 g/L 7 days later. The reticulocyte count peaked at 17.4% on the fifth day, and the jaundice had resolved by 14 days. Re-assay 6 weeks later confirmed G6PD deficiency.

Direct Orally Active Anticoagulant Drugs (DOACs)

A number of orally active direct thrombin and Xa inhibitor drugs (dabigatran, rivaroxaban, apixaban and edoxaban) are used for prevention and treatment of thrombosis. Such drugs have a much broader therapeutic window than warfarin and offer the prospect of fixed drug dosing without the need to monitor coagulation. Antidotes include andexanet (reverses epixaban and rivaroxaban) and idaracizumab (reverses dabigatran).

CASE HISTORY (4)

You are asked to see a 36-year-old female with an acutely swollen calf. Clinical diagnosis is a distal DVT. She has no complicating problems.

HOW SHOULD SHE BE TREATED?

Initially, the diagnosis should be confirmed by venous compression ultrasonography (sensitivity 97% for proximal and 73% for calf veins). An acutely swollen leg has a range of causes:
- Deep vein thrombosis
- Ruptured Baker cyst
- Rupture of the head of gastrocnemius
- Acute knee injury
- Haematoma
- Infection (e.g. cellulitis)

ACTION

If a DVT is confirmed:
- Give SC LMW heparin
- Commence a DOAC (e.g. apixaban or rivaroxaban) or warfarin

This can be managed in outpatients with good nursing and laboratory support.
If the DVT is complex (i.e. iliofemoral):
- Admit
- Give IV unfractionated heparin or LMW heparin
- Commence a DOAC or warfarin

There is an increasing move to outpatient management of VTE.

You are called about a 36-year-old male with an acute right lower limb ischaemia due to an arterial thrombosis. He has a family history of thrombosis. There has been improvement in the ischaemic area over 24 h. The patient is on IV heparin infusion and is being monitored by the vascular surgeons. In view of the family history, the doctor wonders whether the male should be investigated for thrombophilia. The doctor has already sent off a standard thrombophilia screen and asks if this is all that you need.

You tell him that thrombophilia is uncommon in arterial disease, but there are a number of risk factors for arterial thrombosis. You suggest that he requests:

- Plasma homocysteine
- Lipid profile
- Plasminogen activator inhibitor

Finding a cause in arterial disease is less likely than in venous thrombosis.

Progress. No evidence of thrombophilia was found in this patient, but he is a smoker and his cholesterol was 7.4 mmol/L with risk factors for atherosclerosis. His lifestyle issues were addressed by the cardiac rehabilitation nurse specialist and he was started on a statin.

You are asked to see a 60-year-old female with a right leg DVT, who is on unfractionated heparin. She has been in hospital for 5 days and started warfarin therapy 48 h previously. She has now developed a cold, painful leg on the left that is pulseless. You are told that her platelet count has been falling since starting heparin.

WHAT IS THE MOST LIKELY DIAGNOSIS TO CONSIDER?

This would be a good picture for **heparin-induced thrombocytopenia (HIT) with thrombosis** of the artery. The classic features are progressive platelet decline and new thrombosis. **HIT** is a clinical diagnosis and is diagnosed in any patient on heparin whose platelet count falls significantly.

ACTION

- Stop *all* heparin (including heparin flush)
- Contact a haematologist
- Alternative forms of anticoagulation are not required for the DVT in this female because she is on warfarin, the INR is 2.0 and heparin was about to be discontinued

HIT is due to an immune induction of antiheparin/PF4 antibodies, which bind to and activate platelets via an Fc receptor. This results in a prothrombotic state with low platelets. There is usually a previous history of heparin exposure.

Note:

- Fatal thrombosis, both venous and arterial, can arise if heparin is not stopped immediately
- **HIT** can occur after SC heparin use. It is becoming increasingly common with the use of heparin prophylaxis

Progress. This patient has left acute ischaemic lower limb and required surgical removal of the thrombus in her popliteal artery. She fortunately made a good recovery, although she still has a swollen, painful right leg (from the DVT) and ischaemic pain in the left leg after exertion.

Splenomegaly, Splenectomy and Hyposplenism

CASE HISTORY (1)

A 55-year-old male presented with a 3-month history of discomfort in the left side of his abdomen. The discomfort is present most of the time and now seems to be getting worse.

He has had rheumatoid arthritis for many years, but his condition has stabilised on methotrexate therapy and occasional use of diclofenac for pain in his knees.

On examination, he looks pale and has evidence of rheumatoid arthritis in his hands, with ulnar drift and palmar subluxation of the metacarpophalangeal joints (MCPJs). He has rheumatoid nodules in both elbows. Both knees are deformed. Examination of his abdomen shows a large spleen.

Investigations show a normochromic normocytic anaemia with low platelets and a neutropenia. The diagnosis is **Felty syndrome** in a patient with rheumatoid arthritis.

Felty syndrome consists of splenomegaly and neutropenia in a patient with rheumatoid arthritis. A normochromic, normocytic anaemia of chronic disease is usually present, although iron-deficient and rare haemolytic (Coombs-positive) anaemias are seen. Hypersplenism causing a pancytopenia may occur.

Spleen size can be assessed by abdominal palpation or by imaging, for example, ultrasound. Computed tomography, MRI and PET scans are also used to delineate the cause, for example, lymphoproliferative disease.

There are many causes of splenomegaly, with the most frequent showing geographical variation. In temperate climates malignant blood diseases, portal hypertension, haemolytic anaemias and infective endocarditis account for most cases, whereas in tropical countries malaria, leishmaniasis and the haemoglobinopathies are prevalent.

INFORMATION

Causes of Splenomegaly

- Malignant haematological disease, for example, acute or chronic leukaemia, malignant lymphoma
- Myeloproliferative disorders, for example, PV, myelofibrosis (often massive)
- Haemoglobinopathies, for example, β-thalassaemia major, Hb, H, SC or E disease
- Haemolytic anaemias, for example, hereditary spherocytosis
- Congestive splenomegaly, for example, portal hypertension (cirrhosis)
- Inborn errors of metabolism, for example, Gaucher disease
- Autoimmune rheumatic disorders: for example, SLE, rheumatoid arthritis (Felty syndrome)
- Infections:
  1. Viral, for example, infectious mononucleosis
  2. Bacterial (any bacteria), occasionally – remember infective endocarditis
  3. Protozoal, for example, malaria, kala-azar
- Miscellaneous (rare), for example, amyloid, tropical splenomegaly

Enlargement of the spleen from any cause can be complicated by **hypersplenism.** This is characterised by:

- Splenomegaly
- Pancytopenia
- Normal or hypercellular bone marrow

PATHOPHYSIOLOGY OF HYPERSPLENISM

Mature red cells, neutrophils and platelets 'pool', or are trapped, in the sinusoids of the large spleen and prematurely destroyed.

CAUSES OF HYPOSPLENISM

- Congenital absence
- Splenectomy: surgical or by irradiation
- Splenic atrophy, for example, coeliac disease, chronic inflammatory bowel disease
- Splenic infarction, for example, HbSS
- Splenic infiltration

REMEMBER

Surgical splenectomy might be carried out because of:

- Trauma
- Treatment: e.g. hereditary spherocytosis, idiopathic thrombocytopenic purpura or myelofibrosis

Splenic function can be assessed by:

- Peripheral blood film- look for abnormal red cells:
  1. Acanthocytes (spiky red cells)
  2. Target cells (like an archery target)
  3. Pappenheimer bodies (iron granules)
  4. Howell–Jolly bodies (nuclear DNA fragments)
- Differential interference microscopy of blood: increased pitted red cell (red cells with sub-membrane vacuoles) count
- Radioactive spleen scan

The functional size of the spleen can be assessed by scanning with a scintillation counter following the injection of radiolabelled (^{99m}Tc), heat-damaged, autologous red cells. These cells are removed from the circulation solely by the spleen.

Progress. In this patient with rheumatoid arthritis, Felty syndrome was confirmed as the cause of the splenomegaly. Over the following year, he developed recurrent infections with a persistent, refractory neutropenia and eventually had a splenectomy.

CASE HISTORY (2)

A 6-month-old baby male of Nigerian parents was admitted to the emergency department, collapsed and unconscious. The family was travelling to the airport by taxi and diverted the car to hospital when the baby became suddenly unwell. Twelve hours before admission the child had been seen at a different emergency department with a short history of poor feeding, irritability and diarrhoea. He was noted to be febrile but not thought to be seriously unwell.

On examination, the child was noted to be pale, with a GCS of 5. He was febrile at 39.5°C, with a firm spleen extending to below the umbilicus. The results of his blood count and blood film were:

Blood count:
- Haemoglobin 24 g/L
- Mean cell volume 76 fL
- White cell count 30.5 × 10⁹/L
- Platelets 27 × 10⁹/L
- Reticulocytes 7.0%

Blood film:
- Polychromasia
- Very reduced platelets
- Nucleated red cells
- Occasional elongated sickle cells
- Diplococci both within neutrophils and macrophages, and free in the plasma

Subsequent investigations demonstrated *S. pneumoniae* on blood culture.

DIAGNOSIS

Sickle-cell anaemia with pneumococcal sepsis.

Haemoglobin electrophoresis showed:

- HbS: 90%
- HbF: 8%
- HbA$_2$: 1.8%

REMEMBER

Prevention of pneumococcal sepsis in babies with sickle-cell anaemia is dependent on maternal antenatal haemoglobinopathy. At-risk pregnancies need to be identified and screened:

- Haemoglobinopathy screening of cord blood samples
- Institution of penicillin prophylaxis by 8 weeks of age

Progress. This baby presented moribund with splenomegaly, severe anaemia and thrombocytopenia. The reticulocytosis/polychromasia and nucleated red cells suggested a haemolytic anaemia. Haemoglobin electrophoresis subsequently confirmed HbSS. The sickle-cell mutation affects the β-globin gene and only assumes clinical importance 4 months after birth when foetal haemaglobin (HbF) levels drop and the β-globin gene is activated.

The thrombocytopenia was almost certainly related to DIC secondary to the bacterial infection. Severe hyposplenism is a characteristic feature of sickle-cell anaemia and is established by 4 to 6 months. Pneumococcal sepsis secondary to hyposplenism is a common cause of death in children <3 years old with sickle-cell anaemia.

The gross splenomegaly and severe anaemia were due to acute splenic sequestration of sickled red cells within the spleen, which often accompanies pneumococcal sepsis in this age.

Overwhelming postsplenectomy infection (OPSI) is the most feared complication of hyposplenism.

REMEMBER

- The greatest risk of OPSI following splenectomy is in the first 2 years, but the increased risk is life-long
- The mortality rate with OPSI due to *S. pneumoniae* is 50% despite treatment

---

PATHOPHYSIOLOGY

- Decreased antibody synthesis
- Decreased phagocytosis of opsonised bacteria

The Major Pathogens Involved in OPSI

- *S. pneumoniae* (>80%)
- *Haemophilus influenzae* type B
- *Neisseria meningitidis*

These are all encapsulated bacteria – the spleen is a vital first line of defence against encapsulated organisms. Severe infections in the hyposplenic patient can also occur in malaria and babesiosis (mosquito and tick bites, respectively) and following dog bites with *Capnocytophaga canimorsus*.

REMEMBER

- Following vaccination, check adequacy of antibody response
- Repeat antibody levels at 5 years post vaccination and give booster doses if appropriate

PREVENTION OF OPSI

This depends on:

- Identification of the patient at risk
- Education of the patient about the risks of infection, dog bites and tropical travel
- Issue of a 'postsplenectomy' card and leaflet to the patient
- Life-long prophylactic antibiotic therapy, for example, penicillin V 250 mg × 2 daily
- Vaccination with a pneumococcal polysaccharide conjugate vaccine and the Hib vaccine
- Meningococcal conjugate (ACWY) series and monovalent meningococcal serogroup B vaccine series

Blood Transfusion

The Blood Transfusion department supplies red cells, platelets and plasma products, such as FFP, cryoprecipitate and human albumin.

The efficient and safe provision of blood products depends on good communication between you and the laboratory, and accurate patient identification.

ALWAYS

- Provide complete and accurate patient identification on the blood sample and request form
- Tell the blood transfusion department how much of what blood product is required and the urgency of the clinical situation

NEVER

- Take blood from more than one patient at a time
- Prelabel the blood sample tube

REMEMBER

When you request blood, always make clear the urgency of the clinical situation:
- Very urgent: there is a life-threatening haemorrhage and blood is required in 1–5 min:
  1. Action: No pretransfusion compatibility test. The laboratory will issue group 0 Rh(D)-negative blood
- Urgent: blood required in 5–10 min:
  1. Action: ABO and Rh(D) group on patient sample. The laboratory will issue ABO and Rh(D) group-compatible blood
- Nonurgent: blood required in 30–60 min:
  1. Action: Full pretransfusion compatibility test. The laboratory will issue fully compatible blood

To provide compatible red cells for transfusion, the following procedures are undertaken by the blood transfusion laboratory:
- ABO and Rh(D) blood group:
  - Major haemolytic transfusion reactions usually result from the transfusion of ABO-incompatible blood
  - The Rh(D) antigen is very immunogenic, and the development of anti-D must be avoided in females of childbearing age
- Antibody screen: excludes the presence of clinically significant red cell alloantibodies in the patient's plasma. These might result in an acute or delayed haemolytic transfusion reaction
- Selection of appropriate donor units: wherever possible, blood of the same ABO and Rh(D) group as the patient is selected and will be negative for the appropriate antigen if an alloantibody has been identified
- Cross-match: the patient's plasma is reacted with the donor red cells in vitro. Incompatibility is indicated by agglutination or haemolysis

A full compatibility procedure is always completed, but this can be retrospective if the clinical demand for blood is urgent.

CASE HISTORY (1)

You are asked to see a 72-year-old male with myelodysplasia, who receives regular blood transfusions. One unit of blood was given uneventfully, but 15 min into the second unit, he began to shiver, felt unwell, and developed a pyrexia and tachycardia.

A febrile transfusion reaction to human leukocyte antigen (HLA) or granulocyte antigens is common in multitransfused patients but cannot be safely distinguished from a haemolytic transfusion reaction due to red cell antibodies without appropriate laboratory tests.

ACTION

- Stop the transfusion immediately:
  - Replace giving set
  - Keep IV line open with 0.9% saline
- Check patient identification:
  - Wrist band
  - Compatibility form
  - Compatibility label on unit of blood
- Take appropriate samples:
  - Blood count
  - Blood cultures
  - Blood transfusion sample
  - Urine for Hb
- Take samples and a relevant unit of blood to the laboratory
- Inform haematology medical staff of the problem
- The laboratory will:
  - Check laboratory documentation
  - Repeat ABO Rh(D) group, antibody screen and cross-match on pre- and post-transfusion samples in parallel
  - Carry out a DAT (Coombs' test; see Fig. 11.2) to exclude the presence of alloantibodies on the patient's red cells

OUTCOME

The red cell alloantibody was identified.

Diagnosis: Haemolytic Transfusion Reaction

Monitor renal function, urine output, Hb concentration and check coagulation screen.

A major ABO incompatibility can be life-threatening, with acute kidney injury and DIC:

- Monitor as above
- Insert urinary catheter and monitor urine output
- Give IV fluids to maintain urine output (>1.5 mL/h per kg)
- Refer to renal unit
- Report to Serious Hazards of Blood Transfusion (SHOT), a confidential enquiry into major blood transfusion errors in the UK

Progress. An error in the collection of the blood from the laboratory led to the wrong blood being given to this patient. The error was reported to the hospital as a serious event. The patient maintained his normal BP and his symptoms settled, requiring no further treatment for this.

A major review of blood transfusion procedures was instituted. Fortunately, with the prompt treatment, this male had no serious problems.

PRESENTATION OF OTHER ACUTE COMPLICATIONS OF BLOOD TRANSFUSION

- Nonhaemolytic (febrile) transfusion reactions. These are due to the presence of leucocyte antibodies in a multiply transfused person acting against donor leucocytes in red cell concentrate, leading to release of pyrogens. Leucocyte-depleted blood is now used in many countries, so the febrile reaction is not often seen
- Breathlessness:
  - Acute volume overload
  - Transfusion-related acute lung injury (TRALI): characterised by dyspnoea, fever, cough and lung shadowing on CXR
- Urticaria or anaphylaxis: reaction to plasma proteins
- Collapse or hypotension: major ABO incompatibility-infected blood product
- Cardiac arrhythmia:
  - Hypocalcaemia
  - Hyperkalaemia
  - Rapid transfusion with 'cold' blood

REMEMBER

There are other longer-term complications of blood transfusion, including:

- Post-transfusion purpura (PTP)
- Viral infection: hepatitis C, hepatitis B, HIV (*Note:* donor blood in many countries is checked for these), cytomegalovirus (CMV)
- Iron overload (multiple transfusions)
- Graft-versus-host disease

CASE HISTORY (2)

A 64-year-old male with known severe chronic liver disease, who is on the liver transplant list, has been admitted on a number of occasions with haematemesis due to variceal bleeding. Endoscopic banding of the varices has been undertaken and he is on propranolol therapy.

He is admitted on this occasion with a large haematemesis.

On examination, he is cold and pale, with a pulse rate of 120/min and a BP of 80/50.

He is in hypovolaemic shock and needs urgent resuscitation with fluid and blood, and vasoconstrictor therapy with terlipressin before urgent endoscopy.

MANAGEMENT OF MASSIVE HAEMORRHAGE (FIG. 11.13)

- Communicate nature and urgency of the situation to the laboratory
- Predict requirements for blood and blood products; always try to think ahead
- Monitor:
  - Volume replacement
  - Haemostatic parameters
  - Serum calcium: blood is preserved with citrate–phosphate dextrose solution, which chelates calcium

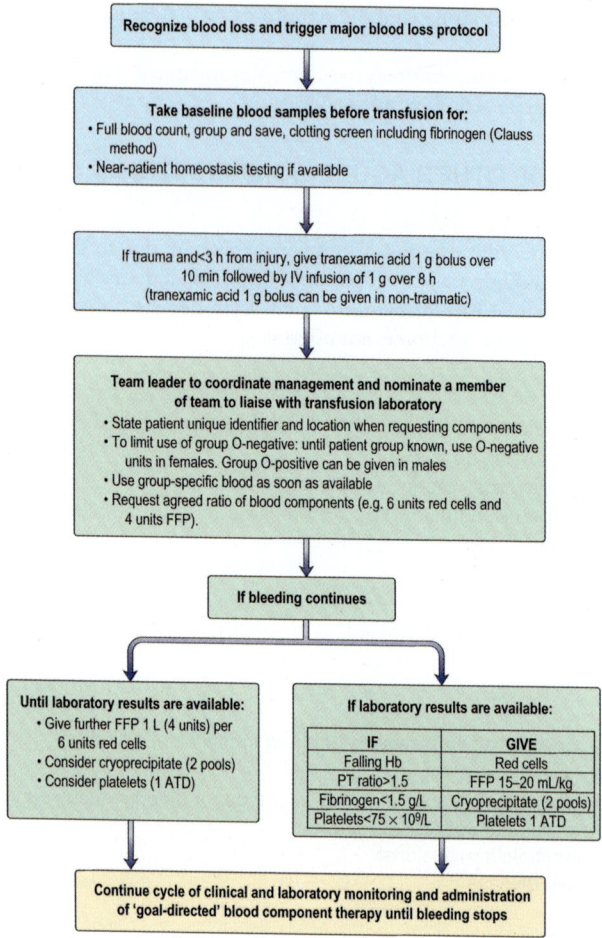

Fig. 11.13 Algorithm for the management of major haemorrhage. ATD, Adult therapeutic dose; FFP, fresh frozen plasma; PT, prothrombin time. (From Norfolk D. 2013. Handbook of Transfusion Medicine, The Stationery Office, with permission. Available at www.transfusionguidelines.com.)

- Maintain intravascular volume
- Avoid:
  - Hypovolaemia
  - Acute kidney injury
  - Disseminated intravascular coagulation
  - Cardiac arrhythmias
- Use:
  - Saline/colloid solutions
  - Group O Rh(D) negative blood
  - ABO Rh(D) group-compatible blood until fully compatible blood is available

REMEMBER

Give blood through a blood warmer to minimise hyperkalaemia and cardiac arrhythmias.

CHECK FOR FAILURE OF HAEMOSTASIS

- Initially at beginning of emergency
- Every 5 units of blood given
- Whenever additional blood products (platelets, FFP, cryoprecipitate) are given

INVESTIGATIONS

Anticipate haemostatic failure. Check:
- Full blood count
- Prothrombin/INR
- Activated partial thromboplastin time Fibrinogen concentration
- Fibrinogen degradation products or fibrin D-dimers

CAUSES OF HAEMOSTASIS FAILURE

- Disseminated intravascular coagulation: secondary to hypovolaemic shock with additional liver failure, infection or tissue trauma
- Dilutional coagulopathy
- Stored blood depleted of coagulation factors and containing few platelets

ACTION

- Request platelets to maintain platelet count $>50 \times 10^9/L$ or if sequential platelet counts are falling progressively
- Request cryoprecipitate (10 units) if fibrinogen concentration <1.0 g/L
- Request FFP (10–20 mL/kg) if PT/INR and partial thromboplastin time with kaolin (PTTK) prolonged

REMEMBER

- Fresh frozen plasma takes 30 min to unfreeze
- Platelets might need to be delivered from regional transfusion centres

Progress. This patient was given 9 units of blood and also underwent balloon tamponade as he was exsanguinating. He could not be resuscitated.

Haematological Oncology

This umbrella term covers a huge range of disorders. Some present dramatically and require urgent treatment; at the other end of the spectrum, there are diseases that are indolent and chronic, often requiring no therapy. You should be able to recognise the low-grade (nonurgent) and high-grade (urgent) disorders, and refer to your haematology department. (Outside normal hours do not be afraid to talk to the haematology registrar/consultant on call.)

WHAT MAIN GROUPS OF DISEASE ARE THERE?

- Leukaemias can be acute (short duration, serious, rapidly fatal if not treated) or chronic. They generally have elevated WCC and other features. These are marrow-/blood-based diseases
- Lymphomas are lymph node-based, sometimes involving blood and marrow. Some need urgent treatment and others can be sorted out at leisure

■ Myeloma is a low-grade, highly destructive disorder caused by malignant plasma cells, often presenting with bone pain, kidney injury and hypercalcaemia

CASE HISTORY (1)

A 63-year-old cleaner is admitted to MAU with pyrexia and a cough productive of sputum. Her general health has been reasonable until now.

On examination, she has chest signs suggestive of pneumonia. In addition, she has generalised lymphadenopathy and a three-fingerbreadth spleen. Scarring over her trunk is, she claims, due to shingles 4 months earlier.

An FBC shows mild anaemia (Hb 106 g/L), normal platelets and an elevated WCC of 25×10^9/L. The haematology technician phones to say that most of the white cells are lymphocytes and there are smear cells on the film.

REMEMBER

A smear cell is an artefact induced by making the blood film (the CLL cells are fragile and burst). There are no smear cells actually circulating in the patient's blood.

WHAT DO YOU NEED TO ESTABLISH NOW?

■ Whether this is an acute or chronic disease
■ If urgent treatment is required
■ What steps you would need to take to make a diagnosis

KEY FEATURES

■ Older patient
■ Fairly well
■ Shingles
■ Active infection
■ Lymphadenopathy/splenomegaly
■ High WCC with smear cells

This must be CLL, the most common leukaemia in adults (Fig. 11.14). It is a slowly progressive disorder and is an incidental finding or presents with an infective complication. Shingles is a fairly common presenting feature.

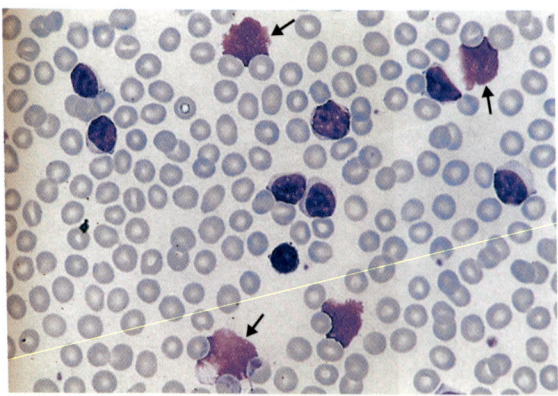

Fig. 11.14   Blood film in chronic lymphocytic leukaemia showing numerous smear cells (*artefacts*; *arrows*).

Chronic lymphocytic leukaemia is a disease mainly of the B lymphocytes (95%, the remaining 5% are T lymphocytes) – determined by checking cell markers. There is a reduction in immuno-globulin synthesis, leading to the infective complications.

OTHER FEATURES

- Possibly, decreased Hb and platelets (depends on disease stage)
- Haemolytic anaemia (red cell autoantibodies)
- Other autoimmune complications

MANAGEMENT

On Day of Admission

Start IV antibiotics as per local guidelines (e.g. cefuroxime 750 mg × 3, erythromycin 500 mg × 4); rehydrate if necessary. Refer to the Haematology department next day.

The prognosis in CLL is very variable and the disease may remain stable for several years. Many patients (approximately 30%) with CLL never need any treatment at all and lead normal lives.

Long-Term Treatment

Observation; the patient might require oral chemotherapy at a later stage (e.g. chlorambucil). Rituximab, in combination with chemotherapy, is first-line therapy.

CASE HISTORY (2)

You are called to see a 43-year-old accountant in the emergency department. This male went to see his doctor suffering from excessive tiredness. You are presented with an anxious, pale male, who has bruising over his lower limbs and arms. Temperature is 39°C. He is admitted urgently to the MAU, where further examination reveals no other signs.

WHAT TESTS WOULD YOU ARRANGE?

- Full blood count, U and Es
- Blood cultures
- Mid-stream urine
- Chest X-ray

The Hb is 60 g/L, WCC 90 × 10^9/L and platelets are 30 × 10^9/L. Renal function is normal and the CXR shows minimal increased shadowing at the right base.

REMEMBER

Do not wait until the next morning – the patient may succumb before then!

IS THIS AN ACUTE OR CHRONIC DISORDER?

A short history in an ill patient with severe anaemia and thrombocytopenia indicates an acute disorder.

You must ask what the white cells are, morphologically. If they are neutrophils (neutrophilia), this might reflect an underlying infection; this is unlikely with such a high WCC.

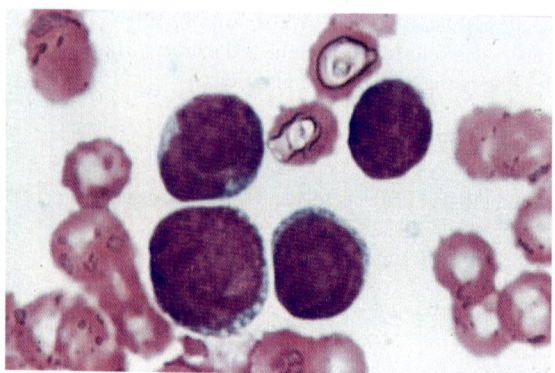

Fig. 11.15   Bone marrow in acute myeloid leukaemia showing numerous large leukaemic blasts.

However, the technician looks at the blood film and tells you they look like blasts.

REMEMBER

Blasts are primitive white cells present in bone marrow in small numbers. They are never seen in peripheral blood in health.

This suggests an **acute leukaemia** (Fig. 11.15). In a patient of this age, AML is most likely (if he were a child, acute lymphoblastic leukaemia would be more likely).

INVESTIGATIONS

- Specific diagnostic tests (performed by haematology department)
- Peripheral blood film examination (Are there Auer rods? If so, their presence confirms AML, as are not all that common)
- Bone marrow aspirate and biopsy
- Cell marker analysis (determines pattern of antigens on white cells)
- Cytogenetic studies on marrow blasts: several karyotypic abnormalities are diagnostic
- Other tests, for example, HLA typing

You should aim to perform only the initial treatment steps: IV fluids, empirical (blind) therapy for infection (send blood and urine cultures first), and then notification of haematology staff as soon as possible.

CASE HISTORY (3)

A 72-year-old former butcher is currently on the orthopaedic ward with a collapse of one of his lumbar vertebrae. The orthopaedic trainee is concerned because some results have come back that she wishes to discuss with you.

The patient has mild anaemia with an elevated WCC (26×10^9/L, mainly neutrophils). The ESR is 120 mm/h. Blood film comment: red cell rouleaux.

There is mild renal impairment and hypercalcaemia (corrected calcium is 3.21 mmol/L).

The patient appears quite uncomfortable and has pain in the lower back pain, left rib cage, right humerus and right thigh. His general health was excellent until about 4 months ago when he developed anorexia and mild weight loss. His wife, who is present, is concerned, as he is forgetful and confused at times (this has been much worse over the past 1–2 weeks).

WHAT POSSIBLE DIAGNOSES ARE THERE?

Although not in extremis, this male is very unwell:

- An ESR of 120 mm/h suggests serious underlying pathology (an ESR of 120 could be due to serious infection, autoimmune disease, rheumatoid disease or malignancy)
- Red cell rouleaux, renal impairment and hypercalcaemia in a patient with bone disease suggest either a primary bone disorder (such as myeloma) or possible infiltration by malignancy, for example, carcinoma

If outside working hours, there is little else you can request. Your main objective is to treat the symptoms, for example, rehydrate, start antibiotics if you think infection is present, and correct the elevated calcium level. Alert the haematology team.

WHAT TO CHECK AS SOON AS POSSIBLE

- Blood film
- Immunoglobulin levels/serum protein electrophoresis/immunofixation
- Repeat biochemistry to check renal function and calcium level
- Send urine for Bence-Jones protein and plasma for free immunoglobulin light chains
- Blood cultures if febrile
- Mid-stream urine
- Arrange skeletal survey (plain radiology of skull, spine, pelvis, femora)

RESULTS IN THIS CASE

- Elevated total IgG with reduced IgA and IgM
- Serum IgG M paraprotein (paraprotein is monoclonal immunoglobulin produced by the malignant clone of plasma cells)
- Bence-Jones protein present: kappa light chains
- Widespread lytic lesions throughout skeleton
- Subsequent bone marrow aspirate showed infiltration by abnormal plasma cells (Fig. 11.16)

Diagnosis

Multiple myeloma.

The patient should be referred for specialist advice regarding treatment for his myeloma. He also needs bisphosphonate treatment for his bone disease and orthopaedic referral for possible

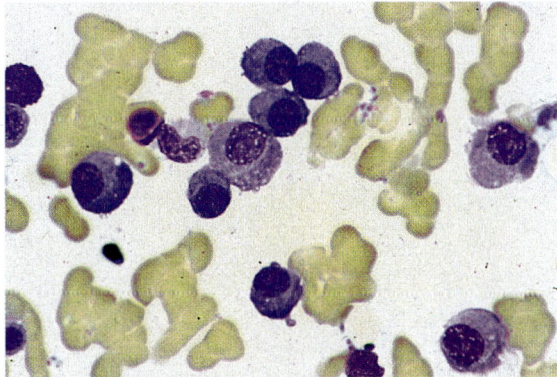

Fig. 11.16 Bone marrow aspirate in myeloma showing large numbers of plasma cells.

kyphoplasty, which involves inflating a balloon in the affected vertebral body and filling this with methyl methacrylate cement in order to restore the vertebral shape.

CASE HISTORY (4)

A 50-year-old bank manager is admitted with weight loss, sweats and splenomegaly.
Initial investigations show mild anaemia, WCC 200 × 10⁹/L and platelets 600 × 10⁹/L.

WHAT FURTHER INFORMATION DO YOU REQUIRE?

- White cells: are they blasts? No – there are neutrophils, eosinophils, basophils and early (i.e. immature) granulocytes (e.g. promyelocytes, myelocytes)
- How large is the spleen? Palpable to umbilicus (ultrasound = 24 cm)

Biochemical Screen

- Normal, apart from elevated serum uric acid level

Reexamine the Patient Yourself

Are there any other abnormal findings?
- There is no lymphadenopathy
- Liver edge is palpable
- Chest is clear
- Fundi: nothing abnormal

WHAT IS THE UNDERLYING DIAGNOSIS?

There are several significant findings: very high WCC, splenomegaly with weight loss and sweats. Could the patient have an underlying infection/neoplasm producing these features (i.e. reactive process)? Yes, but it is much more suggestive of an underlying primary blood disorder such as **CML** because the WCC is very high with the whole spectrum of granulocytic cells present (Fig. 11.17). If the blood picture were 'reactive', a neutrophilia would be more likely.

WHAT SINGLE INVESTIGATION WILL CONFIRM THE DIAGNOSIS?

Cytogenetic analysis of peripheral blood white cells or bone marrow white cells.

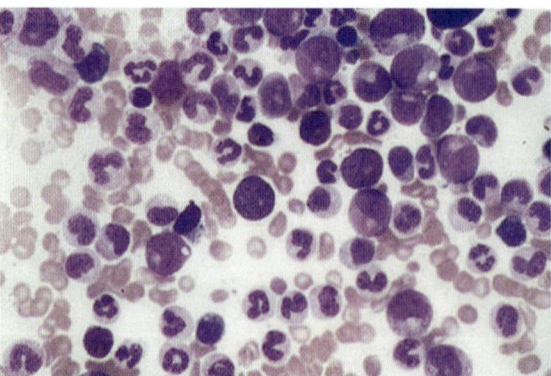

Fig. 11.17 Blood film in chronic myeloid leukaemia. Note the large numbers of granulocytic cells, in particular neutrophils, at all stages of development.

The Philadelphia chromosome will be present (translocation of DNA between chromosomes 9 and 22) in most cases (95%) of CML.

> **REMEMBER**
>
> Philadelphia chromosome is present in some acute leukaemias, but this patient does not have features of acute leukaemia; the bone marrow will confirm this.

DOES HE NEED URGENT REFERRAL TO THE HAEMATOLOGY TEAM?

Unless the patient is very unwell or has features of leucostasis (blood sludging in the lungs or brain due to a high WCC), there is no immediate need for urgent referral. You should, however, alert the haematology team, who should take over the patient's care the next day. Leucostasis can result in:

- Confusion
- Visual disturbance
- Cough and dyspnoea

FEATURES SUGGESTIVE OF ACUTE LEUKAEMIA/HIGH-GRADE LYMPHOMA

- Acute onset
- Unwell patient
- Dramatic presentation
- Extensive infection and/or bruising
- Gum swelling
- Fundal haemorrhage
- Coagulopathy
- Blasts/immature cells in peripheral blood
- Auer rods (neutrophil granules join up to produce these rod-like structures, which are pathognomonic of AML

FEATURES SUGGESTIVE OF CHRONIC/LOW-GRADE HAEMATOLOGICAL MALIGNANCY

- Less dramatic onset
- Patient who is not particularly unwell
- Previous infection (e.g. chest infection or herpes zoster)
- Absence of blasts in blood
- Abnormal peripheral blood cells: lymphocytes with abnormal morphology or immature granulocytes. Generalised lymphadenopathy present for months

Refer all patients suspected of having acute leukaemia to the haematology team as soon as possible, for specialist management.

> **REMEMBER**
>
> The WCC does not have to be high to diagnose acute (or chronic) leukaemia. In many cases acute leukaemia may present with normal or low WCC.
>
> Not all patients with acute leukaemia are ill at presentation.

IS IT LYMPHOMA OR LEUKAEMIA? (FIG. 11.18)

- Leukaemias generally involve bone marrow and blood. Lymph nodes and other organs might be involved
- Lymphomas originate in lymphoid tissue (lymph nodes, spleen), sometimes spill over into blood and might involve marrow (especially low-grade lymphomas)
- High-grade lymphoma and acute lymphoblastic leukaemia are very similar
- Low-grade lymphomas and chronic lymphoid leukaemias are similar

Progress. This patient with CML was referred to the haematologists who treated him with imatinib. He achieved a complete haematological response.

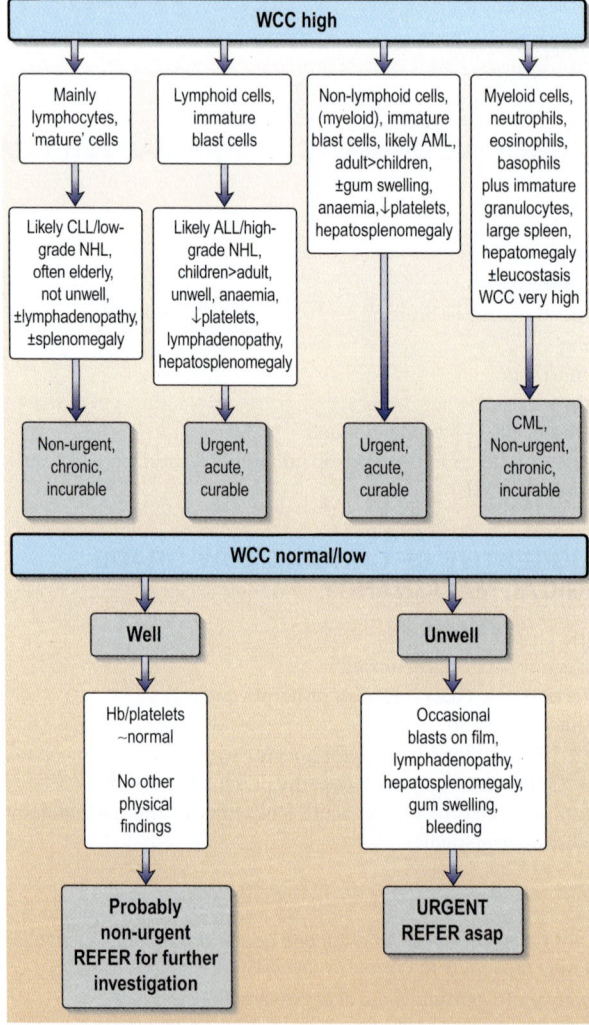

Fig. 11.18 Summary of suspected haematological malignancy. ALL, Acute lymphoblastic leukaemia; AML, acute myeloid leukaemia; CLL, chronic lymphocytic leukaemia; NHL, non-Hodgkin lymphoma.

Anaemia in Rheumatoid Arthritis, Chronic Kidney Disease and Liver Disease

ANAEMIA IN RHEUMATOID ARTHRITIS

CASE HISTORY

A 53-year-old female with rheumatoid arthritis was admitted for investigation of anaemia.

On examination, she has typical features of rheumatoid arthritis in her hands and arms. Her hands are grossly deformed and swollen, with redness over the MCPJs. She has tender, subcutaneous nodules on her elbows. All these features are indicative of an acute flare-up of her condition.

Investigations showed an Hb of 92 g/L, MCV of 84 fL, WBC of 11.4×10^9/L and platelets 490×10^9/L. Serum vitamin B_{12}, folate and ferritin were checked and found to be normal.

There are several possible causes for this anaemia:

- Bleeding (e.g. due to NSAIDs): the patient denies obvious GI bleeding. If she had been bleeding chronically, her MCV would probably have been reduced (iron deficiency). This female's MCV is normal, making chronic blood loss unlikely
- Poor diet: can induce folate deficiency, but we know her folate level is normal
- Autoimmune causes: for example, pernicious anaemia (she has rheumatoid arthritis and might possibly have pernicious anaemia, another associated autoimmune disease). However, her vitamin B_{12} level is normal
- Felty syndrome: rheumatoid arthritis, splenomegaly and neutropenia. This female has no features of this disorder
- Infiltrations, myelodysplasia: difficult to exclude these in the absence of additional information, for example, bone marrow. In myelodysplasia and marrow infiltration due to carcinoma in the presence of reduced Hb, it is likely (but not always the case) that the blood film would show morphological abnormalities such as 'tear-drop' red cells, nucleated red cells, hypogranular neutrophils or immature white cells. This female's blood film simply showed RBC rouleaux
- Renal impairment or liver disease: again, morphological abnormalities are usually present on the film, and the biochemical screen will assess liver and renal function
- Drug-induced anaemia: several mechanisms, for example, haemolysis. There are no features suggesting this. Remember the bone marrow suppressive effect of gold and azathioprine

This female's ESR was found to be >100 mm/h with a high CRP. Her rheumatoid disease was very active (flare-up), and 3 months before admission her Hb was 110 g/L. The drop in Hb has coincided with the flare-up: a common finding, especially in patients with rheumatoid arthritis.

A major diagnostic pitfall in the assessment of anaemia in patients with inflammatory disease is in the determination of iron status. Patients can be iron-deficient (confirmed by bone marrow aspirate stained for iron, the 'gold standard') yet have a normal serum ferritin, an acute-phase protein that rises to normal (or greater than normal) in patients with inflammation.

ASSESSMENT OF IRON STATUS IN PATIENTS WITH INFLAMMATORY DISORDERS

- Ferritin: likely to be misleading for the reasons given above
- Serum iron/total iron binding capacity (TIBC): there might be a reduction of both in chronic disease. These tests are seldom performed now because they are unreliable. Ferritin is the preferred assay
- Bone marrow: will determine iron status, but is expensive, painful and to be avoided if possible

■ Serum transferrin receptor assay: the number of transferrin receptors on red cells rises in iron deficiency but remains normal in secondary anaemia. This test is replacing bone marrow aspirate in diagnosis of iron deficiency in patients such as this

This female had normal transferrin receptor levels, confirming anaemia of chronic disease. She failed treatment with sulfasalazine and methotrexate. She was therefore treated with etanercept SC, a fully humanised p75 TNF-α receptor IgG fusion protein, with a good response in her joints and the ESR. She is now attending the rheumatology clinic for follow-up.

ANAEMIA IN CHRONIC KIDNEY DISEASE (CKD)

The kidney is the body's major site of erythropoietin (EPO) production. In renal disease, EPO levels fall, leading to chronic anaemia.

Additional Factors in Development of Anaemia in CKD

■ Reduced RBC lifespan
■ Iron deficiency (blood loss in dialysis tubing or GI tract)
■ Folate loss due to dialysis

What Features Should You Look For?

■ Low Hb
■ Normal MCV
■ Reticulocytes normal or reduced: low Epo reduces RBC production
■ Bizarre RBC shape on blood film: burr cells

Management

Generally, EPO replacement given at dialysis improves the Hb in these patients (50–100 units/kg × 3 per week IV). Alternatively, darbepoetin alfa can be given weekly. The patient might also require additional iron and folic acid. The Hb should be kept within the range of 100 to 120 g/L.

ANAEMIA IN LIVER DISEASE

Complex and Multifactorial

Patients with chronic liver failure generally have moderate anaemia.

The red cells are often macrocytic and can have abnormal shapes–target cells and spur cells–owing to membrane abnormalities.

Vitamin B_{12} levels are normal or high; folate levels are often low, owing to poor dietary intake.

■ Bleeding produces a hypochromic, microcytic picture
■ Alcohol causes macrocytosis, sometimes with leucopenia and thrombocytopenia due to bone marrow suppression
■ Hypersplenism results in pancytopenia
■ Cholestasis can often produce abnormal-shaped cells and also deficiency of vitamin K
■ Haemolysis accompanies acute liver failure and jaundice
■ Aplastic anaemia is present in up to 2% of patients with acute viral hepatitis
■ A raised serum ferritin with transferrin saturation (> 60%) is seen in hereditary haemochromatosis

Anaemia in Cancer

CASE HISTORY

A 55-year-old female, who underwent a right mastectomy 10 years earlier, presents with a subcapsular fracture of the left humerus. This had followed minimal trauma sustained when she slipped on the floor in the supermarket. It was thought that she might have disseminated bony metastases.

The contributory information provided by the blood count is:

- Haemoglobin 86 g/L
- Mean cell volume 76 fL
- White cell count 14.7 × 10⁹/L
- Platelets 64 × 10⁹/L
- Reticulocytes 2.0%
- Nucleated red cells
- Occasional myelocytes noted 4/100 WBCs
- Rouleaux +
- Platelets clumped ++

INFORMATION

Rouleaux

The tendency of red cells on the blood film to stack up like a 'pile of coins' relates to an increase in plasma proteins, particularly fibrinogen, as part of the acute-phase response.

This patient has a microcytic anaemia with rouleaux formation on the blood film. The anaemia of chronic disorder is common in disseminated malignancy and many other inflammatory and infective illnesses.

FURTHER INVESTIGATIONS

- Blood:
  - Serum alkaline phosphatase 247 IU/L
  - C-reactive protein 80
  - Serum calcium 2.9 mmol/L
- Imaging:
  - X-ray of shoulders showed humeral fracture
  - Skeletal survey showed bony metastases in thoracic spine and pelvis

Diagnosis

Carcinoma of the breast with bony secondaries.

ANAEMIA OF CHRONIC DISORDER: PATHOPHYSIOLOGY

- Functional iron deficiency
- Reduced sensitivity to EPO
- Reduced red cell lifespan

This patient has a raised total WCC with nucleated red cells and immature granulocytes seen on the blood film. This is a **leucoerythroblastic picture;** such cells are normally confined to the bone marrow. Bone marrow infiltration by disseminated malignancy disrupts the normal mechanisms controlling release of haemopoietic cells into the blood.

Leucoerythroblastic Anaemia

Causes include:

- Acute haemolysis
- Severe infection
- Severe hypoxia
- Bone marrow infiltration:
- Carcinoma
- Myeloma
- Lymphoma
- Tuberculosis
- Myelofibrosis
- Osteopetrosis

> **REMEMBER**
>
> Most blood count analysers cannot distinguish nucleated RBCs (nRBCs) from white cells and might give an inappropriately high WCC when nRBCs are present. Ask for the blood film to be reviewed.

The reticulocyte count is not increased and no red cell fragmentation is present on blood film review. Microangiopathic haemolytic anaemia (MAHA), which sometimes complicates disseminated breast, prostate or gastric carcinoma, is not likely to be a feature in this patient. Microangiopathic haemolytic anaemia results from mechanical disruption of red cells in small blood vessels and can be complicated by chronic DIC, with a coagulopathy, reduced fibrinogen concentration, elevated fibrin breakdown products and thrombocytopenia.

> **REMEMBER**
>
> Before accepting that a patient is thrombocytopenic:
> - Ask for the blood film to be reviewed
> - Repeat the blood count: fibrin formation or a small clot in the sample will result in a low platelet count

This patient has thrombocytopenia. The aetiology of thrombocytopenia in disseminated malignancy is complex and can be due to:

- Bone marrow infiltration
- Folate deficiency secondary to anorexia
- Cytotoxic chemotherapy
- Disseminated intravascular coagulation

However, a review of the blood film in this patient reveals that the thrombocytopenia is spurious – platelets are clumped on the blood film. Platelet clumping is a common phenomenon related to the EDTA anticoagulant that blood is collected into.

Progress and Management. This patient was treated symptomatically with NSAIDs and started on bisphosphonates. She was referred to the oncology department for a multidisciplinary team (MDT) for discussion of further management.

Infection/Sepsis

BACTERIAL SEPSIS

This results in a characteristic constellation of changes in the blood, which provide confirmatory evidence of sepsis and, in occasional patients with occult infection, may direct appropriate investigations.

- Neutrophil leucocytosis: increased numbers of neutrophils
- Immature granulocytes (= left-shift): occasional promyelocytes, myelocytes
- Toxic granulation: coarse neutrophil granulation
- Döhle bodies (white cells containing large RNA inclusions that are seen in, for example, sepsis, malignancy and pregnancy)

REMEMBER

A neutrophil leucocytosis may reflect processes other than infection:

- Tissue ischaemia:
  1. Myocardial infarct
  2. Sickle-cell crisis
- Inflammation:
  1. Rheumatoid arthritis
  2. Vasculitis
- Endocrine disease:
  1. Thyrotoxicosis
  2. Cushing disease
  3. Postsplenectomy
- Steroid therapy

POSSIBLE ACCOMPANIMENTS OF UNCONTROLLED SEPSIS

- A falling WCC/neutropenia
- Granulocyte vacuolation
- Bacteria visible on the stained blood film
- Thrombocytopenia
- Disseminated intravascular coagulation

Anaemia is common in bacterial sepsis and is usually related to the acute-phase response. Occasionally, haemolysis and red-cell fragmentation accompany DIC, and severe haemolysis might complicate *C. welchii* septicaemia with spherocytosis on the blood film.

Further Reading

Microcytic and Macrocytic Anaemia

British Committee for Standards in Haematology, 2014. Guidelines for the diagnosis and treatment of cobalamin and folate disorders. Br. J. Haematol. 166 (4), 496 513.

Camaschella, C., 2015. Iron deficiency anemia. N. Engl. J. Med. 372 (19), 1832–1843.

NICE CKS 2023. Anaemia - B$_{12}$ and Folate Deficiency.

NICE CKS 2023. Anaemia - Iron Deficiency.

Sickle-Cell Disease

NICE CKS 2023. Sickle Cell Disease.

Piel, F.B., et al., 2017. Sickle cell disease. N. Engl. J. Med. 376 (16), 1561–1573.

Elevated White Blood Cell Count

Stock, W., Hoffman, R., 2000. White blood cells 1: non-malignant disorders. Lancet 355 (9212), 1351–1357.

Platelet Disorders

Imbach, P., Crowther, M., 2011. Thrombopoietin receptor agonists for primary immune thrombocytopenia. N. Engl. J. Med. 365 (5), 734–741.

Provan, D., Newland, A., 2002. Fifty years of idiopathic thrombocytopenic purpura (ITP): management of refractory ITP in adults. Br. J. Haematol. 118 (4), 933–944.

Blood Transfusion

Joint United Kingdom (UK) Blood Transfusion and Tissue Transplantation Services Professional Advisory Committee Guidelines transfusionguidelines.org.

Murphy, M.F., Roberts, D.J., 2022. Practical Blood Transfusion. Wiley–Blackwell, Oxford.

Haematological Oncology

Devereaux, S., Cuthill, K., 2017. Chronic lymphocytic leukaemia. Medicine 45, 292–296.

Longo, D.L., 2017. Imatinib changed everything. N. Engl. J. Med. 376 (10), 982–983.

CHAPTER 12

Dermatology

A Swollen Red Leg

CASE HISTORY

The emergency department doctor asks you to come and see a 50-year-old male who is unwell and has a red, swollen leg. He thinks he needs anticoagulation for a possible deep vein thrombosis (DVT).

On arrival, you check if this was of sudden onset or a chronically swollen leg. You ask if there is a past history of DVT or whether there are any risk factors, such as a long car journey, air travel, immobility, or a family history of clotting disorders. You also ask about any recent illness, for example, heart failure or blood disorder.

WHAT SHOULD YOU DO NEXT?

You do a full medical examination.

On examination, the patient weighs 102 kg and has a temperature of 38°C. The leg is indeed red, swollen, hot and tender below the knee. You note a small ulcer on the medial side of the leg above the ankle. The dorsalis pedis pulse is palpable.

WHAT IS YOUR DIAGNOSIS?

Cellulitis, probably due to streptococci gaining entry via the venous ulcer.

Differential Diagnosis

- Deep vein thrombosis
- Ruptured Baker cyst
- Lipodermatosclerosis
- Acute allergic contact dermatitis: for example, to dressings
- Necrotising fasciitis: black necrotic areas within cellulitic area

INFORMATION

Lipodermatosclerosis
- Hot, red and woody hard 'atrophic' skin
- Long-standing venous disease
- Can mimic cellulitis but the patient is well, there is no pyrexia, and it may be bilateral

INVESTIGATIONS
- Consider streptococcal titres: antistreptolysin O titre (ASOT), anti-DNase B (ADB)
- Wound swab if obvious broken skin
- Blood culture if systemically unwell (rarely positive)

417

HOW DO YOU TREAT?

Flucloxacillin 0.5-1 g × 4 daily, having ascertained that he is not allergic to penicillin. Oral therapy should be for 7-10 days. When the cellulitis is severe commence IV flucloxacillin 1-2 g × 4 daily. Always follow local guidelines.

Progress. The patient's leg improved with antibiotics and he was discharged after 3 days. He was given compression stockings for his venous hypertension and referred to a dietitian for advice on weight reduction.

Leg Ulceration

Take a full history of associated diseases (diabetes mellitus, rheumatoid arthritis, past history of DVT, varicose veins, heart disease, hypertension, vasculitis, sickle cell, scleroderma).

Causes and Signs

- Venous hypertension:
  - Ulcer: chronic and recurrent, site – internal malleolus
  - Oedema
  - Venous eczema
  - Skin discoloration: atrophie blanche (stellate scarring with telangiectasia), erythema, haemosiderin pigmentation
  - Skin texture: lipodermatosclerosis
- Arterial disease:
  - Ulcer: punched out; site – often lateral or higher up on leg (painful)
  - Pulses: absent dorsalis pedis or posterior tibial
  - Cool leg
- Vasculitis: nonblanching purpura
- Neuropathic: sensory signs of decreased sensation present, particularly over pressure areas on feet; common in diabetics

INVESTIGATIONS

- General: full blood count (FBC), urea and electrolytes (U and Es), liver biochemistry, auto-antibodies (vasculitis), blood sugar, vitamin B_{12}, *Treponema pallidum* enzyme immunoassay (neuropathic ulcer)
- Venous: Doppler ultrasound – always perform before compression bandaging
- Arterial: Doppler ultrasound, digital subtraction angiography

Management

- **Venous ulcers:** elevation, exercise, compression dressings. Antibiotics if infected (always check Doppler pressures before considering compression, as many ulcers have mixed venous and arterial aetiology). Adequate analgesia
- **Arterial ulcers:** investigate arterial supply, dressings with *no* compression. Adequate analgesia
- **Vasculitic ulcers:** vasculitic screen, for example, antineutrophil cytoplasmic antibody (ANCA), antinuclear antibody (ANA), rheumatoid factor
- **Neuropathic ulcers:** keep ulcer clean and remove pressure or trauma from affected area
Note: Operating on varicose veins rarely helps venous insufficiency problems.

Contact your hospital's tissue viability nurse for assistance with dressings and compression bandaging, and for arranging longer-term community nursing follow-up.

> **INFORMATION**
>
> **Compression Bandages**
>
> Four-layer bandaging provides high levels of graduated compression with pressure decreasing up the leg.
>
> Eighty percent of ulcers can be healed within 6 months.

Generalised Rash or Eruption

Erythroderma means red skin. By definition, it is the term used when >90% of the skin is involved. Erythroderma is not an extensive maculopapular rash.

> **CASE HISTORY**
>
> A 63-year-old male presents to the emergency department unwell, shivering and red all over. He has suffered with chronic plaque psoriasis for 40 years and has been managed on topical therapy only. He smells of alcohol and admits to being a heavy drinker.
>
> **Examination** reveals **erythroderma** and multiple tiny pustules over the trunk. He has a pyrexia of 39.5°C and is clinically dehydrated.

HISTORY AND CLINICAL EXAMINATION

Take a comprehensive history of onset, past history, previous skin disease, family history, medication, occupation and other systemic symptoms. These include chills, flu-like symptoms and itching and burning of the skin. A full skin examination, including nails, mouth, genitals, scalp and hair, should be performed, as well as a general examination of lymph nodes and organomegaly.

Differential Diagnosis

- Eczema.
- Psoriasis
- Drug eruption
- Idiopathic
- Cutaneous T-cell lymphoma (mycosis fungoides, Sézary syndrome)
- Pemphigus foliaceus

ARE THERE ANY COMPLICATIONS YOU SHOULD LOOK OUT FOR?

- High-output cardiac failure from increased blood flow
- Hypothermia from heat loss
- Fluid loss
- Hypoalbuminaemia
- Increased basal metabolic rate, that is, catabolic
- Capillary leak syndrome in very severe cases of psoriasis: can give rise to acute respiratory distress syndrome (ARDS).
  (*Note:* this can be seen in severe drug rash).

Management

- Bed rest
- Rehydrate, plenty of fluids orally or IV
- Keep warm (space blankets)
- Moisturize the skin
- Refer all cases to dermatology urgently
- Regular (hourly) observations, for example, BP, pulse, fluid input/output chart, core temperature, weight

Investigate for cause and treat as appropriate, according to primary skin disease.

INVESTIGATIONS

- Full blood count
- Urea and electrolytes
- Liver biochemistry
- Chest X-ray (CXR)
- Culture of blood, skin, urine, sputum if pyrexial
- Skin biopsy

Progress. This patient was treated initially with IV glucose/saline with added potassium, then oral fluids. His core temperature fell to 37.2°C, so he was kept warm with space blankets in a heated room. He remained unwell for 2 weeks but then gradually improved.

Pruritus

Differentiate between a visible rash that is itchy and 'normal-looking' skin (with no rash other than scratch marks) that is itchy.

CASE HISTORY

A 19-year-old male presents with a 6-week history of an itchy skin, which has been 'driving him mad', especially at night-time, and he cannot sleep. There is nothing relevant in his past medical history or social history. He had bad asthma as a child.

On examination, he had multiple small red papules on the trunk, around nipples, wrists and axillae, and on the penis. These were accompanied by marked excoriations. No burrows were seen. A few lesions were seen on the soles of the feet.

Diagnosis

Scabies. The diagnosis of scabies was made on clinical grounds. Burrows are not always present but the distribution of nonspecific papules (occasionally vesicles) is highly suggestive. Sites commonly involved are axillae, nipples, penis, wrists, palms, soles and web spaces. The face/head is spared in adults. Scabies can be confirmed by skin scraping and microscopy.

CAUSES OF PRURITUS

Diseases of the Skin Associated With Pruritus

- Eczema (Fig. 12.1)
- Scabies
- Urticaria
- Psoriasis

- Lichen planus
- Dermatitis herpetiformis
- Pemphigoid

Systemic Diseases Associated With Pruritus

- Hypothyroidism
- Iron deficiency
- Advanced chronic kidney disease
- Liver disease (especially primary biliary cholangitis and hepatitis C)
- Lymphoma/myeloproliferative disease
- Coeliac disease

General Management of Urticaria

Treat the primary skin disease and refer to Dermatology.

- Eczema: moisturisers and topical corticosteroids
- Psoriasis: tar, vitamin D_3 ointments, mild to moderate topical steroids, dithranol (causes staining)
- Urticaria: nonsedating antihistamines
- Lichen planus: potent topical steroids/oral steroids
- Systemic diseases: see individual disease for treatment

INVESTIGATIONS

- Primary skin diseases: most cases can be diagnosed on clinical grounds but scrapings for direct microscopy (scabies), punch biopsy (+ immunofluorescence) and serum IgE for atopic disease are helpful
- Systemic diseases: FBC, U and Es, liver biochemistry, iron, folate, vitamin B_{12}, TFTs, auto-immune hepatitis screen, including mitochondrial antibodies, endomysial/gliadin antibodies. Consider serum immunoglobulins/protein electrophoresis/CXR in selected cases

Progress

- Scabies: malathion was given to the patient. He was told to be careful in applying malathion all over his body, including crevices of his body and webs of his fingers. This should be washed off after 24 h. Sexual contacts (if known), even if asymptomatic and without rash, should be given two treatments 7 days apart
- Repeated scabies prescriptions can lead to irritant dermatitis. Patients should be warned that the itching can go on for 1 month after successful treatment of scabies.

This patient's scabies was treated successfully and his symptoms resolved over the course of several weeks.

Eczema

CASE HISTORY

A 6-year-old male presents with his mother to his general practitioner (GP) reporting a 2-year history of itchy skin rashes. His mother explains that the rash often flares up, becoming red and inflamed, particularly on the backs of his knees, the creases of his elbows, and on his face. She mentions that the flares seem to worsen with changes in weather and after consuming certain foods, such as dairy and eggs. His sleep is frequently disturbed due to the itchiness, and he has been missing school because of the discomfort and the noticeable lesions on his skin. There is a family history of asthma and allergic rhinitis.

WHAT IS THE MOST LIKELY DIAGNOSIS?

He most likely has atopic eczema, which is supported by his chronic, itchy rash in typical distribution areas, a family history of atopy, and triggers that exacerbate his symptoms.

WHAT ARE THE COMMON TRIGGERS FOR ATOPIC ECZEMA?

Common triggers include irritants (soaps, detergents), allergens (dust mites, pet dander, pollen), foods (dairy, eggs, nuts), environmental factors (weather changes, stress) and infections.

INVESTIGATION

Investigations are not routinely required for the diagnosis of eczema but may be considered to rule out other conditions or if there is suspicion of a secondary infection. Potential investigations include:
- Skin swabs for bacterial culture when infection is suspected
- Allergy testing if there is a history suggestive of allergic triggers
- Blood tests to rule out other conditions in atypical cases

HOW CAN THE SEVERITY OF ATOPIC ECZEMA BE ASSESSED?

Severity can be assessed by the impact on quality of life, including sleep disturbance and psychological well-being, the extent and frequency of flares, and response to treatment.

INFORMATION

Eczema, also known as atopic dermatitis, is a common inflammatory skin condition characterized by pruritus, redness, and vesicular lesions (Fig. 12.1). It often follows a relapsing-remitting course and is associated with other atopic disorders. Management includes skin care, trigger avoidance, and pharmacotherapy. Patient education and support are integral to improving outcomes and quality of life.

Management

Management of atopic eczema includes both nonpharmacological and pharmacological strategies. Education on trigger avoidance and skincare is essential. A stepped approach should be used, where mild eczema may only require emollients, while more severe cases may need topical corticosteroids

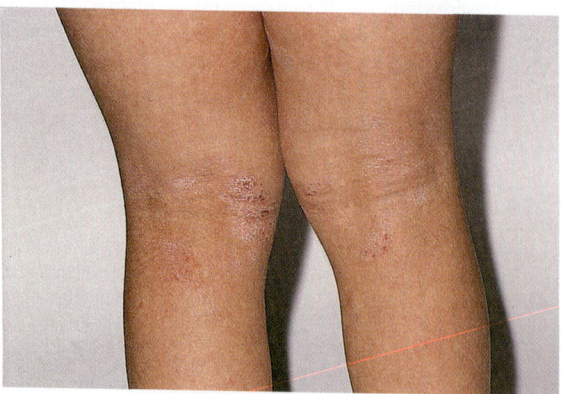

Fig. 12.1   Eczema.

or even systemic treatment. Antibiotics may be prescribed if there is evidence of a secondary bacterial infection. Regular follow-up is important to reassess and adjust the management plan.

REMEMBER

Eczema is a chronic condition that requires a long-term management strategy.

Patient education on skincare and trigger avoidance is key to successful management.

The treatment plan should be individualized based on the severity and patient response.

Progress. Over the past month, following the initial consultation, the patient's eczema has improved with the use of a regular emollient regimen and a moderate-potency topical corticosteroid during flare-ups. His mother reports that his sleep has improved and that there are fewer days of school missed. She has also started to implement dietary changes by reducing the intake of known triggers.

Psoriasis

CASE HISTORY

A 35-year-old female visits her GP with a history of persistent, scaly, red patches on her elbows and knees that have been present for several months. She reports the patches are itchy and sometimes painful, especially at night. She has tried over-the-counter moisturizers without much improvement. There is a family history of psoriasis; her father also had skin and joint problems.

INFORMATION

Psoriasis is a systemic inflammatory disorder with predominantly skin and joint manifestations. It is characterised by a chronic, relapsing-remitting course. Management is tailored to individual needs, severity, and impact on quality of life. Topical treatments are often first-line, with systemic therapies reserved for more severe cases. Regular monitoring and multidisciplinary care are important for optimal outcomes.

WHAT IS THE MOST COMMON FORM OF PSORIASIS THAT THIS PATIENT IS EXPERIENCING?

She is most likely experiencing chronic plaque psoriasis, given the description of persistent, scaly, red patches on typical extensor surfaces.

INVESTIGATION

While the diagnosis of psoriasis is primarily clinical, certain investigations may be considered, such as:

- Skin biopsy: In atypical cases or when the diagnosis is uncertain
- Joint assessment: If there are symptoms suggestive of psoriatic arthritis

WHAT ARE THE KEY CONSIDERATIONS WHEN PRESCRIBING TOPICAL TREATMENTS FOR PSORIASIS?

Key considerations include the severity and extent of skin involvement, patient preference, cosmetic acceptability, practical aspects of application, and the potential side effects of the treatments.

HOW CAN PSORIASIS IMPACT A PATIENT'S QUALITY OF LIFE?

Psoriasis can significantly impact a patient's physical appearance, self-esteem, and social interactions. It can also affect sleep and cause psychological distress, including anxiety and depression.

Management

Management includes education about psoriasis, its course, and potential triggers. Topical therapies with a potent corticosteroid and vitamin D analogue have been initiated. Lifestyle modifications, such as stress reduction techniques, smoking cessation, and maintaining a healthy weight, have been advised. Regular follow-ups are scheduled to monitor treatment response and adjust the management plan accordingly.

> **REMEMBER**
>
> Psoriasis is a chronic condition with systemic implications. Patient education and support are crucial for long-term management. Treatment efficacy should be balanced with the potential for side effects. Monitor patients regularly for the development of psoriatic arthritis.

Progress. After an initial consultation, this patient was prescribed a potent topical corticosteroid and a vitamin D analogue, which she applies as instructed. At a 4-week follow-up, she reports a 50% improvement in the appearance of the plaques, with reduced itching and discomfort. Her sleep quality has improved, and she feels more confident. She has also been seeking support from psoriasis support groups, which she finds helpful in managing her condition.

Urticaria and Angio-Oedema

Urticaria or **hives** is characterised by short-lived dermal swelling (weals) anywhere on the body (Fig. 12.2). These usually itch and, except in some subtypes, resolve without bruising within 24 hours (often within 10–20 min). They can form bizarre serpiginous or annular-shaped lesions. The latter show central clearing, not central necrosis as seen in erythema multiforme.

Angio-oedema is a deeper form of swelling affecting the dermis and subcutis, usually involving the mucous membranes, for example, eyes, lips, tongue, genitals and much less commonly the larynx and gastrointestinal tract. It is generally not itchy but can be painful and disappears within 72 hours. It may occur in isolation or with urticaria (45% of cases).

The incidence of urticaria/angio-oedema is about 15% in a person's lifetime and both conditions are more common in atopics.

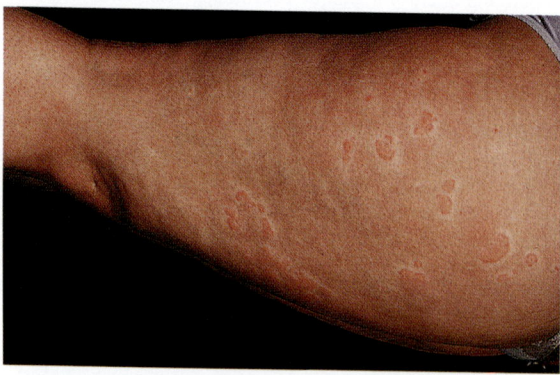

Fig. 12.2 Urticaria.

A 22-year-old female presents to the emergency department with a 6-hour history of a florid raised red rash all over the body. It is very itchy and distressing and has caused swelling around her eyes and her right hand. Previous medical history was of atopic eczema as a child and mild hay fever.

On examination, she had red, raised weals all over her body and periorbital swelling.

Diagnosis

Urticaria with angio-oedema.

CLASSIFICATION OF URTICARIAS

Acute

By definition, this lasts <6 weeks. Few cases have an identifiable allergen. They are IgE-mediated. In the most severe form, there is an anaphylactic reaction but this is fortunately very rare.

- Acute idiopathic urticaria and angio-oedema: account for >90% of urticaria. A good history should exclude an allergic cause. Viral infections will sometimes set off an acute urticaria
- Acute allergic urticaria: drug reactions, insect bites and foods (e.g. peanuts or seafood) can cause this type of reaction, as well as contact urticaria caused by, for example, latex or tomatoes. A history of an almost immediate reaction (seconds to minutes) after contact with an allergen should alert the clinician to this form

Chronic

By definition, this persists for >6 weeks. Only 2% to 4% of cases have an identifiable cause and extensive investigation is not indicated. Some cases are auto-immune, and functionally significant IgG (which acts against the high-affinity IgE receptors on mast cells) can be demonstrated in the patient's serum. In a few individuals, an acute illness (hepatitis, brucellosis), focal sepsis (e.g. dental abscess), or dermatophyte or parasitic infections can precipitate a reaction but this is very rare.

Physical

Reproducible wealing occurs in response to a specific physical stimulus, for example, friction, pressure, cold, heat, water, sun. The diagnosis might be suspected from the patient's history or the site of urticaria, that is, pressure sites in cases of dermographism or delayed pressure urticaria.

General Management

- Explanation of condition and likelihood of not identifying specific cause
- Avoidance of nonspecific factors, for example, aspirin, NSAIDs, opiates
- H_1 antihistamines (nonsedating or combination of daytime nonsedating H_1 blockers and sedating H_1 blocker at night); 90% of cases will respond to a nonsedating antihistamine, e.g. loratadine 10 mg daily
- Immunosuppression:
  - Short-term: a short, 7-day course of oral prednisolone 30 mg daily may be started in the emergency department to settle an attack quickly (especially if angio-oedema is prominent) while waiting for antihistamines to work
  - Long-term/chronic urticaria: corticosteroids, IV immunoglobulin, ciclosporin. For very severe cases, refer to the dermatology department

Preferred Regimens If No Contraindications

- Loratadine 10 mg daily or cetirizine 10 mg daily or fexofenadine 180 mg daily (all nonsedating antihistamines)
- Sedative antihistamines, for example, hydroxyzine 25–50 mg at night

Refer: to dermatology department if no response to antihistamines.

Refer: to type 1 allergy clinic (usually different to dermatology) *only* if allergic urticaria is suspected from history.

Management of Severe Angio-Oedema

- Adrenaline (epinephrine): 1:1000 (1 mg/mL) IM. Adult dose 0.5–1.0 mL
- Intravenous chlorphenamine: 10–20 mg (max. 40 mg/24 h)
- Intravenous hydrocortisone succinate: 100–300 mg

Home (Injectable Adrenaline) Pens

These should never be prescribed lightly and then only after full investigation in an allergy clinic, when relevant allergens have been proven and where a genuine anaphylactic reaction has occurred. They are most commonly used in those severely allergic to nuts. Injectable adrenaline pens are *not* appropriate for isolated severe cutaneous urticaria or angio-oedema.

Patients/parents need to attend an allergy clinic to be instructed in both when and how to use the pens and, indeed, how frequently, if the first injection gives only temporary relief (two pens should be prescribed).

Adrenaline (epinephrine) 1:1000 (1 mg/mL) is available in preloaded injections to deliver a dose of 0.3 or 0.5 mg (adult) or 0.15 mg (paediatric), and injections should be carried out by the patient.

Progress. This patient was given prednisolone 30 mg daily for 7 days and started on loratadine 20 mg daily. The nature of the complaint was explained to her; no specific antigen was identified. She was seen by her doctor after 4 days and was completely free of symptoms. She continued with loratadine for 1 month.

Hereditary Angio-Oedema (HAE)

Skin lesions may develop and laryngeal obstruction can occur. Lesions appear as deep swellings with associated enlarging oedematous borders that last up to 2 to 4 days. Urticaria does not occur as part of HAE. Patients generally suffer from recurrent attacks of painful angio-oedema, which can be precipitated by minor trauma, emotional upset, infections and temperature change. Involvement of the gastrointestinal tract can cause severe acute pain and simulate a surgical emergency. Recurrent abdominal pain often occurs and starts in childhood. Hereditary angio-oedema is inherited in an autosomal dominant fashion with either a functional or absolute deficiency of C1 esterase inhibitor (C1-INH). Eighty percent of cases give a positive family history (e.g. of sudden death). Acquired forms are seen in systemic lupus erythematosus (SLE) or lymphoma.

> **REMEMBER**
>
> **Hereditary Angio-Oedema (HAE)**
> Patients can develop laryngeal obstruction requiring urgent treatment.

Management

Patients are unresponsive to antihistamines, which can exacerbate the condition, systemic steroids and adrenaline (epinephrine). Refer all patients for management; the acute treatment of choice in A and E is IV (C1-INH) concentrates. If unavailable, fresh frozen plasma can be used. Most cases/families already diagnosed will know where local supplies of C1-INH are to be found. Icatibant (a bradykinin antagonist) and ecallantide (a kallikrein inhibitor) are also of benefit in acute attacks.

In adults, chronic treatment or 'prophylaxis' with lanadelumab, a recombinant fully human monoclonal antibody, produces sustained inhibition of kallikrein and is now the treatment of choice.

Cutaneous Adverse Drug Reaction (ADR)

The true incidence is unknown, as many go unreported, but the skin is the most commonly affected organ, involved in 30% of reported ADRs.

Preexisting disease (SLE, chronic lymphocytic leukaemia, HIV), advancing age (polypharmacy, reduced renal and hepatic clearance) and sensitivity to other drugs (e.g. penicillins: 10% cross-reactivity with cephalosporins) can all increase susceptibility to the development of ADRs.

CASE HISTORY (1)

A 24-year-old male developed a severe sore throat and a fever. He was seen by his doctor, who diagnosed a streptococcal sore throat and prescribed amoxicillin. Two days later, he presented with a macropapular rash (Fig. 12.3).

On examination, he was noted to have cervical lymphadenopathy and a small palpable spleen. Infectious mononucleosis (glandular fever) was diagnosed with a Monospot test and the amoxicillin was stopped.

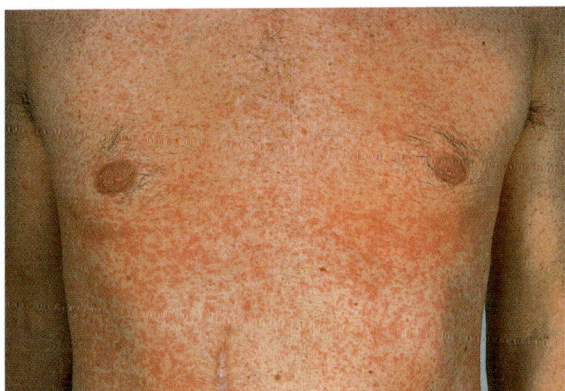

Fig. 12.3 Maculopapular rash following amoxicillin therapy in patient with infectious mononucleosis.

REMEMBER

Never use amoxicillin in a patient unless glandular fever has been excluded.

CASE HISTORY (2)

A 54-year-old doctor presented with a 1-year history of early morning stiffness of her hands and Raynaud's. She had self-medicated with a number of NSAIDs, which had helped to ease the pain and stiffness. She was seen by a rheumatologist, who found a slight deformity of her fingers but no other signs of rheumatoid arthritis. In view of the long history, she was prescribed sulfasalazine as a disease-modifying drug. A month later, she developed a severe, itchy, morbilliform rash all over her body. This settled on stopping the sulfasalazine, which contains a sulfonamide and 5-aminosalicylic acid (ASA).

Progress. Both cases resolved on stopping the drugs.

REMEMBER

Always discuss the harm/benefit ratio of drugs with your patient. Also, review their current drug therapy and check for interactions.

CLASSIFICATION

- Type A: augmented (~80% of all ADRs) – exaggerated responses to known effects of the drug. Predictable and dose-related, for example, skin necrosis after extravasation of vincristine, alopecia due to cytotoxic agents, cheilitis due to retinoids, urticaria triggered by opiates causing mast cell degranulation
- Type B: unpredictable/bizarre – idiosyncratic and therefore more difficult to diagnose

Physiology

There are a number of mechanisms, but the pathogenesis of many cutaneous ADRs remains unknown.

Cutaneous ADRs can also be categorised morphologically into three groups:
1. Skin reactions specific to drugs
2. Rashes potentially caused by drugs
3. Established skin disease exacerbated by drugs

SKIN REACTIONS SPECIFIC TO DRUGS

Fixed drug eruptions are very rare. They develop within 24 hours of drug ingestion and usually affect localised areas showing sharply demarcated, round, red, oedematous (and sometimes bullous) plaques that become violaceous or hyperpigmented with time. Lesions recur at the same site on reexposure to the drug.

Pigmentation Caused by Drugs

- Long-term amiodarone or chlorpromazine: purple/slate-grey pigmentation on sun-exposed sites
- Long-term minocycline: blue/black pigmentation of skin, nails, buccal mucosa, scars (may be irreversible)
- Mepacrine: reversible yellow skin pigmentation
- Bleomycin: flagellate erythema then hyperpigmentation of trunk

RASHES POTENTIALLY CAUSED BY DRUGS

There are many different reaction patterns and only a few common ones are considered here.

Maculopapular/Exanthematic Eruptions

This is the most common type of cutaneous ADR. It is thought to be a cell-mediated reaction (may also be immune complex) involving CD8 T cells (Table 12.1). There are widespread, symmetrical, itchy eruptions. Macules and papules may become confluent and develop into a sheet-like erythema, sometimes with fever and eosinophilia. When due to a drug, the rash usually begins on the trunk. Suspect a viral aetiology if it starts on the face and moves down, and if there is associated lymphadenopathy and conjunctivitis. After withdrawal of the drug, the rash usually settles over 2 weeks.

Note: if this eruption has progressed rapidly over 24 hours it may herald the onset of the following:

Erythroderma. More than 90% of the skin surface is erythematous and inflamed. Ten percent of cases are drug-induced (e.g. sulfonamides, sulfonylureas, penicillins, barbiturates, allopurinol, gold, mercury, arsenicals).

Toxic Epidermal Necrolysis (TEN). The development of vesicles and/or bullae and skin tenderness raises this possibility (this might then be followed by 'sheeting off' of the epidermis). Mucosal involvement also suggests TEN.

Anticonvulsant Hypersensitivity Syndrome. This is not just a severe ADR from an anticonvulsant but a distinct syndrome that, if undiagnosed, can lead to death if patients are changed to a different anticonvulsant that cross-reacts. The rash normally starts 2 to 4 weeks after starting any of the aromatic anticonvulsants (carbamazepine, phenytoin, phenobarbital, primidone). The rash is a nonspecific maculopapular eruption that may involve mucosal surfaces and occasionally pustulates. The distinguishing clinical features from a 'normal' ADR are any of the following:

- Fever
- Hepatosplenomegaly/lymphadenopathy
- Conjunctivitis/periorbital oedema
- Arthralgia
- Pharyngitis
- Severe malaise.

TABLE 12.1 ■ **Pathogenesis of Some Cutaneous ADRs (Hypersensitivity Reactions)**

Type	Examples
Type 1 Immediate, IgE-mediated hypersensitivity	Urticaria and anaphylaxis due to penicillins
Type II Cytotoxic	Allergic thrombocytopenic purpura
Type III Immune complex formation	Morbilliform maculopapular rash Serum sickness Vasculitis, e.g. allopurinol and penicillin
Type IV Cell-mediated	Allergic contact dermatitis to topical medicaments Erythema multiforme, toxic epidermal necrolysis Lichenoid drug eruption

ADRs, Adverse drug reactions.

Blood tests may show:

- Eosinophilia
- Lymphocytosis with atypical lymphocytes
- Raised hepatic transferases

If the drug is not stopped immediately, the patient may progress to multiorgan failure and need intensive care. *All* aromatic anticonvulsant drugs must be avoided in the future because further exposure is likely to lead to an even more severe reaction. Sodium valproate is a reasonable alternative.

Photosensitivity

(See Box 12.1.) Reactions range from erythema to blistering and characteristically spare the submental area, finger webs, under eyebrow area and triangle of skin behind the ear lobe.

Lichenoid Eruption

(See Box 12.1.) This is similar to idiopathic lichen planus but often more widespread and rarely involves mucous membranes.

Spectrum of Erythema Multiforme, Stevens–Johnson Syndrome and Toxic Epidermal Necrolysis

The classification of these diseases is confusing in the literature.

Erythema Multiforme. Ten percent of cases are drug-related (the majority are postinfectious, for example, herpes simplex virus, and mycoplasma). They are mild and self-limiting and usually resolve within 2 to 4 weeks. They are characterised by target lesions of a central dusky erythema (sometimes with blistering), a pale oedematous ring and a peripheral erythematous ring. These usually occur acrally (extremities) and symmetrically on extensor surfaces. They involve palms and soles. Mucosal involvement may be present but is mild and limited to one mucosal surface, for example, the oral cavity.

Stevens–Johnson Syndrome (SJS; Also Called Erythema Multiforme Major). This is a more severe and extensive eruption. Widespread atypical target lesions appear on the trunk, in which epidermal necrosis results in the formation of blisters and epidermal detachment involving <10% of the body surface area. At least two mucosal surfaces are involved (oral, ocular, genital). Mucosal lesions are often more prominent than skin lesions. Systemic toxicity may occur. Steven–Johnson syndrome usually resolves within 6 weeks.

Stevens–Johnson Syndrome/TEN Overlap. When the extent of epidermal detachment is between 10% and 30% of the body surface area, in the presence of other features of SJS, this is considered an SJS/TEN overlap. The skin lesions are often necrotic blisters rather than target lesions, and mucosal lesions are prominent and severe.

Toxic Epidermal Necrolysis. This is of sudden onset (usually evolves over 24–48 h) with widespread morbilliform or confluent dusky erythema and skin tenderness. This is followed by widespread blistering (necrolysis) of the skin with histological evidence of full-thickness epidermal necrosis, subepidermal separation and a sparse or absent dermal infiltrate. The Nikolsky sign is positive. Mucous membrane involvement is usually severe, including ocular, genital, oral, nasopharynx and GI tract; mortality is 20% to 30%.

Adverse prognostic factors include:

- Age >60 years
- Area of involved skin >50%

- Plasma urea >17 mmol/L
- Neutropenia <1.0 × 10^9/L
- Idiopathic nature of TEN

If extensive:

- Ventilation may be required
- Contact ICU, dermatology and ophthalmology urgently

Treatment of TEN

- Early high-dose immunosuppression may help but remains controversial (IV immunoglobulin is also commonly used).
- Analgesia (opiate)
- Dressings/human skin bank/autologous skin grafts
- Eye protection and review for scarring
- Pressure-relieving bed
- Intensive therapy unit supportive therapy

REMEMBER

- All cases of TEN should be considered to be drug-induced and suspected drug(s) should be stopped immediately
- The most common drugs responsible are sulfonamides, penicillins, anticonvulsants and NSAIDs

ESTABLISHED SKIN DISEASE EXACERBATED BY DRUGS (SEE BOX 12.1)

- Psoriasis: can be destabilised by lithium and possibly beta-blockers and antimalarials
- Acne: can be aggravated by progesterone-containing contraceptives, lithium and corticosteroids

BOX 12.1 ■ Common Drug Associations

Maculopapular Eruption

- Antibiotics
- (Penicillins, sulfonamides)
- Anticonvulsants
- (Carbamazepine, phenytoin)
- NSAIDs

Photosensitivity

- Thiazides
- Sulfonamides
- Amiodarone
- Tetracycline
- Nalidixic acid

Lichenoid Eruption

- Gold
- Beta blockers
- Quinine/antimalarials
- Thiazides
- Allopurinol

- Rosacea: worse with topical steroids
- Perioral dermatitis: caused and exacerbated by topical steroids

DIAGNOSIS OF ADRS

The key elements to a diagnosis are a meticulous drug history and a high index of suspicion.

- Exclude other causes by history and examination
- Take a careful drug history: remember to ask about over-the-counter preparations, for example, laxatives, tonics, cough medicines, vitamins and complementary treatments
- Establish the start and stop dates of medication and relationship to onset of the rash
- When the eruption begins 7 to 21 days after the first administration of a drug or within 48 hours if the drug has caused a similar reaction in the past, this is highly suggestive of an ADR
- The timing is incompatible with an ADR if the drug was started after the onset of cutaneous or mucous membrane signs. If the onset is within 24 hours of the first dose, or more than 21 days after stopping the drug, a drug aetiology is doubtful. If there are several drugs, each should be considered as a potential cause
- Consult drug information for previous reports

INVESTIGATIONS

These are of little help!

- Blood eosinophilia (may be found in toxic erythema but is non-specific)
- Biopsy 'may suggest but not prove a drug aetiology':
  - Lots of eosinophils: common
  - Lichenoid pattern: rare
  - Systemic lupus erythematosus pattern: rare
  - Vasculitis: sometimes
- Blood level of drug (may be useful to check for overdosage)
- If a fixed drug eruption is suspected, rechallenge may be helpful (in other situations it is rarely justifiable for fear of precipitating a more severe reaction)
- Patch testing is helpful in patients with suspected allergic contact dermatitis (type IV hypersensitivity reactions) but *cannot* be used for systemic ADRs

TREATMENT

- Withdraw drug(s): symptomatic treatment with oral antihistamines, topical steroids and moisturisers
- Severe reactions (SJS and TEN) require supportive therapy and monitoring of infection, fluid balance and temperature. Patients may need ITU. Use of systemic immunosuppression may be considered if patients are seen within the first 24 hours of onset
- Dressings: leave on
- Support mattress
- Opiate analgesia
- Give written information to patient and doctors to ensure no repeat exposure

Fig. 12.4 can be used as a guide to referral.

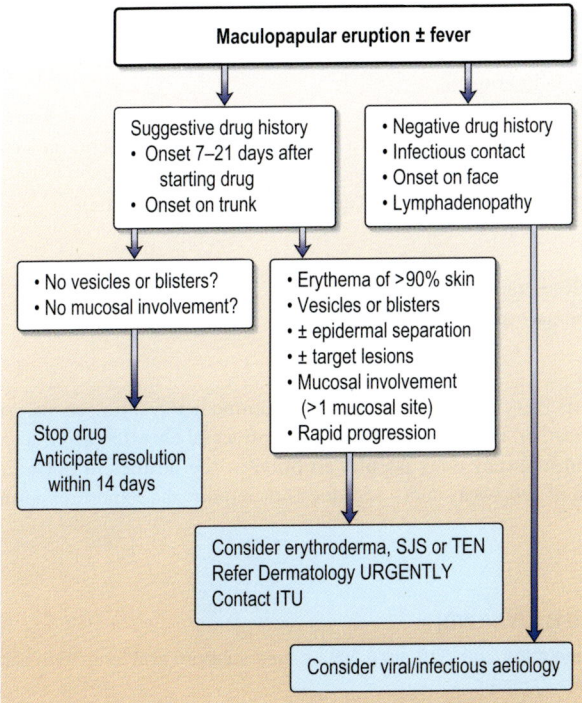

Fig. 12.4 When to refer to a dermatologist in the case of an adverse drug reaction. SJS, Stevens–Johnson syndrome; TEN, toxic epidermal necrolysis.

Sun-Induced Rash

CASE HISTORY

A 24-year-old arrived in the emergency department with blisters on her face and arms. She had fallen asleep on the beach in the sun. She had applied factor 4 sunscreen and was surprised that she had developed an itchy rash. **On examination**, she had papules and a few vesicles over the exposed areas.

REMEMBER

- Always take a drug history in somebody who is photosensitive (e.g. doxycycline, amiodarone)
- Always keep SLE and porphyrias in mind for any photosensitivity case where diagnosis is not obvious

WHAT IS THE DIAGNOSIS?

This is **polymorphic light eruption**, which occurs in 10% to 20% of the population. The rash appears some hours after the exposure and can last for several hours or a few days following exposure. The rash may be papular or papulovesicular. This patient also had evidence of sunburn – remember, factor 4 does not protect for very long.

DIFFERENTIAL DIAGNOSIS

Common

- Polymorphic light eruption
- Sunburn
- Sunscreen allergy leading to photo contact dermatitis (presents as eczema rather than papules/vesicles)
- Drug-induced photosensitive rash (e.g. doxycycline, amiodarone)

Rare

- Photosensitive eczema
- Lupus erythematosus (all forms)
- Porphyrias
- Actinic prurigo
- Solar urticaria (very rare): gives rise to a rash immediately after sun exposure.

Note: 'prickly heat' or 'heat rash' (miliaria) is incorrect labels often given to polymorphic light eruption. This is an intensely itchy papular eruption in the flexures in hot humid conditions. It is due to blockage of the sweat ducts and does not require sun exposure; neither is it found on sun-exposed skin.

INFORMATION

Ultraviolet A and B (UVA/UVB)

- Medium wavelengths 280–310 nm (UVB): cause sunburn and long-term skin changes, for example, ageing/cancer
- Long wavelengths 310–400 nm (UVA): do not cause sunburn (unless high doses through glass) but do cause photodermatoses. Also contribute to long-term skin damage
- Sunscreen preparations protect against UVB: the sun protection factor (SPF) number gives an indication of the amount of time that a person is protected against burning compared to unprotected skin. Most sunscreens also protect against UVA by utilizing reflectants or chemical absorbers

---

Most sunscreens are insufficiently applied (and not reapplied after bathing), and so do not give the protection suggested by the SPF factor.

HOW WOULD YOU TREAT THIS PATIENT?

No treatment was necessary for this patient because she was virtually asymptomatic. She was given a leaflet on sun exposure and told that her type of rash usually tended to improve over the summer period.

Refer: to the dermatology department if the condition is not controlled by the use of sunblock and advice to increase sun exposure slowly in spring/early summer.

If the rash becomes worse each year, consider desensitizing with low-dose psoralens + UVA (PUVA) each spring or short bursts of oral prednisolone (e.g. 30 mg daily for 1 week) for an attack.

Erythema Nodosum

Erythema nodosum is a hypersensitivity reaction to various antigens (e.g. drugs, infectious agents and unknown antigens), producing an inflammation in the dermis and subcutaneous layer (panniculitis).

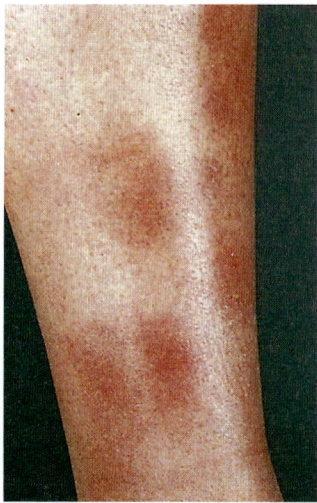

Fig. 12.5 Erythema nodosum.

It presents with painful, tender, dusky blue–red nodules, usually on the shins and lower limbs (Fig. 12.5).

CASE HISTORY

A 16-year-old female presents to the emergency department with her mother. She has painful red lumps on her shins and arthralgia. Walking has become painful. She is otherwise well, with no relevant previous medical history.

On examination, she has tender, red/purple lumps on her shins but no other signs. The clinical picture was of erythema nodosum.

Make the Diagnosis

- Spontaneous onset over days; evolution over a few days or weeks
- Single or multiple deep, bruise-like nodules 1–10 cm in diameter (better felt than seen)
- Tender and warm to touch
- Predominantly affecting limbs (shins or lower limbs)
- No age or sex limitation (but young females are more common)
- Sometimes associated with arthralgia
- Always do a CXR looking for hilar lymphadenopathy or tuberculosis

WHAT IS THE CAUSE?

- Drugs:
  - Oral contraceptives
  - Aspirin and other NSAIDs
  - Sulphonamides
- Infection:
  - Streptococcal
  - Tuberculosis
  - Leprosy (patient from endemic area)
  - Chlamydia (rare)

- Sarcoidosis
- Inflammatory bowel disease
- Idiopathic (most common)
- Pregnancy

Initial Treatment

- Aspirin 600 mg as required (unless this is the identified cause of the erythema nodosum)
- Bed rest if severe
- Tubigrip support bandages
- If severe symptoms and/or cutaneous ulceration consider using dapsone or steroids (e.g. prednisolone 30 mg daily decreasing course)

Note: Monitor for haemolytic anaemia and avoid dapsone if there is a glucose-6-phosphate dehydrogenase (G6PD) deficiency.

WHEN SHOULD SHE BE REFERRED?

- Recurrent or unresolving symptoms
- Ulceration
- Sarcoidosis/tuberculosis/leprosy/inflammatory bowel disease suspected
- Systemically unwell patient

Progress. This patient went home with her mother, reassured that her illness would settle. After 7 days with occasional aspirin therapy, she was much better and was able to restart school. Her CXR showed hilar lymphadenopathy. With erythema nodosum, this is characteristic of sarcoidosis.

She returned to the hospital after 6 months for a follow-up CXR, which was normal.

Shingles

Varicella zoster virus causes a primary infection – chickenpox, usually in children.

The virus remains latent in dorsal root and cranial nerve ganglia, and reactivation results in shingles.

> **CASE HISTORY**
>
> A 75-year-old male presents to his GP with severe right-sided chest pain for the previous 2 days. In the past 24 hours, he has noted a rash on the right side of his chest, in the distribution of T5 to T6.

WHAT DO YOU THINK THE LIKELY DIAGNOSIS IS?

Shingles.

WHAT QUESTION WOULD YOU LIKE TO ASK THE PATIENT?

Have you had chickenpox?

> **REMEMBER**
>
> Not everyone who has antibodies to varicella zoster virus remembers having the primary disease.
>
> All people over the age of 65 years should have prophylactic varicella inoculation.

WHAT INVESTIGATIONS MIGHT YOU PERFORM?

The disease is usually diagnosed clinically. It can be confirmed by examination of the vesicular fluid under an electron microscope to look for herpes virus. Serology can also be performed.

HOW WOULD YOU MANAGE THE PATIENT?

If admitted to hospital this patient should be nursed in a side room and only by nurses who are known to have antibodies against varicella-zoster virus. If he were to remain at home, he must avoid contact with people who have no history of having had chickenpox.

As the patient has had the rash for less than 3 days, he should be commenced on aciclovir. Alternative CV agents active against varicella zoster virus include famciclovir or valaciclovir (may reduce incidence of chronic pain compared to aciclovir). The usual adult dose of aciclovir for treatment of shingles is 800 mg × 5 daily by mouth or 5-10 mg/kg × 3 daily if given intravenously.

> **REMEMBER**
> - Modification of the dose of aciclovir might be required if the patient has renal impairment
> - Patients should be prevailed upon not to scratch their lesions, as this can predispose to secondary infection. Calamine lotion can help
> - Patients are likely to require analgesia

Progress. The patient was admitted to hospital because he lives on his own and he was started on aciclovir. Twenty-four hours later, he developed a high fever. A nurse noticed that one of the lesions had an inflamed area around it.

WHAT DO YOU THINK HAS HAPPENED? HOW WOULD YOU MANAGE THE PATIENT?

Secondary infection of the shingles lesions has occurred. The most likely pathogens to cause this are *Streptococcus pyogenes* or *Staphylococcus aureus*. Swabs should be taken and sent to microbiology for microscopy, culture and sensitivity, and blood cultures should also be taken. The patient was commenced on IV benzylpenicillin (active against *Strep. pyogenes*) and IV flucloxacillin (active against *S. aureus*), and switched to oral therapy after 3 days. His infected area settled, but on discharge after 6 days he still had a painful area of shingles on his chest with some new lesions. His aciclovir was therefore continued for 10 days.

He was also given amitriptyline 10 mg at night for pain. He remained unwell for 3 weeks, but after 2 months his pain had settled and he made a full recovery.

> **INFORMATION**
> Ophthalmic herpes is infection of the 1st division of the Vth nerve and can lead to corneal scarring and secondary panophthalmitis. Ramsay Hunt syndrome is due to herpes infection of the geniculate ganglia. It causes a facial palsy with vesicles on the pinna of the ear. Postherpetic neuralgia is a burning, continuous pain in the area of the previous eruption. It is common in the elderly and accompanied by depression. It is difficult to treat.

Skin Lesions (see Box 12.2)

CASE HISTORY 1

A 30-year-old female has become increasingly concerned about a mole on her right thigh (Fig. 12.6). Over the past 6 months, she has observed that the mole has grown in size, with portions appearing darker and others lighter. The mole's shape is asymmetrical, and the edges are notched. Occasionally, the mole has been itchy and has bled without significant trauma.

BOX 12.2 ■ Clinical Criteria for the Diagnosis of Malignant Melanoma

ABCDE Criteria (United States)

- Asymmetry of mole
- Border irregularity
- Colour variegation
- Diameter >6 mm
- Elevation

The Glasgow Seven-Point Checklist

Major Criteria

- Change in size
- Change in shape
- Change in colour

Minor Criteria

- Diameter >6 mm
- Inflammation
- Oozing or bleeding
- Mild itch or altered sensation

From Kumar, P., Clark, M., eds., 2017. Agnosis, ninth ed. Elsevier, Edinburgh; Box 31.8.

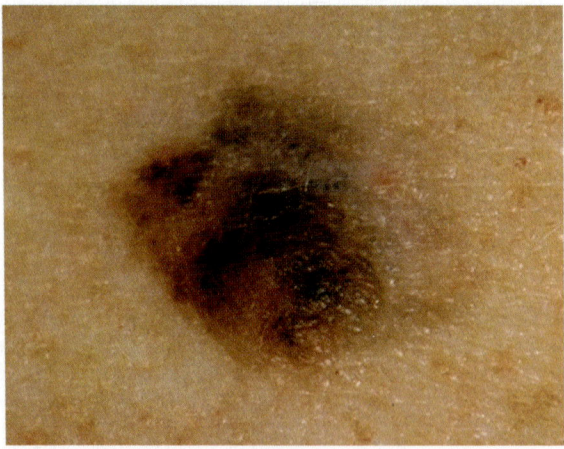

Fig. 12.6   Case 1's skin lesion. (From Peter, C.N., 2024. Plastic Surgery, fifth ed. Tumors of the hand, Fig. 16.18, Elsevier INC, Philadelphia, PA.)

WHAT IS THE SIGNIFICANCE OF BRESLOW THICKNESS IN MELANOMA?

Breslow thickness refers to the depth of the melanoma in the skin. It's a critical prognostic factor; the thicker the melanoma, the greater the risk for metastasis.

INVESTIGATION

- Complete skin examination with particular attention to the size, shape, colour and evolution of pigmented lesions
- Dermoscopic evaluation to identify specific melanoma features
- Excisional biopsy with histopathology to confirm diagnosis and assess prognostic features like Breslow thickness and ulceration
- Imaging studies, such as lymphoscintigraphy, may be indicated for sentinel lymph node mapping

CAN YOU DESCRIBE THE MANAGEMENT PLAN FOLLOWING A DIAGNOSIS OF EARLY-STAGE MELANOMA?

Management includes wide local excision with margins appropriate to the Breslow thickness, sentinel lymph node biopsy for melanomas over 1 mm thickness, regular follow-up for early detection of recurrence or new primary melanomas, and patient education on the importance of sun protection.

WHAT ARE THE FOLLOW-UP RECOMMENDATIONS FOR A PATIENT DIAGNOSED WITH STAGE IA MELANOMA?

Follow-up typically involves regular skin examinations by a healthcare provider, which may be every 3 to 12 months depending on the patient's risk factors, and patient education on self-examination techniques.

INFORMATION

Melanoma is a potentially aggressive form of skin cancer originating from melanocytes. Key warning signs include changes in an existing mole or the appearance of a new pigmented lesion that follows the Asymmetry, Border, Colour, Diameter, Evolving (ABCDE) rule. Risk factors include fair skin, high sun exposure, family history of melanoma, and the presence of numerous or atypical moles. Treatment success and prognosis are significantly better when melanoma is detected and treated early.

Management

Wide excision of the primary melanoma with appropriate margins to ensure complete removal.

Sentinel lymph node biopsy for staging and to guide further treatment. Education on sun safety, including using a broad-spectrum sunscreen, wearing protective clothing and seeking shade.

Regular dermatologic follow-up to monitor for local recurrence, new primary lesions, and systemic spread. Psychological support to cope with the cancer diagnosis and its implications.

REMEMBER

Melanoma can be life-threatening if it spreads; early diagnosis and treatment are key.

Regular skin self-examination and professional skin evaluations are important, especially for high-risk individuals. Comprehensive sun protection measures are essential to prevent melanoma and other skin cancers.

Progress. Her GP referred her for an urgent dermatological assessment due to the suspicious changes. The dermatologist performed a detailed examination using dermoscopy, which revealed irregular pigmentation and structure suggestive of melanoma. An excisional biopsy was conducted with a narrow margin, and the pathology report confirmed malignant melanoma with a Breslow thickness of 0.9 mm. She underwent a wider excision with a 1 cm margin and a sentinel lymph node biopsy. Fortunately, the biopsy showed no evidence of metastasis, classifying her melanoma as Stage IA. She has been advised to attend regular follow-up appointments every 3 months for skin checks and to practice strict sun protection.

CASE HISTORY 2

A 65-year-old male with a history of kidney transplantation presents with a persistent rough, scaly patch on his right ear that has been slowly enlarging over the past 6 months (Fig. 12.7). He reports that the lesion occasionally bleeds when he scratches it and is tender to touch.

WHAT IS THE LIKELY DIAGNOSIS?

Squamous cell carcinoma.

WHAT ARE THE TREATMENT OPTIONS FOR SQUAMOUS CELL CARCINOMA?

Treatment options include surgical excision, Mohs micrographic surgery, cryotherapy for small lesions, radiation therapy and systemic therapy for advanced cases.

INFORMATION

Squamous cell carcinoma (SCC) is a common skin cancer associated with cumulative UV exposure, especially in fair-skinned individuals. It can be more aggressive in immunocompromised patients. The risk of metastasis, while generally low, is higher for lesions on the lips and ears. Prognosis is good with early detection and appropriate treatment.

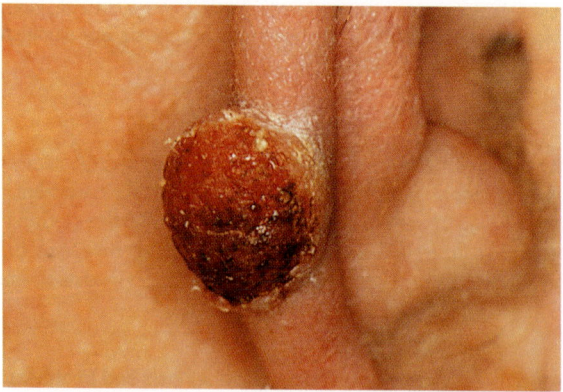

Fig. 12.7   Case 2's skin lesion. (From Zenith. 2050. Medical Assisting Module A Textbook, second ed. Integumentary System, Fig. 1.26, Elsevier INC, St. Louis, MO.)

WHAT ROLE DOES IMMUNOSUPPRESSION PLAY IN THE RISK AND PROGNOSIS OF SCC?

Immunosuppression can lead to an increased risk of developing SCC, potentially more aggressive behaviour, and a higher likelihood of recurrence and metastasis.

INVESTIGATION

- Clinical examination with palpation of regional lymph nodes
- Punch or shave biopsy for histopathological diagnosis
- For advanced cases, imaging such as CT or MRI may be required to assess local invasion and metastasis

Management

- Early and complete excision of the lesion with histopathological margin assessment
- Regular postoperative surveillance due to increased risk of recurrence, particularly in immunocompromised individuals
- Education on the importance of self-examination and immediate reporting of new or changing lesions
- Skin protection against UV radiation with lip balms containing SPF

REMEMBER

Squamous cell carcinoma often arises in sun-exposed areas and may present as a nonhealing ulcer or a scaly patch.

Early intervention can prevent local invasion and reduce the risk of metastasis.

Education on UV protection and the importance of regular skin checks is vital for patients with a history of SCC.

CASE HISTORY 3

A 52-year-old female presents with a small, shiny, pearly bump on the side of her nose that she first noticed a year ago (Fig. 12.8). The bump has slowly grown and sometimes crusts over and bleeds slightly. She has a history of using tanning beds in her 20s and 30s and recalls occasional sunburns.

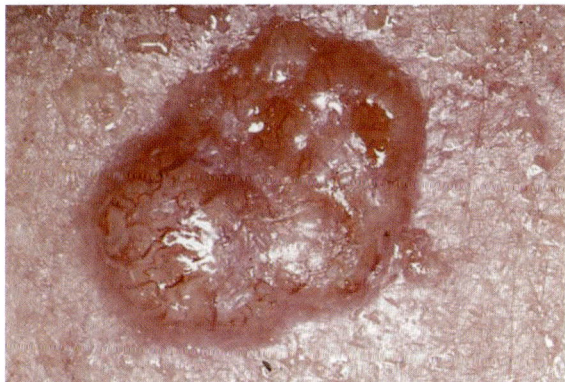

Fig. 12.8 Case 3's skin lesion. (From Peter, C.N., 2024. Plastic Surgery, fifth ed. Tumors of the hand, Fig. 16.14, Elsevier INC, Philadelphia, PA.)

WHAT ARE THE DIFFERENT CLINICAL SUBTYPES OF BASAL CELL CARCINOMA?

The clinical subtypes include nodular, superficial, morpheaform (sclerosing) and pigmented BCC.

> **INFORMATION**
>
> Basal cell carcinoma (BCC) arises from the basal cells of the epidermis and is strongly related to UV radiation exposure. It commonly presents as a pearly nodule, often on the head and neck. Risk factors include fair skin, sun exposure and immunosuppression. While BCC has a very low risk of metastasis, it can cause significant local destruction. Prevention includes minimizing UV exposure and routine skin examinations.

WHY IS MOHS SURGERY PARTICULARLY USEFUL FOR BCC ON THE FACE?

Mohs surgery allows for the precise removal of cancerous cells layer by layer while conserving as much healthy tissue as possible, which is particularly important in cosmetically sensitive areas like the face.

ARE THERE NONSURGICAL TREATMENTS FOR BCC, AND IF SO, WHAT ARE THEY?

Yes, nonsurgical options include topical treatments like imiquimod or 5-fluorouracil for superficial BCC, photodynamic therapy and radiation therapy, usually reserved for patients who cannot undergo surgery.

Management

Surgical excision or Mohs micrographic surgery is the treatment of choice, particularly for facial BCCs. Patient education on the importance of avoiding tanning beds and protecting skin from sun exposure. Regular follow-up due to the potential for new BCCs to develop over time.

> **REMEMBER**
>
> - Basal cell carcinoma is the most common and least aggressive form of skin cancer
> - It rarely metastasizes but can cause significant disfigurement if not treated
> - Regular skin examinations are important for early detection, especially for individuals with a history of BCC or extensive UV exposure
> - Investigation box
> - Dermoscopic assessment to distinguish BCC from other skin lesions
> - Biopsy (usually shave or punch) for histopathological confirmation
> - Rarely, imaging may be used for extensive lesions to assess for deeper invasion

Progress. After an initial evaluation, her GP referred her to a dermatologist, suspecting BCC. The dermatologist noted the classic appearance of a nodular BCC with a translucent border and overlying telangiectasia. A biopsy confirmed the diagnosis. She was treated with Mohs micrographic surgery to ensure complete cancer removal while preserving as much healthy tissue as possible. The procedure was successful, and she now has regular skin checks every 6 months to monitor for new lesions.

Further Reading

A Swollen Red Leg

Thomas, K.S., Crooke, A.M., Nunn, A.J., et al., 2013. Penicillin to prevent recurrent leg ulceration. N. Engl. J. Med. 368, 1695–1703.

Urticaria and Angio-Oedema

Longhurst, H.J., 2017. Kallikrein inhibition for hereditary angioedema. N. Engl. J. Med. 376, 788–789.

Sun-Induced Rash

Lehmann, P., 2011. Sun exposed skin disease. Clin. Dermatol. 29, 180–188.

Pruritus

Menter, A., Korman, N.J., Elmets, C.A., et al., 2011. Guidelines of care for the management of psoriasis and psoriatic arthritis: section 6. J. Am. Acad. Dermatol. 65, 137–174.

Schneider, L.C., 2017. Ditching the itch with anti-type 2 cytokine therapies for atopic dermatitis. N. Engl. J. Med. 376, 878–879.

Eczema

NICE, CKS, 2023. Eczema. NICE.

Cutaneous Adverse Drug Reaction

Eshki, M., Allanore, L., Musette, P., et al., Twelve-year analysis of severe cases of drug reaction with eosinophilia and systemic symptoms, Arch. Dermatol. 145, 67–72.

Litt, J.Z., 2017. Drug Eruption and Reaction Manual, twenty-third ed. CRC Press, Boca Raton.

Shingles

Cohen, J.L., 2013. Herpes zoster. N. Engl. J. Med. 369, 255–263.

Skin Lesions

NICE, CKS, 2023. Skin cancers – recognition and referral. NICE.

CHAPTER 13

Infectious Diseases

Viral Infections

These produce a variety of specific and nonspecific effects on the blood that might be helpful diagnostically.

Nonspecific Effects

These are common to many viral illnesses:
- Mild neutropenia and thrombocytopenia
- Occasional reactive lymphoid cells on blood film

Specific Effects

- **Glandular fever** is produced by Epstein–Barr virus infection. Similar features are seen in cytomegalovirus (CMV) infection and also in toxoplasmosis. The reactive lymphocytosis must be distinguished from malignant lymphoid proliferation.
- **Parvovirus B19** causes Fifth disease and specifically infects erythroid progenitor cells, resulting in transient erythroid hypoplasia and failure of red cell production This is of no consequence in otherwise healthy individuals, but in those with chronic haemolytic anaemia, it causes a sudden fall in the haemoglobin (Hb) concentration, with absent reticulocytes. Urgent blood transfusion can be life-saving.

Sepsis and Septic Shock

Sepsis is characterized by life-threatening organ dysfunction in response to an infection. Septic shock is a severe subset of sepsis with a higher risk of mortality, indicated by circulatory, cellular and metabolic abnormalities.

Septic shock is defined as sepsis that has circulatory, cellular and metabolic abnormalities profound enough to increase mortality substantially (see Chapter 1).

> ### CASE HISTORY
>
> A 70-year-old female was admitted to hospital with fever, confusion and hypotension. She lived on her own and was unable to give a history.
> **On examination**, she was clinically dehydrated and confused and had cold, clammy peripheries. Pulse rate 108/min, respiratory rate 22/min.
> She was also hypotensive with a BP of 90/50 mmHg and had a temperature of 39°C.
> **Likely diagnosis:** Sepsis.

WHAT ARE THE MOST COMMON CAUSES OF SEPSIS IN PATIENTS PRESENTING FROM THE COMMUNITY?

The most common organisms isolated are *Escherichia coli*, *Staphylococcus aureus*, *Streptococcus pneumoniae* and *pyogenic streptococci* – especially group A *streptococci*. *Neisseria meningitidis* should not be forgotten as a possible cause of community-acquired sepsis.

In hospital, coagulase-negative staphylococci can also cause sepsis in immunosuppressed patients with IV lines in situ. Wounds, the respiratory tract (especially in ventilated patients) and the urinary tract (in catheterised patients) are other sources of sepsis in hospitalised patients.

WHAT FACTORS PREDISPOSE TO SEPSIS?

In both Gram-positive and Gram-negative septicaemia, impaired host defences, surgery or instrumentation (including intravenous cannulae, urinary catheters and mechanical ventilation) predispose to septicaemia (Box 13.1).

WHAT IS THE DIFFERENTIAL DIAGNOSIS OF SEPTIC SHOCK?

Noninfective disorders, such as acute myocardial infarction, pulmonary embolism or drug reactions, must be excluded (see Chapter 1). Toxic shock (e.g. toxic shock syndrome) can also present in a similar manner.

BOX 13.1 ■ Predisposing Factors for Sepsis

Gram-Negative Sepsis
- Urinary tract infections
- Hospital-acquired pneumonia, especially ventilator-associated
- Preexisting abdominal sepsis, biliary tract infections
- Severe burns
- Obstetric or neonatal infections
- Meningococcal septicaemia

Gram-Positive Sepsis
- IV catheters
- Skin/wound infections
- Bone and joint infections
- IV drug usage
- Respiratory tract infections/pneumonia
- Obstetric or neonatal infections
- Meningitis, endocarditis

WHAT WOULD BE YOUR INITIAL MANAGEMENT OF THIS FEMALE, AND WHAT INVESTIGATIONS WOULD YOU DO?

Quick SOFA

Designed to identify high-risk patients for in-hospital mortality with suspected infection outside the ICU:

- Respiratory rate ≥22/min
- Altered mentation (GCS ↓)
- Systolic BP ≤100 mmHg

If >2, contact the intensive care unit (ICU).

Sequential Organ Failure Assessment Score (SOFA)

This patient required supportive therapy (e.g. fluid replacement) because she was dehydrated; oxygen was given and inotropes. Broad-spectrum antibiotics were started after blood and urine cultures had been taken. The antibiotic therapy varies according to local hospital policy and the likely focus of infection.

The National Early Warning Score 2 (NEWS 2) system and the NEWS thresholds and triggers are shown in Figs. 13.1 and 13.2.

INVESTIGATIONS

- To confirm the diagnosis of sepsis and identify the causative organism, a series of investigations should be promptly carried out. These tests serve to establish the extent of the infection, assess organ function and guide appropriate antibiotic therapy
- **Full blood count (FBC):** An increased white cell count (WCC) count may signal an infection, while a differential can help identify the type of cells that are elevated, which can suggest specific types of infection
- **Urea and electrolytes (U and Es):** For kidney function assessment, and can indicate dehydration or acute kidney injury, which are common complications of sepsis
- **Blood Sugar and Liver Biochemistry:** Sepsis can cause liver dysfunction and alter blood sugar levels
- **Serum Lactate:** Elevated lactate levels may indicate tissue hypoxia and can be a marker of the severity of sepsis
- **Erythrocyte sedimentation rate (ESR)/C-reactive protein (CRP):** These are markers of inflammation in the body and can be elevated in sepsis
- **Blood Cultures:** Blood samples are cultured to detect the presence of bacteria or fungi in the blood, which can confirm the diagnosis of sepsis and identify the causative pathogen
- **Blood Gases:** This test measures oxygen and carbon dioxide levels in the blood and can provide information on lung function and the body's acid-base balance
- **Urine for Microscopy, Culture, and Sensitivity:** A urine test can identify the presence of bacteria and white blood cells, indicating a urinary tract infection, a common source of sepsis
- **Sputum Culture:** If the patient produces sputum, it should be cultured to identify respiratory pathogens
- **Swabs of infected-looking lesions:** If there are any wounds or skin lesions, swabs should be taken for culture to identify the presence of bacteria and guide antibiotic therapy
- **High Vaginal Swab in Females:** This may be necessary if there are signs of gynaecological infection or if the patient has recently given birth or had a miscarriage
- **Nucleic Acid Amplification Test (NAAT):** This test can rapidly detect genetic material from pathogens and can be particularly useful for identifying difficult-to-culture organisms
- **Chest X-ray (CXR):** An X-ray of the chest can identify pneumonia or other lung conditions that may be causing sepsis
- **Electrocardiogram (ECG):** An ECG can rule out cardiac causes of the patient's symptoms, such as a heart attack

Physiological parameter	3	2	1	Score 0	1	2	3
Respiration rate (per minute)	≤8		9–11	12–20		21–24	≥25
SpO₂ Scale 1(%)	≤91	92–93	94–95	≥96			
SpO₂ Scale 2(%)	≤83	84–85	86–87	88–92 ≥93 on air	93–94 on oxygen	95–96 on oxygen	≥97 on oxygen
Air or oxygen?		Oxygen		Air			
Systolic blood pressure (mmHg)	≤90	91–100	101–110	111–219			≥220
Pulse (per minute)	≤40		41–50	51-90	91–110	111–130	≥131
Consciousness				Alert			CVPU
Temperature (°C)	≤35.0		35.1–36.0	36.1–38.0	38.1–39.0	≥39.1	

Fig. 13.1 The National Early Warning Score (NEWS) system. CVPU, confused, responds to voice, responds to pain, unresponsive. (From Royal College of Physicians, 2017. National Early Warning Score (NEWS) 2: standardising the assessment of acute-illness severity in the NHS. Updated report of a working party, Royal College of Physicians, London.)

NEW score	Clinical risk	Response
Aggregate score 0–4	Low	Ward-based response
Red score Score of 3 in any individual parameter	Low–medium	Urgent ward-based response*
Aggregate score 5–6	Medium	Key threshold for urgent response*
Aggregate score 7 or more	High	Urgent or emergency response**

*Response by a clinician or team with competence in the assessment and treatment of acutely ill patients and in recognising when the escalation of care to a critical care team is appropriate.
**The response team must also include staff with critical care skills, including airway management.

Fig. 13.2 The National Early Warning Score 2 (NEWS2) thresholds and triggers. (From Royal College of Physicians, 2017. National Early Warning Score (NEWS) 2: standardising the assessment of acute-illness severity in the NHS. Updated report of a working party. Royal College of Physicians, London.)

Management

The choice of antibiotics is critical in the management of sepsis and should be guided by the most likely source of infection, local resistance patterns, and any known patient allergies. Common initial choices include broad-spectrum cephalosporins, such as cefuroxime, cefotaxime or ceftriaxone, or a combination of a broad-spectrum penicillin with a β-lactamase inhibitor like piperacillin/ tazobactam. If MRSA or other resistant organisms are suspected, vancomycin or another appropriate antibiotic may be added until culture results are available.

If a **urinary tract infection** is thought to be the likely source, a broad-spectrum cephalosporin is often appropriate (e.g. cefuroxime) or a quinolone (e.g. ciprofloxacin).

If there is no obvious focus of infection, blind therapy must be broad-spectrum and cover streptococci, staphylococci and coliforms.

Suitable choices are:

- A broad-spectrum cephalosporin, for example, IV cefuroxime or IV cefotaxime or IV ceftriaxone
- Metronidazole in addition if an anaerobic infection is considered likely
- A broad-spectrum penicillin with β-lactamase inhibitor (e.g. piperacillin/tazobactam); gentamicin in addition if the patient is very ill
- A carbapenem (e.g. imipenem, although this is a restricted antibiotic in many hospitals)

ANTIBIOTIC USAGE

'Start Smart'

- Do not start antibiotics in absence of clinical evidence of bacterial infection
- Take a thorough allergy history
- Note local guidelines
- Take a blood culture before therapy
- Document on drug chart and notes: clinical indication, duration or review/stop dates, route and dose

'Focus'

Review clinical diagnosis and continuing need for antibiotics by 48 hours.

Options are:

- Stop
- Switch IV to oral antibiotics
- Change to more appropriate antibiotic
- Continue
- Change to outpatient antibiotic therapy

REMEMBER

- If you give gentamicin, you will need to monitor serum levels. Combining it with a cephalosporin can potentiate its nephrotoxicity
- Cefuroxime, ceftriaxone and cefotaxime have fairly good activity against staphylococci and streptococci, as well as against many Gram-negative rods; they have poor activity against *Pseudomonas* spp. Ceftazidime has poor activity against streptococci and staphylococci but excellent activity against *Pseudomonas* spp. and other Gram-negative organisms. No cephalosporins are active against *Enterococcus* spp
- Cephalosporins are associated with *Clostridium difficile* diarrhoea and should be avoided if possible
- If a patient develops sepsis while in hospital, it is possibly due to resistant organisms, for example, methicillin-resistant *S. aureus* (MRSA) or resistant Gram-negative rods
- If MRSA infection is considered likely and the patient is very sick, add IV vancomycin while awaiting culture results

A urine sample was obtained from this patient. Microscopy found it to contain 1000 WCC/mm^3 and ++ bacteria

Management (Sepsis Six)

1. High-flow oxygen (if hypoxic)
2. Blood cultures and consider source control
3. Intravenous antibiotics
4. Intravenous fluid resuscitation
5. Check haemoglobin and serial lactates
6. Hourly urine output measurement

Progress. The patient, with a high clinical risk score, was transferred to the ICU. She was treated with IV cefuroxime and gentamicin. Cultures confirmed *E. coli* is sensitive to the antibiotics provided. She responded well to treatment and recovered.

> **REMEMBER**
>
> Always consult hospital guidelines or seek microbiological advice for antibiotic usage, and be informed about local resistance patterns, particularly for urinary tract infections.

IN YOUR HOSPITAL, DO YOU KNOW THE APPROXIMATE PERCENTAGE OF ORGANISMS CAUSING URINARY TRACT INFECTIONS THAT ARE SUSCEPTIBLE TO COMMONLY USED ANTIBIOTICS?

In many areas, approximately 50% of *E. coli* causing urinary tract infection are resistant to amoxicillin and 20% to 30% are resistant to trimethoprim. More than 90% are susceptible to cefuroxime, ciprofloxacin and gentamicin. You need to know local resistance patterns.

Malaria

> **CASE HISTORY**
>
> A 20-year-old student returns from a 6-week backpacking tour of Africa. Two weeks after his return, he goes to the emergency department complaining of fever, headache and malaise of 7 days' duration.
>
> **On examination**, the patient is thin and febrile with a temperature of 38°C. There are no other abnormal findings.

WHAT FURTHER QUESTIONS DO YOU WANT TO ASK THIS PATIENT?

In addition to a comprehensive medical history, it is critical to gather specific information about his travel itinerary, including:

- Exact locations visited in Africa
- Vaccinations received before travel
- Adherence to antimalarial prophylaxis: type of medication and regularity of intake
- Instances of insect bites, particularly mosquito bites
- Exposure to individuals with apparent illness
- Dietary habits during travel, focusing on consumption of potentially contaminated food or water
- Engagement in unprotected sexual activities

BOX 13.2 ■ Causes of Febrile Illness in Travellers Returning from the Tropics and Worldwide

WHO advises that fever occurring in a traveller 1 week or more after entering a malaria risk area and up to 3 months after departure is a medical emergency.

Low-/Mid-Income Countries (LMICs)

- Malaria
- Schistosomiasis
- Dengue
- Tick typhus
- Typhoid
- Tuberculosis
- Dysentery
- Hepatitis A
- Amoebiasis

Worldwide

- Influenza
- Pneumonia
- Upper respiratory tract infection
- Urinary tract infection
- Traveller's diarrhoea
- Viral infection
- Sexually transmitted diseases

Specific Geographical Areas

- Histoplasmosis
- Brucellosis

- Differential diagnosis considerations, including common infections or sexually transmitted infections (STIs)

Differential diagnosis is shown in Box 13.2.

REMEMBER

Travel history does not exempt the patient from other common infections, such as influenza, common colds or STIs, which can be contracted during holidays.

Investigations

Start with simple, cheap and relatively noninvasive investigations whenever possible. Perform other investigations as appropriate, depending on symptoms, signs and results of initial investigations, for example, imaging (CT scan, ultrasound or MRI), aspiration or needle biopsy.

INVESTIGATIONS

- **Full blood count:** To check for anaemia or signs of infection
- **Routine Blood Chemistry:** To assess kidney and liver function
- **Urine Analysis:** To evaluate kidney function and look for signs of infection
- **Blood Cultures:** To identify potential bloodstream infections
- **Stool Cultures:** To rule out gastrointestinal infections
- **Chest X-ray:** To detect any respiratory conditions
- **Thick and thin blood films:** Repeat these three times to check for malarial parasites
- **Serology:** Store blood for serology and retake samples after 2 weeks to monitor for changes

Diagnosis

Thick and thin blood films showed that this patient had malaria with a 5% parasitaemia. His malaria was due to *Plasmodium falciparum*. This is a serious infection and requires immediate emergency treatment in an ICU.

HOW WOULD YOU MANAGE THE PATIENT?

For severe *P. falciparum infection*, which exhibits resistance to chloroquine, the first-line treatment is intravenous artesunate (at 2.4 mg/kg). If unavailable, intravenous artemether or quinine sulphate should be administered until the patient can be switched to oral treatment. Regular blood sugar monitoring is crucial due to the risk of hypoglycaemia with quinine, and cardiac monitoring is ideal given its potential cardiac effects. Following initial parental treatment, patients should continue treatment with an effective oral antimalarial regimen (such as artemether/lumefantrine, atovaquone/proguanil, or quinine and doxycycline).

Progress. This young male made a full recovery. He admitted that he had not taken his malaria prophylaxis regularly.

Some Features of Severe *falciparum* Malaria

CNS:
- Cerebral malaria (coma, convulsion)

Renal:
- Haemoglobinuria (blackwater fever)
  - Oliguria
  - Uraemia (acute tubular necrosis)

Blood:
- Severe anaemia (haemolysis and dyserythropoiesis)
- Disseminated intravascular coagulation (DIC): haemorrhage

Respiratory:
- Acute respiratory distress syndrome

Metabolic:
- Hypoglycaemia (particularly in children)
- Metabolic acidosis

Gastrointestinal/liver:
- Diarrhoea
- Jaundice/splenic rupture

Other:
- Shock: hypotension
- Hyperpyrexia

Beware

The parasite count in *falciparum* malaria may underestimate the severity of the infection due to parasite sequestration. It is crucial to take a diagnosis of falciparum malaria seriously, regardless of the parasite count, and manage accordingly.

Pyrexia of Unknown Origin (PUO)

Pyrexia of unknown origin (sometimes called fever of unknown origin [FUO]) is best defined as a fever persisting for more than 2 weeks with no clear diagnosis despite intelligent and intensive investigation.

Not all cases of PUO are due to infection. Approximately two-thirds of cases with recent-onset PUO are due to infection, compared with only about one-third of cases with long-standing PUO. Other causes include malignancy and autoimmune rheumatic disorders (Box 13.3).

CASE HISTORY

A 25-year-old male is seen in the emergency department, at the request of his doctor, with a history of fever, anorexia and malaise. He had returned the previous week from a month's backpacking trip around India, where he had lost 5 kg in weight. The emergency department doctor asks you to see this patient with PUO. The preliminary blood investigations by the general practitioner (GP) were normal.

On examination, the patient was found to be febrile with a temperature of 39.5°C. He had no lymphadenopathy or pallor of mucous membranes.

Blood pressure 110/70; pulse 90; heart sounds normal.

Chest: clinically clear.

Examination of abdomen: slight generalised tenderness. Liver, kidneys and spleen not palpable. Examination of CNS unremarkable.

WHERE WOULD YOU MANAGE THIS PATIENT?

Admit to a medical assessment unit (MAU) side room until an infectious aetiology has been ruled out.

BOX 13.3 ■ Causes of Pyrexia of Unknown Origin (PUO)

- Infections
- Neoplasms, especially lymphomas, renal cell carcinoma
- Autoimmune rheumatic disease
- Vasculitides, for example, giant cell arteritis
- Others, for example, granulomatous disease, drug reactions, factitious

Infective Causes

General

- Abscesses, for example, liver, abdomen, pelvis, ear, sinus or dental infection
- Infective endocarditis
- Urinary tract infection

Specific

Bacterial:

- *Mycobacterium tuberculosis*
- *Salmonella typhi* or *S. paratyphi*
- *Brucella* spp.

- Leptospirosis
- Lyme disease

Viral:

- Epstein–Barr
- Hepatitis
- Cytomegalovirus
- HIV
- Dengue fever

Protozoal:

- Malaria
- Amoebiasis
- Leishmaniasis
- Toxoplasmosis
- Trypanosomiasis

Rickettsial:

- Typhus
- Q fever

Chlamydophila:

- Psittacosis

WHAT QUESTIONS SHOULD YOU SPECIFICALLY ASK WHEN YOU SEE A PATIENT WITH PUO (IN ADDITION TO ROUTINE QUESTIONS)?

- Full travel history, including exactly where the patient has been and the type of accommodation stayed in
- Vaccination/prophylaxis history
- Contact with animals/sick people
- Occupation: exactly what does the patient do?
- Water exposure: occupational/recreational
- Food history: eating shellfish or reheated/raw foods, drinking dirty water
- Risk behaviour: IV drug usage, unprotected sexual contact
- Factors that might predispose to infection

WHAT INITIAL INVESTIGATIONS SHOULD YOU PERFORM IN A PATIENT PRESENTING WITH PUO?

Perform minimally invasive tests before highly invasive and expensive ones. It is always worth repeating previously performed tests (see Investigations box).

INVESTIGATIONS

- Full blood count
- C-reactive protein/ESR
- Urea and electrolytes
- Liver biochemistry
- Blood cultures – repeated
- Urine analysis and microscopy, culture and sensitivity
- Chest X-ray
- Sputum (if producing any) for microscopy, culture and sensitivity and for acid-fast bacilli
- Stools for ova, cysts and parasites, and culture and sensitivity
- Store serum for future serological tests if required
- Wounds: take swabs for culture
- Screen for autoimmune rheumatic disorders
- Additional investigations in this male because of travel abroad: thick and thin blood films for malaria

Results in This Patient

- White cell count: slightly raised at $12,000 \times 10^9$/L
- Alanine aminotransferase (ALT): 92 IU/L (normal range 5–40 IU/L)
- Alkaline phosphatase: 190 IU/L (normal range 25–115 IU/L)
- All other initial investigations normal

WHAT SHOULD YOU DO NOW?

- Recheck his travel history
- Recheck his risk factors for hepatitis and HIV
- Send blood for viral markers for hepatitis
- Arrange a liver ultrasound

The ultrasound shows a **liver abscess** in the right lobe and, in view of his travel history, an amoebic abscess is a strong possibility. Fortunately, you had sent off an amoebic complement fixation test (CFT) sample and you ring the reference laboratory urgently. The test is positive (usually positive with an amoebic liver abscess).

Management

Treat with metronidazole (e.g. 500–750 mg × 3 daily for 10 days) followed by a luminal agent (e.g. paromomycin for 7 days) to clear the luminal infection, even if a stool microscopy is negative. Aspiration of the abscess under ultrasound or CT guidance is required only if the cyst is at risk of rupture or medical therapy fails.

REMEMBER

- Take a careful history: *always repeat*
- Examine the patient thoroughly: *always repeat*
- Initial investigations often give a clue to the diagnosis: often need repeating
- Be patient and do not give antibiotics until diagnosis is made, unless the patient is very sick
- Perform invasive and/or expensive investigations only when appropriate, for example, echo, CT scan/MRI, bone marrow and culture, lymph node/liver biopsy

---

Progress. This patient responded quickly to therapy, with loss of pain and improvement in appetite, becoming apyrexial after 4 days. A repeat ultrasound 3 weeks later still showed a small residual cavity.

Epstein–Barr Virus

Epstein–Barr Virus (EBV) is known to cause infectious mononucleosis, commonly referred to as glandular fever. It primarily affects teenagers and young adults and is transmitted through saliva or aerosols.

CASE HISTORY

A 19-year-old college student presents to his doctor with a 1-week history of severe sore throat, fever and extreme fatigue.

On examination, the patient is found to have a fever of 38.8°C, and cervical, axillary and inguinal lymphadenopathy.

The tonsils appear enlarged and the pharynx erythematous; palatal petechiae are present.

The spleen is just palpable.

WHAT IS THE LIKELY DIAGNOSIS IN THIS PATIENT?

Given the patient's age, short duration of fever, generalized malaise, lymphadenopathy and intense sore throat, infectious mononucleosis or glandular fever is the probable diagnosis. While *streptococcal* sore throat can clinically resemble infectious mononucleosis, it typically does not present with hepatosplenomegaly or lymphadenopathy in the inguinal and axillary regions. Other conditions that present similarly include cytomegalovirus infections and toxoplasmosis, though with a milder sore throat. Viral hepatitis and HIV seroconversion may also present with glandular fever-like symptoms. Lymphomas and leukaemia can sometimes manifest in a similar manner.

HOW WOULD YOU CONFIRM THE DIAGNOSIS?

An FBC should be ordered, which often reveals a mononuclear lymphocytosis with atypical lymphocytes in over two-thirds of cases. Mild neutropenia is common, and platelet counts may be slightly reduced. Serum aminotransferases are typically elevated. The presence of heterophile antibodies that agglutinate sheep red blood cells, identified through the Paul–Bunnell test, is indicative during the second week of infection. The Monospot test, a rapid screening tool, confirms glandular fever in approximately 85% of patients. For Paul–Bunnell-negative cases of 'glandular fever' or atypical presentations, Epstein–Barr virus-specific antibodies can be sought, although these tests are not routinely performed. Consultation with a local virology laboratory is recommended for further information if necessary.

TREATMENT

Treatment is generally supportive, with recommendations to avoid contact sports while splenomegaly persists. Paracetamol is useful for alleviating sore throat and fever. In cases where tonsillar swelling poses discomfort, local topical anaesthetic spray may be beneficial, typically discontinued within 1 to 2 weeks.

REMEMBER

Approximately 90% of patients with infectious mononucleosis who receive ampicillin or amoxicillin develop a rash. If the diagnosis remains uncertain, if *streptococcal* sore throat or a secondary *streptococcal* infection is suspected, start IV benzylpenicillin while awaiting culture and serology results. For nonadmitted patients, high-dose oral penicillin is an alternative.

Progress. This student's sore throat and fever settled after 5 to 6 days, but he still felt unwell for a further 3 weeks.

Helminthic Infections/Parasitic Infections

CASE HISTORY

A 35-year-old male, who recently returned from a hiking trip in a tropical region, presents with abdominal discomfort, diarrhoea, and noticeable weight loss over the past 2 weeks. He mentions consuming local street food and drinking untreated water from streams during his trip.

WHAT ARE THE MOST COMMON HELMINTHIC INFECTIONS ENCOUNTERED IN TRAVELLERS RETURNING FROM TROPICAL REGIONS?

Common infections include hookworm, *Ascaris lumbricoides* (roundworm), *Trichuris trichiura* (whipworm) and *Strongyloides stercoralis*.

INVESTIGATION

Stool ova and parasite examination are the mainstays of diagnosis for most helminthic infections.

A full blood count may show eosinophilia. Serological tests can help diagnose certain infections like strongyloidiasis.

HOW CAN HELMINTHIC INFECTIONS BE PREVENTED WHILE TRAVELING?

Preventive measures include avoiding contaminated food and water, practicing good hand hygiene, wearing protective footwear and considering prophylactic medications if appropriate.

INFORMATION

Helminthic infections are a group of parasitic diseases caused by various species of worms.

Transmission often occurs through contact with soil contaminated by human faeces or ingestion of contaminated food or water. These infections are more prevalent in areas with poor sanitation and are a significant cause of morbidity in developing countries.

WHAT ARE THE TYPICAL CLINICAL FEATURES OF SOIL-TRANSMITTED HELMINTHIASIS?

Symptoms can range from asymptomatic to abdominal pain, diarrhoea, malnutrition, and in severe cases, anaemia, and protein-energy malnutrition.

Management

Initial management involves symptomatic relief and hydration. Anthelmintic medications, such as albendazole or mebendazole, are commonly used, with the choice of drug depending on the specific infection. Supportive care, including treatment of anaemia and nutritional deficiencies, may be necessary. Education regarding proper sanitation and hygiene practices is crucial to prevent reinfection.

REMEMBER

Helminthic infections can be asymptomatic; always consider travel history in the differential diagnosis. Untreated water and food are common sources of infection. Many helminthic infections have similar clinical presentations, necessitating laboratory confirmation for accurate treatment.

Further Reading

Epstein–Bar Virus

NICE, CKS, 2023. Glandular fever (infectious mononucleosis). NICE.

Sepsis and Septic Shock

NICE, CKS, 2023. Sepsis. NICE.

Pyrexia of Unknown Origin

WHO. Infectious diseases. Available from: http://www.who.int/topics/infectious_diseases/en.

Malaria

NICE, CKS, 2023. Malaria. NICE.

The Returning Traveller

WHO. WHO guidelines. Available from: www.who.int/topics/infectious_diseases/en/.
WHO. Treatment of malaria. Available from: www.who.int/malaria/publications/atoz/9789241549127/en/.

General Information

British Infection Association British Infection Association. Available from: britishinfection.org.
Centers for Disease Control and Prevention (USA). Available from: www.cdc.gov.

CHAPTER 14

Sexually Transmitted Infections

HIV/AIDS

CASE HISTORY

A 35-year-old male with a new HIV-positive diagnosis has been experiencing general malaise and weight loss over the last 6 months. He presents with a persistent cough that has worsened over the past 2 weeks. Examination reveals a high temperature, increased pulse and respiratory rate, accompanied by signs of oral candidiasis. He is not currently on any medication.

WHAT ARE THE LIKELY DIAGNOSES AND THE IMMEDIATE MANAGEMENT?

Pneumocystis jirovecii pneumonia commonly has an insidious onset, often with worsening shortness of breath and deteriorating exercise tolerance; the cough is usually nonproductive.

- Examination of the chest can yield few signs other than tachypnoea and tachycardia. Fine inspiratory crackles might be heard
- The chest X-ray (CXR) is often normal or shows little, although bilateral perihilar interstitial shadowing with a bat-wing appearance is the characteristic abnormality
- High-resolution CT of the lungs shows a characteristic ground glass appearance, even when there is little to see on the plain CXR
- Oxygen saturation characteristically falls on exercise. Arterial blood gas analysis might show hypoxia with a normal carbon dioxide and pH
- The diagnosis is made on broncho-alveolar lavage

The introduction of highly active antiretroviral therapy (ART) in HIV-infected people has led to a significant decline in *Pneumocystis* infection and it is most commonly seen in those not previously recognised as HIV-infected. *Pneumocystis* infection occurs most frequently in the context of significant immunosuppression, when the CD4 count is <200 cells/mm^3. There may be clinical markers of poor immune function, such as candidiasis, as in this patient.

Primary prophylaxis is recommended in those who are aware of their HIV status if their CD4 count falls into this range. Cotrimoxazole (trimethoprim and sulfamethoxazole) is first line. This intervention alone has reduced the incidence of *Pneumocystis* infection in HIV-infected populations. *Pneumocystis* pneumonia is an AIDS defining diagnosis.

HOW WOULD YOU TREAT THIS PATIENT?

Intravenous cotrimoxazole (trimethoprim 15–20 mg/kg per day plus sulfamethoxazole 75 mg/kg per day) is the preferred first-line treatment, although a significant proportion of patients will develop allergy. Intravenous pentamidine or dapsone plus pyrimethamine can also be used.

Treatment is given for 3 weeks. Systemic corticosteroids (IV methylprednisolone 40 mg × 4 daily for 5 days) are added in severe cases (PO$_2$ <8 kPa). Patients with *Pneumocystis* infection can develop respiratory failure and require ventilatory support. Pneumothorax is a further complication of *Pneumocystis* infection.

If the organism is not cleared by treatment, secondary prophylaxis (usually cotrimoxazole) is recommended. This can be withdrawn later if the patient starts ART and the CD4 count remains consistently >200 cells/mm^3.

Initiation of therapy in a patient not already on ART should be discussed with a specialist physician.

WHAT OTHER CHEST CONDITIONS ARE ASSOCIATED WITH HIV?

Tuberculosis

Tuberculosis (TB) is caused by *Mycobacterium tuberculosis (MTB)*, which has a high pathogenicity. It can develop relatively early in the course of HIV infection. It is particularly common in those who have lived in areas of the world with a high incidence of MTB, for example, sub-Saharan Africa. Pulmonary infection presents with a cough (usually productive) and chest pain, but in the context of HIV infection the presentation is often insidious and nonspecific, with fever, sweats, malaise and weight loss. History of contact with MTB should always be sought, along with details of any previous antituberculous therapy, because in such patients there is a risk of multidrug-resistant tuberculosis (MDRTB). There might be generalised lymph node enlargement or hepato-megaly in addition to signs in the chest. In some cases, pulmonary infection is coupled with CNS involvement – either TB meningitis or tuberculoma. The chest radiological changes are few and are frequently atypical, showing lower zone changes without cavitation. Other radiological find-ings include hilar lymphadenopathy, pleural effusion or lobar consolidation.

In patients with HIV, the usual immunological reactions to MTB might be blunted or absent, making diagnosis more difficult. Mantoux tests are rarely helpful because immunosuppressed patients do not produce a normal delayed hypersensitivity reaction. Granuloma formation can be compromised, leading to atypical histological changes. Sputum smears may be negative in up to 50% of those with culture-proven TB. Urine lipoarabinomannan (LF-LAM) is detected in some patients with active TB, providing a result in 30 min. The sensitivity of the test is low but is higher in HIV patients with low CD4 cell counts. Diagnosis relies heavily on clinical suspicion backed by positive cultures from, for example, sputum, broncho-alveolar lavage, blood, bone marrow and lymph nodes, as appropriate.

Treatment of TB in HIV-coinfected patients presents specific challenges and requires input from a specialist physician. Treatment is similar to that for HIV-negative patients, although inter-mittent and short-course regimens are not advised.

Therapy should be initiated with four drugs – for example isoniazid, rifampicin, pyrazinamide and ethambutol – for 2 months. Once sensitivities are confirmed, pyrazinamide and ethambu-tol can be withdrawn and the other two drugs continued for 4 months, although this might be extended in some circumstances. The drug–drug interactions between antiretroviral and antituber-culous medications are complex and are a consequence of enzyme induction or inhibition. There are interactions between rifampicin derivatives and the protease inhibitor class of antiretroviral agents, leading to an increase in rifampicin toxicity and reduced protease efficacy. The nonnucleo-side reverse transcriptase class also interacts variably with rifampicin, requiring dose alterations. Additionally, there are overlapping toxicities between ART regimens and antituberculous drugs: in particular, hepatotoxicity, peripheral neuropathy and gastrointestinal side effects.

> **REMEMBER**
>
> When the suspicion of TB is great enough to start antituberculous therapy, the case *must* be notified to the local consultant in communicable disease control (CCDC).
>
> Paradoxical inflammatory reactions (e.g. immune reconstitution inflammatory syn-drome [IRIS]), which include exacerbation of symptoms, new or worsening clinical signs and

deteriorating radiological appearances, have been associated with the improvement of immune function. Immune reconstitution inflammatory syndrome is most commonly seen in the first few weeks after initiation of ART in patients recovering from TB and can last several weeks or months. The syndrome does not reflect inadequate TB therapy and is not confined to any particular combination of antiretroviral agents; always exclude new pathology in this situation.

Bacterial Chest Infection

Several respiratory infections are more common in patients with HIV infection: in particular, *Streptococcus pneumoniae*, *Haemophilus influenza* and *Moraxella catarrhalis*. The onset is usually rapid, with a productive cough. Signs of consolidation occur and radiological changes of consolidation or infiltration might be present. Diagnosis is based on sputum and blood cultures, and management is with appropriate broad-spectrum antibiotics (e.g. cefotaxime).

Other Infective Conditions

Cytomegalovirus, *Cryptococcus neoformans*, *Aspergillus fumigatus*, *Histoplasma capsulatum* and *Nocardia asteroides* can all cause fever, cough and dyspnoea in association with advanced HIV infection. The clinical signs and radiological findings are usually nondiagnostic. The diagnosis depends on broncho-alveolar lavage.

MALIGNANCY

The incidence of **Kaposi sarcoma** (KS) has declined significantly since the widespread introduction of ART. This is a vascular tumour associated with human herpes virus type 8 (HHV8). Although most commonly found on the skin, KS can infiltrate the lungs to cause cough and shortness of breath. On examination, other KS lesions are usually found on the skin or in the mouth, but in rare cases, the lungs alone may be involved.

Radiological changes are of diffuse lung infiltration, often with a nodular appearance. Pleural effusion might be present. Lesions are visualised on bronchoscopy. Treatment is with systemic chemotherapy. ART should be initiated if the patient is not already on treatment.

Non-Hodgkin lymphoma can also cause lung infiltration. Patients additionally present with systemic 'B' symptoms. On examination, lymphadenopathy and splenomegaly might be found. Hilar lymphadenopathy seen on the CXR and CT scan indicates widespread lymph node enlargement in the chest and abdominal cavities. The diagnosis is made on the histological appearance of lymph node biopsy. Such lymphomas are often aggressive. Treatment is with chemotherapy.

HOW WOULD YOU MANAGE AN HIV-POSITIVE PATIENT WITH RESPIRATORY SYMPTOMS?

The differential diagnosis in an HIV-infected patient presenting with respiratory symptoms is wide. There is considerable advantage in establishing a specific diagnosis rather than treating symptoms empirically. Factors that have an impact on diagnosis and management include clinical presentation, level of immunosuppression of the individual, lifetime exposure to infective agents and current medication.

REMEMBER

In HIV-Infected Patients
- Common conditions can have unusual presentations
- Uncommon conditions occur more frequently
- Many different conditions can present in similar ways – clinically and radiologically

- Standard investigations that depend on an intact immune system will not be useful
- A tissue or culture diagnosis is frequently required
- Pathology is related to:
  - The degree of immunosuppression
  - The virulence of the organism
  - The microbiological repertoire to which an individual has been exposed
  - The multiple pathology that is frequently encountered
  - The medication that the patient is taking

Assessment

- Full history and examination, including details of travel, previous infections, previous or existing HIV-related pathology, current surrogate marker data (if known), current therapy, including antiretroviral drugs and antimicrobial prophylaxis
- Assessment of the degree of immunosuppression by looking for clinical signs such as oral candidiasis, hairy oral leukoplakia and seborrhoeic dermatitis. Look for pathology in all systems, including examination of the mouth and fundi
- Chest X-ray, exercise oximetry, blood gases, blood cultures, sputum examination for acid-fast bacilli (AFB), and microscopy, culture and sensitivity. Full blood count, liver and renal function.

Treatment

If the patient is clinically immunosuppressed, has a previous AIDS-defining illness or is known to have a CD4 count <200/mm³ *and* has chest X-ray abnormalities, desaturates on exercise, or has a hypoxic blood gas picture suggestive of *Pneumocystis* infection, institute therapy pending bronchoscopy. Organisms will still be found several days into treatment.

REMEMBER

- Drug allergies
- Bone marrow suppression with high-dose co-trimoxazole
- Hypotension/hypoglycaemia with IV pentamidine
- CD4 counts and HIV viral load measurements are altered in the face of any acute infection and might not accurately reflect the underlying situation

If the patient has a history of TB or exposure to TB or has clinical and radiological findings consistent with TB, isolate and investigate. Do not initiate empirical antituberculous therapy without an expert opinion, as this will have long-lasting and far-reaching consequences for the patient and for future management.

If the patient has a sputum smear that is positive for AFB or has culture-proven TB, isolate and start antituberculous therapy with four drugs. Notify and seek expert opinion.

If the patient has clinical or radiological signs of bacterial infection, institute therapy with broad-spectrum antibiotics, for example, amoxicillin or azithromycin.

REMEMBER

If the patient does not respond as detailed:
- Reconsider the diagnosis
- Suspect multiple pathology

HIV and the Skin

- Up to 90% of HIV-positive patients will develop a mucocutaneous disease, sometimes related to drug therapy

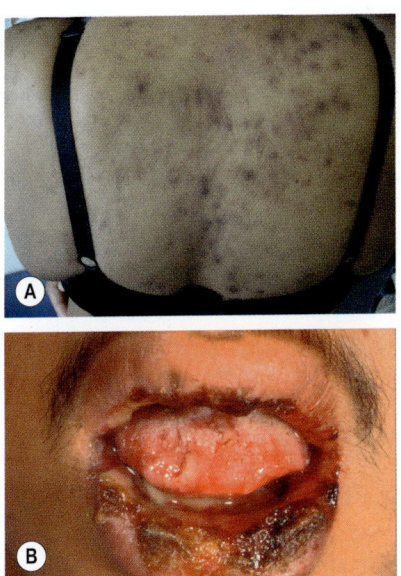

Fig. 14.1   Rashes associated with HIV. (A) Eosinophilic folliculitis – a classical HIV dermatosis; (B) Stevens–Johnson syndrome/toxic epidermal necrolysis is more common in HIV. ([A] Courtesy Dr Michael Arden-Jones. [B] Courtesy Dr David Paige.)

- Between 30% and 40% of people with AIDS will suffer from three different dermatoses
- A rash may be the presenting sign of HIV infection or AIDS (remember that up to 30% receive their diagnosis of AIDS and HIV at the same time, suggesting a large pool of undiagnosed patients)

CASE HISTORY

Two patients with HIV presented to the clinic with different rashes, both of which are more common in HIV patients. One presented with an eosinophilic folliculitis and the other with Stevens–Johnson/toxic epidermal necrolysis (Fig. 14.1A and B).

Progress.   Both patients were referred to the HIV specialist ART.

WHAT DERMATOSES HAVE COMMONLY BEEN THE PRESENTING ILLNESS OF HIV (OR OTHER CAUSES OF IMMUNOSUPPRESSION)?

- Extensive molluscum contagiosum in an adult
- Kaposi sarcoma (KS)
- Extensive seborrhoeic dermatitis or eosinophilic folliculitis
- Pruritic papular eruption (PPE; also called itchy folliculitis) of HIV
- Extensive oro-pharyngeal candida
- Hairy leucoplakia

WHY IS THE SKIN SO FREQUENTLY AFFECTED?

The exact mechanisms are not known but include:
- Immune deficiency: increased infection

- Poor immune surveillance: increased skin tumours
- Post infection: reactive arthritis
- Auto-antibodies: Sjögren syndrome, polymyositis, idiopathic thrombocytopenic purpura, pemphigoid, vitiligo, alopecia areata
- Aberrant immune function TH1–TH2 switch: eczema, pruritus, PPE
- Graft-versus-host disease (GVHD): lichen planus, erythroderma

WHAT TYPES OF RASH ARE SEEN?

There are many different rashes, which can be arbitrarily divided:
- Cutaneous infection
- Opportunistic infection
- Malignancy (basal cell carcinoma [BCC], squamous cell carcinoma [SCC], KS, malignant melanoma)
- Papulo-squamous/inflammatory
- Oral lesions

Antiretroviral therapy has reduced the incidence of all skin lesions.

HOW WOULD YOU DIAGNOSE THE RASHES?

The diagnosis can be difficult, as frequently the rash is very extensive or there is an atypical clinical presentation. You should always have a low index for doing:
- Skin biopsies: both for all the routine stains and for culture of bacteria, fungi, viruses and acid-fast bacilli
- Skin swabs
- Serology screens
- Investigation of other 'organs', for example, blood, stools, sputum, bone marrow. Furthermore, treatment is often problematic, as HIV rashes (even those that are common in immunocompetent people) tend to be resistant to standard therapies, and the use of immunosuppressive drugs is usually contraindicated

---

INFORMATION

Cutaneous Infections in HIV

Bacterial
- Impetigo (*Staphylococcus aureus*), cellulitis/erysipelas (*streptococci*): clinically, these infections tend to look much the same as in immunocompetent individuals; deep-seated ecthyma may be seen

Viral
- Herpes: may present with blisters, often extensive and ulcerative, especially perianally and orally
- Shingles/varicella-zoster virus: often painful, verrucous and extending over more than one dermatome; may be bilateral

Fungal
- Dermatophyte and candidal infections: common in the skin and present typically; often require systemic antifungal therapy for eradication

WHAT OPPORTUNISTIC INFECTIONS OCCUR IN THE IMMUNOCOMPROMISED AND HOW WOULD YOU DISTINGUISH BETWEEN THEM?

INFORMATION

Failure to diagnose scabies (especially crusted scabies) can lead to a high proportion of medical staff becoming infected.

A variety of normally nonpathogenic organisms have been described in AIDS and other immunosuppressed patients. Clinically they are difficult to distinguish:

- Cutaneous cytomegalovirus may present with blisters, ulcers or a necrotic lesion
- Fungi are common culprits and may present with nodules (often deep subcutaneous) or scaly papules (*Cryptococcus* is seen in the UK whereas *Histoplasma* is more common in the US)
- Scabies present typically with itchy papules and burrows in the web spaces, wrists, genitalia and palms/soles. Crusted scabies ('Norwegian scabies') presents atypically with a rather crusted eczematous-looking rash, often centred around the web spaces, and may not be itchy
- Nontuberculous or 'atypical' mycobacteria are a particular problem in advanced AIDS and present with papules, nodules, ulcers or sporotrichosis-like lesions

These infections can be localised to the skin but also present as a systemic infection. Malaise, fever, abdominal pain, headache or diarrhoea may be nonspecifically suggestive of systemic infection. Biopsy and culture are the best ways to diagnose these rashes.

WHAT CAUSES HAIRY LEUCOPLAKIA AND WHAT DOES IT LOOK LIKE?

It is due to the Epstein–Barr virus in an immunosuppressed individual and is almost unique to HIV patients. It is a relatively late sign of HIV disease. Clinically, white plaques appear on the sides of the tongue. Vertical ridging or corrugations are seen within the plaques. Unlike candidal infections, there are no small satellite lesions around the edge and the white material cannot be scraped off to leave raw areas underneath.

WHAT TYPES OF MALIGNANCY OCCUR IN IMMUNOCOMPROMISED PATIENTS?

- The two most common types of skin cancer (basal cell carcinoma [BCC] and squamous cell carcinoma [SCC]) are increased in HIV-positive patients. They look the same as in immunocompetent patients
- Malignant melanoma may be increased in prevalence. The clinical appearance is typical
- Kaposi sarcoma is more common and more severe in AIDS patients (without available ART therapy) than in classical or African KS. It presents as purplish-brown plaques and nodules. The nose, palate and genitalia seem common sites, but remember disease can spread internally. KS is predominantly seen in males who have sex with males with AIDS. There is a strong link between herpes virus type 8 and the development of all types of KS, although other factors might be involved, as not all people with herpes virus type 8 contract KS
- Lymphomas are more common with HIV and may present with lymphadenopathy, pleural effusions, night sweats and weight loss

WHAT ARE THE MORE COMMON 'PAPULO-SQUAMOUS' DERMATOSES ENCOUNTERED IN HIV PATIENTS?

These are:

- Seborrhoeic dermatitis: 80%
- Unexplained pruritus: 40%
- Xerosis (dry skin), ichthyosis: 30%
- PPE: 20%
- Eczema: 10%
- Psoriasis: 5%
- Drug rashes: 20%

In general, these rashes become more common (and severe) with progression of the disease.

Seborrhoeic Dermatitis

There is an itchy, red and scaly eczematous rash in the seborrhoeic areas (sides of nose, around eyes, forehead, scalp, sternum, glans penis). This looks similar to seborrhoeic dermatitis in immunocompetent patients but is often more extensive. It may appear in early 'asymptomatic' HIV disease.

Therapy. Treatments include topical miconazole/hydrocortisone cream, emollients, ketoconazole shampoo. If resistant, consider topical 0.1% tacrolimus ointment, topical lithium and oral antifungal therapy (e.g. itraconazole 100 mg × 2 daily for 2 weeks).

Pruritus and Xerosis

These often go together and the aetiology is unclear. Again, they may be early manifestations of advanced HIV disease.

Therapy. Emollients, bath oils and aqueous cream as soap substitute. Sedating antihistamines (e.g. hydroxyzine or chlorphenamine). Consider 0.5% menthol in aqueous cream or crotamiton. Phototherapy if resistant.

Pruritic Papular Eruption (PPE); Also Called Itchy Folliculitis

This is a unique papular and (at times) pustular eruption centred on hair follicles. It is intensely itchy and usually involves the upper trunk, back and proximal arms. Papules tend to arise, grow in size, frequently have the top scratched off and then recede as other new lesions arise. In African–Caribbean patients, lesions are often larger and more frequently involve the face. Skin biopsy reveals a lymphohistiocytic infiltrate around blood vessels and hair follicles, often accompanied by eosinophils.

The so-called unique HIV rash, 'eosinophilic folliculitis', is probably a variant of PPE.

Pruritic papular eruption tends to appear in more advanced HIV disease and becomes worse as CD4 counts fall.

Therapy. Medium-strength topical steroids, oral antihistamines and low-dose long-term antibiotics (as used in acne) may help. Isotretinoin or psoralen and ultraviolet A (PUVA) is effective for resistant cases.

Eczema

The prevalence of eczema is probably increased in HIV patients, reflecting the eosinophilia and high IgE levels that are commonly seen. It looks similar to eczema in immunocompetent patients.

Therapy. As for normal eczema.

Psoriasis

The prevalence of psoriasis is increased in HIV (5% vs. 2% in the normal population); 30% may get psoriatic arthropathy (vs. 5% of normal psoriatics). The disease can be typical with red, scaly plaques on elbows and knees, and scaling in the scalp. However, psoriasis occasionally becomes severe and widespread in advanced HIV patients. They may become erythrodermic or develop pustular psoriasis, especially on the soles of the feet. When the latter happens, there is clearly an overlap with reactive arthritis.

Therapy. Topical steroids, calcipotriol (a synthetic vitamin D_3 analogue) and tar compounds will help mild cases. Ultraviolet B (UVB) or PUVA is useful for more advanced disease. Although there is some in vitro evidence that phototherapy may promote HIV replication, this has not been shown to be a problem in clinical practice.

Oral drugs for severe disease include acitretin or antiretroviral drugs.

The other drugs used in 'normal' psoriasis include methotrexate, ciclosporin and hydroxyurea. Biological agents are now being used.

Vaginal Discharge

CASE HISTORY

A 25-year-old female presents to her general practitioner with a 3-days history of vaginal discharge that is white and curdy in appearance. She reports associated vulval itching and superficial soreness but denies any dysuria or abdominal pain. Her last menstrual period was two weeks ago, and she is currently using a copper intrauterine device (IUD) for contraception. She has no relevant past medical history and is not taking any medications.

WHAT ARE THE MOST COMMON CAUSES OF ABNORMAL VAGINAL DISCHARGE?

The most common causes include bacterial vaginosis, characterized by a fishy-smelling, thin, grey/white homogeneous discharge, and vaginal candidiasis, presenting with an odourless, white, curdy discharge often accompanied by vulval itching and soreness.

INFORMATION

Normal physiological discharge is typically clear or white, nonoffensive, and varies with the menstrual cycle. Abnormal discharge may have a change in colour, consistency, volume or odour and can be associated with symptoms such as itching or soreness. Management strategies should be tailored based on whether the cause of discharge is infective or noninfective.

HOW DOES THE PH LEVEL ASSIST IN DIAGNOSING THE CAUSE OF VAGINAL DISCHARGE

Vaginal pH testing is a useful diagnostic tool. A pH higher than 4.5 suggests bacterial vaginosis or trichomoniasis, while a pH of 4.5 or less is typical of vaginal candidiasis.

INVESTIGATION

Perform a speculum examination to inspect the cervix and vagina. Collect swabs for Gram staining and culture to exclude other causes if indicated. Test the pH of the vaginal discharge.

WHEN SHOULD A FEMALE PATIENT WITH VAGINAL DISCHARGE BE REFERRED TO A GENITO-URINARY MEDICINE (GUM) CLINIC?

Referral to a GUM clinic is advised for females at high risk of a sexually transmitted infections (STIs) or with characteristic features of trichomoniasis, cervicitis or pelvic inflammatory disease, to facilitate screening for infections and partner notification.

Management

Empirical antibiotic treatment for suspected bacterial vaginosis or vaginal candidiasis is appropriate after ruling out STIs or other causes. If symptoms are recurrent or persistent, further investigation and referral may be required. Provide advice on personal hygiene and safe sexual practices, and reassure the patient if discharge is physiological.

REMEMBER

The nature of physiological discharge can vary throughout the menstrual cycle. A detailed clinical history is crucial to differentiate between infective and noninfective causes. Diagnosis should not solely rely on self-reported symptoms; examination and investigations are often necessary.

Urethritis

CASE HISTORY

A 24-year-old male reports to the clinic with a 2-day history of a burning sensation during urination and a milky discharge from the penis that he noticed this morning. He has had two new sexual partners in the past 6 months and admits to inconsistent condom use. He denies any recent history of catheterization or urethral instrumentation.

WHAT ARE THE CLASSIFICATIONS OF URETHRITIS IN MALES?

Urethritis is classified as gonococcal urethritis, nongonococcal urethritis (NGU) or persistent/recurrent urethritis, which occurs 30 to 90 days after treatment for acute NGU and typically has no identifiable cause.

INVESTIGATION

Test for Chlamydia trachomatis and gonorrhoea using a first-void urine sample for nucleic acid amplification testing (NAAT). For possible trichomoniasis, arrange a urethral swab and/or first-void urine for culture and/or microscopy. Consider additional STI screening including syphilis and HIV.

WHAT EMPIRICAL TREATMENT IS RECOMMENDED FOR SUSPECTED CHLAMYDIAL INFECTION WITH URETHRITIS?

Doxycycline 100 mg twice a day for 7 days is recommended. Alternatives include azithromycin 1 g on the first day followed by 500 mg daily for 2 additional days, or ofloxacin 200 mg twice daily or 400 mg once daily for 7 days.

WHEN SHOULD SEXUAL PARTNERS BE NOTIFIED IN CASES OF URETHRITIS?

All recent sexual partners should be notified and advised to attend a GUM clinic for assessment and treatment. Contact tracing should cover all partners within the previous 4 weeks.

Urethritis is inflammation of the urethra, often caused by STIs. Nongonococcal urethritis has no identifiable cause in over 50% of cases; if an organism is identified, *C. trachomatis* and *Mycoplasma genitalium* are most likely. Persistent urethritis has no identifiable cause but may be linked to *M. genitalium* or *Trichomonas vaginalis*.

Management

Offer referral to a GUM clinic or other local specialist sexual health service for all males with suspected urethritis. If referral is not possible, empirically treat for chlamydial infection, screen for other STIs, and advise on safe sexual practices. Follow up 1 to 2 weeks after treatment to assess for symptom resolution and ensure contact tracing has been carried out.

Progress. The patient's symptoms and sexual history raise suspicion for urethritis, likely of infectious origin. He is referred to a GUM clinic for further evaluation and management, including testing for STIs.

REMEMBER

1. Up to 25% of urethral infections may be asymptomatic
2. Sexual history is essential to assess STI risk
3. Noninfective causes of urethritis may include trauma or chemical irritation

Anogenital Warts

CASE HISTORY

A young male in his early twenties seeks medical advice for growths in the anogenital area. He reports no significant pain but mentions occasional irritation and discomfort, especially during physical activities that involve friction.

INVESTIGATION

Clinical examination is usually sufficient for diagnosis. A biopsy is reserved for atypical lesions or when diagnosis is uncertain. Screening for other STIs is essential, especially in younger individuals.

WHAT ARE ANOGENITAL WARTS, AND WHAT CAUSES THEM?

A: Anogenital warts, also known as condylomata acuminata, are benign growths in the genital and anal areas caused by human papillomavirus (HPV), typically genotypes 6 and 11.

INFORMATION

Anogenital warts are the most common viral STI, with a peak prevalence at 20 to 24 years.
They are not always indicative of recent infidelity due to the long latency period of HPV.
Human papillomavirus vaccines have contributed to a decrease in the incidence of genital warts.

HOW ARE ANOGENITAL WARTS TRANSMITTED?

The primary mode of transmission is sexual contact, but they can also spread through perinatal contact, from hand warts, and potentially through nonsexual means.

Management

Treatments for anogenital warts include self-applied creams like podophyllotoxin or imiquimod, ablative methods like cryotherapy, or no treatment as warts can spontaneously resolve. Referral to a sexual health specialist is suggested for diagnosis confirmation and comprehensive management. Treatment in primary care is only advised if referral is not possible and the primary care provider has the necessary resources. Clear information about the condition, its treatment, and implications should be provided to the patient.

> **REMEMBER**
>
> Anogenital warts are typically asymptomatic and may resolve spontaneously. Smoking cessation and condom use may improve treatment outcomes. High-risk HPV types associated with anogenital warts can coexist with types causing cancer.

Further Reading

British HIV Association. Available from: bhiva.org.
British HIV Association, World Health Organisation. Available from: who.int/hiv/pub.
Melhuish, A., Lewthwaite, P., 2018. Natural history of HIV and AIDS. Medicine 46, 356–361.
NICE, CKS, 2023. HIV and AIDS. NICE.
Yarchoan, R., Uldrick, J.S., 2018. HIV associated cancer and related diseases. N. Engl. J. Med. 378, 1029–1045.

HIV and the Skin

Rodgers, S., Leslie, K.S., 2011. Skin infections in HIV-infected individuals in the era of ART. Curr. Opin. Infect. Dis. 24, 124–129.

Vaginal Discharge

NICE, CKS, 2023. Vaginal discharge. NICE.

Urethritis

NICE, CKS, 2023. Urethritis. NICE.

Anogenital Warts

NICE, CKS, 2023. Warts – anogenital.

CHAPTER 15

Care of the Elderly and Palliative Care

Blackouts

This implies either altered consciousness, with or without falling, or sometimes a visual disturbance.

CASE HISTORY

An 86-year-old female is brought into the emergency department with a 'blackout'. She had been found on the floor but had regained consciousness on the way to hospital.
On examination, pulse and BP were normal and there was no abnormality found on neurological examination.

WHAT SHOULD YOU ASCERTAIN FROM THE HISTORY?

- Any previous episodes
- What the patient was doing at the time (e.g. micturition, change in posture, coughing)
- Symptoms preceding blackout:
- Chest pain or palpitations, suggesting cardiac cause
- Aura, suggesting epilepsy
- Witness history: any witness(es) to give a description of the blackout

Differential Diagnosis

Common causes include neurological or cardiovascular events.

EPILEPSY IN THE ELDERLY

- Focal fits or a focal origin of generalised seizures are common in the elderly (accounting for 80% of fits in this age group)
- Postictal confusion, headache and focal signs (Todd paresis) are common
- Thirty-five percent to fifty percent of fits in the elderly are caused by vascular disease
- Twenty percent of patients with stroke have seizures within the first year
- Elderly persons are more susceptible to pharmacological causes of fits, for example, neuroleptics, tricyclics, and alcohol withdrawal
- An electroencephalography (EEG) can be useful, but a normal or nondiagnostic EEG does not rule out epilepsy
- Do not forget hypoglycaemia as a cause of fits
- Anticonvulsant drugs should be started after the first fit if a vascular or structural cause is suspected
- Pallor suggests a cardiac cause
- Tonic–clonic contractions or incontinence suggest epilepsy
- Was there a history of head turning or tight neckwear? This suggests carotid sinus syndrome
- Was there a period of drowsiness after the blackout? This suggests epilepsy but might also occur in cardiac causes

REMEMBER

Epilepsy might be secondary to reduced cardiac output.

INVESTIGATIONS

- Full blood count (FBC), urea and electrolyte (U and Es), glucose, thyroid function tests (TFTs), Ca^{2+}
- Electrocardiogram (ECG)
- Twenty-hour tape if ECG abnormal or history suggestive of cardiac cause
- Electroencephalography and/or CT scan if history suggests epilepsy
- Specialist intervention: carotid sinus massage – undertaken if carotid sinus syndrome suspected (**Note:** contraindications for massage include the presence of a carotid bruit and history of carotid territory neurological events)

CARDIOVASCULAR CAUSES OF BLACKOUTS

- Arrhythmias (brady- or tachy-) can be difficult to diagnose and sometimes require repeated 24-hour tapes or 2- to 3-week 'event recorders'
- Myocardial infarction (MI) can be pain-free in older people
- Aortic stenosis typically causes exertional syncope, also shortness of breath on exertion and angina
- Hypertrophic cardiomyopathy is diagnosed on echocardiogram
- Postural hypotension
- Carotid sinus syndrome is an underdiagnosed cause of unexplained blackouts. It is caused by an exaggerated response of baroreceptors in the carotid sinus and requires specialist investigation by carotid sinus massage with close observation. There are three variants. (1) The **cardio-inhibitory variant** is diagnosed by >3-s asystole on massage; (2) the **vasopressor variant** is diagnosed by a 50-mm Hg drop in BP or systolic BP drop to <90 mm Hg.(3) up to one-third of cases are mixed
- Vasovagal syncope occasionally presents for the first time in older people. Consider if there is a long history of 'funny turns'

TREATMENT

In this patient, an ECG, chest X-ray (CXR) and blood tests were normal. It was thought that the blackout could be due to an **arrhythmia,** so a 24-hour tape ECG was performed. This showed episodes of tachycardia and bradycardia, with two episodes of sinus arrest, compatible with the **sick sinus syndrome**.

Progress. This patient was fitted with a pacemaker/DDD and has had no further attacks.

Falls in the Elderly

CASE HISTORY

A 79-year-old male was brought into the emergency department following a fall. He was taking atenolol 100 mg daily, aspirin 75 mg daily and bendroflumethiazide 2.5 mg daily.

    On examination, he was well. His pulse was normal but his BP was low at 90/50; he had no abnormal neurological signs. He had symptomatic **postural hypotension** on standing up.

WHAT QUESTIONS SHOULD YOU ASK?

- What was he doing when he fell, for example, was there a postural element?
- What does he remember about the fall?
- Did he lose consciousness?
- What happened immediately before the fall?
- Were there any preceding symptoms?
- Was there a witness?
- Were there any physical hazards, for example, wet floor, carpet edge?
- Had he fallen before?

These features can help distinguish pathological causes (intrinsic) from those with a major external factor (extrinsic), although in practice, most falls are multifactorial. Falls or 'collapse' can be seen as a final common pathway for many frequently encountered diseases in the elderly.

EXAMINATION AFTER FALLS

Full physical examination, especially:

Cardiovascular:
- Blood pressure, including postural changes after 1–3 minutes
- Evidence of heart failure or rhythm disturbance
- Murmur.

Musculoskeletal:
- Arthritis: acute or chronic, and evidence of joint instability
- Muscle wasting, especially quadriceps.

Neurological:
- Focal signs; don't forget cerebellar/brainstem
- Hearing or visual impairment

Gait: observation of the patient standing from sitting (with arms folded) and walking (with turns) provides a good assessment of risk for falling.

Frailty: the Fried Frailty score assesses:
- Slowness in walking
- Exhaustion
- Weakness (decreased hand grip strength)
- Physical inactivity (low energy expenditure)
- Weight loss (body mass index [BMI] <18.5 or >5% weight loss in the last year)

Score of 3 or more defines frailty.

ORTHOSTATIC HYPOTENSION

This is defined as a >20-mm Hg drop in systolic BP on standing or during head-up tilt:

- Common in the elderly: occurs in up to 30% of healthy older people and it is not clear why some develop symptoms
- 'Physiological' changes in elderly: decreased baroreceptor sensitivity increases risk of postural hypotension
- 'Pathological' changes: for example, sepsis with vasodilatation, poor left ventricular function, neurological disease affecting reflex pathways
- Pharmacological causes: beta-blockers, vasodilators, antiparkinsonian drugs, sedatives, neuroleptics, diuretics

INVESTIGATION OF FALLS

- Blood pressure and heart rate measurement with patient lying flat, standing upright or at 45 degrees on tilt table after 1, 3 and 5 minutes
- Full blood count for evidence of infection, anaemia
- Urea and electrolytes, creatinine for evidence of dehydration, renal impairment (estimated glomerular filtration rate [eGFR] is calculated)
- Blood glucose for hypo-/hyperglycaemia
- Thyroid function test for subclinical hypothyroidism
- Chest X-ray for infection, tumour
- Electrocardiogram for ischaemia, arrhythmias, silent MI
- Heart beat monitoring (beat-to-beat variation) for autonomic neuropathy
- Mid-stream urine (MSU) for infection

MANAGEMENT OF FALLS

- Review medications and withdraw exacerbating drugs if possible
- Treat medical factors, for example, sepsis
- Assessment and reduction of osteoporosis risk
- Advice to patients
- Drug treatment occasionally used in patients with persistent disabling symptoms:
  1. Fludrocortisone 100–200 µg at night. Watch for fluid retention and hypokalaemia
  2. If still symptomatic, add a sympathomimetic agent, for example midodrine

Progress. In this patient with postural hypotension, the atenolol was stopped and a careful watch was kept on his BP (he had his own BP machine) over the following few weeks. He should stay on aspirin and bendroflumethiazide. His BP stabilised at 115/80 and therefore no further medication was required.

ADVICE FOR PATIENTS WITH POSTURAL HYPOTENSION

- Get out of bed in stages
- Pause between positional changes
- Wear leg support tights during the day; take them off at night
- Raise head of bed
- Avoid alcohol

Benign Paroxysmal Positional Vertigo (BPPV)

CASE HISTORY

A 72-year-old retired schoolteacher presents to the clinic with a one-week history of episodes of dizziness. These episodes occur when she turns her head to the right, especially when lying down or getting out of bed. She reports that the spinning sensation lasts for less than a minute and is sometimes accompanied by nausea. There is no history of hearing loss or tinnitus. Her past medical history is significant for hypertension, managed with amlodipine, and type 2 diabetes controlled by diet.

WHAT IS THE MOST LIKELY DIAGNOSIS FOR EPISODIC DIZZINESS PROVOKED BY HEAD MOVEMENT?

The symptoms described are indicative of benign paroxysmal positional vertigo (BPPV), a condition where loose calcium carbonate crystals in the semicircular canals of the inner ear move when the head's position changes, triggering brief episodes of vertigo.

INFORMATION

- Benign paroxysmal positional vertigo is the most common cause of vertigo in the elderly and is generally not associated with hearing loss
- The condition is caused by the dislodgment of otoconia into the semicircular canals, typically the posterior canal
- The Epley manoeuvre is effective in treating posterior canal BPPV and can be performed in the office setting
- Patient education is crucial for managing expectations and handling recurrent episodes

---

WHICH CLINICAL MANOEUVRE CAN BE USED TO DIAGNOSE BPPV?

The Dix-Hallpike manoeuvre is commonly used to diagnose BPPV. It involves rapidly moving the patient from sitting to a supine position with their head turned and observing for characteristic nystagmus, which confirms the presence of BPPV.

INVESTIGATION

- **Dix-Hallpike manoeuvre:** To elicit nystagmus and vertigo, confirming BPPV
- **Imaging:** Not required for diagnosis of BPPV but may be necessary to exclude other conditions if the presentation is atypical or if neurological symptoms are present
- **Audiology testing:** Not routinely necessary unless there's a history suggestive of hearing loss

---

WHAT IS THE PATHOPHYSIOLOGY BEHIND BPPV?

Benign paroxysmal positional vertigo occurs when otoconia detaches from the utricle and migrates into the semicircular canals, especially the posterior canal. Head movements cause these particles to shift, leading to abnormal fluid displacement and stimulation of hair cells, which send false signals of head movement to the brain, resulting in vertigo.

MANAGEMENT

Initial management of BPPV includes the following steps:

Educate the patient about the condition, reassuring them about the benign nature of BPPV.

Offer a particle repositioning manoeuvre, such as the Epley manoeuvre, to move the dislodged crystals out of the semicircular canal.

Instruct the patient on home exercises, such as Brandt-Daroff exercises, if they prefer self-management or if symptoms persist after the repositioning manoeuvre.

Advise on safety measures to prevent falls and injuries during episodes of vertigo.

Progress. After undergoing the Epley manoeuvre in the clinic, the patient reports an immediate improvement in symptoms. She is given instructions on how to perform Brandt-Daroff exercises at home and advised to return if her symptoms persist. At a follow-up appointment 4 weeks later, she reports only one mild episode of dizziness, which resolved with self-administered exercises. She is satisfied with the control over her symptoms and feels confident in managing potential recurrences.

Delirium

Delirium, commonly known as a 'acute confusional state,' is a critical medical condition characterized by a sudden onset of confusion, commonly seen in general medical settings. It is akin to 'brain failure,' where there is a notable impairment in attention and alterations in perception and mood.

CASE HISTORY

Consider a 76-year-old female admitted with confusion and hallucinatory episodes. Despite signs of pulmonary consolidation, her vital signs are normal. This case exemplifies the challenge of diagnosing delirium, which often goes unrecognized in hospitals. It is prevalent, affecting 10% to 20% of inpatients, with rates increasing to 60% among the elderly. Delirium is associated with higher morbidity and mortality, underscoring the necessity for prompt recognition and management.

CORE FEATURES OF DELIRIUM

- Impaired consciousness and attention
- Global cognitive dysfunction
- Psychomotor abnormalities
- Sleep-wake cycle disturbances
- Emotional dysregulation

DIAGNOSIS

An acute onset and fluctuating course are valuable diagnostically. Delirium represents an acute generalised impairment of cognitive function. The primary feature is disorientation in time and place (more rarely, person). A well patient should know the day of the week, the month and the

---

BOX 15.1 ■ **Delirium: Diagnostic Criteria (Derived from DSM-5)**

- Disturbance of consciousness:
  1. Clarity of awareness of environment
  2. Ability to focus, sustain or shift attention
- Change in cognition:
  1. Memory deficit, disorientation
  2. Language disturbance, perceptual disturbance
- Disturbance develops over a short period (hours or days)
- Fluctuation over course of day

---

year (people who are well can occasionally get the date and time wrong). They should know that they are in hospital, its name and location, and the name of the ward. Other psychoses do not affect orientation.

Abnormal cognition: memory loss, disorientation, poor language and poor speech, all refer to the variable level of attention seen in delirium.

Abnormal perception: visual or auditory hallucinations, paranoid delusions, misperception are commonly present, so the patient may mistake a curtain movement in a dimly lit ward as a threatening person, resulting in extreme fear and agitation, especially at night.

Persecutory delusions: are the most common and may make patients refuse food, drink and medicines because they believe that they are being poisoned. Alternatively, these delusions can cause aggression, as patients defend themselves against a perceived threat.

Confusional Assessment Method (CAM), which is based on the DSM criteria (Box 15.1).

CONFUSIONAL ASSESSMENT METHOD (CAM) CRITERIA

Need points 1 and 2:

Acute onset + fluctuating course: this history is usually obtained from the family/carer or from the nurse caring for a patient who is already in hospital.

Inattention: is the patient easily distractible or does he/she have difficulty keeping track of what is being said?

… and either 3 or 4:

Disorganised thinking: is the patient incoherent? Is the conversation irrelevant?

Altered level of consciousness: the patient might be hyperactive, hypoactive/lethargic or semiconscious.

REMEMBER

Hyperactive delirium is characterized by agitation, delusions, hallucinations, wandering and aggression.

Hypoactive delirium is characterized by lethargy, slowness with everyday tasks, excessive sleeping and inattention.

Fluctuating presentation and disturbed sleep/wake cycle may conceal abnormalities during the day.

Emotional disturbance (fear, perplexity, apathy, depression) is common in delirium.

PREDISPOSING FACTORS

Delirium can emerge in individuals with existing vulnerabilities – such as the very young or old, those with brain injuries, or preexisting cognitive impairments – when combined with triggering factors like new medications, surgical procedures or environmental changes.

HOW WOULD YOU INVESTIGATE THIS PATIENT?

- Corroborative history from family/partner (duration of history, drug history, past medical and psychiatric history, alcohol/drug use)
- An EEG shows excess slow waves in 90% (with the exception of drug withdrawal states) and may show sharp waves and spikes in status epilepticus. It is used occasionally as a confirmatory test if there is doubt about the clinical diagnosis
- Investigations
- Look for infections (MSU, CXR, blood and sputum cultures, lumbar puncture if indicated)
- Urea and electrolytes (hyponatraemia)
- Calcium
- Blood sugar
- Liver and cardiac enzymes
- E (silent myocardial infarct)
- Computed tomography brain scan ('silent' parietal infarct; predisposing brain disease/damage)
- Second-line investigations
- Therapeutic drug levels (anticonvulsant, lithium)
- Endocrine (TFTs)
- Vitamin deficiency (thiamine, nicotinic acid, B_{12})
- Illicit drug screen

INVESTIGATIONS

A thorough history from family or carers, physical examination, and targeted investigations are crucial. These may include blood tests for infections, metabolic imbalances and imaging studies to rule out intracranial causes.

MANAGEMENT

Supportive Care

Ensure a safe and quiet environment to reduce overstimulation. A well-lit room with a clock and calendar can help with orientation.

Maintain a consistent schedule for the patient, including regular sleep-wake times and meal times.

Encourage the presence of familiar objects and visits from family members, as long as they are not overstimulating for the patient.

Assist with mobility and self-care activities to prevent complications such as pressure ulcers and deep vein thrombosis.

Monitor nutritional and fluid intake to prevent malnutrition and dehydration.

Address any sensory impairments, such as providing glasses or hearing aids, to aid in reorientation and reduce confusion.

Pharmacological Interventions

Pharmacotherapy is generally reserved for patients who are severely agitated, distressed or pose a risk to themselves or others.

Antipsychotic medications, such as haloperidol or atypical antipsychotics (e.g. olanzapine, quetiapine), may be used to manage agitation and psychotic symptoms. These should be used at the lowest effective dose and for the shortest duration possible.

Benzodiazepines like lorazepam may be considered for delirium due to alcohol withdrawal or when antipsychotics are contraindicated. Caution is advised as they can potentially worsen delirium in some cases.

Cholinesterase inhibitors have been explored for delirium treatment, particularly when the underlying cause is suspected to be related to a decrease in central cholinergic neurotransmission.

Monitoring and Follow-Up

Regularly assess the patient's mental status, looking for improvements or worsening of delirium symptoms.

Adjust the management plan as the patient's condition evolves.

Plan for a transition of care, which may include arranging for home care services or rehabilitation if necessary.

Prognosis. The prognosis is contingent on the resolution of the underlying condition and the individual's baseline health. Cognitive function may lag in recovery, necessitating careful monitoring.

TREATMENT FOR DRUG-INDUCED DELIRIUM

Immediate cessation of the offending agent is the first step. Supportive care and targeted treatments for specific causes, like oxygen therapy for carbon monoxide poisoning, form the cornerstone of management. In cases of withdrawal, a careful replacement of the drug class may be necessary.

PREVENTING DELIRIUM

Delirium prevention entails avoiding known precipitating drugs, optimizing the patient's environment and addressing sensory impairments.

Differential Diagnosis

Dementia: Delirium has an acute onset and fluctuating course, while dementia is characterized by a more gradual decline in cognitive function.

Psychiatric disorders: Delirium is reversible, whereas psychiatric disorders often have a chronic course.

Substance intoxication or withdrawal: Certain substances can cause confusion and altered mental status similar to delirium.

Metabolic disturbances: Electrolyte imbalances and organ dysfunction can lead to delirium-like symptoms.

Infections: Systemic infections can cause delirium due to the inflammatory response and effects on the central nervous system.

Neurological conditions: Structural brain abnormalities and acute neurological events can result in delirium.

Medication side effects: Some medications can induce delirium-like symptoms as a side effect.

Sleep deprivation: Prolonged lack of sleep can impair cognitive function and contribute to delirium.

Pain: Severe pain can lead to agitation and confusion resembling delirium.

Endocrine disorders: Hormonal imbalances can affect brain function and contribute to delirium.

Dementia

Definition

Dementia is defined by the Royal College of Physicians as global impairment of higher cortical functions, including memory:

- The capacity to solve problems of day-to-day living
- The performance of learned perceptuomotor skills
- The correct use of social skills
- The control of emotional reactions in the absence of gross clouding of consciousness

Dementia encompasses a decline in cognitive function beyond what might be expected from normal ageing. It affects memory, problem-solving abilities, the execution of complex tasks, social interaction skills and emotional control. These changes occur in the absence of significant impairment to consciousness.

CASE HISTORY

An 89-year-old male with a 6-month history of deteriorating short-term memory and increasing confusion is referred to the emergency department because of self-neglect. He has become even more confused over the previous 24 h. He was diagnosed as having **dementia** and referred to the care of the elderly team.

REMEMBER

Differentiate between delirium and dementia. However, delirium often occurs in patients already diagnosed with dementia, as seen in this case.

- Dementia is often irreversible and progressive and has a number of causes
- Assessment: this is performed using the 10-point abbreviated mental test (AMT) (see Box 15.2) or Clock-drawing test (Fig. 15.1)
- Although screening tests are useful in demonstrating the presence of deficits in cognition, they cannot be used for making the diagnosis of dementia or identifying the underlying cause. This requires imaging (CT or MRI scan) and, in some patients, assessment by a clinical psychologist and/or a psychiatrist. A history of progressive decline in memory or cognition over 6 months is significant.

BOX 15.2 ■ Abbreviated Mental Test (AMT)

Total score 10 (1 point for each item)
- Age
- Time (to nearest hour)
- Address for recall
- Year
- Where do you live (town or road)?
- Recognition of two persons
- Date of birth (day and month)
- Year of the start of the First World War
- Name of present leader of the country
- Count backwards from 20 to 1

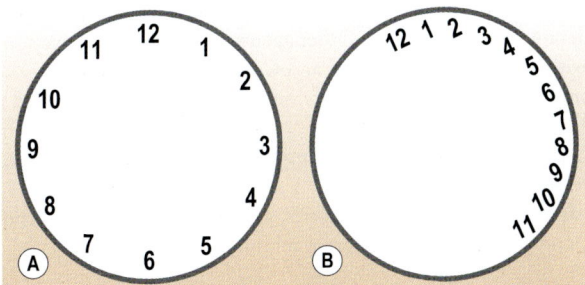

Fig. 15.1 Clock drawing test. (A) Normal; (B) Abnormal – inappropriate spread.

BOX 15.3 ■ Examples of Treatable Causes of Dementia-Like Syndrome

- Hypothyroidism
- Vitamin B$_{12}$ deficiency
- Folate deficiency
- Recurrent hypoglycaemia
- Alcohol excess
- Depression ('pseudodementia')
- Subdural haematoma
- Normal pressure hydrocephalus

INVESTIGATIONS

Initial Investigation for Dementia

- Full Blood Count (FBC) and film
- Urea and Electrolytes (U and Es)
- Random Blood Glucose
- Liver Biochemistry
- Thyroid Function Tests (TFTs)
- Vitamin B$_{12}$ and Folate levels
- Syphilis Serology
- Chest X-ray (CXR)
- Electrocardiogram (ECG)
- Brain imaging (CT/MRI scan) or positron emission tomography (PET) scan

CAUSES

The common causes of dementia include Alzheimer disease (AD), vascular dementia, Lewy body dementia and Creutzfeldt–Jakob disease, but other conditions can produce a dementia-like syndrome (Box 15.3).

MANAGEMENT

- **Alzheimer disease:** although there is no cure, research on acetylcholine esterase inhibitors has shown that in selected patients with mild to moderate AD, the decline can be slowed down. The National Institute for Health and Care Excellence (NICE) has produced guidance on use of donepezil, rivastigmine, memantine and galantamine in patients with mild to moderate AD by specialists. Other agents/drugs that may have some modest benefit in patients with AD include vitamin E and *Ginkgo biloba* extract

- **Vascular dementia:** treat the risk factors, such as hypertension. Aspirin also has a role in preventing further strokes.
- As dementia progresses, the management focus changes to care provision for patients plus support for carers
- **Lewy body dementia:** avoid antipsychotics, as they can increase confusion. Some of these patients respond to acetylcholine esterase inhibitors

---

REMEMBER

Pharmacological management of AD is initiated by a specialist (psychiatrist, neurologist or geriatrician):

- Donepezil 5–10 mg daily
- Rivastigmine 3–12 mg daily
- Galantamine 8–24 mg daily
- Memantine 5–20 mg daily

Progress and Management. This patient's previous history of hypertension and two small strokes suggested vascular dementia. The diagnosis was confirmed by an MRI. The care of the elderly team arranged for full support in the community, and he was continued on his treatment for hypertension. He is being assessed regularly to see if pharmacological treatment for his dementia is required.

REMEMBER

In all types of dementia, it might be necessary to use pharmacological agents to control agitation and other behavioural disturbances, but it is important to remember that patients with Lewy body dementia are very susceptible to the side effects of antipsychotic drugs.

Depression

Depression is common in old age. Community studies have revealed a prevalence of 11.3% for depressive symptoms and 3% for depression in the UK. Studies of elderly hospital inpatients have shown that up to 33% have depression. It is common in the elderly with chronic physical illnesses, such as stroke, and it can also be the presentation of an occult physical illness, such as hypothyroidism, hypercalcaemia or carcinoma of the lung. Physical illness is the biggest risk factor for depression in old age.

REMEMBER

Whereas the clinical features of depression in old age can be the same as in younger patients, somatic complaints, delusions and decline in cognition ('pseudodementia') are more frequently noted in the elderly.

CASE HISTORY

A senior nurse noted that an 83-year-old male with a cerebrovascular accident (CVA) is eating poorly and is losing weight. On direct questioning, the patient admits to being depressed and feels he has no future.

Examination showed no abnormality, apart from slight residual neurological signs from his CVA.

ASSESSMENT

- Geriatric Depression Scale (Table 15.1), shorter version, is a reliable and valid screening instrument for depression in the elderly. A score <5 indicates probable depression
- Physical examination and investigations to detect/exclude physical causes of depression, such as hypothyroidism, hypercalcaemia and malignancy. In a patient with a normal physical examination, the recommendation is that FBC, U and Es, liver biochemistry, vitamin B_{12}, Ca^{2+}, TFTs and CXR are performed

In this patient these blood tests and the CXR showed no abnormality.

REMEMBER

Always ask the patient about suicidal thoughts/intent.

TABLE 15.1 ■ **Geriatric Depression Scale**

Choose the best answer for how you have felt over the past week:

1.	Are you basically satisfied with your life?	Yes/No
2.	Have you dropped many of your activities and interests?	Yes/No
3.	Do you feel that your life is empty?	Yes/No
4.	Do you often get bored?	Yes/No
5.	Are you in good spirits most of the time?	Yes/No
6.	Are you afraid that something bad is going to happen to you?	Yes/No
7.	Do you feel happy most of the time?	Yes/No
8.	Do you often feel helpless?	Yes/No
9.	Do you prefer to stay at home, rather than going out and doing new things?	Yes/No
10.	Do you feel you have more problems with memory than most?	Yes/No
11.	Do you think it is wonderful to be alive now?	Yes/No
12.	Do you feel pretty worthless the way you are now?	Yes/No
13.	Do you feel full of energy?	Yes/No
14.	Do you feel that your situation is hopeless?	Yes/No
15.	Do you think that most people are better off than you are?	Yes/No

The following answers count as 1 point:

A total score >5 indicates probable depression

1.	No	–
2.	Yes	–
3.	Yes	–
4.	Yes	–
5.	No	–
6.	Yes	–
7.	No	–
8.	Yes	–
9.	Yes	–
10.	Yes	–
11.	No	–
12.	Yes	–
13.	No	–
14.	Yes	–
15.	Yes	–

From Sheikh, J.I., Yesavage, J.A., 1986. Geriatric Depression Scale (GDS), Clin. Gerontol. 5, 165–173.

MANAGEMENT

Significantly depressed patients can be treated successfully with drugs. Drugs commonly used for treating depression in older people include:

- Citalopram: a selective serotonin reuptake inhibitor (SSRI), 10–20 mg daily
- Mirtazapine: a presynaptic alpha-2 antagonist is particularly useful in patients with poor appetite, 15 mg daily, increased according to response to 45 mg daily
- Venlafaxine: a serotonin and noradrenaline reuptake inhibitor, 75–150 mg daily

Severely depressed patients with or without suicidal ideation need urgent referral to a psychiatrist for further assessment.

Progress and Treatment. Management of this patient consisted of multidisciplinary support in the community with short-term use of mirtazapine daily to help his depression.

Nonspecific Presentation of Illness in the Elderly

Many illnesses in the elderly population can present in a nonspecific manner. Taking a detailed and informative history can be very difficult because underlying memory loss due to dementia can be exacerbated by an acute medical problem (delirium). Information regarding the previous medical, mental, functional and social conditions is needed to make an accurate assessment of the patient's current state.

History obtained from the patient should be augmented by information from the patient's doctor, district nurse, carers, relations and neighbours, if necessary, particularly if the patient is confused.

These problems are highlighted in the following case. The National Early Warning Score (NEWS) is a simple physiological scoring system that can be used at the bedside. It identifies patients at risk of deterioration and who may require more specialised care.

CASE HISTORY (1)

Mr S. is 85 years old and lives alone in a bungalow. His neighbours noticed that he had failed to collect the milk from the front door for 2 days. They called the family doctor, who found Mr S. sitting in a chair with grossly swollen feet. In his letter referring the patient to hospital, the doctor confirmed that Mr S. had been on salbutamol and ipratropium inhalers for 5 years. However, he had not visited the surgery for some time.

On arrival at hospital, Mr S. was very confused and unable to give a detailed history. His abbreviated mental test (AMT) score (see Box 15.2) was 3 out of 10.

On examination, he had a low-grade temperature of 37.6°C and appeared breathless on minimal exertion, with central cyanosis, and had signs of congestive heart failure: high JVP, an enlarged liver and leg swelling up to the groin.

A CXR showed signs of left **heart failure** and there was left basal shadowing suggestive of **left lower lobe pneumonia** (Fig. 15.2).

It was not clear how long he had been confused or how mobile he had been before these problems. His next of kin was a younger brother who lived far away. He was contacted by telephone and confirmed that the patient was not married and had been able to go out to the local shops (a quarter of a mile away) until 3 weeks ago. He also commented that the patient had been mildly confused and needed some help in running his own affairs for several years but was self-caring and did not need help at home.

TREATMENT

Mr S. was started on antibiotics – amoxicillin 500 mg × 3 daily – bendroflumethiazide 2.5 mg daily and enalapril 2.5 mg × 2 daily for his pneumonia and heart failure. He was also found to

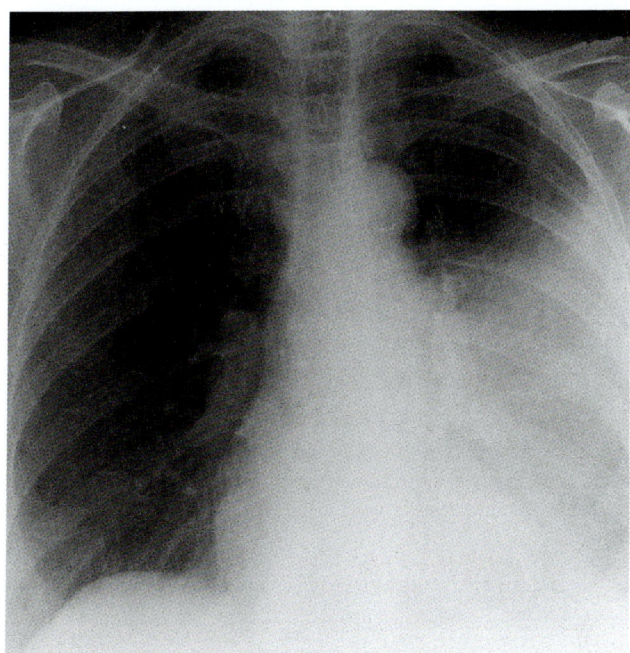

Fig. 15.2 Chest X-ray showing lobar pneumonia. (From Feather, A., Randall, D., Waterhouse, M., 2021. Kumar and Clark's Clinical Medicine, tenth ed. Respiratory Disease, Fig. 28.28, Elsevier Ltd, Edinburgh.)

be hypothyroid and was started on levothyroxine 25 µg initially. His general condition gradually improved and his AMT rose to 7 out of 10.

Progress. With the help of the physiotherapist, Mr S. was able to get back on his feet using a Zimmer frame. A home visit was successful, and he returned to his bungalow with daily home-care support and follow-up in the day hospital, with adjustment of his medication, to maintain his mobility.

> **REMEMBER**
>
> All elderly persons presenting to hospital with nonspecific complaints should have full physical examinations and investigations that include FBC, U and Es, liver biochemistry, Ca^{2+}, phosphate, TFTs, ECG, MSU and CXR, plus any other investigations as indicated by the findings on examination.

> **CASE HISTORY (2)**
>
> A 79-year-old male was admitted after having an unexplained fall. He was mildly confused, but on direct questioning denied any symptoms.
>   **On examination**, he had a tachycardia of 100 beats per minute (bpm), normal heart sounds and a clear chest. An ECG revealed a raised ST segment in leads II, III and AVF, which is an acute inferior myocardial infarct (STEMI). He had a raised serum troponin.

- Any illness in old age can present with any of the so-called 'giants' of geriatric medicine, that is, confusion, falls/instability and incontinence
- In addition, some illnesses present atypically. Examples of this include:
  - 'Silent' MI
  - Pneumonia without pyrexia or rise in white cell count (WCC)
  - 'Silent' peptic ulcer perforation, that is peptic, ulcers might perforate with little or no pain but the patient becomes nonspecifically unwell, anorexic and bed-bound

DIAGNOSIS

This patient has had a 'silent' MI.

MANAGEMENT

Aspirin 300 mg and clopidogrel 300 mg were given. He was assessed urgently by the cardiac team, who felt that, despite his age, he should be treated urgently with percutaneous coronary intervention (PCI). He responded well, with a fall in the ST segment to normal, without any complications of treatment.

Progress. The patient was discharged, given post-MI drug treatment, and was followed up by the cardiac rehabilitation nurse.

DRUG THERAPY AND ASSESSMENT OF POSTACUTE CORONARY SYNDROME (ACS)

Extensive clinical trial evidence has been gathered in post-MI patients, demonstrating that a range of pharmaceuticals is advantageous in reducing mortality over the following years. Therefore, after MI, most patients should be taking most of the following medications:
- Aspirin 75 mg daily
- An adenosine diphosphate (ADP)-receptor blocker, e.g. clopidogrel
- An oral beta-blocker to maintain heart rate <60 bpm
- Angiotensin-converting enzyme (ACE) inhibitors or angiotensin receptor blockers, particularly if left ventricular ejection fraction (LVEF) is <40%
- High-intensity statins with target low-density lipoprotein (LDL) cholesterol <1.8 mmol/L
- An aldosterone antagonist, if there is clinical evidence of heart failure and LVEF is <40%; the serum creatinine is <221 μmol/L (males) or <177 μmol/L (females); and the serum potassium is <5.0 mEq/L

> **REMEMBER**
>
> Older patients often do well with active treatment of STEMI (fibrinolysis or PCI).

Appropriate Assessment Scales

The Royal College of Physicians has produced a list of useful assessment scales/tools for the day-to-day management of the elderly. The following scales are recommended:
- **Barthel Index:** for activities of daily living (ADL) (Table 15.2)
- **Mini-Mental State Examination (MMSE):** cognitive screening test for dementia and delirium
- **Geriatric Depression Scale:** screening instrument test for depression (see Table 15.1)

TABLE 15.2 ■ Barthel Index

Item	Categories
Bowels	0 = incontinent (or needs to be given an enema)
	1 = occasional accident (once per week)
	2 = continent
Bladder	0 = incontinent/catheterised, unable to manage
	1 = occasional accident (max. once every 24 h)
	2 = continent (for over 7 days)
Grooming	0 = needs help with personal care
	1 = independent face/hair/teeth/shaving (implements provided)
Toilet use	0 = dependent
	1 = needs some help but can do something alone
	2 = independent (on and off, dressing, wiping)
Feeding	0 = unable
	1 = needs help cutting, spreading butter, etc.
	2 = independent (food provided in reach)
Transfer	0 = unable – no sitting balance
	1 = major help (one or two people, physical), can sit
	2 = minor help (verbal or physical)
	3 = independent
Mobility	0 = immobile
	1 = wheelchair independent (includes corners)
	2 = walks with help of one (verbal/physical)
	3 = independent (may use any aid, e.g. stick)
Dressing	0 = dependent
	1 = needs help, does about half unaided
	2 = independent, includes buttons, zips, shoes
Stairs	0 = unable
	1 = needs help (verbal, physical), carrying aid
	2 = independent
Bathing	0 = dependent
	1 = independent (may use shower)

- ■ **Waterlow Score:** for risk quantification for pressure ulcers (Table 15.3)
- ■ **Philadelphia Geriatric Center Morale Scale:** for quality of life (Table 15.4); provides a multidimensional approach to assessing the psychological state of older people, that is, well-being/life satisfaction/quality of life

Other scales, for example, Braden, Walsall and Maelor, are also available.

The Barthel Index should be used as a record of what a patient does (not as a record of what the patient could do). The main aim is to establish the degree of dependence on any help, physical or verbal. A need for supervision means that the patient is not independent. Performance over the preceding 24 to 48 hours is used when completing the Barthel Index, but longer periods of assessment might be more relevant. A patient's performance should be established using the best available evidence. Ask the patient or carer but also observe what the patient can do. The use of aids to be independent is allowed. Direct testing is not needed. Unconscious patients score '0' throughout.

Stroke

This is the sudden onset of focal neurological symptoms caused by interruption of the vascular supply to the brain (ischaemic stroke) or intra-cerebral haemorrhage (haemorrhagic stroke).

TABLE 15.3 ■ Waterlow Pressure Ulcer Risk Assessment

Build/Weight for Height		Visual Skin Type		Continence		Mobility		Sex/Age		Appetite	
Average	0	Healthy	0	Complete	0	Fully mobile	0	Male	1	Average	0
Above average	2	Tissue paper	1	Occasionally incontinent	1	Restricted/ difficult	1	Female	2	Poor	1
		Dry	1	–		–		14–18	1	Anorectic	2
Below average	3	Oedematous	1	Catheter/ incontinent of faeces	2	Restless, fidgety	2	50–64	2	–	–
		Clammy	1	–		–		65–75	3	–	–
		Discoloured	2	–		Apathetic	3	75–80	4	–	–
		Broken/spot	3	Doubly incontinent	3	Inert/ traction	4	81+	5	–	–

Special risk factors		Assessment value	
1. Poor nutrition, e.g. terminal cachexia	8	At risk	10
2. Sensory deprivation, e.g. diabetes, paraplegia, cerebrovascular event	6	High risk	15
3. High-dose antiinflammatory or steroid in use	3	Very high risk	20
4. Smoking 10+ per day	1	–	–
5. Orthopaedic surgery/fracture below waist	3	–	–

The Waterlow assessment is mainly used in acute hospital settings in order to highlight patients at risk of pressure sores who will require special nursing care, including aids, and to prevent the development of pressure sores.

CASE HISTORY

A 78-year-old male presents with a reduced conscious level, Glasgow Coma Score (GCS) of 12, weakness of the right arm and leg, and inability to speak. His daughter thinks that he has had a stroke. She also says that her father has been well and is still working 2 days a week.

INFORMATION

Each year in England, about 100,000 (1.6–2 per 1000) people have a first stroke. Stroke is the most common cause of severe disability in adult life. There are 64,000 deaths attributed to first or recurrent strokes, which makes it the third most common cause of death in the UK.

Paramedics and members of the public are encouraged to make the diagnosis of stroke on a history and simple examination (FAST test):

- Face – sudden weakness of the face
- Arm – sudden weakness of one or both arms
- Speech – difficulty speaking/slurred speech
- Time – the sooner the treatment can be started, the better
! Stroke is a medical emergency and prompt treatment can improve prognosis.

QUESTIONS YOU NEED TO ADDRESS

- Is it a stroke?
- What type of stroke?
- What part of the brain is affected?

TABLE 15.4 ■ **Philadelphia Geriatric Center Morale Scale**

–	High Morale Response	Low Morale Response
Do little things bother you more this year?	No	Yes
Do you sometimes worry so much that you can't sleep?	No	Yes
Are you afraid of a lot of things?	No	Yes
Do you get mad more than you used to?	No	Yes
Do you take things hard?	No	Yes
Do you get upset easily?	No	Yes
Do things keep getting worse as you get older?	No	Yes
Do you have as much pep as you had last year?	No	Yes
Do you feel that as you get older you are less useful?	No	Yes
As you get older, are things … than you thought?	Better	Worse or same
Are you as happy now as you were when you were younger?	No	Yes
How much do you feel lonely?	Not much	A lot
Do you see enough of your friends and relatives?	Yes	No
Do you sometimes feel that life isn't worth living?	No	Yes
Do you have a lot to be sad about?	No	Yes
Is life hard much of the time?	No	Yes
How satisfied are you with your life today?	Satisfied	Not satisfied

From Lawton, M.P., 1975. The Philadelphia geriatric center morale scale: a revision, J. Gerontol. 30, 85–89; Royal College of Physicians, 1992. Report of A Joint Workshop with the Royal College of Physicians and the British Geriatrics Society Standardised Assessment Scales for Elderly People. Royal College of Physicians, London.

- What is the prognosis?
- Are there complications to treat or prevent?

PATHOLOGY

- Eighty to ninety percent of strokes are ischaemic, that is due to thrombosis or embolism
- Ten to twenty percent are the result of primary cerebral haemorrhage or aneurysm rupture

COMMON SOURCES OF EMBOLI

- Carotid artery and aortic arch atheroma
- Intra-cardiac sources, for example, left atrium in atrial fibrillation (AF), left ventricle mural thrombus, left-sided heart valves
- Vertebral artery atheroma or dissection

UNCOMMON CAUSES OF THROMBOTIC STROKE

- Giant cell arteritis
- Other vasculitides
- Haematological disorders, for example, polycythaemia vera, hyperviscosity syndrome

TYPICAL SIGNS OF A STROKE

The typical signs of a stroke are listed in Table 15.5.

TABLE 15.5 ■ Clinical Deficits Associated With Different Vascular Territories of the Brain

Anatomical Location	Common Neurological Deficits
Left middle cerebral artery	Right-sided weakness, involving face and arm >leg with expressive, receptive or mixed dysphasia
Right middle cerebral artery	Left-sided weakness, face and arm >leg, visual and/or sensory neglect or inattention of left side, denial of disability (anosognosia)
Lateral medulla (posterior inferior cerebellar artery and/or parent vertebral artery)	Ipsilateral Horner syndrome, Xth nerve palsy (due to infarction of nucleus ambiguus), facial sensory loss (trigeminal nerve), limb ataxia with contralateral spinothalamic sensory loss
	Typically, patients are vertiginous and unable to feed by mouth due (mainly) to failure of laryngeal closure during swallowing and ineffective coughing
	Cervical radiculopathies may occur due to involvement of radicular branches of the vertebral artery
Posterior cerebral artery	Homonymous hemianopia with variable additional deficits due to involvement of parietal and/or temporal lobe
Internal capsule	Motor, sensory or sensorimotor loss, involving face, arm and leg to a roughly similar extent
	There may be profound dysarthria due to involvement of corticobulbar fibres but the patient should not be dysphasic or have other cortical-type deficits, such as dyslexia or dysgraphia
Bilateral paramedian thalamus (30% of population have a single common arterial stem supplying medial aspect of both thalami)	Coma or disturbed vigilance at presentation, ophthalmoplegia (internal and/or external), ataxia and memory impairment
	Some patients require ventilation
Carotid artery dissection	Ipsilateral Horner syndrome due to compression of the sympathetic plexus around the carotid artery; the same process can also affect the lower cranial nerves (Xth and XIIth most obvious clinically) in the carotid sheath, or the VIth nerve in the cavernous sinus
	If ipsilateral cerebral infarction follows (due to hypoperfusion or embolisation), the clinical picture can mimic a brainstem event; in this way, carotid artery dissection can mimic vertebral artery dissection

FEATURES OF A STROKE INVOLVING THE BRAINSTEM

- Hemiplegia/quadriplegia
- Ataxia/vertigo/tinnitus
- Dysphagia
- Dysarthria
- Gaze paresis
- Temperature control disturbance
- Altered respiratory pattern

IS YOUR DIAGNOSIS OF A STROKE CORRECT?

Most strokes are easily diagnosed clinically, but errors do occur. Not all acute neurological impairments are due to stroke and other conditions can be misdiagnosed as stroke.

Unusual symptoms and signs should make you question the diagnosis, for example:

- Papilloedema
- Persistent headache

- Fluctuating signs
- Unexplained fever
- History of trauma to head or neck

EXAMPLES OF STROKE-MIMICS

- Todd paresis secondary to epileptic fit
- Space-occupying lesions:
  - Primary tumours, metastases
  - Subdural haematoma
  - Cerebral abscess
  - Venous sinus thrombosis
  - Carotid or vertebral artery dissection
- Infections:
  - Meningitis
  - Encephalitis
- Metabolic disturbance:
  - Hypo-/hyperglycaemia
  - Hypo-/hypernatraemia
  - Chronic kidney disease
- Intoxication/overdose:
  - Alcohol
  - Drugs, for example, sedatives and tricyclics. (**Note:** focal neurological signs are common with tricyclic overdose)
- Hypotension:
  - Hypovolaemia
  - Cardiac dysrhythmia
  - Cardiogenic shock
  - Old neurological deficits, for example, previous stroke

STROKE MANAGEMENT (FIG. 15.3)

Clinical Problems Associated With a Stroke (See Table 15.5)

Neurological Deficit

Early Management of a Stroke

- Thrombolytic treatment with IV alteplase (tPA): needs to be given in <4.5 h (ideally 90 min) of onset of stroke, once haemorrhage has been excluded on scanning. It can be considered between 4.5 h and 9 h if there is evidence of the potential to salvage brain tissue on CT/MRI perfusion. Tenecteplase is an alternative agent. Endovascular thrombectomy is performed after thrombolytic treatment in many units
- Aspirin: 300 mg and clopidogrel 75 mg after CT scanning (to rule out haemorrhage), if fibrinolysis is not being used
- Hydration and/or feeding: early nasogastric (NG) or percutaneous endoscopic gastrostomy (PEG) feeding improves outcome in stroke patients who have unsafe swallowing
- Treatment of hyperglycaemia with insulin regimen initially
- Paracetamol for pyrexia: if present
- Prevention of complications:
  - Chest infection: attention to swallowing and chest physiotherapy
  - Deep vein thrombosis (DVT). Thrombo-embolic deterrent (TED) stockings have been shown not to be helpful. Prophylactic low-molecular-weight (LMW) heparin (if haemorrhage has been ruled out) should be used early

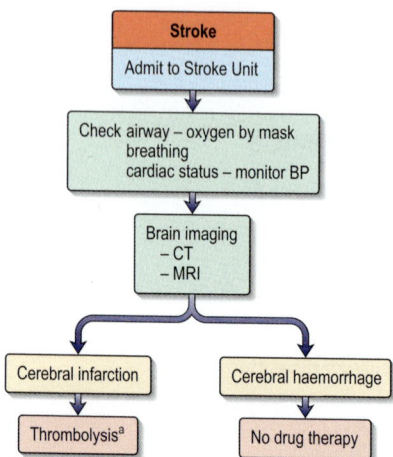

Fig. 15.3 Management of stroke. [a]Thrombectomy is being performed after thrombolysis in many units. (From Kumar, P., Clark, M., eds., 2011. Medical Management & Therapeutics. Saunders/Elsevier, Edinburgh; Fig. 20.20.)

- Pressure ulcers
- Contractures
- Rapid treatment of infection (most commonly chest and urinary tract)
- Hypertension: BP often rises in acute stroke but usually settles. Lowering of BP is only necessary in the early stage for severe hypertension. Persistently raised BP requires treatment for its secondary prevention benefits
- Support and interventions for the patient and family: stroke is a major life event, and both the patient and family need information and support

Dysphagia and Aspiration. These can occur in up to 50% of patients at presentation. Patients will need further assessment by a Speech and Language Therapist (SALT), and sometimes further investigation by videofluoroscopy.

If the patient's conscious level is impaired, don't assess the swallow until it improves.

Skin Condition

- Are there any pressure ulcers?
- Are there any areas of skin at risk?

Bladder Function

- Incontinence can result from the neurological problem or from immobility
- Catheterisation is required only if the patient is incontinent and there is a risk of pressure ulcers

REMEMBER

The specific symptoms and signs detected will depend on site of the lesion. Some 75% of strokes occur in middle cerebral artery territory; 15% are in the vertebrobasilar territory (see Table 15.5).

HOW WOULD YOU INVESTIGATE AND TREAT THIS PATIENT?

A CT scan (MRI not available) was performed approximately 3 hours after the onset of the stroke. This showed a middle cerebral artery thrombus.

The National Stroke Guidelines state that fibrinolytic therapy should be commenced; fibrinolytic therapy is indicated in patients with a cerebral infarct due to a thrombus, which occurred less than 4.5 hours ago. Therapy should be given as soon as possible, however, to allow the damaged brain to recover. A CT scan in the first 24 hours after an infarct might appear normal; if so, it will need to be repeated if MRI cannot be performed. Haemorrhage can usually be seen. An MRI scan shows an infarct early in the diagnosis.

INVESTIGATIONS

- Full blood counts
- Urea and electrolytes
- Random blood glucose
- Electrolyte sedimentation rate (ESR)
- Electrocardiogram
- Chest X-ray
- Computed tomography or MRI scan of brain

MAJOR RISK FACTORS FOR STROKE

- Smoking
- Hypertension
- Peripheral vascular disease
- Diabetes
- Atrial fibrillation
- Hypercholesterolaemia
- Previous stroke
- Coronary artery disease

REMEMBER

Poor Prognostic Signs in Stroke

- Reduced conscious level on admission
- Gaze paresis
- Early and persisting urinary incontinence
- Sensory inattention
- Preexisting disability
- Previous cognitive impairment

FURTHER MANAGEMENT – REHABILITATION

- Physiotherapy to maximise functional recovery and prevent contractures
- Occupational therapy for functional assessment, aids and adaptations
- Speech and Language Therapist for assessment and management of speech and swallowing problems
- Continuing medical review

Poststroke care and rehabilitation in Stroke Units have been shown to reduce mortality and early disability.

SECONDARY PREVENTION AFTER STROKE

- Hypertension: if persisting at 28 days after stroke, this should be treated according to British Hypertension Society Guidelines
- Antiplatelet agents: aspirin 75 mg daily and clopidogrel 75 mg daily should be started. Dipyridamole MR 200 mg is used if clopidogrel 75 mg daily is contraindicated or not tolerated
- Anticoagulation: given in patients with ischaemic stroke who make a reasonable recovery and have AF, mitral valve disease or a prosthetic heart valve, or are within 3 months of MI
- Carotid endarterectomy: if carotid stenosis of 70%–90% is present in patients who are not severely disabled by their stroke. Early investigation and surgery should be performed within 1 week
- Statins: for those with cholesterol >3.5 mmol/L
- Smoking cessation: refer to antismoking clinic

Progress. This patient improved a few hours after the fibrolytic therapy. Two days later, he was able to stand with help. With physiotherapy and speech therapy, he became fully ambulant in 6 days and his speech was improving. At assessment, 3 months later, he was living an independent life.

Heart Disease in the Elderly

CASE HISTORY

A 78-year-old male with long-standing AF was admitted with tiredness and breathlessness. He also complained of indigestion and recent falls.
   Examination revealed a radial pulse of 96, apical rate of 110 irregular, a raised JVP, swollen ankles and crackles up to both lung mid-zones.
   He was taking digoxin 125 µg daily and aspirin 75 mg daily.

WHAT INVESTIGATIONS WOULD YOU DO?

- Full blood count
- Urea and electrolytes
- Liver biochemistry
- Thyroid function tests
- Troponins
- Electrocardiogram
- Chest X-ray

Investigations revealed AF with no R wave progression on his ECG, suggesting a possible **acute myocardial infarct.**

His CXR showed pulmonary oedema (Fig. 15.4A). The FBC showed a haemoglobin (Hb) of 98 g/L with a mean corpuscular volume (MCV) of 70 fL, suggesting an iron deficiency anaemia, possibly related to his aspirin intake.

LEARNING POINTS

- Cardiac failure in the elderly may present with nonspecific symptoms such as tiredness and falls
- Aspirin, even at low dose, can be associated with occult gastrointestinal (GI) blood loss

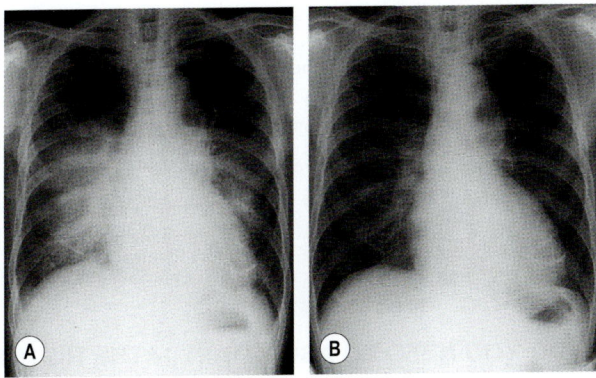

Fig. 15.4 A pair of chest X-rays taken from a patient before (A) and after (B) treatment of acute pulmonary oedema. The chest X-ray taken when the oedema was present demonstrates hilar haziness, Kerley B lines, upper lobe venous engorgement and fluid in the right horizontal interlobar fissure. These abnormalities are resolved on the film taken after successful treatment.

- Always check compliance in older people, especially if the patient thinks that the medication is not effective
- Benefits have been shown for anticoagulation of elderly patients in AF up to age 85, but contraindications (e.g. falls or GI haemorrhage) are more common in this population. In this case the microcytic anaemia would need to be investigated before starting anticoagulants
- Risks of anticoagulation in the over-85s are high and no study has shown a benefit in this age group
- Angiotensin-converting enzyme inhibitors should be used in hypertension in the elderly, starting with a low dose, and renal function closely monitored due to increased risk of renal impairment

ACUTE MI

The management principles of heart disease in the elderly are the same as those in young people, with a few exceptions.

Age alone is not a contraindication to thrombolysis/PCI in acute MI; in fact, the greatest benefits are seen in older patients. However, other comorbidities causing contraindications are more common in older people.

Acute MI may present silently (with no pain), more commonly in the elderly.

Treatment

This patient was given diuretic therapy with furosemide 40 mg orally daily. This helped his breathlessness and his ankles became less swollen. His CXR improved (Fig. 15.4B). As his presentation was over a few days, he was not given fibrinolytic therapy. He was started on an ACE inhibitor with enalapril 2.5 mg.

Endoscopy was performed, and he was found to have gastric and duodenal erosions due to his aspirin intake. The aspirin was stopped. Colonoscopy showed no lesion.

Progress. Three weeks later he was feeling much better. He was given iron therapy and started on anticoagulation with apixaban.

Transient Ischaemic Attack (TIA)

This is a transient episode of neurological dysfunction caused by focal brain, spinal cord or retinal ischaemia without acute infarction. The arbitrary time of <24 hours is no longer used; the criteria depend on having no demonstrable lesion on imaging.

CASE HISTORY

A 68-year-old male presents to the emergency department with weakness of the right arm and leg, expressive dysphasia and a facial palsy. While he is being examined, his symptoms and signs start to improve and have resolved by the time he returns from the X-ray department. A diagnosis of a TIA is made.

WHAT POINTS DO YOU NEED TO ASCERTAIN IN THE HISTORY?

- Previous similar episodes, especially recently
- Previous episodes of amaurosis fugax (sudden transient loss of vision in one eye)
- History of palpitations, hypertension, diabetes, high cholesterol or stroke
- Smoking history
- Current and previous medication
- Functional status: mental and physical

WHAT ARE THE MAJOR ASPECTS OF THE EXAMINATION?

- The neurological examination
- Blood pressure
- Pulse rate and rhythm
- Presence of cardiac murmurs, carotid bruits
- Papilloedema, visual field deficit, signs of retinal emboli

INVESTIGATIONS

- Full blood count
- Erythrocyte sedimentation rate
- Urea and electrolytes
- Blood sugar
- Cholesterol
- Electrocardiogram/24-h tape in selected patients
- Chest X-ray
- Computed tomography head
- Echocardiogram in patients with suspected valvular disease or mural thrombus
- Carotid duplex ultrasonography in patients with carotid territory TIAs

SHOULD YOU ADMIT THIS PATIENT?

Updated National Stroke guidelines for the UK recommend that a patient with a TIA should be admitted to hospital if he/she cannot be assessed and investigated in a neurovascular clinic within 24 hours of TIA.

Other reasons for admission:

- Doubt over diagnosis, for example, need to exclude space-occupying lesion
- Multiple TIAs in a short time: these patients should also be fast-tracked to carotid endarterectomy
- Identification of pathology requiring immediate intervention, for example, cardiac arrhythmia
- Background disability with poor social circumstances

HOW WOULD YOU MANAGE A CASE OF TIA?

- Aspirin and clopidogrel 300 mg loading doses followed by 75 mg daily
- Anticoagulation with apixaban in patients with AF
- Statins for those with hypercholesterolaemia (cholesterol >3.5 mmol/L)
- Treatment of risk factors, for example, hypertension
- Smoking cessation
- Advice not to drive for 1 month following the event

FURTHER MANAGEMENT – CAROTID ENDARTERECTOMY

Carotid endarterectomy is recommended for patients with TIAs and minor strokes who have 70% to 90% stenosis of the relevant carotid artery and who are otherwise fit, with no major persisting disability.

Investigation and treatment should be performed within 1 week. Magnetic resonance (MR) angiography is required prior to surgery. Carotid endarterectomy has a 1% to 2% perioperative stroke risk in the most experienced hands but reduces the incidence of stroke by 75% over the next 2 to 3 years.

The **ABCD² score** can help to stratify stroke risk in the first 2 days (Table 15.6).

Note: asymptomatic carotid stenosis is associated with a lower stroke risk but benefit from surgery is not proven.

PROGNOSIS AFTER UNTREATED TIA OVER 4 YEARS

- Twenty-five percent dead
- Twenty-five percent stroke
- Ten percent MI

Progress. This patient had a carotid endarterectomy performed 6 days after his admission to hospital. He made a good recovery; at 6-month review, he was still taking treatment for stroke prevention and had started on an exercise programme.

TABLE 15.6 ■ **ABCD² Score in the Stratification of Stroke Risk**

Parameter	Score
Age >60 years	1
BP >140 mm Hg systolic and/or diastolic >90 mm Hg	1
Clinical features	–
Unilateral weakness	2
Isolated speech disturbance	1
Other	0
Duration of symptoms (min)	
>60	2
10–59	1
<10	0
Diabetes	1
A score of <4 is associated with a minimal risk, whereas >6 is high risk for a stroke within 7 days of a TIA	

TIA, Transient ischaemic attack.
From Feather, A., Randall, D., Waterhouse, M., eds., 2020. Kumar and Clark's Clinical Medicine, tenth ed. Elsevier, Edinburgh; Box 26.33.

Hypothermia

INFORMATION

Hypothermia is defined as a core body temperature of <35°C. It is associated with many clinical conditions, and in most patients, aetiology is multifactorial.

CASE HISTORY

An 89-year-old female is found lying on the floor by her carer. On arrival at the emergency department, she is noted to be very drowsy and confused with a rectal temperature of 34°C.

AETIOLOGICAL FACTORS

- Exposure to cold
- Impaired thermoregulation
- Impaired shivering thermogenesis
- Low metabolic heat production
- Impaired temperature perception
- Drugs, for example, phenothiazines, hypnotics, alcohol
- Hypothyroidism
- Intercurrent illness

CLINICAL FEATURES

These vary with the degree of hypothermia. Whereas those with a core temperature of 33°C to 34°C can be confused and have slow cerebration, those with a temperature of 30°C are more likely to be drowsy and have muscular stiffness.

Some patients with hypothermia have features such as slow relaxing reflexes, which are suggestive of hypothyroidism.

The ECG can show changes such as sinus bradycardia, slow AF, prolonged PR interval and 'J' waves (commonly seen in leads V_3–V_4) (Fig. 15.5).

Complications of hypothermia include pancreatitis, oliguria, cardiac arrhythmias (particularly during rewarming) and aspiration pneumonia.

INVESTIGATIONS

- Full blood count
- Urea and electrolyte
- Glucose
- Amylase
- Liver biochemistry
- Calcium
- Arterial blood gases
- Electrocardiogram
- Chest X-ray
- Thyroid function tests

This patient was found to be grossly hypothyroid with a TSH of 14.3 mU/L and a T_4 of 4 pmol/L.

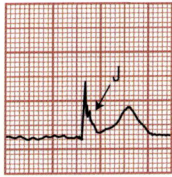

Fig. 15.5   Electrocardiogram showing J *waves*.

HOW WOULD YOU MANAGE THIS PATIENT?

She was managed as follows:
- Nursing with space blanket in a warm room (allowing temperature to rise by 0.5°C/h)
- Oxygen: remember that patients with COPD might require 24% oxygen
- Intravenous fluids (through blood warmer)
- Triiodothyronine 5–10 µg slowly IV 12-hourly for her severe hypothyroidism

A severely hypothermic patient will require admission to intensive care unit (ICU) for positive pressure ventilation, central venous pressure (CVP) line and ECG monitoring.

Progress. This patient made a slow but steady recovery and was discharged home on levothyroxine 125 µg daily with a follow-up appointment.

Pressure Ulcers

Pressure ulcers are common. Ill elderly people are most at risk of developing pressure ulcers. The reported prevalence rates vary widely – on average, 5% to 10% of this group.

> **CASE HISTORY**
>
> A 78-year-old female with a right hemiplegia from a previous stroke was brought to the emergency department, having fallen at home. She had been on the floor for at least 24 h because she was unable to get up.
>   **On examination**, she was conscious and aware of her surroundings. There were no specific abnormalities on physical examination, apart from evidence of a right hemiparesis. When examining her, you notice a dusky area over the right hip overlying the greater trochanter.

RISK FACTORS FOR DEVELOPING PRESSURE ULCERS

- Low/excessive body weight
- Poor nutritional state
- Motor deficit/immobility
- Sensory deficit
- Presence of intercurrent illness
- Incontinence: bladder/bowel
- Use of certain medications, for example, long-term prednisolone, sedatives and analgesics, which reduce sensation and hence stimulation to move

OTHER PATIENTS AT SPECIAL RISK

- Those undergoing surgery, particularly orthopaedic
- Those with neurological disease
- Those with spinal cord injury, including cord compression
- Those receiving palliative care

WHY DO PRESSURE ULCERS OCCUR?

Pressure greater than the mean capillary pressure (25–32 mm Hg) will occlude blood vessels and lead to anoxia of the skin. Hard surfaces can generate pressures of >100 mm Hg; damage to the skin therefore results from the pressure applied and the length of time exposed to the pressure. In addition to pressure, shearing force is another significant factor.

Pressure ulcers can be graded into superficial (grades 1 and 2) and deep (grades 3 and 4).

CLINICAL ASSESSMENT

Document pressure ulcers fully:
- Site, size and grade of pressure ulcer
- Condition of the surrounding skin
- Presence/absence of infection

Photography is a good method of recording pressure ulcers and monitoring change.

Perform a general examination of the patient with special regard to:
- Nutritional state, including body weight
- Full neurological examination
- Abdominal examination, especially bladder and bowel

HOW WOULD YOU INVESTIGATE?

Investigations will be directed by the physical examination, but special attention should be paid to those in the Investigations box.

INVESTIGATIONS

- Full blood count: presence of anaemia will delay wound healing
- Albumin: marker of nutrition; low albumin will delay wound healing
- Blood sugar: hyperglycaemia delays healing
- Wound swabs: for culture and sensitivity
- Blood cultures: if concern about septicaemia
- X-ray of the underlying bone: to rule out osteomyelitis if the wound is deep, overlies a bony prominence and has been present for some time

HOW WOULD YOU MANAGE PRESSURE ULCERS?

Prevention is definitely better than cure and all at-risk patients require immediate assessment.

REMEMBER

- Pressure ulcers can develop in 1–2 h
- Beware of leaving patients on hard trolleys or X-ray tables for too long

- Relief of pressure with appropriate support mattress and/or cushion for chair
  - Low-risk patients: a soft overlay to the mattress may be adequate
  - High-risk patients: an alternating pressure support system, for example, special pressure-relieving mattresses
- Appropriate dressings for wounds. **Note:** dry dressings should not be used on moist wounds Examples of dressings include:
  - Hydrocolloid for superficial granulating wounds

- Alginates for exuding or bleeding wounds
- Treatment of infection (cellulitis or associated septicaemia), when present, with appropriate systemic antibiotics
- General management of the patient:
  - Pain relief
  - Treatment of medical conditions, including anaemia
  - Review of drug treatment: NSAIDs and steroids delay wound healing
  - Review of nutrition, including use of supplements, such as vitamin C and zinc
  - Management of incontinence
- Severe pressure ulcers often require surgical debridement and skin grafting by plastic surgeons, when noninfected

Most hospitals have tissue viability specialist nurses to advise on prevention and treatment of pressure ulcers. For quantification of risk, these nurses can use the Waterlow score or Norton Scale.

Progress. This patient was admitted to the MAU and the tissue viability nurse was contacted to assess her pressure areas. Despite immediate treatment, she developed a pressure ulcer over her right hip.

Urinary Tract Infection and Incontinence

CASE HISTORY

An 80-year-old female with mild dementia presented with 24 h of increasing confusion and drowsiness. She had a 3-day history of urinary incontinence and diarrhoea. She was taking codydramol for arthritis.

Examination revealed a female with confusion, with no knowledge of her surroundings or time of day. Her GCS score was 12. Examination of her abdomen was normal, but rectal examination showed constipation with faecal impaction and overflow diarrhoea. A urine sample was offensive and positive to Stix testing for nitrites, leucocytes, blood and protein.

PARTICULAR POINTS TO NOTE IN THE HISTORY

- Urinary tract infection (UTI) in the elderly can present with nonspecific symptoms, such as confusion, drowsiness or falls
- Recurrent UTIs should be investigated (>3 in a female, >1 in a male) with renal tract ultrasound, including assessment of postmicturition bladder volume
- New urge incontinence may be precipitated by infection, leading to an unstable bladder
- Infection can be precipitated by obstruction: most commonly caused by constipation or prostatic hypertrophy
- Drug history for precipitating causes: drugs causing constipation, diuretics, sedatives

EXAMINATION

Examination of this patient included:
- Full physical examination for coexisting causes of confusion, for example, chest infection
- Rectal examination, to assess for constipation/overflow (prostatic enlargement in males)
- Neurological examination, to exclude neurological causes of urinary retention and constipation

HOW WOULD YOU TREAT THIS PATIENT?

- Treat symptomatic infection with oral antibiotics following local guidelines, for example:
  - Trimethoprim 200 mg × 2 for 3–5 days is a good first-line treatment. Use parenteral antibiotics only if the patient is very ill or vomiting
- Treat constipation: enemas and laxatives. Stop codydramol. Repeat residual volumes after constipation is treated, as this patient's constipation was likely to be due to the codeine in codydramol. The latter was replaced by paracetamol

Progress. This patient's confusion and drowsiness improved with successful treatment of her UTI. Her faecal impaction was relieved by the enemas, but she is still inclined to constipation, and this is treated symptomatically with Macrogol.

Arteritis

CASE HISTORY

An 82-year-old widower was admitted with left-sided temporal headache of 3 days' duration. He is known to have type 2 diabetes (on insulin), visual impairment due to macular degeneration, hypertension and an old left hemiparesis. He lives alone in a house and has one son who lives far away.

MEDICAL ASSESSMENT

On examination, the patient had signs of an old left hemiparesis and a peripheral neuropathy (probably due to long-standing diabetes) and visual impairment. His BP was 150/80 on losartan therapy. In addition, it was noted that the left temporal artery was pulsatile but tender.

Investigations revealed a significantly elevated ESR (>100 mm in 1 h).

A clinical diagnosis of **temporal arteritis** was made. A temporal artery biopsy showed:

- Cellular infiltrate of CD4 and T lymphocytes
- Macrophages in the vessel wall
- Granulomatous inflammation of the intima and media
- Breaking up of the internal elastic lamina
- Giant cells, lymphocytes and plasma cells in the internal elastic lamina

His response to steroids was very good, although he remained tired and slightly frailer than previously

HOW WOULD YOU ORGANISE HIS DISCHARGE?

The patient needs a multidisciplinary assessment before discharge to ensure his safety. His son should also be contacted, with the patient's permission.

General Points for Discharge Planning

Discharge planning of an elderly person should start as early as possible after admission. Once the person's medical problems have been accurately diagnosed and treated, his/her potential for returning home should be assessed by a multidisciplinary team (MDT) of professionals, taking into account the elderly person's views.

> **REMEMBER**
>
> A competent adult has a right to decide whether he/she wishes to go home, even if this decision is against the advice offered by member(s) of the MDT.

The MDT review includes:
- Assessment by a physiotherapist to assess the patient's mobility, transfers and ability to climb stairs
- Assessment by an occupational therapist to assess independence and safety in ADL, kitchen assessment and/or a home visit
- Social work assessment that will take into account the assessments of other professionals to quantify his/her needs for care on discharge
- Assessment by a SALT, a dietitian or a psychologist in some cases
- Referral to a district nurse, for example, for treatment of leg ulcers, monitoring of diabetic control, monitoring of medication
- Discussion with a general practitioner (GP) about on-going medical care

Following discharge, it might be possible to continue further rehabilitation or monitoring of medical or nursing care in a day-hospital setting.

Progress. This patient was keen to go home, even though he was still frail. He required full support at his house, with community nurses managing his insulin therapy. His headaches disappeared on steroid therapy, which was reduced, making his diabetes easier to manage. He continues to improve.

Parkinson Disease (PD)

CASE HISTORY

An 80-year-old male with a history of hypertension presents with a fall. He has had numerous falls recently and, on questioning, said he had slowed down generally.

You immediately notice a tremor in his left arm, a lack of facial expression and a monotonous voice. You suspect a diagnosis of PD.

FEATURES OF PD

- Akinesia/bradykinesia:
  - Poor initiation of movement
  - Slowing of repetitive movements
  - Fatigue
- Rigidity:
  - Lead pipe *and/or*
  - Cogwheel (if tremor is present)

- Tremor: 70% of patients present with tremor, usually unilateral:
  - Rest tremor
  - Three to seven Hertz
  - Absent in 30% at presentation
- Postural instability is usually a late feature of idiopathic PD
- Response to levodopa (L-dopa) suggests idiopathic PD

REMEMBER

- The disease is often asymmetrical at presentation
- Depression is a common association, often missed

CLINICAL DIAGNOSIS OF PD

Parkinson disease is a clinical diagnosis; there are no diagnostic tests. Diagnosis requires two cardinal features, including:

- Akinesia/bradykinesia of the upper body
- Asymmetrical onset with resting tremor
- Clear response to L-dopa

WHAT IS THE DIFFERENTIAL DIAGNOSIS OF PD?

- Essential tremor:
  - Isolated tremor, can affect the head (Yes/Yes or No/No pattern)
  - Becomes more prominent with increasing age
  - Autosomal dominant inheritance
  - Responds to alcohol, beta-blockers
- Arteriosclerotic parkinsonism:
  - History of cerebrovascular disease and hypertension common
  - Wide-based, short-stepped gait: *marche* à petit pas
  - Upper part of body not affected
  - Limited/transient response to L-dopa
- Drug-induced parkinsonism:
  - Antipsychotic drugs, especially depot preparations
  - Metoclopramide: acute
- Rarer causes of parkinsonism:
  - Multiple system atrophy, Shy–Drager parkinsonism: autonomic failure and dementia
  - Steele–Richardson–Olszewski parkinsonism: loss of voluntary conjugate deviation of gaze, and pseudobulbar dysarthria

---

REMEMBER

When to Question a Diagnosis of PD

- Poor response to L-dopa
- Early instability
- Pyramidal or cerebellar signs
- Early autonomic failure, for example, postural hypotension, incontinence
- Dementia early in course of disease
- Voluntary downward gaze palsy

HOW WOULD YOU MANAGE THIS PATIENT?

- This patient was started on L-dopa as first-line treatment (e.g. cobeneldopa), as it is useful in the elderly. Dose requires titration, depending on improvement and side-effects of medication, for example, postural hypotension, nausea, hallucinations
- Synthetic dopamine agonists (ropinirole, pramipexole) are less effective but might be useful in early disease. Hallucinations and somnolence are common side-effects but are tolerated by approximately 46% of very elderly patients. They may need to be used with domperidone to avoid GI side effects. Other dopamine agonists have ergot side effects and are poorly tolerated by the elderly
- The monoamine oxidase inhibitor (MAOI-B) selegiline should be avoided in patients with postural hypotension or hallucinations
- Catechol-O-methyl transferase (COMT) inhibitors (e.g. tolcapone, entacapone) are used as adjuncts to L-dopa
- Apomorphine SC infusion is used in specialist centres

The frequency of this patient's falls improved with PD therapy, but nevertheless, exercise and balance training was started. He was referred to an MDT to assess the need for walking aids and changes in the home environment.

Progress. The patient was commenced on cobeneldopa and was able to return home with community support.

Drugs as a Cause of Illness, Admission to Hospital and Delayed Discharge

Individuals over the age of 65 make up approximately 18% of the population but represent 25% to 30% of drug expenditure. Approximately 87% of the elderly take one prescribed medication and one-third of this group take three or more drugs.

Age-associated increases in the incidence of adverse reactions have been well described for certain groups of drugs, for example, benzodiazepines.

The most frequently used classes are cardiovascular drugs, analgesics, GI preparations and sedatives (Table 15.7).

TABLE 15.7 ■ **Drugs That Are More Likely to Produce Adverse Effects in the Elderly**

Drug	Adverse Effects
Benzodiazepines	Sedation, drowsiness, confusion, ataxia
NSAIDs	Gastric erosions, fluid retention, renal impairment and drug interaction, e.g. diuretics
Opiates	Sedation, confusion, constipation
Antimuscarinic	Urinary retention, glaucoma
Antiarrhythmics	Confusion, urinary retention, thyroid problems
Antipsychotics	Confusion, sedation, tardive dyskinesia, malignant hyperthermia
Diuretics	Dehydration, hyponatraemia, hypo- or hyperkalaemia, postural hypotension, renal impairment, gout
Antibiotics	Renal failure, diarrhoea, auditory complications

CASE HISTORY (1)

A 75-year-old female was admitted to the MAU with a severe cough and purulent sputum. She was known to have chronic obstructive pulmonary disease (COPD) and this was thought to be an infective exacerbation.

On examination, she was tachypnoeic but not cyanosed. Examination of her chest showed diffuse wheeze with some basal crackles. Her oxygen saturation was 92%.

She was started on amoxicillin 500 mg × 3 daily, in addition to nebulised salbutamol and ipratropium, with a good response.

A few days later, she developed watery diarrhoea, which was bad enough to require IV fluids. Her stool analysis was positive for *Clostridium difficile* toxin. She was prescribed a 10-day course of metronidazole 400 mg × 3 daily. Apart from transient nausea, she made a good recovery from her diarrhoea and was able to go home after 6 days.

CASE HISTORY (2)

A 71-year-old female was admitted with malaise, fatigue, weight loss and a general feeling of being unwell.

On examination, she looked anxious, underweight and tremulous with a tachycardia.

In the past, she had suffered from AF and was taking amiodarone 200 mg once daily.

Investigations revealed thyrotoxicosis (thought to be due to amiodarone) with undetectable thyroid stimulating hormone (TSH) <0.05 mU/L and very high free triiodothyronine (T_3) (10 pmol/L and thyroxine [T_4] 35 pmol/L).

The amiodarone was stopped, and her cardiologist contacted about alternative therapy for her AF. She was started on antithyroid therapy (carbimazole 10 mg × 3 daily) and steroids (prednisolone 40 mg once daily). Her response was slow, and she remained an inpatient for 2 weeks before her condition was brought under control. She was seen in the endocrine clinic for dose adjustment of her carbimazole.

CASE HISTORY (3)

A 79-year-old female with a background of type 2 diabetes and ischaemic heart disease was admitted to the MAU with uncontrolled diabetes and progressive shortness of breath. She was taking gliclazide 160 mg × 2 daily and coamilofruse (5 mg amiloride, 40 mg furosemide) one tablet in the morning. A few weeks prior to admission, she complained of back pain and her doctor prescribed diclofenac 50 mg × 3 a day (an NSAID).

On examination, she was in acute left ventricular failure with a tachycardia, raised venous pressure, gallop rhythm and basal crackles. She was treated acutely with oxygen, IV furosemide 50 mg and buccal glyceryl trinitrate 2 mg repeated every 20 min. There was no evidence of an acute ischaemic episode or chest infection.

Progress. The NSAID was stopped. The dose of furosemide was doubled to 80 mg daily with 2.5 mg of amiloride. Her symptoms settled gradually over the next few days and her furosemide was then reduced without recurrence of her left ventricular failure. Her diabetes is well controlled on gliclazide with a glycated haemoglobin (HbA_{1c}) of 6.5% (48 mmol/mol).

REMEMBER

NSAIDs cause fluid retention and can precipitate heart failure in susceptible individuals (e.g. patients with diabetes, hypertension or renal failure).

Do Not Attempt Resuscitation (DNAR) Decision-Making

CASE HISTORY (1)

A fit, elderly, 72-year-old male presents with an acute MI. If he has a cardiac arrest, would you resuscitate him?

CASE HISTORY (2)

A 75-year-old female presents with hypercalcaemia secondary to disseminated lung carcinoma. You treat her hypercalcaemia aggressively. A nurse asks whether the patient should be recorded for resuscitation or not.

WHAT WOULD YOU SAY?

Cardiopulmonary resuscitation (CPR) is an everyday practice in most hospitals. Despite success in selected patients, there is a consensus that CPR might be inappropriate (e.g. in terminal illness) or ineffective (e.g. very severe pneumonia) in some. Age alone is not a contraindication to CPR.

All decisions should be made by senior medical staff after discussion with the patient (if competent), other members of the team and family/carers (if the patient lacks mental capacity).

WHAT PRINCIPLES MIGHT GUIDE YOU TO DECIDE TO WITHHOLD CPR?

- Likely effectiveness of CPR: only 6%–15% of patients who undergo CPR leave hospital alive. A number of factors predict a poor outcome from CPR attempts. These include:
- A high level of dependency, including housebound lifestyle
- Significant comorbidities
- Patient's wishes: these can be ascertained in advance, or from advance directives and living wills. Mentally competent patients who express their wishes about treatment, including CPR, must have those wishes respected. The guidance also recommends that a patient can refuse to accept a DNAR order made by a clinician and that, under the Human Rights Act, doctors must respect this decision and record the change. If a patient is not mentally competent to decide whether to accept CPR, the doctor must consult family/carers and/or the family doctor to ascertain what the patient's wishes would have been. The doctor then uses this information to 'act in the patient's best interest'. **Note:** there is no provision in law in England and Wales for relatives to make medical decisions, including CPR, on behalf of an adult
- Quality of life: this is the most difficult aspect to address. It includes quality of life as it is now and also as it would be after a CPR attempt, which might be worse. Difficulties arise because it involves professionals making value judgements about other people's lives

REMEMBER

- If no DNAR decision is documented, the patient is for resuscitation
- Any DNAR decision made should be communicated to all members of the healthcare team involved with the patient
- Do not attempt resuscitation decisions should be reviewed if appropriate (i.e. not necessarily in terminal illness)

Case 1. It would be appropriate to resuscitate this patient if it aligned with his wishes. Many patients recover from an MI, even if elderly.

Case 2. It would be approrpiate to have a DNAR discussion with this patient as she is suffering from disseminated cancer.

Palliative Care

CASE HISTORY 1

A 68-year-old patient with a history of metastatic lung cancer presents with symptoms indicative of progression to the terminal phase of illness. The patient has been experiencing increased breathlessness, fatigue, and a reduced ability to engage in daily activities. They express a growing realization of their approaching end of life and a desire to discuss care preferences and expectations.

WHAT ARE THE KEY COMPONENTS OF PALLIATIVE CARE?

Palliative care is an active, holistic approach that includes pain and symptom management, psychological support, social care, spiritual care, and support for the family and carers. It aims to improve the quality of life for patients and their families facing life-threatening illness.

HOW CAN YOU DETERMINE IF A PATIENT IS ENTERING THE TERMINAL PHASE OF THEIR ILLNESS?

Signs that a patient may be entering the terminal phase include a day-by-day deterioration, reduced mobility, increased fatigue without an apparent cause, reduced oral intake, altered level of consciousness, and a patient's expression or realization that they are dying.

WHAT IS ANTICIPATORY PRESCRIBING IN PALLIATIVE CARE?

Anticipatory prescribing involves identifying and prescribing medications in advance for symptoms that are likely to occur as the patient approaches the end of life. This ensures that new or developing symptoms can be treated promptly without delay.

CASE HISTORY 2

A 55-year-old individual with a diagnosis of advanced pancreatic cancer presents with severe, persistent abdominal pain that has progressively worsened over several months. The patient describes the pain as a deep, gnawing sensation that radiates to the back and is exacerbated by eating. They report significant weight loss, fatigue, and decreased appetite. The patient's medical history is notable for chemotherapy and radiotherapy, which provided temporary relief from symptoms but were ultimately unsuccessful in halting disease progression.

WHAT IS THE WHO ANALGESIC LADDER AND HOW IS IT APPLIED IN PALLIATIVE CARE FOR CANCER-RELATED PAIN?

The WHO analgesic ladder is a framework for managing cancer pain that recommends a stepwise approach to analgesia, starting with nonopioids like NSAIDs for mild pain, adding weak opioids for moderate pain, and progressing to strong opioids for severe pain. Adjuvant medications may be used at any step for specific types of pain.

WHAT ARE COMMON BARRIERS TO EFFECTIVE PAIN MANAGEMENT IN PALLIATIVE CARE?

Common barriers include inadequate pain assessment, patient reluctance to report pain, fears of opioid addiction, side effects of medications, and healthcare provider knowledge gaps regarding pain management in palliative care.

HOW CAN BREAKTHROUGH PAIN BE MANAGED IN PALLIATIVE CANCER CARE?

Breakthrough pain should be managed by ensuring the patient has access to immediate-release opioids that can be taken in addition to regular analgesic doses. The dose for breakthrough pain is typically a fraction of the total daily opioid dose and should be adjusted based on the patient's response.

CASE HISTORY 3

A 68-year-old individual with a history of advanced nonsmall cell lung cancer presents with progressive dyspnoea. The patient reports a worsening sensation of breathlessness over the past few weeks, which now occurs even at rest. They describe associated symptoms of anxiety and occasional wheezing. The patient has a past medical history significant for hypertension and a 30-pack-year smoking history. They have been on palliative chemotherapy, which has now been stopped due to disease progression and declining performance status.

WHAT IS DYSPNOEA, AND HOW DOES IT DIFFER FROM BREATHLESSNESS IN THE CONTEXT OF PALLIATIVE CARE?

Dyspnoea is a subjective symptom of discomfort or difficulty in breathing, while breathlessness is an objective, observable sign. In palliative care, dyspnoea is often multifactorial, with anxiety frequently contributing to the sensation of breathlessness.

WHAT ARE THE COMMON CAUSES OF DYSPNOEA IN CANCER PATIENTS?

Dyspnoea in cancer patients can arise from direct causes like primary lung cancer or lung metastases, indirect effects of cancer, such as pleural effusion, superior vena cava syndrome, and nonmalignant causes including pneumonia, COPD, heart failure and anxiety.

HOW SHOULD DYSPNOEA BE ASSESSED IN A PALLIATIVE CARE SETTING?

Dyspnoea assessment should include a thorough history of the symptom's features (severity, timing, onset), associated physical symptoms (cough, sputum, wheeze), psychological symptoms (anxiety), and the impact on the patient's quality of life. An appropriate examination should also be conducted to determine the cause of dyspnoea.

MANAGEMENT

Management of dyspnoea in palliative care should be tailored to the underlying cause and the patient's stage of illness. It includes nonpharmacological strategies like room cooling, relaxation and breathing techniques. Pharmacological interventions may involve opioids, such as immediate-release oral morphine, benzodiazepines for acute anxiety and bronchodilators for wheezing due to airway obstruction.

REMEMBER

Remember that managing dyspnoea in palliative care is not just about pharmacological treatments; addressing psychological, social, and spiritual needs is equally vital. Regular reassessment of dyspnoea and its impact on quality of life is crucial for optimal patient care.

CASE HISTORY 4

A 63-year-old patient with metastatic breast cancer is experiencing intractable nausea and vomiting. Despite antiemetic treatment, their symptoms persist, impacting their ability to maintain hydration and nutrition. The patient's current medication regimen includes opioids for pain management and adjuvant chemotherapy. They report a significant decrease in quality of life due to the constant discomfort and social withdrawal resulting from their symptoms.

WHAT FACTORS SHOULD BE CONSIDERED WHEN ASSESSING A PATIENT WITH NAUSEA AND VOMITING IN A PALLIATIVE SETTING?

Factors include the patient's history, examination findings, medication review, and potential causes like drugs, metabolic disturbances, gastric stasis or anxiety. Investigations for reversible causes, such as renal failure or hypercalcaemia, may also be necessary.

HOW DOES THE CHOICE OF ANTIEMETIC VARY ACCORDING TO THE CAUSE OF NAUSEA AND VOMITING?

Antiemetics should be chosen based on the suspected underlying cause. For example, haloperidol is useful for drug-induced vomiting, whereas cyclizine may be better suited for nausea due to vestibular disturbances or raised intracranial pressure.

MANAGEMENT

Management involves identifying reversible causes and selecting appropriate antiemetics based on the underlying mechanism. Simple measures, such as ensuring access to a bowl, tissues, and water, and dietary modifications can be helpful. Pharmacological interventions include prokinetics like metoclopramide, antipsychotics like haloperidol, and antimuscarinics like hyoscine butyl bromide.

REMEMBER

Remember to review the patient's medication regimen and consider potential drug interactions. Always consider the patient's and family's preferences, prognosis, and the balance of symptom relief against potential side effects of treatment.

CASE HISTORY 5

A 78-year-old patient with advanced lung cancer is in the terminal phase of their illness. The healthcare team has noticed an accumulation of respiratory secretions, leading to a prominent gurgling sound during breathing, known as the 'death rattle'. This symptom has become distressing for the patient's family, although the patient appears to be unbothered due to decreased consciousness.

WHAT ARE THE COMMON CAUSES OF THE ACCUMULATION OF SECRETIONS AT THE END OF LIFE?

Secretions may accumulate due to decreased ability to clear them, such as from reduced coughing or swallowing. Other causes include increased mucus production from chest infections, pulmonary oedema or bronchorrhoea, as well as factors like gastric reflux or aspiration.

HOW CAN NOISY RESPIRATORY SECRETIONS BE MANAGED CONSERVATIVELY?

Repositioning the patient on one side with the upper body elevated can help with postural drainage. Ensuring adequate explanation to family members about the nature of the secretions and that the patient is not in distress can also be important.

WHEN SHOULD PHARMACOLOGICAL TREATMENT BE CONSIDERED FOR MANAGING SECRETIONS?

Pharmacological treatment with antimuscarinic drugs, like glycopyrronium bromide or hyoscine butyl bromide, can be considered if conservative measures are ineffective, and the secretions are causing distress to the patient or their family.

> **INFORMATION**
>
> Inform families that the patient is unlikely to be distressed by noisy secretions due to reduced consciousness at the end of life. Educate them on the purpose and effects of antimuscarinic medications, if used, and the importance of repositioning to help manage secretions.

Further Reading

General

British Geriatrics Society. Available from: https://www.bgs.org.uk.

Falls in the Elderly

Rodriguez-Mañas, L., Fried, L.P., 2015. Frailty in the clinical scenario. Lancet 385, 67.

Delirium

Folstein, M.F., Folstein, S.E., McHugh, P.R., 1975. Mini-mental state: a practical method for grading cognitive state of patients for the clinician. J. Psychiatr. Res. 12, 189–198.
HELP website. Available from: http://hospitalelderlifeprogram.org.
Marcantonio, E.R., 2017. Delirium in hospitalized older adults. N. Engl. J. Med. 377, 1456–1466.
NICE, CKS, 2023. Delirium. NICE.

Dementia

Mini-Mental State Examination. Available from: http://en.wikipedia.org/wiki/Mini%E2%80%93mental_state_examination.
National Institute for Health and Care Excellence, 2018. Dementia: assessment, management and support for people living with dementia and their carers, NICE Guideline 97, www.nice.org.uk.
NICE, CKS, 2023. Dementia. NICE.
Scheptens, P., 2016. Alzheimer's disease. Lancet 388, 505–517.

Stroke

Baird, A.E., 2018. Paving the way for improved treatment of acute stroke with tenecteplase. N. Engl. J. Med. 378, 1635–1636.

Hughes, T., 2011. Stroke on the acute medical take. Clin. Med. 10, 68–72.

Langhorne, P., Bernhardt, J., Kwakkel, G., 2011. Stroke care 2. Lancet 377, 1693–1702.

Rothwell, P.M., Algra, A., Amarenco, P., 2011. Stroke care 1. Lancet 377, 1681–1692.

Royal College of Physicians Stroke Programme. Available from: https://www.rcplondon.ac.uk/stroke.

Hypothermia

Morrison, G., 2017. Management of acute hypothermia. Medicine 45, 135–138.

Pressure Ulcers

National Institute for Health and Care Excellence, 2006. Nutrition support for adults, Clinical Guideline 32. Available from: www.nice.org.uk.

Reddy, M., Gill, S.S., Rochon, P.A., 2006. Preventing pressure ulcers; a systematic review. J. Am. Med. Assoc. 296, 974–984.

Parkinson's Disease

Bressman, S., Saunders-Pullman, R., 2019. When to start levodopa therapy for Parkinson's disease. N. Engl. J. Med. 380, 389–390.

Kalia, L.V., Lang, A.E., 2015. Parkinson's disease. Lancet 386, 896–912.

DNAR Decision-Making

Resuscitation Council (UK). Available from: https://www.resus.org.uk.

Palliative Care

NICE, CKS, 2023. Palliative Care – Dyspnoea. NICE.

NICE, CKS, 2023. Palliative Care – General issues. NICE.

NICE, CKS, 2023. Palliative Care – Nausea and Vomiting. NICE.

NICE, CKS, 2023. Palliative Care – Pain. NICE.

NICE, CKS, 2023. Palliative Care – Secretion. NICE.

Note: Page numbers followed by "*f*" indicate figures, "*t*" indicate tables, and "*b*" indicate boxes.

A

Abbreviated Mental Test, 478*b*, 478, 482–483
ABCD² score (stroke risk), 495, 495*t*
Abdominal pain, 140
  case study, 140*b*
  diagnosis of, 142
  investigations for, 141
  management of, 141
Abnormal liver biochemistry, 157, 158*t*
Abscess
  prognosis of, 133
  treatment of, 133
Acetaminophen overdose, 15
Acetylcholine esterase inhibitors, 480
Acetylcysteine, adverse reactions to, 17
Acid–base changes, 92, 93*f*
Acquired bleeding disorders, 374
Acute abdominal pain
  of gradual onset, 152
  of sudden onset, 152
Acute breathlessness, 78
  assessment of, 78
  case study, 78*b*
  causes of, 79*b*
  diagnosis of, 79
Acute chest syndrome, 387
  pathophysiology, 387
  treatment, 387
Acute coronary syndrome, 40, 45, 88, 484
  case study, 40*b*
  classification, 45
Acute haemolysis, 390*b*, 393
  in glucose-6-phosphate dehydrogenase, 390,
    392*t*
Acute heart failure, 183–184
  case study, 184*b*
  causes of, 183–184
  diagnosis of, 184
Acute kidney injury, 192
  definition of, 193
  diagnosis of, 193
  KDIGO classification of, 193*t*
  RIFLE criteria for, 194*t*
Acute leukaemia, 368, 406
  features of, 409
Acute myocardial infarction, 42*f*, 492
  enzyme profile in, 42*f*
  troponin profile in, 42*f*

Acute respiratory distress syndrome, 9
  case study, 9*b*
  causes of, 10
  experimental methods, 11
  key features of, 9, 10*f*
  management of, 9, 11
  outlook of, 11
  pathophysiology of, 10
  results, 9
Acute respiratory failure, in patient with COPD,
    arterial blood gas abnormalities in, 94
Addison disease, 337
Adenosine, 31
Adrenal mineralocorticoid production, 340–341
Adult advanced life-support algorithm, 41*f*
Adult basic life support, 39*f*
Alcohol, case study, 170*b*
Alcohol Dependency Unit, 164
Alemtuzuma, 255
Allopurinol, 203
Alteplase, 45
Amiodarone, 329, 504*b*
Amoxicillin, 482–483, 504*b*
Anaemia, 196
  cancer, 413
  causes of, 411
  chronic kidney disease and, 412
  classification, 355*b*
  definition of, 355
  drug-induced, 411
  leucoerythroblastic, 414
  liver disease, 412
  pernicious, 411
  rheumatoid arthritis, 411
Anagrelide, 369
Analgesic, acute painful sickle-cell crises, 386
Anaphylactic shock, 8
Anaphylaxis, 7
  case study, 7*b*
  diagnosis of, 7
  management of, 8
  prevention of, 9
ANCA-positive vasculitis, 200
Androgens, 361
Angio-oedema, 424
Angiotensin receptor blockers, 484
Angiotensin-converting enzyme inhibition, 47,
    186*f*, 187, 293, 484

Antibiotics, 405, 482–483
Antibiotic therapy, indications for, 127
Anticoagulant drugs
    orally active, 394
    overdosage, 379
Anticonvulsant drugs, 469
Antiglobulin (Coombs') tests, 362*f*, 391, 400
Antimicrobial prophylaxis, 66
Antineutrophil cytoplasmic antibody, 199, 200*f*
Anxiety, acute, 272
Aortic dissection, 89
    causes of, 43
Aortic regurgitation, 63
Aortic stenosis, 61, 71*f*, 71*t*
Aortic valve disease, 62*f*
    pulse patterns, 62*f*
Apomorphine, 503
Arrhythmias, 13, 31, 32*f*, 470
Arterial and central venous pressure, 178
Arterial blood gas
    abnormalities in, 94
    sampling, 92
Arterial ulcers, 418
Arteriosclerotic parkinsonism, 502
Arteritis, 500
    assessment of, 500
    case study, 500*b*
Arthritis, 374*f*
Ascites, 163
Ascitic fluid, 163
    diagnosis of, 163
    management of, 164
Ascitis, 163
Aspergillus fumigatus, 459
Assessment scales, 484
Asthma, 81, 83
    arterial blood gas abnormalities in, 94
    causes of, 82*f*
    discharge, 84
    high dependency unit, indications
        for, 84
    treatment of, 84
    triggers of, 82*f*
Atheromatous renovascular disease, 187
Atopic eczema, 422
Atrial fibrillation, 32, 33*f*
    case study, 32*b*
    HAS-BLED Score for bleeding risk on oral
        anticoagulation in, 34*t*
    management of, 33
    prevalence and risks of, 32
    VASc scoring system for, 34*t*
Atrial tachycardia, 28
Atrioventricular nodal reentry
        tachycardia, 28

Autoimmune haemolytic anaemia,
        361, 363*b*
    diagnosis of, 362
    management of, 363
Autoimmune rheumatic disease, 175, 290
Avascular necrosis, femoral head, 388*f*
Azathioprine, 203, 363, 367*b*, 368, 411

B
B$_{12}$ deficiency
    causes, 358
Back pain
    acute, 299, 301
    severe, 302
Bacterial chest infection, 459
    HIV/AIDS and, 459
Bacterial sepsis, 415
Balloon tamponade, 167
Barrett oesophagus, 144
Barthel Index, 484, 485*t*
Bell's palsy, 220*f*, 220
Bendroflumethiazide, 482–483
Benzodiazepine overdose, 15*b*
Biochemical screen, 408
Bisphosphonates, 407–408, 414
Blackouts, 469
    cardiovascular causes, 470
    case study, 469*b*
    investigations of, 470*b*
    treatment of, 470
Bladder function, 490
Bleeding disorders, 373. *See also*
        Haematemesis/melaena
    acquired, 374
    case study, 373*b*
    inherited, 374*f*–375*f*, 374
    investigations of, 375
Blood dyscrasia, 175
Blood pressure, 13
Blood transfusion, 399
    case study, 400*b*–401*b*
    complications of, 401*b*, 401
    outcome, 400
BODE Index, 99*t*
Bone marrow pathology, 369*f*, 369
Bowel ischaemia, 191
Bradycardia, 35
    diagnosis of, 36
    management of, 36
Brain
    abscess, 236
    neurological deficits, 488*t*
Brainstem, stroke, 488
Breathlessness, 81
    case study, 82*b*

Broad-complex tachycardia, 30f
Bronchiolitis
  case study, 90b
  diagnosis of, 90–91
  management of, 91
  risk factors for, 91
Bronchus, carcinoma of, 122b, 122
  case study, 122b
  categories of, 126
  complications of, 125
  diagnosis of, 122, 125
  investigations for, 123
  management of, 125
Busulfan, 369

C
Calcium-channel blockers, 55
Capnocytophaga canimorsus, 398
Carbimazole, 504b
Cardiac arrest, 38
Cardiac pain, 88
Cardio inhibitory variant, 470
Cardiogenic shock, 48
Cardiomyopathy, 69
Cardiopulmonary resuscitation, 505
  principles, 505
Cardiovascular causes, blackouts, 470
Cardiovascular diseases, 175
Carotid endarterectomy, 492, 495
Carotid sinus syncope, 24
Catechol-O-methyl transferase inhibitors, 503
Cefuroxime, 405
Cervical myelopathy, causes of, 249
Chest conditions, HIV/AIDS and, 458
Chest pain, 40
  acute coronary syndrome and, 88
  approach to, 88
  cardiac markers, 40
  cardiac pain and, 88
  causes of, 43
  functional, 90
  investigations of, 90
  musculoskeletal, 90
  oesophageal, 89
  pericarditis and, 88
Cheyne–Stokes respiration, 22
Chloroquine, 392t
Cholangitis, acute, 173
Cholecystitis, 171
Chronic haematological malignancy, 409
Chronic kidney disease, 195
  anaemia, 412
  classification of, 197t
  diagnosis of, 377
  features of, 196

Chronic kidney disease (Continued)
  management of, 196
  multidisciplinary approach to, 198f
  signs of, 197f
  symptoms of, 197f
Chronic lymphoblastic (lymphocytic) leukaemia,
    360b, 404f, 404, 410f
Chronic myeloid leukaemia,
    408f, 408
  investigations of, 408
  diagnosis of, 408
  referral, 409
Chronic obstructive pulmonary disease
    (COPD), 97
  ambulatory management of, 98
  case study, 97b, 99b
  considerations in, 99
  follow-up in chest clinic, 102
  management of, 100
  oxygen therapy in, 100, 101f
  prognosis of, 99
Chronic respiratory failure, in patient
    with COPD, arterial blood gas
    abnormalities in, 94
Ciclosporin, 203
Ciprofloxacin, 156, 392t
Citalopram, 482
Clarithromycin resistance, 106
Clock-drawing tests, 478, 479f
Clopidogrel, 492, 495
Clostridium difficile, 504b
Coamilofruse, 504b
Cocaine, 20
  case study, 20b
  clinical features of, 21f, 21
  management of, 21
Coeliac disease, 148
Colitis, acute, 138
Colon cancer, 150
  case study, 150b
  development risks for, 150
Community-acquired pneumonia
  antibiotic choices for, 105
  management of, 105
  moderate, 105
  severe, 105
  uncomplicated mild, 105
Confusional Assessment Method,
    475
Congestive cardiac failure, 33
Constipation, 135
  case study, 135b
  causes of, 136
  treatment of, 136
  urinary tract infection, 500

Coombs' tests, 362*f*, 391, 400
Cor pulmonale, 67
    management of, 67
    pathophysiology of, 67
    prognosis of, 68
Corticosteroids, 363
Cortisol, 361*b*
Cotrimoxazole, 392*t*, 457
Cough, 80
    acute, 80
    assessment of, 80
    case study, 80*b*
    chronic, 81
    diagnosis of, 80
    investigations of, 81*b*
    syncope, 24
Crohn disease, 140
    and ulcerative colitis, 140*t*
Cryptococcus neoformans, 459
Crystal arthritis, 295
CURB-65 criteria, CAP and, 103, 104*b*
Cushing syndrome, 327
Cutaneous adverse drug reaction, 427
Cytomegalovirus, 459

D
Dabigatran, 394
Dapsone, 391*b*, 392*t*, 457
Deep vein thrombosis, 116, 380*b*, 395
    ultrasonography for, 119
Delirium, 474
    case study, 474*b*
    Confusional Assessment Method, 475
    diagnosis of, 474
    investigations of, 476*b*
    management of, 476
Delirium tremens, 262
    case study, 262*b*
Dementia, 259, 478
    Abbreviated Mental Test, 478*b*
    case study, 478*b*
    causes of, 259, 260*b*
    definition of, 478
    diagnosis of, 259
    investigations of, 479*b*
    management of, 261, 479
Dementia-like syndrome, 479*b*, 479
Depressed consciousness, causes of, 9
Depression, 264, 480
    assessment of, 481
    case study, 480*b*
    diagnosis of, 266
    management of, 266, 482
Dermatomyositis, 299
Diabetes insipidus, 351

Diabetes mellitus, 311
    management of, 322
    in pregnancy, 326
Diabetic ketoacidosis, 313
Dialysis, 201, 202*f*
Diarrhoea, 136
    case study, 137*b*–138*b*
    diagnosis of, 137
    management of, 137
Diclofenac, 386, 396*b*, 504*b*
Digoxin, 35
    heart conditions, 492*b*
Dilated cardiomyopathy, 69
    management of, 69
Dimercaprol, 392*t*
Diplopia, 211
    causes of, 213*b*
Direct oral anticoagulants, 76
Disseminated intravascular coagulation, 377
    case study, 378*b*–379*b*
    causes of, 378
    diagnosis of, 378
    management of, 378
    surgical cause, 380
Distributive shock, 5
Diuretic therapy, 180
Dizziness, 37
Do Not Attempt Resuscitation decision-making, 505
Döhle bodies, 415
Donepezil, 479
Dopamine agonists, 503
Drug-induced, anaemia, 411
Drug-induced conditions, parkinsonism, 502
Drug-induced illness, elderly, 503, 503*t*
    case study, 504*b*
Dual-chamber pacemaker, 26, 36
Duodenal ulcer disease, case study, 145*b*
Dysphagia, 134, 490
    case study, 134*b*
    diagnosis of, 135
    management of, 135

E
Ecstasy, 22
    clinical features of, 21*f*, 22
    treatment of, 22
Eczema, 421, 422*f*
    atopic, 422
    case study, 421*b*
    diagnosis of, 422
    management of, 422
Electrocardiogram, 38*f*
Electrolytes, 175, 178, 201
    case study, 176*b*
    clinical assessment of, 175

Emboli, 487
Empyema, 116
Enalapril, 493
Encephalitis, 229
Endoscopic retrograde cholangiopancreatography, 159–160
   complications of, 160
   investigations of, 161*b*
Enterohaemorrhagic *Escherichia coli*, 154
Epilepsy, elderly, 469, 470*b*
Epstein-Barr virus, 454
   infection, 162
Erythema nodosum, 127
Erythroderma, 419
Erythromelalgia, toes, 365, 366*f*
Erythromycin, 405
Essential thrombocythaemia, 369*f*–370*f*, 369
Essential tremor, Parkinson disease, 502
Etanercept, 412
Ethambutol, 458–459
Exacerbation, acute, 97
Extradural haemorrhage, 238

F
Faecal occult bloods, 147
   investigations for, 147
Falls, elderly, 470
   case study, 470*b*
   examination, 471
   investigations of, 472
   management of, 472
   questions for, 471
Familial adenomatous polyposis, 150
Fava beans *(Vicia faba)*, 391–392
Favism, 391–392
Felty syndrome, 396*b*, 396, 411
Femoral head, avascular necrosis, 388*f*
Ferritin, 357*b*, 357, 411
Fibrinogen degradation products, 378
Fibrinolysis, 45
Fibrinolytic therapy, 491
Filgrastim, indications for, 127
Fits and faints, 242
Flash pulmonary oedema, 185
Flexi-sigmoidoscopy, 150
Fludarabine, 363
Fludrocortisone, 472
Fluid
   balance, 175, 178
   challenge, 175
   replacement, 183*t*
   status, 177*t*
Folate deficiency, 411
Folinic acid, 360
Food bolus obstruction, 134

Food poisoning, 154
   case study, 154*b*
   diagnosis of, 154
   investigations of, 154*b*
   management of, 155
Functional bowel disease, 151
   case study, 151*b*
   management of, 152
Furosemide, 504*b*

G
Galantamine, 479
Gallstones, clinical presentation of, 159*f*
Gamma hydroxybutyric acid
   clinical features of, 22
   treatment of, 23
Gastric cancer, case study, 146*b*
Gastro-oesophageal reflux disease (GORD), 142
   case study, 143*b*
   investigations of, 143*b*, 143
   management of, 143
Gastroenterology, 131
Gastrointestinal haemorrhage, 166*f*
Giants geriatric medicine, 484
Ginkgo biloba, 479–480
Glandular fever, 368, 444
Glatiramer acetate, 255
Gliclazide, 504*b*
Glomerulonephritis, acute, 198
Glucose-6-phosphate dehydrogenase (G6PD), 390
   acute haemolysis in, 391, 392*t*
   assessment of, 393
   case study, 390*b*
   clinical features of, 392
   definition of, 390
   diagnosis of, 390, 391*t*, 392
   investigations of, 390*b*
   laboratory features of, 392
   treatment of, 393
Glyceryl trinitrate, 504*b*
Goodpasture disease, 200
Gradual loss of vision, 217
Granulation, 415
Granulocytes, immature, 415
Guillain-Barré syndrome, 255

H
Haematemesis, 164–165
Haematological malignancy, 409, 410*f*
Haematological oncology, 403
   case study, 404*b*–406*b*
   diagnosis of, 407
   disease groups, 403
   features of, 404

Haematological oncology *(Continued)*
  long-term treatment of, 405
  management of, 405
Haematuria
  without albuminuria, 205
  cause, 205
Haemoglobin electrophoresis, 389*f,* 389
Haemolysis
  acute, 390*b*, 391, 392*t*, 393
  aspirin, 391*b*, 392*t*
  features of, 361
Haemolytic anaemia, 360
  case study, 360*b*
  chronic, 391
  features of, 361
  investigations of, 361*b*
  management of, 363
  microangiopathic, 414
  red cell, 361
Haemolytic transfusion reaction, 399*b*, 400
Haemolytic uraemic syndrome, features of, 155
Haemophilia, 374*f*–375*f*
Haemophilus influenzae, 398, 459
Haemoptysis, 85
  case study, 85*b*, 87*f*
  colour of blood, 86
  conditions in, 86
  management of, 87
Haemorrhage, 390*b*, 401, 402*f*
Haemostasis, failure, 403
  causes of, 403
  investigations of, 403*b*
Haloperidol, 476
Headaches, 244
  causes of, 247*b*
Heart disease, elderly, 492
  case study, 492*b*
  investigations of, 492
Heart failure, 482
Helicobacter pylori infection
  metabolism of urea by, 145*f*
  tests for, 144
  treatment of, 145
Helminthic infections, 455
Heparin, 381*b*
  bleeding disorders, 380
  induced thrombocytopenia with thrombosis, 395
  thrombosis, 381
Hepatic encephalopathy, 161
Hepatitis B, 158*t*
Hereditary angio-oedema, 426
Hereditary nonpolyposis cancer of colon, 150
  diagnostic criteria for, 151*b*
Hernia repair, 372
Hiccups, 133

Hiccups *(Continued)*
  case study, 133*b*
  causes of, 133
High-grade lymphoma, features of, 409
Highly active antiretroviral therapy, 457
Histoplasma capsulatum, 459
HIV/AIDS, 457
  assessment of, 460
  bacterial chest infection, 459
  case study, 457*b*
  chest conditions, 458
  diagnosis of, 457
  malignancy, 459
  management of, 457
  treatment of, 457
Hives, 424
Hospital-acquired pneumonia
  case study, 107*b*–108*b*
  diagnosis of, 108
  management of, 108
  organisms in, 108
Humerus, osteomyelitis, 388*f*
Hydroxocobalamin, 359–360
Hydroxycarbamide, 369, 386
Hydroxyzine, 386
Hypercalcaemia, 341
  and bronchial carcinoma, 125
Hypercholesterolaemia, 204
Hyperkalaemia, 188
  causes of, 188, 190*b*
Hypernatraemia, 179*t*, 180
  causes of, 180
Hyperosmolar hyperglycaemic state, 317
Hyperparathyroidism, 196
Hypersplenism, 396*b*, 396
  causes of, 397
  pathophysiology of, 396
Hypertension, 70
Hyperthermia, 14
Hyperthyroidism, 329
Hyperventilation, 85
  case study, 85*b*
Hyperventilation syndrome, 85
Hypocalcaemia, 344
Hypoglycaemic coma, 319
Hyponatraemia, 179*t*
  causes of, 180*b*
Hypopituitarism, 348
Hyposplenic prophylaxis, 385
Hyposplenism, 396. *See also* Overwhelming
       postsplenectomy infection
Hypotension
  after intubation, 97
  orthostatic, 471
  postural, 472

Hypothermia, 14, 496
  aetiological factors, 496
  case study, 496*b*
  features of, 496, 497*f*
  investigations of, 496*b*
  management of, 497
Hypothyroidism
  case study, 336*b*
  treatment of, 337
Hypovolaemic shock, 401*b*, 403

I

Ibuprofen, 386
Idiopathic thrombocytopenic purpura, 372
Immune thrombocytopenic purpura, 371
Immunoglobin A, 200
Immunosuppressive therapy, 290
Infection, 415
Infectious diseases, 175
Infective endocarditis, 64
Inflammatory bowel disease, extragastrointestinal
  manifestations of, 138, 141*b*
Inflammatory disorders, iron status, 411
Inherited bleeding disorders,
  374*f*–375*f*, 374
Inherited platelet disorder, 373
Inherited thrombocytopenia, 371*b*
Intercostal tube, management of, 121
Intravascular haemolysis
  cause of, 393*t*
  evidence to show, 390, 391*t*
  features of, 392
Iron deficiency anaemia, 147
  case study, 147*b*
Iron status, inflammatory disorders, 411
Isotope renography, 187

J

Jaundice, 159
  case study, 417*b*
  investigations of, 417*b*

K

Kaposi's sarcoma, 459
Kidney disease, 175

L

L-dopa, 503
Laxatives, 386
Lead displacement, 37
12-lead ECG, 27
Left lower lobe pneumonia, 482*b*, 483*f*
Legionnaire disease, 106
Leg ulceration, 418
  causes of, 418

Leg ulceration *(Continued)*
  investigations of, 418*b*
  management of, 418
  signs of, 418
Legs, weakness of, and bronchial carcinoma, 125
Leucoerythroblastic anaemia, 414
Leukaemia, 403. *See also* Acute leukaemia
Levothyroxine, 482–483
Lewy body dementia, 479
Lipid-lowering drugs, 55
Lipodermatosclerosis, 417
Liver disease
  acute, 162, 162*t*
  anaemia, 412
  bleeding, 376
Liver failure, 169
Liver function tests, 157
Lorazepam, 477
Low urinary output, 181
  case study, 181*b*
  causes of, 182
  management of, 182
Low urine output, 181–182
Low-grade haematological malignancy, 409
Lung abscess, 109
  case study, 109*b*, 109*f*
  diagnoses of, 109
Lung cancer, radiological manifestations of,
  123*f*–124*f*, 123
Lung disease, polycythaemia and, 366
Lymphoblastic leukaemia, acute, 410*f*
Lymphomas, high-grade, features of, 403, 409

M

Macrocytic anaemia, 355
  case study, 358*b*
  causes of, 358
  diagnosis of, 359
  investigations of, 358*b*, 359
  management of, 359
Macroscopic haematuria, 205
Maculopapular rash, 427*f*
Magnetic resonance angiography, 187
Magnetic resonance imaging, 214
Malaria, 390, 449
  diagnosis of, 450
  investigations of, 450
Massive haemorrhage, management of, 401, 402*f*
Mechanical ventilation, 97
Megaloblastic anaemia, 358*b*
Melaena, 164
Memantine, 479
Meningitis, 232
  case study, 232*b*
  causes of, 235*b*

Meningococcal meningitis, 231
Meningococcal septicaemia, 370*b*
Metabolic acidosis, 93
Metabolic alkalosis, 94
Metabolic bone diseases, 306
Metabolic disease, 175
Metabolic hypoglycaemia, 25
Methotrexate, 358*b*, 360, 396*b*, 412
Methylene blue, 392*t*
Microangiopathic haemolytic anaemia, 414
Microcytic anaemia, 357
Micturition syncope, 24
Middle East respiratory syndrome coronavirus
        (MERS-CoV), 102
Mini-Mental State Examination, 142
Mirtazapine, 482
Mitoxantrone, 255
Mitral valve disease, 63
Mobitz type II atrioventricular block, 26*f*
    second-degree heart block, 26
Monoamine oxidase inhibitor, 503
Monospot test, 367*b*
Moraxella catarrhalis, 459
Morphine, 386
Movement disorders, 250
Multidrug-resistant tuberculosis, 458
Multiple myeloma, diagnosis of, 407
Multiple sclerosis, 253*f*, 253
Multisystem vasculitis, 198
    diagnose of, 199
Musculoskeletal examination, 283*f*
Mycoplasma pneumonia, 106
Myelodysplasia, 411
Myeloid leukaemia, acute, 406*f*, 406, 409, 410*f*
Myeloma, 404, 407*f*
    multiple, diagnosis of, 407
Myeloproliferative disorder, 369*b*, 369
Myocardial infarction, 51, 54, 484

N
Nalidixic acid, 392*t*
Naphthalene, 391*b*, 392*t*, 394
Narrow-complex tachycardia, 27*f*
Natalizumab, 255
National Institute for Health and Care Excellence
        (NICE) guidelines, 479–480
Neisseria meningitidis, 398
Nephrotic syndrome, 203–204
    management of, 204
Nerve root irritation, 89
Neurally mediated syndromes, 26
Neurological conditions, deficits, stroke, 488*t*, 489
Neuropathic ulcers, 418
Neutropenia, management of patients with, after
        chemotherapy, 126

Neutrophil leucocytosis, 415*b*, 415
New oral disease-modifying drugs, 255
Nitrofurantoin, 392*t*
Nocardia asteroides, 459
Non-Hodgkin lymphoma, 410*f*, 459
Nonacute diarrhoea, causes of, 137
Nonalcoholic fatty liver disease, 168
Non-steroidal anti-inflammatory drugs (NSAIDs),
        60, 504
Noninfective disorders, 445
Nonspecific illness, elderly, 482
    case study, 482*b*–483*b*
Norton Scale, pressure ulcers, 499

O
Oesophageal, 89
Oesophageal cancer, 135
Oesophageal rupture, 89
Oesophageal varices, 167*f*
Olanzapine, 476
Opiate dependence, 274
Orthostatic hypotension, 25, 471
Osmotic diuresis, 180
Osteoarthritis, 281
Osteomyelitis
    case study, 304*b*, 304
    diagnosis of, 304
    humerus, 388*f*
Osteoporosis, 302
Overdose, management of, 14
Overwhelming postsplenectomy infection,
        398*b*, 398
    pathophysiology of, 398
    prevention of, 399
Oximeters, 92
Oxygen dissociation curve, 95*f*, 95

P
Pacemakers
    classification of, 36
    complications of, 37
    erosion, 37
    syndrome, 37
Papilloedema, 214*f*
Paracetamol (acetaminophen) poisoning, 15
    acetylcysteine for, 17
    antidotes, 17
    case study, 15*b*
    investigations of, 15*b*
    management of, 16
    physical examination, 16
    treatment of, 17
        nomogram, 16*f*, 16
Paraganglioma, 346
Parasitic infections, 455

Parkinson disease, 252, 501
  case study, 501*b*
  diagnosis of, 502*b*, 502
  features of, 501
  management of, 503
Parvovirus B19, 444
Patient wishes, cardiopulmonary
        resuscitation, 505
Patient-controlled analgesia, 386
Pentamidine, 457
Peptic ulcer disease, 144
  alarm features of, 144
  case study, 144*b*
Pericardial disease, 59
  aetiology of, 60*t*
  management of, 60
Pericarditis, 88
Pernicious anaemia, 358, 411
Phaeochromocytoma, 346
Phenothiazines, 496
Philadelphia chromosome, 409*b*, 409
Philadelphia Geriatric Center, Morale Scale,
        485, 487*t*
Platelet count, elevated, 368
  case study, 368*b*
  causes of, 368
  complications of, 370
  management of, 369
Platelet disorders, 370
  case study, 370*b*, 372*b*–373*b*
  diagnosis of, 373
  inherited, 373
  management of, 373
Plateletpheresis, 369
Pleural effusion, 114
  case study, 114*b*–115*b*, 116*f*
  causes of, 115
  clinical signs of, 114
  diagnosis of, 114
Pleurisy, 89
Pneumococcal sepsis, 398
  prevention, 398*b*
  sickle-cell anaemia with, 398
Pneumocystis jirovecii pneumonia, 457
  diagnosis of, 106
  treatment of, 107
Pneumonia, 102
  assessment of, 103, 104*b*
  case study, 103*b*–104*b*, 104*f*–105*f*, 106*b*–108*b*
  diagnosis of, 106, 107*f*, 125
  investigations of, 103*b*
  severe, arterial blood gas abnormalities in, 94
  treatment of, *P. jirovecii* infection, 107
  viral respiratory epidemics, 102
  viral respiratory pandemics, 102

Pneumothorax, 119
  case study, 119*b*, 120*f*, 121*b*
  diagnoses of, 121
  management of, 120
    after aspiration, 120
Poisoning
  cardiovascular support, 13
  case study, 12*b*
  examination of, 12
  management of, 13
  paracetamol (acetaminophen), 15
  physical signs of, 12*f*, 12
  respiratory support, 13
Polycythaemia, 363
  apparent/relative, 366
  case study, 363*b*
  causes, 363, 364*f*
  diagnosis of, 365
  investigations of, 365*b*
  long-term complications of, 367
  management of, 366
  secondary, 366
Polycythaemia vera, 364*f*, 364
  criteria for, 365*b*
  features of, 365
Polymyalgia rheumatica, 297
Polymyositis, 299
Postural hypotension, 470, 472
Pott's disease, 304
Pramipexole, 503
Prednisolone, 504*b*
Pressure ulcers, 497
  assessment of, 498
  case study, 497*b*
  causes of, 498
  investigations of, 498*b*, 498
  management of, 498
  risk factors of, 497
Primaquine, 391*b*, 392*t*
Prochlorperazine, 386
Proctoscopy, 149
Prosthetic valve endocarditis, 66
Pruritus, 420
  case study, 420*b*
  causes of, 420
  diagnosis of, 420
Pseudomembranous colitis, 152
  case study, 152*b*
  diagnosis of, 152
  investigations of, 153
  management of, 153
  prevention of, 153
Psoriasis, 423
Pulmonary embolism, 116
  case study, 116*b*, 117*f*

Pulmonary embolism *(Continued)*
　diagnosis of, 117
　investigations of, 118
　treatment of, 119
Pulmonary haemorrhage, 200
Pulmonary hypertension, 66
Pulmonary oedema, acute, 492, 493*f*
Pyodermagangrenosum, 141*f*
Pyrazinamide, 458–459
Pyrexia of unknown origin, 452
Pyrimethamine, 392*t*, 457

Q
Quality of life, 505
Quinine, 392*t*
Quinolone, 392*t*

R
Radionuclide ventilation/perfusion scanning, 118
Rash/eruption, generalized, 419
　case study, 419*b*
　complications of, 419
　diagnosis of, 419
　management of, 420
Reactive arthritis, 294*f*, 294
Rectal bleeding, 149
　case study, 149*b*
　management of, 149
Red eye, 218
Referred pain, 89
Renal disease, 377
Renal tract imaging, 194
Renal unit referral, 194, 195*b*
Renal/ureteric colic, 207
　aetiology of, 208
　case study, 207*b*
　diagnosis of, 208
　management of, 208
Renovascular disease, 184
　features of, 184
　management of, 185
Repeated lumbar puncture, 215
Respiratory acidosis, 93
Respiratory alkalosis, 93
Respiratory arrest, signs of impending, 95
Respiratory disorders, 78
Respiratory failure, 92
　case study, 96*b*
　management of, 94
　treatment of, 95
Rhabdomyolysis, 191
Rheumatoid arthritis, 286, 396*b*
Rifampicin, tuberculosis and, 458–459
Right ventricular infarction, 50
Right-sided endocarditis, 66

Rituximab, 363
Rivastigmine, 479–480
Romiplostim, 372*b*
Ropinirole, 503
Rouleaux, 411, 413*b*
Royal College of Physicians, 484–485

S
Salicylate overdose, 18
　case study, 18*b*
　clinical features of, 19
　management of, 19
　　challenges in, 19
Sarcoidosis, 127–128
　bilateral hilar lymph node enlargement in, 128*f*
　case study, 127*b*–129*b*
　extrapulmonary manifestations of, 128
Secondary polycythaemia, 366
Selegiline, 503
Self-poisoning, 11
Sengstaken–Blakemore tube, 167
Sepsis, 415, 444
　definition of, 5
　diagnosis of, 445
　lactate level in, relationship of, 6*t*
　management of, 4*f*, 6–7
　predisposing factors for, 445*b*
　signs of, 6
　symptoms of, 6
Septic arthritis, 305
　case study, 305
Septic shock, 444
　case study, 5*b*
　cause of, 5
　pathophysiology of, 5
Septicaemia, 231
Sequential Organ Failure Assessment Score, 5, 446
Serum transferrin receptor assay, 357, 412
Severe acute asthma, 82
Severe acute respiratory syndrome (SARS), 102
Severe brain injury, 240*b*
Severe hypercalcaemia, 343
Sexually transmitted infections, 457
Shock, 1, 182*t*
　case study, 1*b*, 5*b*
　causes of, 1
　clinical examination of, 2
　diagnosis of, 1
　physiology of, 1, 2*f*
　treatment of, 3, 4*f*
Shy-Drager parkinsonism, 502
Sick diabetic patient, 321
Sick sinus syndrome, 470
Sickle-cell disease, 384
　anaemia with pneumococcal sepsis, 398

Sickle-cell disease *(Continued)*
  avascular necrosis, femoral head, 387, 388*f*
  blood film, 389*f*, 389–390
  case study, 384*b*
  complications of, 387, 388*f*
  diagnosis of, 389*f*, 389
  investigations of, 384*b*–385*b*
  questions for, 385
  treatment of, 386
  types of, 388
Skin condition, 490
Skin lesions, 426–427
Small intestinal mucosa, 148*f*
Small intestinal obstruction
  diagnosis of, 132
  management of, 132
Small-cell lung cancer, 126
  antibiotic regimens, 127
  prognostic factors of, 126
  treatment of, 126
Smoking, 492
Somatostatin, 167
Speech and language therapist, 491
Spinal tuberculous osteomyelitis, diagnosis of, 304
Spirometry, 98
Spleen size, 396
Splenectomy, 396, 397*b*. *See also* Overwhelming
          postsplenectomy infection
Splenomegaly, 396
  case study, 396*b*–397*b*
  causes of, 396
Squamous carcinoma, 135
Staphylococcal pneumonia, 106
Statins, 492, 495
Steele-Richardson-Olszewski parkinsonism, 502
Steroids, 504*b*
Streptococcus pneumoniae, 385, 459
Stridor
  and bronchial carcinoma, 125
  causes of, 81
Stroke, 224, 485. *See also* Transient ischaemic attack
  case study, 486*b*
  causes of, 487
  diagnosis of, 488
  investigations of, 491*b*, 491
  management of, 489, 490*f*
  pathology of, 487
  prognostic signs in, 491*b*
  questions for, 486
  risk factors of, 491
  secondary prevention, 492
  signs of, 487, 488*t*
Subdural haemorrhage, 228
Subphrenic abscess, 133
Suicide and deliberate self-harm, 268

Sulfasalazine, 392*t*
Superior venocaval obstruction, and bronchial
          carcinoma, 125
Supraventricular tachycardia, 28, 30*b*
Swollen red leg, 417
  case study, 417*b*
  diagnosis of, 417
  investigations of, 417*b*
  treatment of, 418
Symptom relief, 142
Syncope, 24
  carotid sinus, 24
  causes of, 24–25
  cough, 24
  diagnosis of, 24
  micturition, 24
Syndrome of inappropriate antidiuretic hormone,
          180, 352
Systemic lupus erythematosus, 289
  features of, 291*f*

T
Tachycardia, 26
  clinical approach, 26
  narrow-complex, 27*f*
  patient admission, 28*t*
  supraventricular, 28, 30*b*
  ventricular, 29, 30*b*
Temporal arteritis, 500
Tension pneumothorax, 121
Terlipressin, 167
Thrombocytopenia, 358, 371. *See also* Idiopathic
          thrombocytopenic purpura
  causes of, 370–371, 371*b*
  microangiopathic haemolytic anaemia, 414
  questions, 371
  with thrombosis, heparin-induced, 395
Thrombocytosis, 368–369
Thrombolysis, 45, 119, 189
Thrombolytic therapy, 45*b*, 45
  contraindications to, 45*b*
Thrombophilia, 381, 384, 395*b*
Thrombosis, 380. *See also* Deep vein thrombosis
  case study, 380*b*–381*b*
  duration and target INRs for, 382,
          382*t*
  investigations of, 380, 381*b*
Thrombosis prophylaxis, 292
Thyroid function, 334
Thyrotoxicosis, 504*b*
Thyroxine, 361*b*
Toes, erythromelalgia, 365, 366*f*
Total iron binding capacity, 411
Transcobalamin II deficiency, 358
Transoesophageal echo-guided approach, 35

Transient ischaemic attack, 226, 494–495
  case study, 494b
  examination, 494
  history taking, 494
  investigations of, 494b
  management of, 495
  prognosis of, 495
Transient visual disturbance, 216b
Transjugular intrahepatic portosystemic shunt, 167
Transthoracic echocardiography, 43
Traumatic brain injury, 237, 238t
Tricyclic antidepressant overdose, 20
  clinical features of, 20
  treatment of, 20
Trimethoprim, 500
Tuberculosis, 110
  case study, 110b–111b, 111f, 113b
  diagnosis of, 110, 125
  management of, 111, 112f
  reactivation development, risk factors for, 111
  results, 112
  treatment of, 110, 113
Tumour necrosis factor, 5
Typhoid, 155
  case study, 155b
  diagnosis of, 156
  management of, 156
Typical angina, 88

U
Ulcerative colitis, 140
  and Crohn disease, 140t
  findings in severe attack of, 138t, 139f
  management of, 139
Upper airways obstruction, 79
  causes of, 80t
Urinalysis, 194
Urinary tract disease, 175, 206, 499
  case study, 206b, 499b
  discovery of, 175
  examination of, 499
  history taking, 499
  investigations of, 207b, 500b
  management of, 207
  treatment of, 500
Urticaria, 424f, 424

V
Valvular heart disease, 61
Vascular dementia, 479
Vascular disease, 201, 203
Vasculitic ulcers, 418
Vasculitis, 289
  diagnosis of, 289
  management of, 289
Vasoconstrictor agents, 167
Vasoconstrictor therapy, 167
Vasopressor variant, 470
Venlafaxine, 482
Venous thromboembolic disease, 382
  warfarin and, 382b, 382
Ventilation failure, and PACO$_2$, 92
Ventricular tachycardia, 29, 30b
Vertigo, 221
Viral infections, 401, 444
Vitamin E, 479–480
Vitamin K deficiency, 376
  analogues, 392t
  causes of, 376b
  management of, 376
Volume replacement, 177
Vomiting, 131
  case study, 131b
  causes of, 132b
  investigations of, 131b, 132f

W
Warfarin
  bleeding disorders, 376
  thrombosis, 381
  venous thromboembolic disease,
    382
Waterlow Score, pressure ulcers, 485,
    486t, 499
Weight loss, 133
  case study, 133b
  investigations of, 134
Wheeze, 81
White blood cell count, elevated, 367
  case study, 367b
  causes, 367b
  investigations of, 368
Wolff–Parkinson–White syndrome, 28